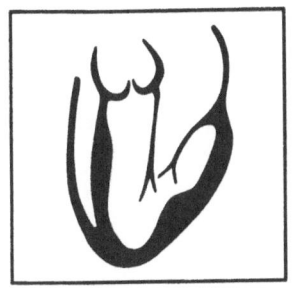

ECHOCARDIOLOGY
SELECTED PAPERS

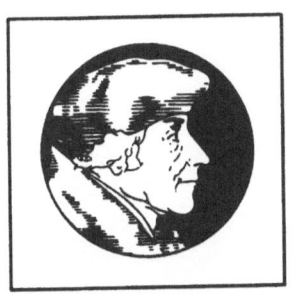

PRESENTED DURING THE THIRD
SYMPOSIUM AT ERASMUS UNIVERSITY,
ROTTERDAM, JUNE 20–22, 1979

INTERUNIVERSITY INSTITUTE OF
CARDIOLOGY, AMSTERDAM

DEVELOPMENTS IN CARDIOVASCULAR MEDICINE

VOLUME 1

ECHOCARDIOLOGY

Edited by

CHARLES T. LANCÉE

Thoraxcenter, Erasmus University, Rotterdam

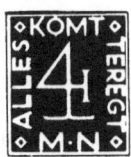

1979

MARTINUS NIJHOFF PUBLISHERS

THE HAGUE / BOSTON / LONDON

The distribution of this book is handled by the following team of publishers:

for the United States and Canada

Kluwer Boston, Inc.
160 Old Derby Street
Hingham, MA 02043
U.S.A.

for all other countries

Kluwer Academic Publishers Group
Distribution Center
P.O. Box 322
3300 AH Dordrecht
The Netherlands

Library of Congress Cataloging in Publication Data   CIP

Main entry under title:

Echocardiology.

    Bibliography: p.
    Includes index.
    1.   Ultrasonic cardiography – Congresses.
2.   Heart – Diseases – Diagnosis – Congresses.
I.   Lancée, Charles T.   II.   Erasmus Universiteit.
RC683.5.U5E25   616.1′2′0754   79–13045

ISBN-13: 978-94-009-9326-6   e-ISBN-13: 978-94-009-9324-2
DOI: 10.1007/ 978-94-009-9324-2

FOREWORD

This Symposium is the third of a series of scientific meetings in the field of echocardiology, held at the Erasmus University Rotterdam.* The series was initiated by Klaas Bom, who organized the first two meetings with great success. These followed the procedure of two days of parallel sessions with invited speakers only.

This time, we decided to broaden the basis of the meeting and have a three-day program of parallel sessions, combining invited papers, free communications and posters.

We decided, however, to maintain one of the most striking features of the last meeting – having the complete proceedings available at the time of the meeting. We confronted the authors-to-be with a very tight schedule in order to make the book a true reflection of the state of the art in echocardiology. As a result, editing time was also very limited and neither terminology nor units have been completely standardized.

This book has three main parts. The first, and largest, part consists of contributions on echocardiology in adults, and is divided into four sections. The first section is a general survey of various applications, whereas the remaining three centre round specific applications, i.e. ischemic disease, left ventricular function and cardiac valves, respectively. The second part contains applications in pediatric cardiology; due to the wide variety of topics covered, no particular subdivision has been made. The last part of the book is devoted to instrumentation, methods and new developments.

This symposium was organized in association with
- Interuniversity Institute of Cardiology, Amsterdam, the Netherlands
- Dutch Society of Ultrasound in Medicine and Biology
- Dutch Heart Foundation, the Hague, the Netherlands
- European Society of Cardiology

Financial support was given by
- Interuniversity Institute of Cardiology, Amsterdam, the Netherlands
- University-fund Rotterdam Foundation, Rotterdam, the Netherlands.

Rotterdam, June 1979   CHARLES T. LANCÉE

---

*The second symposium has been published as: N. Bom (ed.), *Echocardiology*. Martinus Nijhoff Publishers, The Hague/Boston/London, 1977.

ACKNOWLEDGEMENTS

A book of this size is naturally the work of a large team. First of all, I wish to express my gratitude and my admiration for all the lecturers who provided me with their carefully prepared manuscripts, in some cases at very short notice. My colleagues of the organizing committee, Klaas Bom, Jos Roelandt, Hans Rijsterborgh and Paul Hugenholtz were always available for assistance and advice, for which I am very grateful.

I am especially indebted to Mary Rose Hoare who, although educated in the field of computers and mathematics, contributed heavily to the reviewing and correcting of the material.

Furthermore, I have to thank our secretaries, Corrie de Bruijn, Ineke van Lieshout and Ria Willemstein, for their continuous good humour, in spite of the endless stream of rush jobs that goes along with the creation of a book like this.

Thanks are due to Len van der Wal, Olchert Bastiaans, Ad van der Schoot and Adri Duijndam who spent hours on the preparation of the list of contributors.

Finally, I would like to pay a special tribute to my wife Saskia, who not only cheerfully accepted my rather unsocial behaviour during the preparation time of the Symposium, but also stimulated me in every possible way.

CHARLES T. LANCÉE

CONTENTS

B. APPLICATIONS IN ISCHEMIC DISEASE

II. PEDIATRIC ECHOCARDIOLOGY

III. TECHNOLOGICAL ASPECTS OF ECHOCARDIOLOGY

CONTRIBUTORS

Abbate, A.l'., CNR Clinical Physiology Laboratory University of Pisa, Pisa, Italy.

Abitbol, G., Dept. of Cardiology, Fondation A. de Rothschild, Paris, France

Adamec, R., Hôpital Cantonal, Centre de Cardiologie, Geneva, Switzerland.

Alam, M., Henry Ford Hospital, Detroit, Michigan, U.S.A.

Ali, A., Clayton Foundation for Research Laboratory, St. Luke's Episcopal Hospital and Texas Heart Institute, Houston, Texas, U.S.A.

Anliker, M., Institute for Biomedical Engineering, University and ETH, Zurich, Switzerland.

Areias, J.C., University of Porto, Porto, Portugal.

Aubert, A.E., Dept. of Pathophysiology, St. Rafael University Hospital, Leuven, Belgium.

Baker, D.W., Center for Bioengineering, University of Washington, Seattle, Washington, U.S.A.

Bastiaans, O.L., Dept. of Applied Physics, Delft University of Technology, Delft, The Netherlands.

Baudinet, V., University of Liege, Liege, Belgium.

Beppu, S., Research Institute, National Cardiovascular Center, Suita, Osaka, Japan.

Berkhout, A.J., Dept. of Applied Physics, Delft University of Technology, Delft, The Netherlands.

Biamino, G., Dept. of Cardiopneumology, Klinikum Steglitz, FU Berlin, Berlin, Germany.

Bloch, A., Centre de Cardiologie, Hôpital Cantonal Universitaire, Geneva, Switzerland.

Bom, A.H., Thoraxcenter, Erasmus University, Rotterdam, The Netherlands.

Bom, N., Thoraxcenter, Erasmus University, Rotterdam, The Netherlands.

Bonzel, T., Toomey Cardiopulmonary Laboratory and Research Department, St. Joseph's Hospital, Syracuse, New York, U.S.A.

Borzykowsky, J., Hôpital Cantonal, Centre de Cardiologie, Geneva, Switzerland.

Bourdillon, P.D.V., National Heart Hospital and Cardiothoracic Institute, London, England.

Brandestini, M.A., Center for Bioengineering, University of Washington, Seattle, Washington, U.S.A.

Brandon, G., Hôpital Cantonal, Centre de Cardiologie, Geneva, Switzerland.

Bridoux, E., Université de Valenciennes, Valenciennes, France.

Brown, D.J., Cardiac Dept. of Brompton Hospital, London, England.

Brun, P., Groupe de Recherche U 138 de l'I.N.S.E.R.M., Service d'Exploration Fonctionnelle CHU Henri Mondor, Créteil, France.

Bruneel, C., Université de Valenciennes, Valenciennes, France.

Burckhardt, C.B., Central Research Units, F. Hoffmann-La Roche & Co. Basel, Switzerland.

Calleja, H.B., Non-invasive and Hemodynamics Laboratory, Philippine Heart Center for Asia, Quezon City, Philippines.

Casty, M., Institute for Biomedical Engineering, University and ETH, Zurich, Switzerland.

Castro, C.M. De, Clayton Foundation for Research Laboratory, St. Luke's Episcopal Hospital and Texas Heart Institute, Houston, Texas, U.S.A.

Cate, F.J. ten, Thoraxcenter, Erasmus University, Rotterdam, The Netherlands.

Cholot, N., Dept. of Cardiology, Fondation A. de Rothschild, Paris, France.

Choussat, A., Hôpital Cardiologique, CHU Bordeaux, Pessac, France.

Collignon, P., University of Liege, Liege, Belgium.

Convert, C., Hôpital Cardio-vasculaire et Pneumologique Louis Pradel, Lyon, France.

Corya, B., Indiana University School of Medicine, Indianapolis, Indiana, U.S.A.

Dallocchio, M., Hôpital Cardiologique, CHU Bordeaux, Pessac, France.

Davies, A.B., National Heart Hospital, London, England.

Defranould, Ph., Thomson-CSF, ASM Division, Cagnes-sur-Mer, France.

Delannoy, B., Université de Valenciennes, Valenciennes, France.

Delaye, S., Hôpital Cardio-vasculaire et Pneumologique Louis Pradel, Lyon, France.

Denef, B., Dept. of Pathophysiology, St. Raphael University Hospital, Leuven, Belgium.
Didisheim, J.C., Hôpital Cantonal, Centre de Cardiologie, Geneva, Switzerland.
Dillon, J.C., Indiana University School of Medicine, Indianapolis, Indiana, U.S.A.
Distante, A., CNR Clinical Physiology Laboratory and University of Pisa, Pisa, Italy.
Dooley, T.K., University of Washington, Seattle, Washington, U.S.A.
Drobinski, G., Hôpital de la Salpétrière, Paris, France.
Erijman, M., Toor Heart Institute, Beilinson Medical Center, Petah Tiqva, Israel.
Esente, P., Toomey Cardiopulmonary Laboratory and Research Department, St. Joseph's
    Hospital, Syracuse, New York, U.S.A.
Eugène, M., Hôpital de la Salpétrière, Paris, France.
Evans, J.I., Hôpital de la Salpétrière, Paris, France.
Eyer, M.K., Center for Bioengineering, University of Washington, Seattle, Washington, U.S.A.
Fantini, F., Cardiology Unit, University of Florence, Florence, Italy.
Fehr, R., Central Research Units, F. Hoffmann-La Roche & Co., Basel, Switzerland.
Feigenbaum, H., Indiana University School of Medicine, Indianapolis, Indiana, U.S.A.
Feldman, C.L., The Electronics for Medicine Corporation, Sudbury, Massachusetts, U.S.A.
Foale, R.A., National Heart Hospital and Cardiothoracic Institute, London, England.
Folland, E.D., Cardiology Section, Harvard Medical School, Boston, Massachusetts, U.S.A.
Fontan, F., Hôpital Cardiologique, CHU Bordeaux, Pessac, France.
Franklin, D.W., University of Washington, Seattle, Washington, U.S.A.
Garcia, E., Clayton Foundation for Research Laboratory, St. Luke's Episcopal Hospital and
    Texas Heart Institute, Houston, Texas, U.S.A.
Geest, H.de, Dept. of Pathophysiology St. Raphael University Hospital, Leuven, Belgium.
Garcia, J.A., Clayton Foundation for Research Laboratory, St. Luke's Episcopal Hospital and
    Texas Heart Institute, Houston, Texas, U.S.A.
Gensini, G.G., Toomey Cardiopulmonary Laboratory and Research Department, St. Joseph's
    Hospital, Syracuse, New York, U.S.A.
Gentile, R., University of Washington, Seattle, Washington, U.S.A.
Giambartolomei, A., Toomey Cardiopulmonary Laboratory and Research Department, St.
    Joseph's Hospital, Syracuse, New York, U.S.A.
Gibson, D.G., Brompton Hospital, London, England.
Giletti, J., Hôpital Cardio-vasculaire et Pneumologique Louis Pradel, Lyon, France.
Glaser, J., Toor Heart Institute, Beilinson Medical Center, Petah Tiqva, Israel.
Godley, R., Indiana University School of Medicine, Indianapolis, Indiana, U.S.A.
Goldberg, S.J., University of Arizona, Tucson, Arizona, U.S.A.
Goldstein, S., Henry Ford Hospital, Detroit, Michigan, U.S.A.
Gramiak, R., Dept. of Radiology, University of Rochester, Medical Center, Rochester, New
    York, U.S.A.
Grandchamp, P.-A., Central Research Units, F. Hoffmann-La Roche & Co., Basel, Switzerland.
Grimm, J., Medical Policlinic, Department of Internal Medicine, University Hospital Zurich,
    Zurich, Switzerland.
Grosgogeat, Y., Hôpital de la Salpétrière, Paris, France.
Gullace, G., Divisione de Cardiologia, Ospedale Civile di Chiari Brescia, Castrezzato, Italy.
Guntheroth, W.G., Division of Pediatric Cardiology, University of Washington, Seattle,
    Washington, U.S.A.
Gussenhoven, W.J., Thoraxcenter, Erasmus University, Rotterdam, The Netherlands.
Haine, F., Université de Valenciennes, Valenciennes, France.
Hall, R.J., Clayton Foundation for Research Laboratory, St. Luke's Episcopal Hospital and
    Texas Heart Institute, Houston, Texas, U.S.A.
Hanrath, P., Dept. of Cardiology, University Hospital, Hamburg, Germany.
Hayward, R.P., The National Heart Hospital, London, England.
Heil, R.P., Dept. of Pediatric Cardiology, University Children's Hospital, University of
    Tübingen, Tübingen, Germany.
Hess, O.M., Medical Policlinic, Department of Internal Medicine, University Hospital Zurich,
    Zurich, Switzerland.
Hoeks, A.P.G., University of Limburg, Maastricht, The Netherlands.
Hoffmann, H., Central Research Units, F. Hoffmann-La Roche & Co., Basel, Switzerland.
Honkoop, J., Thoraxcenter, Erasmus University, Rotterdam, The Netherlands.
Hübscher, W., Medical Policlinic, University Hospital Zurich, University and ETH, Zurich,
    Switzerland.
Humblet, L., University of Liege. Liege, Belgium.

Ibrahim, Z., Medical Policlinic, University of Tuebingen, Tuebingen, Germany.
Jenni, R., Medical Policlinic, University Hospital Zurich, University and ETH, Zurich, Switzerland.
Kaindl, F., Cardiological Clinic, University of Vienna, Vienna, Austria.
Kalmanson, D., Dept. of Cardiology, Fondation A. de Rothschild, Paris, France.
Kawabori, I., Division of Pediatric Cardiology, University of Washington, Seattle, Washington, U.S.A.
Kesteloot, H., Dept. of Pathophysiology, St. Raphael University Hospital, Leuven, Belgium.
Kisslo, J.A., Duke University Medical Center, Durham, North Carolina, U.S.A.
Klicpera, M., Cardiological Clinic, University of Vienna, Vienna, Austria.
Krajcer, Z., Clayton Foundation for Research Laboratory, St. Luke's Episcopal Hospital and Texas Heart Institute, Houston, Texas, U.S.A.
Krayenbuehl, H.P., Medical Policlinic, University Hospital Zurich, University and ETH, Zurich, Switzerland.
Lakier, J.B., Henry Ford Hospital, Detroit, Michigan, U.S.A.
Lambregts, J.A.C., Dept. of Physiology, Biomedical Center, University of Limburg, Maastricht, The Netherlands.
Lancée, C.T., Thoraxcenter, Erasmus University, Rotterdam, The Netherlands.
Landini, L., CNR Clinical Physiology Laboratory, University of Pisa, Pisa, Italy.
Laporte, J.P., Groupe de Recherche U 138 de l'I.N.S.E.R.M., Service d'Exploration Fonctionnelle, C.H.U., Henri·Mondor, Créteil, France.
Laurent, F., Groupe de Recherche U 138 de l'I.N.S.E.R.M., Service d'Exploration Fonctionnelle, C.H.U., Henri Mondor, Créteil. France.
Lee, P.P.K., Dept. of Radiology, University of Rochester, Rochester, New York, U.S.A.
Ligtvoet, C.M., Thoraxcenter, Erasmus University, Rotterdam, The Netherlands.
Lintermans, J., Service de Cardiologie Pédiatrique, Clinique Universitaire St. Joseph, Herent, Belgium.
Lubsen, J., Thoraxcenter, Erasmus University, Rotterdam, The Netherlands.
Macintosh, P., Dept. of Radiology, University of Rochester, Rochester, New York, U.S.A.
Macpherson, P.C., St. Bartholomew's Hospital, London, England.
Madrazo, A., Henry Ford Hospital, Detroit, Michigan, U.S.A.
Magherini, A., Cardiology Unit, University of Florence, Florence, Italy.
Magilligan, D., Henry Ford Hospital, Detroit, Michigan, U.S.A.
Maseri, A., CNR Clinical Physiology Laboratory, University of Pisa, Pisa, Italy.
Mathur, V.S., Clayton Foundation for Research Laboratory, St. Luke's Episcopal Hospital and Texas Heart Institute, Houston, Texas, U.S.A.
Mayor, Ch., Centre de Cardiologie, Hôpital Cantonal Universitaire, Geneva, Switzerland.
Meldrum, S.J., St. Bartholomew's Hospital, London, England.
Michelassi, C., CNR Clinical Physiology Laboratory, University of Pisa, Pisa, Italy.
Morard, J.-D., Centre de Cardiologie, Hôpital Cantonal Universitaire, Geneva, Switzerland.
Moynihan, P.F., Cardiology Section, Peter Bent Brigham Hospital, Boston, Massachusetts, U.S.A.
Nanda, N.C., Dept. of Cardiology, University of Rochester, Rochester, New York, U.S.A.
Nagata, S., Hospital, National Cardiovascular Center, Suita, Osaka, Japan.
Nimura, Y., Research Institute, National Cardiovascular Center, Suita, Osaka, Japan.
Oddou, C., Groupe de Recherche U 138 de l'I.N.S.E.R.M., Service d'Exploration Fonctionnelle C.H.U. Henri Mondor, Créteil, France.
Orzan, F., Clayton Foundation for Research Laboratory, St. Luke's Episcopal Hospital and Texas Heart Institute, Houston, Texas, U.S.A.
Pachinger, O., Cardiological Clinic, University of Vienna, Vienna, Austria.
Parisi, A.F., Cardiology Section, West Roxbury V.A. Medical Center, Boston, Massachusetts, U.S.A.
Park, Y.-D., Hospital, National Cardiovascular Center, Suita, Osaka, Japan.
Pearlman, A.S., University of Washington, Seattle, Washington, U.S.A.
Pechacek, L.W., Clayton Foundation for Research Laboratory, St. Luke's Episcopal Hospital and Texas Heart Institute, Houston, Texas, U.S.A.
Perrenoud, J.J., Centre de Cardiologie, Hôpital Cantonal Universitaire, Geneva, Switzerland.
Popp, C.I., Cardiology Division, Stanford University, Stanford, California, U.S.A.
Porciuncula, R.L., Non-invasive and Hemodynamics Laboratory, Philippine Heart Center for Asia, Quezon City, Philippines.
Pouget, B., Hôpital Cardiologique, C.H.U. Bordeaux, Pessac, France.

Pourcelot, L.G., Dept. of Biophysics and Nuclear Medicine, C.H.R. Bretonneau, Tours, France.
Probst, P., Cardiological Clinic, University of Vienna, Vienna, Austria.
Ramos, F.P., Non-invasive and Hemodynamics Laboratory, Philippine Heart Center for Asia, Quezon City, Philippines.
Rasmussen, S., Indiana University School of Medicine, Indianapolis, Indiana, U.S.A.
Reneman, R.S., Dept. of Physiology, Biomedical Center, University of Limburg, Maastricht, The Netherlands.
Rickards, A.F., The National Heart Hospital and Cardiothoracic Institute, London, England.
Ridder, J., Delft University of Technology, Dept. of Applied Physics, Group of Acoustics, Delft, The Netherlands.
Righetti, A., Hôpital Cantonal, Centre de Cardiologie, Geneva, Switzerland.
Roelandt, J.R., Thoraxcenter, Erasmus University, Rotterdam, The Netherlands.
Rogé, C., Cardiovascular Research Institute and Dept. of Pediatrics, University of California, San Francisco, California, U.S.A.
Rogers, E., Indiana University School of Medicine, Indianapolis, Indiana, U.S.A.
Rohmer, J., University Hospital, Leiden, The Netherlands.
Roudaut, R., Hôpital Cardiologique, C.H.U. Bordeaux, Pessac, France.
Rubenstein, S.A., Division of Pediatric Cardiology, University of Washington, Seattle, Washington, U.S.A.
Ruissen, C.J., University of Limburg, Maastricht, The Netherlands.
Rijsterborgh, H., Thoraxcenter, Erasmus University, Rotterdam, The Netherlands.
Sahn, D.J., Dept. of Pediatrics, University of Arizona, Health Sciences Center, Tucson, Arizona, U.S.A.
Sakakibara, H., Hospital, National Cardiovascular Center, Suita, Osaka, Japan.
Sam Wann, L., Indiana University School of Medicine, Indianapolis, Indiana, U.S.A.
Schenk, E.A., Pathology Dept., University of Rochester, Rochester, New York, U.S.A.
Schlag, W., Dept. of Cardiopneumology, Klinikum Steglitz FU Berlin, Berlin, Germany.
Schmaltz, A.A., Dept. of Pediatric Cardiology, University Children's Hospital, Tuebingen, Germany.
Schmitz, J.J.F., Dept. of Physiology, Biomedical Center, University of Limburg, Maastricht. The Netherlands.
Schröder, R., Dept. of Cardiopneumology, Klinikum Steglitz FU Berlin, Berlin, Germany.
Silverman, N., Cardiovascular Research Institute and Dept. of Pediatrics, University of California, San Francisco, California, U.S.A.
Simonin, A., Hôpital Cantonal, Centre de Cardiologie, Geneva, Switzerland.
Smeets, F.A.M., University of Limburg, Maastricht, The Netherlands.
Snider, R., Cardiovascular Research Institute and Dept. of Pediatrics, University of California, San Francisco, California, U.S.A.
Snoeckx, L.H.E.H., Dept. of Physiology, Biomedical Center, University of Limburg, Maastricht, The Netherlands.
Somerville, J., The National Heart Hospital and Cardiothoracic Institute, London, England.
Soto, R.C., Non-invasive and Hemodynamics Laboratory, Philippine Heart Center for Asia, Quezon City, Philippines.
Souquet, J., Thomson CSF, ASM Division, Cagnes-sur-Mer, France.
Spitaels, S.E.C., Sophia Children's Hospital, Erasmus University, Rotterdam, The Netherlands.
Stevenson, J.G., Division of Pediatric Cardiology, University of Washington, Seattle, Washington, U.S.A.
Thomin, C., Université de Valenciennes, Valenciennes, France.
Thomson, K., Dept. of Radiology, University of Rochester, Rochester, New York, U.S.A.
Torguet, R., Université de Valenciennes, Valenciennes, France.
Tunstall Pedoe, D.S., St. Bartholomew's Hospital, London, England.
Tynan, M., Hôpital Cardiologique, C.H.U. Bordeaux, Pessac, France.
Verdouw, P.D., Thoraxcenter, Erasmus University, Rotterdam, The Netherlands.
Veyrat, C., Dept. of Cardiology, Fondation A. de Rothschild, Paris, France.
Vidne, B., Toor Heart Institute, Beilinson Medical Center, Petah Tiqva, Israel.
Villeneuve, V.H. de, Sophia Children's Hospital, Erasmus University, Rotterdam, The Netherlands.
Vletter, W.B., Thoraxcenter, Erasmus University, Rotterdam, The Netherlands.
Vogel, J.A., Thoraxcenter, Erasmus University, Rotterdam, The Netherlands.
Voogd, P.J., Dept. of Cardiology, University Hospital, Leiden, The Netherlands.
Vosters, R., Dept. of Obstetrics and Gynaecology, Erasmus University, Rotterdam, The Netherlands.

Waag, R.C., Electrical Engineering Dept., University of Rochester, Rochester, New York, U.S.A.
Wells, P.N.T., Bristol Health District, Dept. of Medical Physics, Bristol General Hospital,
   Bristol, England.
Werf, F. van de, Dept. of Pathophysiology, St. Raphael University Hospital, Leuven, Belgium.
Wessel, H.J., Dept. of Cardiopneumology, Klinikum Steglitz, FU Berlin, Berlin, Germany.
Weyman, A.E., Indiana University School of Medicine, Indianapolis, Indiana, U.S.A.
Wladimiroff, J.W., Dept. of Obstetrics and Gynaecology, Erasmus University, Rotterdam, The
   Netherlands.
Yulde, J.A., Non-invasive and Hemodynamics Laboratory, Philippine Heart Center for Asia,
   Quezon City, Philippines.
Zwieten, G. van, Thoraxcenter, Erasmus University, Rotterdam, The Netherlands.

I

ECHOCARDIOLOGY IN ADULTS

A. GENERAL APPLICATIONS

ECHO-MECHANOCARDIOGRAPHIC ASSESSMENT OF CARDIAC DYNAMICS

A.E. AUBERT, B. DENEF, F. VAN DE WERF, and H. KESTELOOT

INTRODUCTION

Calibrated apexcardiography has become widely accepted as a method for the non-invasive assessment of cardiac performance (1, 2) and as an indirect method for timing intracardiac mechanical events (3, 4, 5). Its intrinsic value can be further increased by simultaneously recording echocardiographic dimensions (6, 7, 8).

The aim of the present study was to compare the morphology of left ventricular pressure (LVP), wall tension (T) and the calibrated apexcardiogram (QLAC), to correlate these signals and to deduce left ventricular function from these data.

METHODOLOGY

A set of acute dog experiments has been performed. During these experiments nine parameters were recorded simultaneously: the ECG, the LVP, recorded with a microtip Gaeltec catheter, its time-derivative, the end-diastolic pressure, the aortic pressure, also measured with a Gaeltec microtip catheter, the phonocardiogram, the QLAC and its time-derivative and finally the M-mode echo. QLAC and the M-mode echo were digitized for further processing using simple computing techniques.

QLAC was recorded with a pixie beam strain gauge. The calibration in pressure units can be performed simply by putting small weights on its surface. This results in a step function that is related to pressure. The derivative of QLAC was calibrated by using an electronic triangular signal. The advantage of calibration in apexcardiography has been pointed out in numerous publications from our group (1, 2, 5).

Recordings were made with the dog in the left recumbent position. The thoracic geometry of the dog is such that the left ventricle can be reached both from a left- and a right-sided approach. Generally QLAC was recorded at the place of maximal displacement on the left side and the M-mode echo from the right side. By changing the angular direction of the echo transducer it was possible to direct the beam either to the left ventricle alone, or through both the right and left ventricles, across the intraventricular septum (7, 8). Contrast echocardiography was performed by injecting a small quantity of CO_2 in order to delineate cardiac structures and dimensions. Figure 1 shows a typical recording.

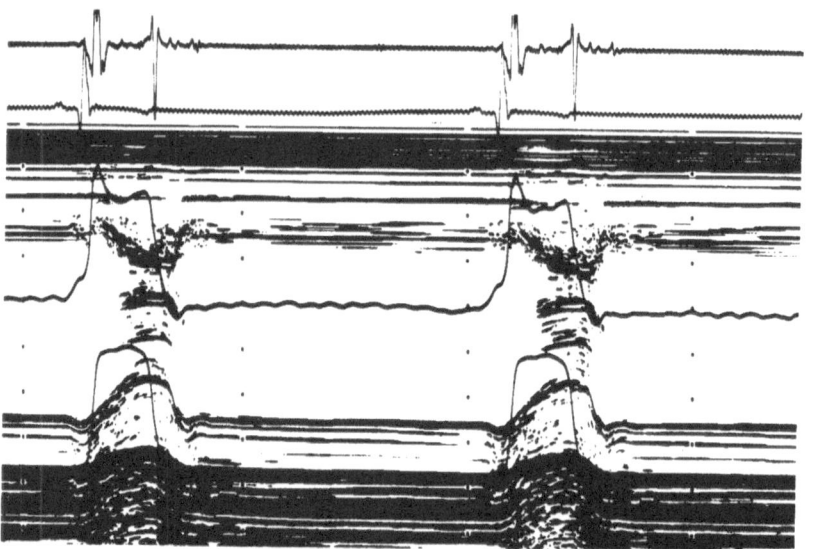

Fig. 1. Echo-mechanocardiogram showing from above: internal phonocardiogram, ECG, QLAC, LVP and LV echocardiogram.

APEXCARDIOGRAPHY AND LVP

As far as the morphology of QLAC and LVP is concerned, a very good correlation has been found during the isovolumic contraction phase (IC) and during isovolumic beats (1, 9). The steep upstroke of QLAC occurs during IC, when only small diameter changes in the left ventricle are apparent. There is also a close correlation during the isovolumic relaxation phase (IR). On the other hand, there are marked differences between the two tracings during the ejection phase (7, 8). (See Fig. 1.) As a general rule the LVP tracing shows a plateau or has a positive slope and QLAC a negative slope in the systolic ejection phase, thus giving an indication that LVP is not the only factor determining QLAC during ejection.

This point raises the question of the genesis of the apexcardiogram. Possible factors affecting QLAC can be divided into three categories: mechanical, geometrical and methodological. *Mechanical factors*: LVP, T, compliance (can influence pressure by opposing more or less resistance to filling), sequence of activation (can influence the time sequence of pressure development during contraction and relaxation), gravity (the position of the patient can affect the contact surface between heart and thoracic wall), work and power generated by the heart (change in flow and peripheral resistance), movements of the heart (rotation and torsion), as well as ballistic forces (although these factors do not play an important role). *Geometrical factors*: orientation of the heart, structure of thoracic wall, contact surface between heart and thoracic wall (influence on location and amplitude of maximal impulse), volume, mass, dimension, geometry of the heart. *Methodological factors*: methods of registration, transducer and its time-constant (optimally

> 3 sec (10)), location of the transducer on the thorax, pressure exerted by the transducer on the thorax.

The next part of this discussion will mainly concentrate on the relation between QLAC, LVP and T.

WALL TENSION

Wall tension, mathematically described by Laplace's law, is in fact a combination of hemodynamical and dimensional data. As a pressure can be defined as a force acting perpendicular to a surface, a tension, in the case of a sphere, can be defined as the force counteracting the pressure in it. This results in an expression for the tension in thick walled bodies: $T = PR/2h$ (P: the pressure, h: wall thickness and R: inner radius). It is more logical to take

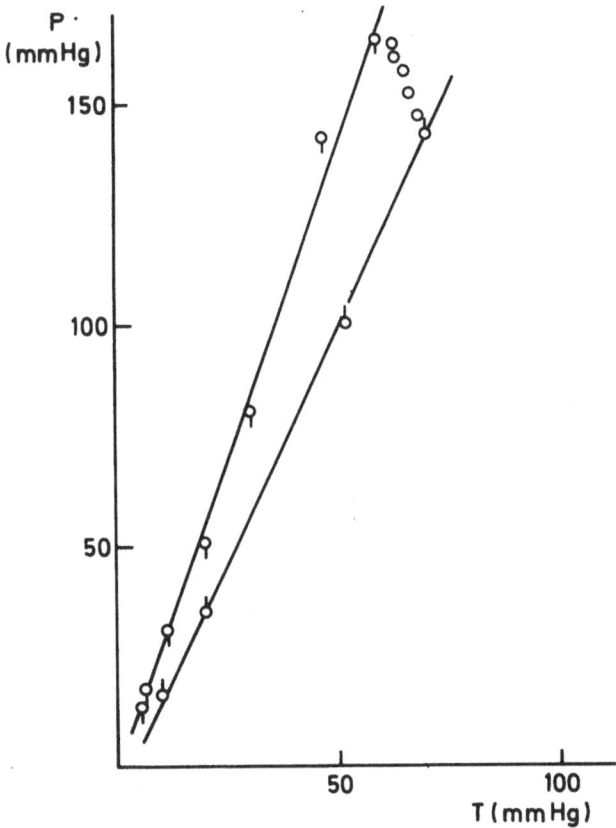

Fig. 2. Correlation between LVP (P) and T.
ð: during IC
o: during systolic plateau
ǫ: during IR.

the inner radius, instead of another parameter, as the pressure exerts force on the inner surface of the heart.

The applicability of mean meridional wall tension as a descriptor of ventricular myocardial function (as a major determinant of myocardial oxygen consumption and hypertrophy) is dependent on the assumption that there are no large local variations in wall force. If this were the case, more complex expressions for the calculation of myocardial tension would have to be used (11).

On the other hand, calculation of the circumferential wall tension requires knowledge of the left ventricular long axis (11). As this dimension is inaccessible by M-mode echo, we restricted ourselves to the calculation of the meridional wall tension.

As only small dimensional changes are apparent during IC and IR it is to be expected that T and LVP are very alike. This is shown on Figure 2: there is an almost perfect correlation during IC and IR.

As far as T is concerned it can be stated that it is proportional to:

1. LVP during IC and IR (dimensions remaining relatively constant),

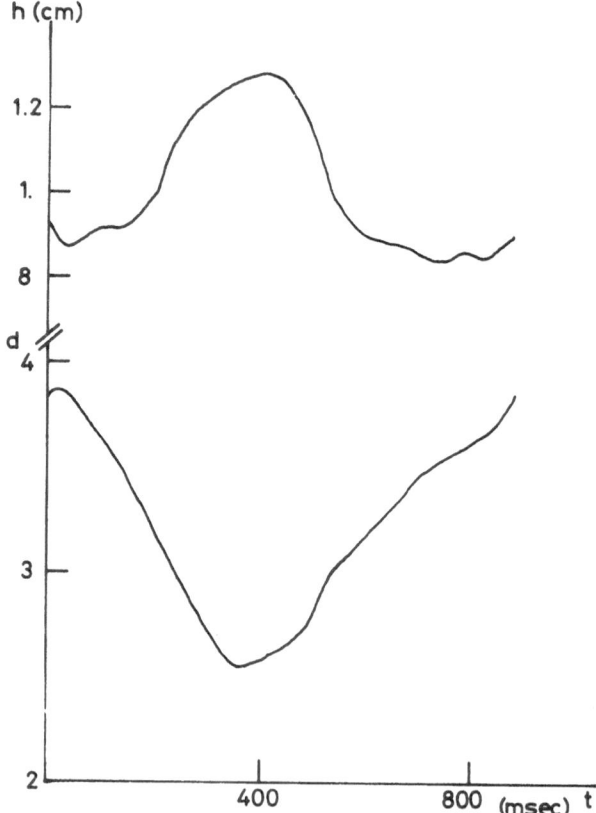

Fig. 3. Upper trace (h): evolution of left ventricular wall thickness. Lower trace (d): instantaneous value of the distance between septum and left posterior wall.

2. Dimensions in diastole (pressure remaining relatively constant except during atrial contraction),
3. LVP and dimensions during ejection.

RESULTS AND DISCUSSION

As pointed out earlier, dimensional changes of the minor diameter and wall thickness can be continuously monitored during a cardiac cycle. This is shown in Figure 3. The lower part shows the ventricular dimension, representing the distance between septum and posterior wall. It varies between 2.6 and 3.9 cm. The upper tracing shows the left ventricular posterior wall thickness. The wall thickness varies between 0.9 and 1.25 cm. It is seen that, as the ventricle expands, wall thickness decreases and vice versa.

Results of combined hemodynamic and M-mode echo data are given in Figure 4 and Figure 5. Figure 4 shows a comparison of QLAC, LVP and T, calculated as above. On inspection there appears to be better agreement between QLAC and T than between QLAC and LVP, especially during the ejection phase; both QLAC and T have a negative slope.

Figure 5 shows the evolution of an acute volume overload by the intravenous injection of 500 ml of Haemaccel (LVP versus left ventricular diameter d). The area of this loop represents the stroke work per unit area of endocardium performed by the region of myocardium that is seen by the

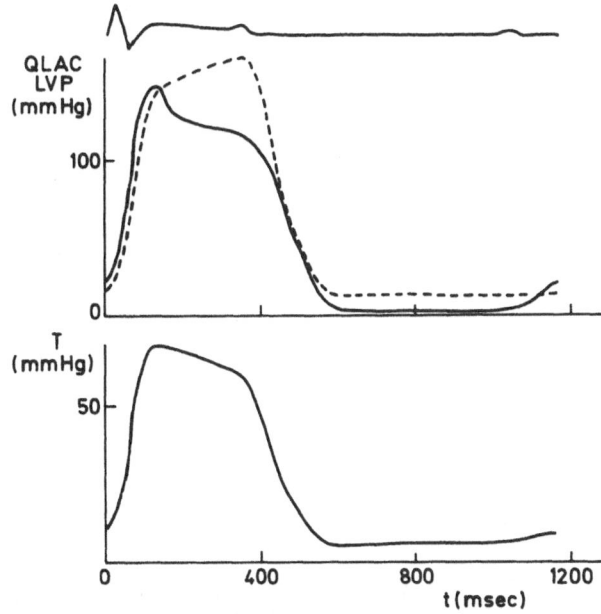

Fig. 4. Digitized and calculated values showing from below: T (full line), QLAC (full line), LVP (dotted line) and ECG.

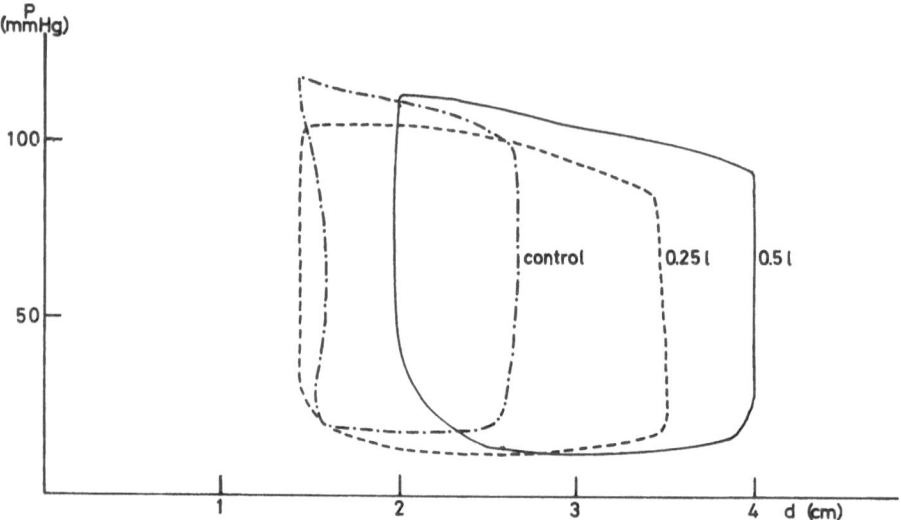

Fig. 5. P–d loops for an acute volume overload: control state (point-dotted line), after the infusion of 0.25 l Haemaccel (dotted line) and after 0.5 l (full line).

echo beam. From Laplace's law, it is clear that T will increase in this case, without a noticeable LVP increase, thus showing that a dilated heart is pumping in an inefficient way needing a high T, at the expense of increased oxygen consumption.

Figure 6 and Figure 7 shows phase or hysteresis loops for LVP and

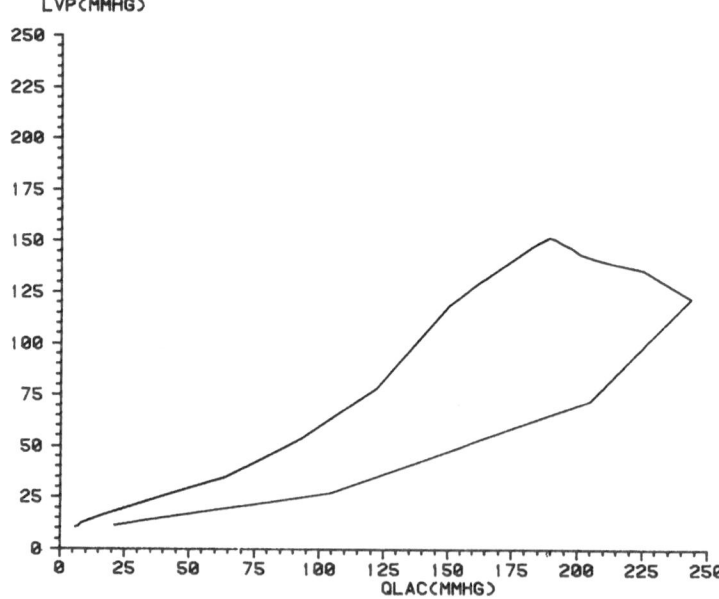

Fig. 6. LVP–QLAC hysteresis loop.

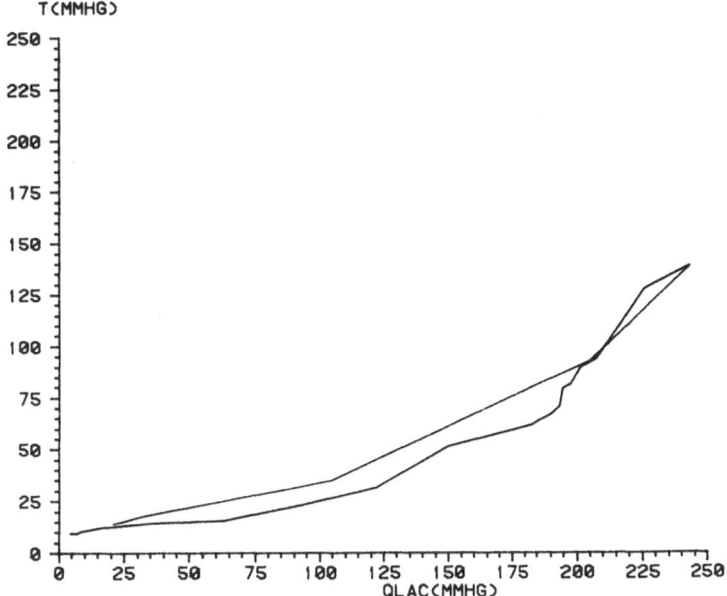

Fig. 7. T–QLAC hysteresis loop, showing a much better correlation than the curve from figure 6.

QLAC, and T and QLAC. The loops are always cycled in a counterclockwise direction.

This approach can indeed be named a phase or hysteresis loop as it shows a phase difference between LVP and QLAC; on the whole, LVP lags QLAC. It confirms previous results from our group (5, 8, 12):

1. A marked synchronism of the onset of systolic rise of QLAC and LVP, because there is a linear relationship between them in that phase (cf. the phase loop of two sinusoids that are in phase results in a straight line).

2. An earlier occurrence of the proto-diastolic nadir on QLAC than on LVP (6, 12), as shown by the ellipsoidal shape in the left corner where the loop closes (cf. the phase loop of two sinusoids out of phase and of unequal amplitude results in an ellipsoid).

From these phase loops it is in principle possible to deduce instantaneous time differences between the two curves. However, practical difficulties arise from the rather distorted shape of the curve, it is difficult to draw an axis of symmetry.

From the comparison between Figure 6 and Figure 7 it appears that T and QLAC are more in phase than are LVP and QLAC. This visual impression can be mathematically confirmed by correlating LVP and QLAC, and T and QLAC. Figure 8 shows the result, which indeed shows a better correlation between the latter pair than between the former pair, and this has been confirmed in numerous experiments. Our previous work (1, 2, 12) had shown the important role of LVP as a determinant of QLAC; highly significant

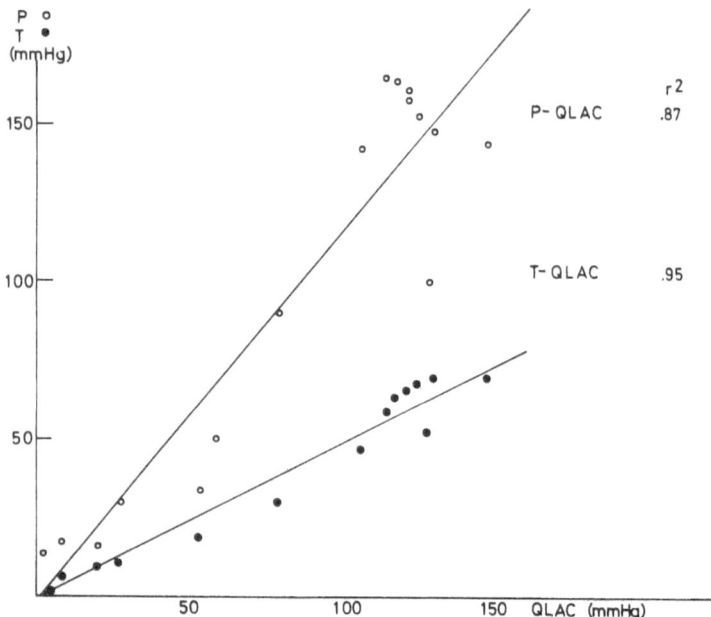

Fig. 8. Correlation between LVP and QLAC (open circles) and between T and QLAC (solid circles).

correlations exist between the height of the first derivatives of QLAC and LVP, both during atrial and during isovolumic contractions. During acute clamping experiments in the ejection phase, nearly identical changes were found in LVP and QLAC (13). Normalized indices of contractility obtained during isovolumic contractions for QLAC and LVP also were significantly correlated (1, 2), however significant discrepancies persisted between QLAC and LVP during the ejection phase.

M-mode echocardiography combined with hemodynamic data can now be used to give a better understanding of externally recorded mechanical events by demonstrating the importance of wall tension; QLAC is proportional to:

1. wall tension or LVP at low LVP,
2. wall tension at higher LVP,
3. wall tension during the systolic plateau phase.

The combination of dimensional and apexcardiography data can also give information on ventricular wall compliance. The slope of QLAC versus ventricular dimension during atrial contraction, both plotted on a logarithmic scale, can be considered as an indicator of ventricular diastolic compliance. Highly significant differences were found between normal hearts on the one hand and hearts with volume or pressure overload and with cardiomyopathies on the other hand (14). These findings further enhance the diagnostic value of a combined mechano-echocardiographic evaluation of heart function.

CONCLUSION

The value of both calibrated apexcardiography and echocardiography for the assessment of myocardial function is enhanced by a combination of the two methods. Our studies indicate that the left apexcardiogram can be considered representative of pressure development in the heart during isovolumic contraction and relaxation, and of wall tension during the left ventricular ejection phase. Uni-directional dimensional changes are considered representative of volume changes of the heart. Thus non-invasive "pressure-volume" loops may be constructed and data can be obtained on left ventricular diastolic compliance.

REFERENCES

1. Kesteloot H, B Denef, J Willems, H de Geest: On the value of the calibrated apexcardiogram in the assessment of left ventricular function. Proceedings of the Meeting on Cardiac Contractility, Bordeaux, 1973, p 173.
2. Denef B, F van de Werf, H De Geest, H Kesteloot: Calibrated apexcardiography and assessment of left ventricular dynamics in man. Eur J Cardiol 4:143, 1976.
3. Benchimol A, E Dimond: The normal and abnormal apexcardiogram. Its physiological variation and its relation to intracardiac events. Am J Cardiol 11:427, 1963.
4. Willems J, H Kesteloot: The left ventricular ejection time. Its relation to heart rate, mechanical systole and some anthropometric data. Acta Cardiol 22:401, 1967.
5. Willems J, H de Geest, H Kesteloot: On the value of apexcardiography for timing intracardiac events. Am J Cardiol 28:59, 1971.
6. Venco A, D Gibson, D Brown: Relation between apexcardiogram and changes in left ventricular pressure and dimensions. Brit Heart J 39:117, 1977.
7. Aubert AE, B Denef, F Van de Werf, H Kesteloot: An experimental study of left ventricular wall stress and its relation to the calibrated apexcardiogram. Transact Eur Soc Card 1:26, 1978.
8. Aubert AE, B Denef, F Van de Werf, H Kesteloot: Cardiac function assessment by simultaneous calibrated apex- and echocardiography. In: Basic and clinical aspects of cardiac dynamics, Baan J, Arntzenius A (eds), Amsterdam Oxford, Excerpta Medica, 1978, p 4.
9. Willems J: The normal apexcardiogram. Arscia Ed., Brussels, 1973.
10. Kesteloot H, J Willems, E van Vollenhoven: On the physical principles and methodology of mechanocardiography. Acta Cardiol 24:147, 1969.
11. Mirsky I: Review of various theories for the evaluation of left ventricular wall stress. Cardiac mechanics. Physiological, clinical, and mathematical considerations. Mirsky I, Ghista D, Sandler H, (eds), New York, J. Wiley, 1974, p 331.
12. Van de Werf F, J Piessens, H Kesteloot, H de Geest: Value of apexcardiography for the timing of left ventricular events in man. Acta Cardiol 33:295, 1978.
13. Kesteloot H: Assessment of left ventricular function by means of calibrated apexcardiography. Archives del Cardiol Mexico 47:499, 1977.
14. Fukumoto T, H Kesteloot: Non-invasive determination of left ventricular diastolic compliance (to be published).

A COMPREHENSIVE APPROACH TO CARDIAC MEASUREMENTS

D.W. BAKER*

The solution to the problem of how to make the most accurate cardiac or cardiovasvular diagnosis has followed an interesting path, led largely by the availability of certain types of instrumentation. Characteristically, when a particular methodology or line of thought starts to become entrenched in the minds of investigators, it becomes increasingly difficult to maintain an objective point of view. In many cases, researchers take up defensive positions to preserve or protect their particular approach.

As new methods or devices appear, followers emerge. Groups tend to compete with other groups using existing methods, and often the methods are viewed as competitive, when in fact they may not be.

The gradual introduction of blood-flow oriented instruments and methods into cardiology is a good example of this. Many clinicians do not understand the methods, the devices, nor the present or future role of blood flow data in a diagnosis. It is as if a new concept suddenly emerged independent of all existing approaches, having no apparent relationship to methods currently in vogue. What seems to be needed in this situation is a basic understanding of cardiac disease in terms of all its various physical forms, along with a unifying concept of the kinds and roles of intrumentation.

For example, if we could clarify the role of blood flow measurements in a given situation, and know when it is important and when it contributes very little, we would not only help the clinician, we would also aid the device developer. The instrumentation researcher is fully aware of the possibilities of combining into one device many modalities or formats (1). For example, the ideal device might include A-Mode, M-Mode, 2D imaging, and pulsed Doppler and tissue signature analysis, all as special modes of the same device, functioning simultaneously or independently. Some of these formats are well established; others are coming into use now, and others are still in the future. At the moment most clinical cardiologists will approach a diagnosis using the tools at hand, generally M-mode; some will use a 2D scanner, and even fewer will use a pulsed Doppler (2). Tissue analysis of the myocardium has not left the research laboratories yet.

As advanced as the new devices are, the cardiologist still is faced with a complex multiparameter diagnostic situation. In many cases, a one-modality non-invasive measurement approach is like tunnel vision. Consider the hypothetical situation shown in Figure 1, involving an infarcted inter-

*University of Washington, Seattle, Washington. Supported by NIH Grant No. HL-07293.

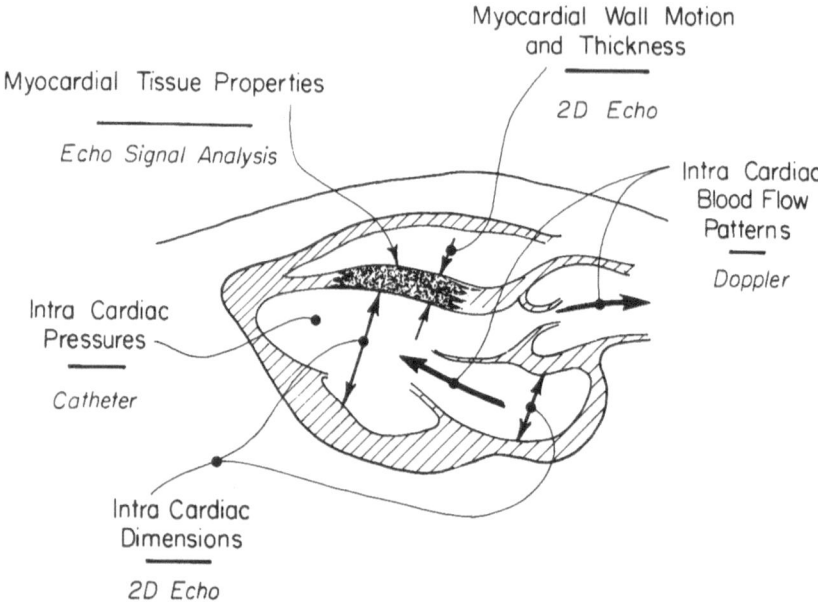

Fig. 1. The physical indicators of a cardiac defect vary in their form and significance. The optimal method for detecting them can vary from situation to situation. Concentration on one approach may lead to low sensitivity and accuracy.

ventricular septum. Many physical aspects of the ejection and filling dynamics will be affected by this situation. Often, the physical parameters characterizing the particular disease state will be interdependent. The sequential order of their change or involvement probably will depend on the specific defect. Their magnitudes also may or may not be independent. Most clinicians would agree, for the example of Figure 1, that the IVS wall motion and thickness would be the most important parameter. Tissue properties of the infarct would be important if we could detect and analyse them. Intracardiac dimensions, stroke volume, blood flow filling, and ejection will all be involved.

One might consider other clinical examples where the relative weighting of the most important parameter or hemodynamic variable is different. For example, small septal defects may manifest themselves more as a blood flow defect than as a detectable anatomical change (3). Regurgitation, along with mitral prolapse, is a blood flow defect not easily detected with M-mode or 2D imaging (4). Aortic stenosis and insufficiency are clearly anatomical or valve defects, yet they often can be more readily detected as a blood flow defect or disturbance (5). If one were to review carefully and objectively all the various cardiac diagnostic problems, one would discover that there appears to be a weighting of the most significant and readily detectable variables or parameters. The match-up between the concepts of "most significant" and "readily detectable" depends on the hemodynamics or physics of the situation and the particular sensitivities or advantages of the instrument modality used.

The logical development and evaluation of instrumentation having multiple capabilities depends heavily on establishing a unifying philosophical framework or approach to the cardiovascular diagnostic problem. From the few simplified examples presented, we can recognize that a disease process exists in a variety of physical forms or states. Ultrasonic energy in the form of a controlled beam is used to probe these states or parameters. Since the output of the instruments is in physical terms, i.e., depth – cm, angle – degrees, two-dimensional images – cm and echo amplitude – volts, there must be a relationship between the physical characteristics of disease and the type or number and magnitude of instrument outputs.

As an example, an infarct has physical dimensions of $x =$ length, $y =$ width, $z =$ thickness. Whether the defect is regular or irregular makes no difference; the infarct still exists in the three dimensions of physical space. If it moves about as the heart contracts, then its location, and possibly its shape, becomes a function of time.

It is not difficult to understand that a complete physical description requires four dimensions. Almost all anatomical defects of the heart exist in four dimensions. Correspondingly, the blood flow patterns associated with a septal defect exist in the dimensions of time and space as well. In fact, all blood flow signals are four-dimensional. Tissue properties are a function of much more than time and space. In this case, one has to consider blood flow to the tissue as well as biochemical and electrochemical parameters. If we return to Figure 1, and consider each parameter as involving an independent set of dimensions as distinct from flow patterns and tissue characteristics, then the number of separate dimensions or variables required to describe the disease state becomes very large. Each instrument modality functions best when concerned with a limited portion or set of these dimensions. For example, echo techniques are best for spatial dimensions, Doppler techniques are best for velocity, i.e., rate of change of position, and echo signal analysis might be best for tissue studies.

As human beings, our sensory capabilities limit our ability to conceive of an entity which has so many variables. To improve our perception requires reducing the number of variables, or order, of this N-dimensional description or space into a lower order of fewer variables. This sequential reduction process can be visualized as a type of communication channel with various kinds of activities distributed along its length. This idea is diagrammed in Figure 2, using ultrasound instrumentation in a cardiovascular diagnosis example. The channel consists of four cascaded operations or steps. Each step is given a name corresponding to the kind of activity involved. These are in sequence, as follows:

- Disease Space -
- Detection Space -
- Analysis Space -
- Display Space -

Each is called a space because of the numerous dimensions or variables existing at each step, which are derived from the original disease entity. The

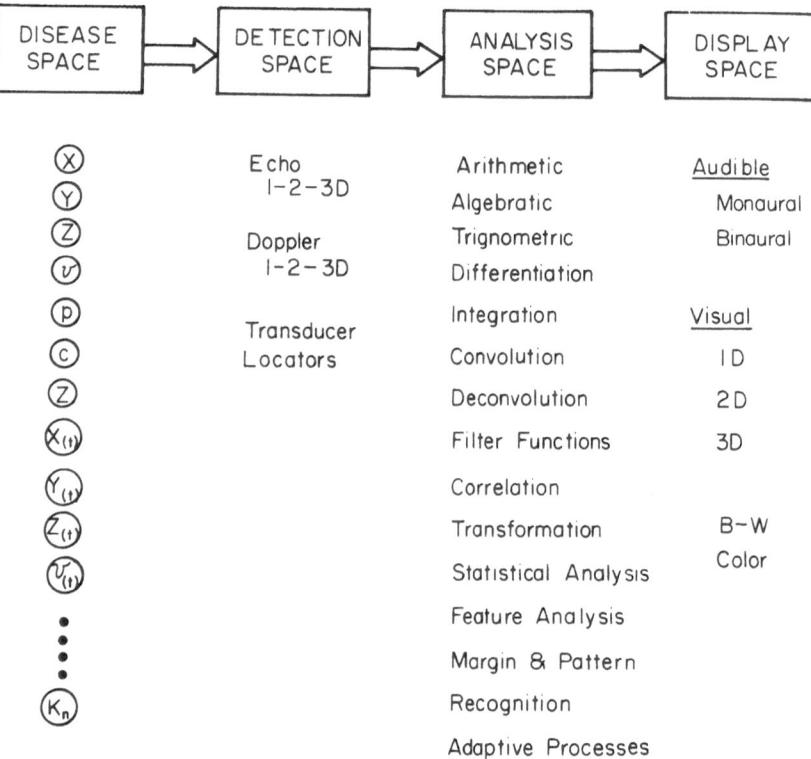

Fig. 2. The diagnostic procedure can be represented by a series of steps or processes. These serve to transform the physical variables of the disease state into a display format which can be readily interpreted by human observers.

form of the original variable changes for each transformation as the information passes step by step toward eventual display for interpretation by the observer.

DISEASE SPACE

The physical manifestation of the disease is called the disease space and has a set of dimensions (variables) of order N set by the particular disease. This is diagrammed as the length of the line on the left of Figure 3. Examples of variables might be: length, width, height, mass, density, velocity, acoustical impedance, velocity of sound, velocity profiles, turbulent intensity.

DETECTION SPACE

The physical characteristics of the disease are probed using beams of ultrasonic energy in echo or Doppler mode. In this step, the dimensions of

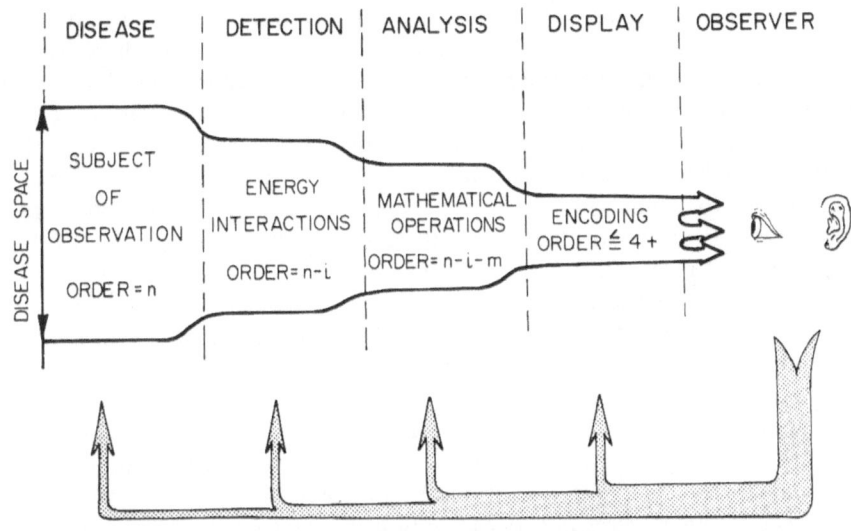

INTERVENTION – OPTIMIZATION

Fig. 3. The physical variables representing the disease state or space can be thought of as moving along a communications channel on their way to being displayed. The width of this channel, which corresponds to the band of information being conveyed, must become narrower to be within the limits of perception of the human observer. Mental processing leads to feedback intended to optimize the entire sequence.

the disease are converted into electrical form by the transducers and associated amplifiers. This step is called the detection space (see Figs. 2 and 3). The order N of the channel may be reduced in this step because the instrument modalities cannot detect all the dimensions or variables of the disease. The output from the detection step cannot yet be interpreted by our senses, because we know only echo amplitude, transit time to an interface and return, or Doppler shift of the echo, etc. If transducer position locators are used, we know the location and direction from which the returns come with respect to external coordinate references.

ANALYSIS SPACE

In the analysis space of the channel, various mathematical operations are performed to the returning signals from the tissue in order to further reduce the number of variables or dimensions of information. Figure 2 lists these operations, which range from simple arithmetic procedures to the yet-to-be developed pattern (or feature) analysis routines. It is in this analysis step that the digital computer finds its place.

DISPLAY SPACE

We require for our sensory inputs some form of display or output device. Display space in the channel sequence represents the final encoding of the disease dimension data into a form we can perceive. These outputs can be both audible and visual. The higher the order, i.e., the more dimensions or variables to be conveyed, the more complex the display will be. For example, the output of an echo-Doppler Duplex scanner, used to evaluate blood flow patterns in conjunction with wall abnormalities in small children, uses a multi-colored M-mode display plus an audible output of the flow signal. An example of this can be found in the paper "M/Q-mode echocardiography – the synthesis of conventional echo with digital multigate Doppler" (see Fig. 4 therein) by Marco Brandestini et al., appearing in this volume (6). That illustration shows the M-mode echo returns as grey scale. Superimposed on the image is blood flow velocity toward the transducer, shown in shades of red. The line on the M-mode image corresponds to the depth of the pulse Doppler sample gate for the audible output.

The entire detection, analysis, and display sequence appears in Figure 3 as a gradually narrowing channel showing the reduction of the order N of the original disease entity (space) for eventual display. The observer usually must intervene in this process in order to optimize the measurement. Manipulation of the transducer and instrument settings to optimize the output displays is readily appreciated by the experienced user. This process becomes more complex when we begin to deal with a multi-parameter disease state.

Referring back to the earlier examples illustrated in Figure 1, we could represent the disease state or space as a disease profile, as in Figure 4. At present, the idea of a disease profile cannot be well defined or calibrated. All we can do is recognize the possibility in the context of an ultrasonic assessment of it.

The disease profile may never be an absolute entity, due to the apparent dependence on how it is measured. The instrument capabilities have to be considered as an influence on the profile shape. Consider, for example, the

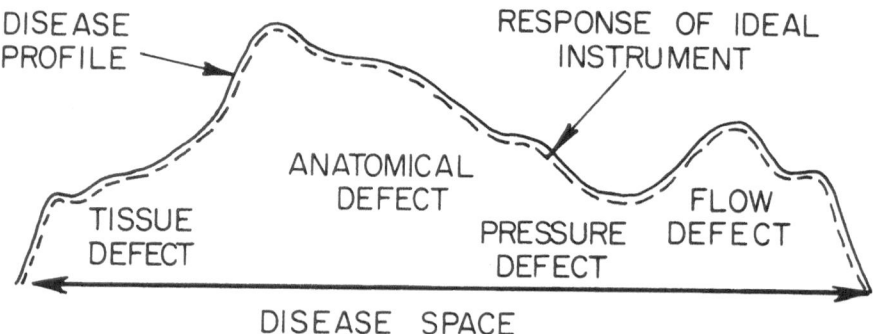

Fig. 4. The state or status of a particular disease process at a given instant in time can be modeled by a profile. The shape of this profile depends on the most significant physical manifestation of the disease, and upon the ability of the measurement methods to detect them. For example, a physical indicator which might be difficult to detect would have a low contribution to the profile; conversely, easily detected, uniquely related parameters will have a high contribution.

possible profile for IHSS, where the tissue anatomical aspects would be heavily weighted, based on our current knowledge of the disease. The pressure and flow aspects would be present but less important. Another example that would have quite a different profile would be mitral prolapse with regurgitation. Here, the flow aspect would have greater weight, with anatomy next, and tissue or pressure of lesser significance. Note, however, that, in establishing these somewhat arbitrary weightings, one must keep in mind the ease with which a particular parameter can be detected by either echo or Doppler techniques. The most we can say at the moment is that a disease profile seems like a workable concept. Further, that it is influenced in some manner by the disease form and by the particular sensitivity of the instruments to the variables or dimensions of the disease.

OPTIMIZATION SPACE

It may be possible to define yet another "space" associated with the optimization of a procedure. If we consider a disease profile as the input information to the communication channel, then optimization would be the process of adapting or modifying the measurement analysis channel in order to match the instrument measurement capability to the input profile. The result is shown as the response of the ideal instrument in Figure 4. Let us assume that the clinician is confronted with a murmur, believed to be associated with either a high membranous VSD or MR, in a pediatric patient. The clinician has an M-mode or 2D scanner. With only these instruments, he will be unable to match the disease profile curve using the detection capabilities available to him. In this instance, use of a Doppler device complementing the imaging would have allowed the clinician to create a more ideal overall measurement response and to optimize the sensitivity of the procedure.

Maximum clinical sensitivity and selectivity for diagnosis of a specific disease is usually determined by good instrument design and use. If an instrument is totally programmable, so that frequency, pulse rate, amplification, beam shape, etc., can be quickly altered, then the best possible recordings might be possible in any given situation. Figure 5 summarizes some of the important performance-controlling parameters of both echo and Doppler instruments. Each of these factors eventually depends upon the tissue characteristics or intrinsic physical limitations. The left column in Figure 5 lists the principal parameter of the device; at the center and to the right are the factors which these parameters most depend upon. For example, image resolution depends upon transducer bandwidth and beamwidth, as well as on tissue dispersion. Velocity ambiguity, i.e., detection of one Doppler shift for one velocity, depends upon several factors. Among these are the velocity of the blood for a given pulse repetition rate, the angle between flow axis and beam, and the transmitted ultrasound frequency. When all these come into play, we usually can find a specific combination of instrument

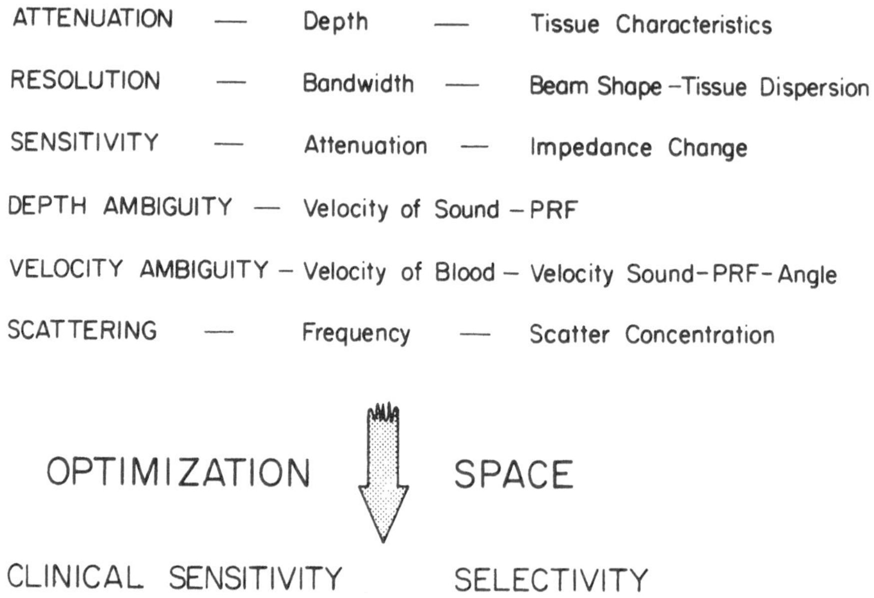

ATTENUATION   —   Depth   —   Tissue Characteristics

RESOLUTION   —   Bandwidth   —   Beam Shape –Tissue Dispersion

SENSITIVITY   —   Attenuation —   Impedance Change

DEPTH AMBIGUITY   — Velocity of Sound – PRF

VELOCITY AMBIGUITY – Velocity of Blood – Velocity Sound–PRF–Angle

SCATTERING   —   Frequency   —   Scatter Concentration

OPTIMIZATION  SPACE

CLINICAL SENSITIVITY   SELECTIVITY

Fig. 5. Optimization of the diagnostic process to improve sensitivity and specificity is largely dependent on the instrument's ability to detect the significant physical variables. This ability is usually governed by physical laws and the physical form of the disease. Maximizing the data often involves trading one instrument characteristic or function for another. For example, good resolution depends on the transducer having broad bandwidth, yet sensitivity to detect small echoes depends on narrow transducer bandwidth.

characteristics which provide the best overall clinical sensitivity and specificity. Optimum adjustment of these characteristics in an echo-Doppler imaging system to match the disease profile, should lead to maximum information transfer to the observer.

CARDIAC DISEASE SPACE

For simplicity, let us divide the cardiac disease space into three broad categories. These are shown as bands of information in Figure 6. Currently, the primary approach to cardiac diagnosis is M-mode echo and 2D imaging, with principal emphasis on the measurement of anatomical dimensions. Blood flow patterns, for lack of experience, understanding, and adequate equipment, are considered by some to be less useful at present.

The possibilities for increased use of flow information remain relatively undeveloped. If we expand upon blood flow detection as an important clinical factor, we can generate the fan-out shown in Figure 7. Here we see the same possibilities for flow velocity as a clinical indicator. Volumetric blood flow quantitation is not considered in this example, because it requires measurement of average velocity over the vessel or orifice lumen, cross-sectional area, and the angle between the sound beam axis and the flow vector. From Figures 7 and 8, we see that the blood flow velocity patterns

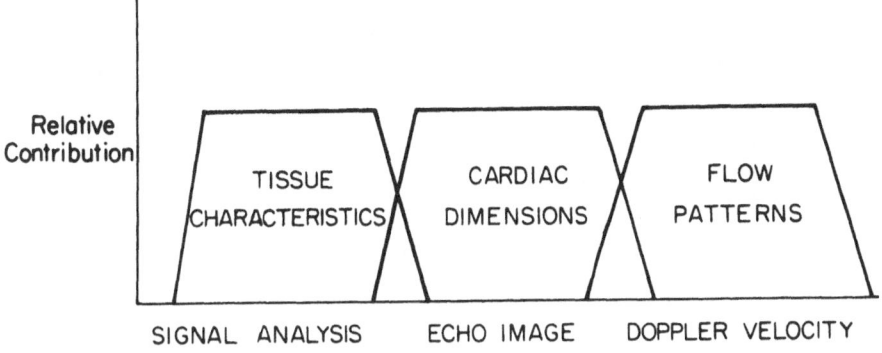

CARDIAC DISEASE SPACE

Fig. 6. The band of information describing the disease state for a specific organ category can be subdivided into sets aligned with particular instrument or analytical methods. Because of instrument limitations, the field of cardiology has had to limit its diagnostic approach to using dimensional data.

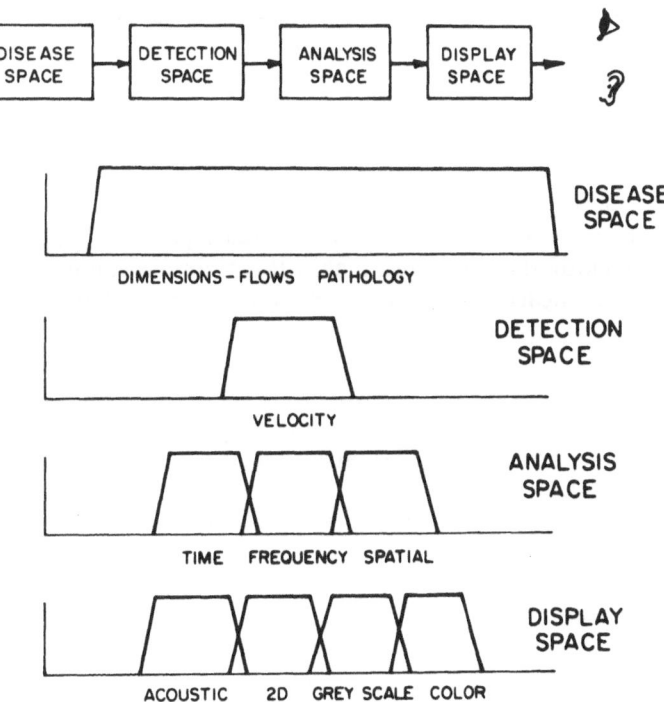

Fig. 7. The potential use of blood flow velocity information can be expanded upon and explained by using a communications channel approach. A separate and independent set can be generated for dimensional as well as tissue measurement.

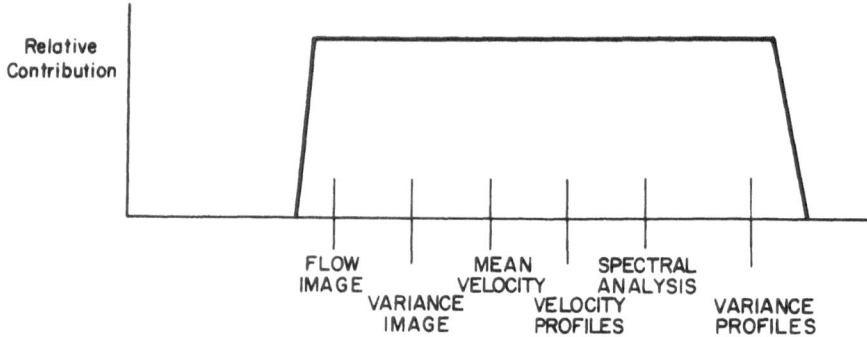

FLOW SPACE

Fig. 8. A closer analysis of flow velocity patterns demonstrates a new subset of data, which can be displayed to show specific features of flow. These, in turn, can be matched to the various physical manifestations of the disease process which are reflection in the blood flow.

can be evaluated and displayed in a variety of ways. This is possible because of the many ways blood flow velocity is altered, due to anatomical as well as physiological defects. Intracardiac shunts and defective valves produce flow disturbances in the form of free jets. These, in turn, produce turbulent wakes in the dimensions of time and physical space. These disturbances can exist at levels which may not lead to the production of low frequency, audible sound production, as in the case of cardiac murmurs. Large patent ductus arteriosus in newborns is a good example of a defect producing flow disturbances but, due to a low pressure drop through the orifice, little or no murmur-type sounds are produced.

Utilizing either single or multigate pulsed Dopplers equipped with a transducer-locating device, we are able to determine the magnitude of the flow velocity along the sound beam axis. If the sample volume is held at one point within the heart, we can determine the temporal characteristics of the mean and instantaneous velocity distribution. By moving the sample volume throughout the intracardiac chamber, while noting the transducer and sample volume position in xyz space, we can determine the spatial extent of the flow disturbance. While not quantitative, the degree to which a flow disturbance is dispersed in the left atrium in mitral regurgitation, for example, is an indicator of the severity of the defect. The principal display outputs in this simple application are the audible Doppler output and the recorded spectral broadening of the detected Doppler shift frequency. Disturbed flow, as in a "jet", sounds harsh, while smooth flow has a tonal quality to its sound.

FLOW SPACE

The manner in which we use blood flow sensing to display disease status depends on the nature of the disease state and the characteristics of the

Doppler technique. A fundamental concept to remember when considering Doppler methods is the fact that the ultrasound scattering process is not directional as compared with the specular reflection process of echo. The magnitude of the Doppler shift will be dependent, however, on the angle between the flow axis and the sound beam axis. All these factors come into play when we wish to investigate the presence and extent of disturbed blood flow within the heart and great vessels. The concept of flow space comes from the fact that the motion of blood through the heart and around the valves is a very complex process. It is easily upset by small anatomical defects. These impart disturbances, in the form of eddys or rotating vortices, which are easily detected by Doppler. Whether true turbulence exists within the heart remains to be proven.

The magnitude and extent of blood flow disturbances appear to bear some relationship to the severity of the defect. Since it is extremely difficult to quantify the volume blood flow in the presence of disturbances, i.e. flow rate through a septal defect, we must, for the moment, look to other flow parameters as a measure of severity. The physical dimensions of a disturbance include velocity, acceleration, vector orientation, and translation, to name a few. All of these vary with time, so we are dealing with a four-dimensional concept that involves many variables.

The various ways we can display flow features are shown in diagrammatic form in Figure 8. The general relationship of each flow display scheme to disease is as follows:

Flow imaging   The actual lumen of the vessel or valve can be shown by a two-dimensional image of those points in the flow which exceed a set threshold velocity. Complete imaging of the value orifices is possible without the problem of specular echo reflection. Recall that many 2D echo images fail to image the orifice because of the varying orientation of the valve leaflets with respect to the sound beam (7).

Variance image   This is a new category of imaging which, potentially, can show in a two-dimensional display whether the flow motion is disturbed or smooth. Disturbed flow causes broading of the Doppler signal spectrum which is detectable. This spectral broadening can be encoded into the image as a color pattern at each point to show degree of disturbance. While this approach is complicated and not fully understood, the feasibility has been established using the digital multigate Doppler system of Brandestini et al. Variance imaging should be useful for imaging jets or other disturbed blood flow patterns.

Mean velocity   This is the only parameter that comes close to most individuals' experience with blood flow. The output of an electromagnetic flowmeter, for example, is the mean velocity over the flow lumen. Doppler techniques can arrive at mean velocity by using a sample volume of the same size as the vessel. Another approach involves scanning a small sample volume over the vessel lumen to determine the velocity profile from which the mean value can be computed. The mean value of velocity is required to compute the volumetric flow rate, for example. It has little value, at the moment, for detection of valve or septal defects.

Velocity profiles   By using either a single small sample volume scanned across the vessel, or a series of fixed sample volumes, we can determine the velocity distribution across the lumen. In a straight tube with smooth, steady flow, this distribution is parabolic. Alterations in lumen geometry, pulsatile flow, and wall defects can all alter this profile. The possibility exists of using profiles as indicators of disease. This approach has been tried in peripheral vessels more than in the heart. Generally, one would consider a velocity profile to be a smooth representation of the instantaneous temporal and spatial velocity pattern.

Spectral analysis   The blood flow signals appearing at the output of a Doppler instrument are a complex spectrum containing a band of frequencies, having many and varying intensities. This occurs because blood flow velocity patterns in the cardiovascular system can become very complicated. Seldom, if ever, will a single velocity exist at any one point. There is always a velocity profile, and flow disturbances, eddies, etc., can be induced by vessel or valve defects. While the relationship between defects and flow disturbances is not well understood, the only practical approach to finding out is through spectral analysis of the Doppler flow signal. To date, the width of the Doppler spectrum which relates to magnitude and range of velocities present in the Doppler sample volume, is the best indicator of flow disturbance. Engineering studies have confirmed this for several situations.

One- and two-dimensional displays based on spectral analysis are being evolved and show promise for clinical application, (8).

Variance profiles   This analysis and display format is similar to those used for velocity profiles. For a Doppler instrument, one in fact generates the data necessary for this display in order to determine the velocity profile. A variance profile in one dimension would show the degree of spectral broadening as a function of vessel lumen diameter. With smooth parabolic flow, one would expect spectral broadening (high variance) near the walls, and low variance in the center. When flow disturbances exist, high variance will exist across the entire lumen. In a two-dimensional version of this display, where magnitude of variance might be assigned a range of colors, one would expect mottled or multi-colored patterns to appear in regions of moderate or high flow disturbance. If done in real-time, this approach would create a type of ultrasonic cine, making flow abnormalities more obvious than current X-ray cine techniques.

TISSUE FEATURE SPACE

It should be apparent that a programmable multi-mode instrument might be able to encode into the two-dimensional image details and features of the tissue characteristics. As we have discussed, there is the possibility of using color displays for showing the fine structure of blood flow patterns in relationship to anatomy; the same possibility exists for tissue. It seems to be limited only by what we can determine via signal analysis: what is the best form in which to display the result? Obviously, one could generate tissue feature patterns which show changes from one region to another. Explaining them may well be another matter. An empirical approach may well produce useful applications before an analytical one.

SUMMARY

The concepts proposed in this paper are intended to provide a philosophical framework in which to work out a better understanding of the diagnostic process using ultrasonic energy forms. The diagnostic-measurements procedure seems to make more sense when viewed as a broad bandwidth communications channel. It would appear that over-emphasis of a one-instrument approach can produce a form of tunnel vision, which is a narrow communications channel. Optimization of the communication channel permits maximum information transfer and transformation for human perception. It seems inevitable that the sensitivity and specificity of a procedure, via better hardware and methods, will be improved by this holistic approach.

REFERENCES

1. Brandestini M: Topoflow – a digital full range Doppler velocity meter. IEEE Transactions on Sonics and Ultrasonics, Vol. SU-25, 287–293, September 1978.
2. Baker Donald W: The present role of Doppler techniques in cardiac diagnosis. In: Progress in Cardiovascular Diseases, Sonnenblick EM (ed), Grune & Stratton, Vol. XXI, p 79–91, September/October 1978.
3. Stevenson, JG: Differentiation of ventricular septal defects from mitral regurgitation by pulsed Doppler echocardiography. Circulation 56:14, 1977.
4. Lorch G, S Rubenstein, D Baker, T Dooley, H Dodge: Doppler echocardiography – use of a graphical display system. Circulation 56:575, 1977.
5. Ward JM, DW Baker, SA Rubenstein, SL Johnson: Detection of aortic insufficiency by pulse Doppler echocardiography. J Clinical Ultrasound 5:5, 1977.
6. Eyer M: A Microprocessor-based digital scan converter and color display system for ultrasonic image presentation. MSEE Thesis, University of Washington, Seattle, Washington, 1978.
7. Strandness DE, Jr, DJ Mozersky, DW Sumner, DW Baker, DE Hokanson,: Non-invasive arteriography: a new approach for arterial visualization. The American Surgeon 38:494, 1972.
8. Felix WR, B Sigel et al.: Pulsed Doppler detection of flow disturbances in arterosclerosis. J Clinical Ultrasound 4:275, 1976.

THE CONTRIBUTION OF DIGITIZED
ECHOCARDIOGRAPHY TO CLINICAL CARDIOLOGY

D.G. GIBSON

INTRODUCTION

The technique of digitization of M-mode records was introduced as a means of taking advantage of the excellent frequency response, 1000/sec, of the standard echocardiograph (1). Its use has been reviewed in detail and reference made to studies in which it has been validated against angiography (2). It is the purpose of the present paper to describe a series of applications in which it gives information not readily available from other methods, and which appear to have clear clinical significance. However, it must be stressed at the outset that the method is limited by the technical quality of the echocardiograms on which it is used. They must be of a standard significantly higher than those from which routine measurements can be made, in being recorded at 100 mm/sec, and in showing clear, continuous endocardial echoes throughout the cardiac cycle.

PEAK RATE OF DIMENSION INCREASE

Once the position of echoes from the left side of the septum and the posterior wall endocardium have been digitized, a continuous trace of left ventricular dimension can be derived, along with its first differential. While the reduction in dimension takes place continuously throughout ejection, the increase during diastole occurs in two clearly defined phases. Following mitral valve opening, dimension increases rapidly, reaching a peak of 10–20 cm/sec. In normal subjects, this early diastolic period ends abruptly 120–200 msec after mitral valve opening, and for the remainder of diastole, the rate of increase of dimension is very much less (1).

In patients with mitral valve disease, this pattern of wall movement is significantly altered (1). In those with mitral stenosis severe enough to require valvotomy, the peak rate of dimension increase is reduced to a mean of 6 cm/sec, and the normal early diastolic period of rapid filling is lost (3). Mitral stenosis can reliably be diagnosed on the basis of these findings, which differ fundamentally in their nature from other echocardiographic criteria used in this condition in that they are not related to abnormal anatomy, but to the physiological consequences of obstruction to left ventricular inflow, and thus directly reflect its severity. Although measurement of the diastolic closure rate of the mitral valve has proved a satisfactory means of detecting rheumatic involvement, it cannot be used to quantify the severity of the haemodynamic disturbance (4). Attempts to measure mitral valve area directly using two-dimensional images initially seemed promising, but this method is subject to uncertainty inherent in attempting to use anything other than the leading edge of an echo for measurement. The apparent thickness of an echo is not clearly related to that of the structure giving rise to it, but also depends on the velocity of sound within it, the possible presence of reverberations, and the gain settings of the instrument. In view of these considerations, it is not surprising that estimates of valve area should prove less than reliable, particularly in the presence of valve calcification. In addition, it is not always clear that the main site of obstruction to flow in rheumatic mitral valve disease is at the level of the valve cusps rather than at that of the chordae or papillary muscles. If the overall effects on left ventricular wall movement are measured, then these effects are automatically taken account of.

Attempts to validate digitized echocardiography against estimates of mitral valve area made at cardiac catheterization proved instructive, since a number of patients were identified in whom there were wide discrepancies between the two methods. Three such have recently been described (5). All had high end-diastolic pressures in the left ventricle, small (less than 2 mm Hg) gradients, near normal calculated mitral valve areas and low ejection fractions. However, echocardiography demonstrated reduced diastolic closure rate and reduced rate of dimension increase. All were severely symptomatic and all have been operated on. Severe mitral stenosis was present in all three, and they have all done well after surgery. At restudy in one, ejection fraction was found to have increased from 35% to 65%, and end-diastolic pressure fallen from 25 to 8 mm Hg. We have concluded that rheumatic mitral stenosis can mimic left ventricular disease, and that standard haemodynamic measurements are unreliable in separating the two. All 3 cases were initially denied operation on the basis of the catheter findings. Anatomical and physiological observations made by echocardiography in association with the clinical findings together constitute a very reliable means of making the diagnosis, and of determining its severity, so that we have abandoned cardiac catheterization in virtually all patients with significant mitral valve disease, whether stenotic or regurgitant. Indeed, we regard use of the procedure as unethical in such circumstances.

Since criteria based on wall movement during filling are not dependent on the anatomy of the mitral valve, they are as appropriate in patients who have undergone mitral valve replacement as in those with naturally occurring mitral valve disease. These results have been described in detail elsewhere (3). It has been possible to assess the performance of a number of currently available mitral valve substitutes including the Starr-Edwards and Bjork-Shiley prostheses and the Hancock xenograft. All are to some extent obstructive, reducing peak rate of dimension increase or prolonging the early diastolic period of rapid filling. Confidence limits were derived for each prosthesis, and used to detect malfunction, either obstructive or regurgitant.

Patients who fail to make expected progress after mitral valve replacement can pose a difficult diagnostic problem, which frequently cannot be resolved clinically. Movement of the prosthesis itself is usually normal, particularly in the presence of a paraprosthetic leak. Left ventriculography may be technically difficult if an aortic prosthesis is also present, or if, as is frequently the case, the patient is severely ill with pulmonary oedema. Digitized echocardiography has proved invaluable in these circumstances: a significant paraprosthetic leak is associated with an increase, and prosthetic obstruction with a reduction in peak rate of dimension increase compared with previous values. The presence of incoordinate left ventricular contraction can also be diagnosed using methods described below. It is now possible to advise surgery in appropriate cases without performing cardiac catheterization. Left ventriculography is undesirable in these severely ill patients in that angiographic dye depresses left ventricular function and aggravates pulmonary oedema by its sodium content. It may also be necessary to trip an aortic prosthesis to enter the ventricle at all thus further increasing the volume load, while at the same time, emergency surgery may be unnecessarily delayed.

Assessment of the pattern of wall movement has also proved helpful in the follow-up of patients who have had conservative operations on the mitral valve. These procedures are being performed increasingly frequently, and unlike with prostheses, the exact haemodynamic result cannot be predicted in individual patients. Examination at the time of discharge, therefore, allows the results of surgery to be assessed, and serves as a base-line for the future (3).

LEFT VENTRICULAR DISEASE

Peak rate of dimension increase may also be reduced in the presence of left ventricular disease, particularly hypertrophy. This was initially demonstrated in patients with hypertrophic cardiomyopathy (6), but more recently has been found to apply in hypertrophy secondary to a variety of causes including hypertension, aortic stenosis, or after aortic valve replacement (7). In all these patients, isovolumic relaxation is characteristically prolonged, so allowing the effects of left ventricular disease to be distinguished from those of mechanical obstruction to left ventricular inflow, where it is either normal or short (8). Abnormalities have also been demonstrated in myotonic muscular dystrophy (9), and untreated hypothyroidism (10). They appear to reflect primary abnormalities of relaxation associated with myocardial disease, and they may well have significant effects on overall cardiac function. They were not previously documented by angiography, although when sought specifically, can readily be demonstrated (11). They are not reflected in either the diastolic closure rate of the mitral valve (6), or in movement of the aortic root, two methods that have been suggested as appropriate for studying left ventricular filling.

SIGNIFICANCE OF WALL MOVEMENT DURING
THE ISOVOLUMIC PERIODS

If plots of left ventricular dimension are available, then wall movement during any specified period in the cardiac cycle can be assessed. Study of the time relations between changes in left ventricular pressure and dimension has demonstrated that energy transfer from myocardium to the circulation is a very efficient process in the normal heart (12). In many patients with left ventricular disease, this is not the case, the main cause of this loss of efficiency being wall movement during isovolumic contraction or relaxation. These two isovolumic periods can readily be timed from the apexcardiogram, direct observation of valve movement and the phonocardiogram (8, 13). It has thus been possible to demonstrate that left ventricular wall movement is coordinate to a high degree in patients with normal ventricular function. This has proved an excellent criterion of normality, unaffected by, for example, the increase in cavity size occurring in athletes, which taken on its own can lead to the erroneous diagnosis of left ventricular disease. In coronary artery disease, abnormal wall movement during isovolumic contraction or relaxation is common, occurring in approximately 85% of patients with symptoms severe enough to warrant coronary arteriography (14). In such patients, digitized echochardiography shows 80% specificity and sensitivity in detecting these abnormalities compared with single plane RAO angiography, analysed using a computer-based method to detect regional wall movement disturbances (14).

Similar abnormalities are also seen after open heart surgery, where they appear to represent the effect of cardiopulmonary bypass, and usually regress either partly or completely within two to three weeks (15). They are also common in acute myocardial infarction (16), and their presence is the major cause of persistance of symptoms after aortic valve replacement (17). They may also be seen in patients with valvular heart disease, even if the large coronary arteries are normal, and appear to be a significant determinant of operative mortality. Conversely, if contraction pattern is coordinate, patients with valvular heart disease withstand operation well, even if ejection fraction is grossly impaired. We have recently studied a group of patients presenting clinically, haemodynamically and angiographically as congestive cardiomyopathy with papillary muscle dysfunction, in whom, rather surprisingly, contraction was coordinate. So far, 10 have been treated surgically, and at operation, the pathology in all was found to be severe dilatation of the mitral ring. Nine patients have survived, with considerable symptomatic improvement. They will be described in detail elsewhere, but it appears that a significant proportion of patients with a clinical diagnosis of congestive cardiomyopathy may benefit from cardiac surgery.

WALL THICKNESS DYNAMICS

Since epicardial as well as endocardial echoes can be defined with instruments of adequate dynamic range, it is also possible to derive continuous measurements of posterior wall thickness. Previous observations of wall dynamics have concentrated on systolic events, and have demonstrated that regional thickening is a sensitive index of contractile activity. However, diastolic events are also worthy of study. In normal subjects, wall thinning during filling takes place more rapidly than thickening during systole, and a period of rapid thinning can be defined, coterminous with rapid filling (18). In patients with coronary artery disease, rapid thinning may precede mitral valve opening, showing that it can be dissociated from rapid filling, and therefore that it is an intrinsic property of relaxing myocardium. Peak thinning rate is also reduced in patients with left ventricular hypertrophy, where it appears to be the cause of the reduction in peak rate of dimension increase, and to reflect the underlying myocardial abnormality. In patients with left ventricular inflow obstruction, particularly those with prosthetic mitral valve replacement, thinning rate may be near normal, and the reduced rate of dimension increase be mediated by reversed septal movement early in diastole. Finally, simultaneous left ventricular pressure and dimension measurements have demonstrated that during the period of rapid wall thinning, the calculated stress-strain curve is horizontal, indicating no change in wall stress with increasing cavity size (19). It appears, therefore, that rapid thinning in the normal subject is the basis of the period of rapid filling, which may be interfered with by myocardial disease, or by asynchronous or delayed relaxation. It appears to be an active process, possibly energized by the previous systole, so that attempts to analyze it in terms of passive elastic models and exponential pressure-volume or stress-strain relations are likely to be unsatisfactory.

EXTENSION TO TWO DIMENSIONS

The methods described above can be extended to two-dimensional images, using a multiple M-mode technique, in which a phased array system is used to record, simultaneously, a series of M-mode echocardiograms, scanning the ventricle from apex to mitral valve ring. The technique has been described in detail elsewhere (20), and allows many regional abnormalities previously demonstrated by angiography to be confirmed by echocardiography. It is also possible to study wall thickness dynamics at all levels of the ventricle.

CONCLUSIONS

Digitized echocardiography thus appears to be a versatile means of studying left ventricular function. Cavity size and peak rates of systolic wall movement can readily be measured. Incoordinate action, both systolic and diastolic can be detected with high specificity and sensitivity. It appears to be the simplest means of studying relaxation and filling, and of detecting abnormalities whether due to mechanical obstruction or myocardial disease. Since valvular disease is of clinical significance mainly insofar as it affects left ventricular physiology, the technique is a valuable adjunct to clinical assessment and anatomical observations made by standard M-mode methods. At Brompton Hospital, this has led to a steady reduction in the number of cardiac catheterizations performed on patients with valvular heart disease, before corrective cardiac surgery. Formal evaluation of the method has indicated annual savings greater than the capital cost of the equipment (21). The method, in allowing incoordinate contraction to be detected has proved a sensitive means of assessing patients with left ventricular disease, in whom surgery might be considered, and has allowed additional indications for operation to be defined. Finally, it is a useful research tool in documenting systolic abnormalities of function, and may well be the means of choice for investigating disturbances of relaxation and filling, which have been little studied by other methods.

REFERENCES

1. Gibson DG, DJ Brown: Measurement of instantaneous left ventricular dimension and filling rate in man, using echocardiography. Brit Heart J 35:1141, 1973.
2. Upton MT, DG Gibson: The study of left ventricular function from digitized echocardiograms. Progress in Cardiovascular Diseases 20:359, 1978.
3. St John Sutton MG, TA Traill, AS Ghafour, et al.: Echocardiographic assessment of left ventricular filling after mitral valve surgery. Brit Heart J 39:1283, 1977.
4. Gustafson A: Ultrasound cardiography in mitral stenosis with particular reference to the relationship to haemodynamic and surgical findings. Acta Medica Scandinavica Supplementum 461:1, 1967.
5. Traill TA, MG St John Sutton, DG Gibson: Mitral stenosis with high left ventricular end-diastolic pressure. Brit Heart J 1979 (in press).
6. Sanderson JE, TA Traill, MG St John Sutton et al.: Left ventricular relaxation and filling in hypertrophic cardiomyopathy: an echocardiographic study. Brit Heart J 40:596, 1978.
7. Gibson DG, TA Traill, RJC Hall et al.: Echocardiographic features of secondary left ventricular hypertrophy. Circulation 56:III–40, 1977.
8. Chen W, D Gibson: Relation of isovolumic relaxation to left ventricular wall movement in man. Brit Heart J 1979 (in press).
9. Venco A, M Saviotti, D Besana et al.: Non-invasive assessment of left ventricular function in myotonic muscular dystrophy. Brit Heart J 40:1262, 1978.
10. Ibrahim Z, S Clarke: Personal communication, 1979.
11. Sanderson JE, DG Gibson, DJ Brown et al.: Left ventricular filling in hypertrophic cardiomyopathy: an angiographic study. Brit Heart J 39:661, 1977.
12. Gibson DG, DJ Brown: Assessment of left ventricular systolic function from simultaneous echocardiographic and pressure measurements. Brit Heart J 38:8, 1976.
13. Venco A, DG Gibson, DJ Brown: Relation between the apexcardiogram and changes in left ventricular pressure and dimension. Brit Heart J 38:117, 1977.
14. Doran JH, TA Traill, DJ Brown et al.: Detection of left ventricular wall movement during isovolumic contraction and early relaxation: comparison of echo- and angiography. Brit Heart J 40:367, 1978.

15. Venco A, MG St John Sutton, DG Gibson et al.: Non-invasive assessment of left ventricular function after correction of severe aortic regurgitation. Brit Heart J 38:1324, 1976.
16. Traill TA: Personal communication.
17. Clarke S, RJC Hall, DG Gibson: Disorders of left ventricular function after valve replacement for aortic incompetence. Trans European Soc Cardiol 1:8, 1978.
18. Traill TA, DG Gibson, DJ Brown: Study of left ventricular wall thickness and dimension changes using echocardiography. Brit Heart J 40:162, 1978.
19. Gibson DG, DJ Brown: Relation between diastolic left ventricular wall stress and strain in man. Brit Heart J 36:1066, 1974.
20. Gibson DG, DJ Brown, RB Logan-Sinclair: Analysis of regional left ventricular wall movement by phased array echocardiography. Brit Heart J 40:1334, 1978.
21. Gibson DG, DJ Brown: Evaluation of the Brompton Hospital Experiment (MS 4595). Department of Health and Social Security, London, 1978.

USEFULNESS OF M-MODE AND CROSS-SECTIONAL ECHOCARDIOGRAPHY FOR ANALYSIS OF RIGHT-SIDED HEART DISEASE

J.A. KISSLO

M-mode echocardiography is useful for the detection of a variety of right-sided heart abnormalities (1). Only recently has two-dimensional echocardiography been used for this purpose. Two dimensional echocardiography is generally superior to M-mode for this purpose because its wide field of view results in easy spatial recognition of right-sided structures such as right atrium, coronary sinus, all three leaflets of the tricuspid valve, right ventricle, pulmonic valve leaflets and proximal pulmonary artery with its bifurcation. This report discusses the echocardiographic approaches to the examination of right-sided cardiac structures.

METHODS

The technique for obtaining M-mode echocardiographic recordings of right-sided structures has been previously described (1). When two-dimensional echocardiography is used, two basic examination planes are suggested (Fig. 1).

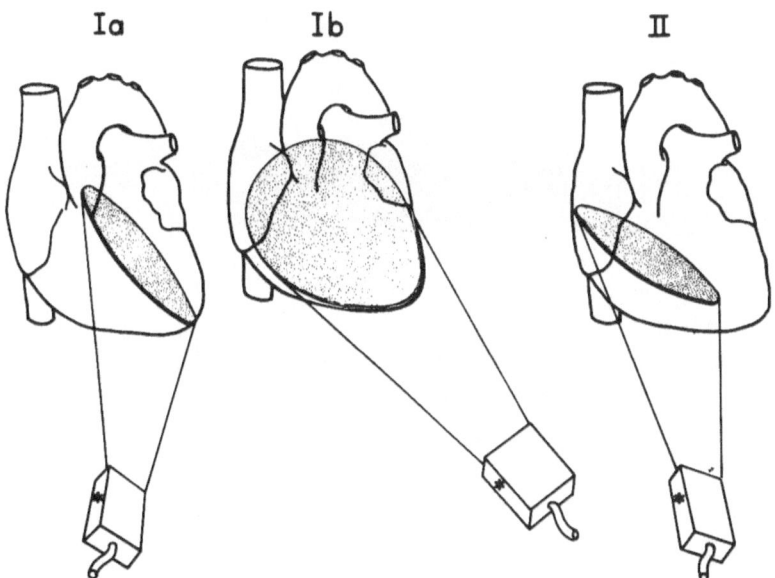

Ia   Ib   II

Fig. 1. Standard planes for examination of the right ventricle. For details, see text.

Charles T. Lancée (ed.), Echocardiology, 37–47. All rights reserved
Copyright © 1979 by Martinus Nijhoff Publishers bv, The Hague/Boston/London

One plane, the apical four chamber view, is obtained by moving the transducer from its normal position for examining the long axis of the left ventricle (Position Ia) to a position over the ventricular apex and rotating clockwise (2). Angling back through the long axis of the heart reveals an image of both ventricles, atrioventricular valves and atria (Position Ib).

A long axis view of the right ventricle (Position II) may be obtained by rotating the transducer slightly counterclockwise from the routine long axis of the left ventricle to obtain right atrium, coronary sinus, tricuspid valve and proximal right ventricle (Fig. 2). Slight superior angulation from this position will reveal the atrial septum (Fig. 3). In panels A and B the tricuspid valve is open in diastole. The right atrium is seen in the upper portions of the scan while the inflow portions are seen in the lower left. Frames C and D show the tricuspid leaflets closed in systole.

Other views of the outflow tract of the right ventricle are obtained by using examination planes similar to those utilized to examine the short axis of the aortic root.

Two-dimensional echocardiographic examples used herein were obtained from dynamically focused phased array imaging systems developed in the Duke University Department of Biomedical Engineering (3, 4). Realtime

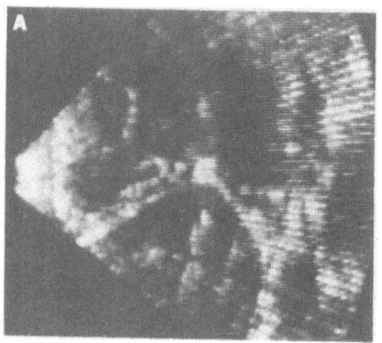

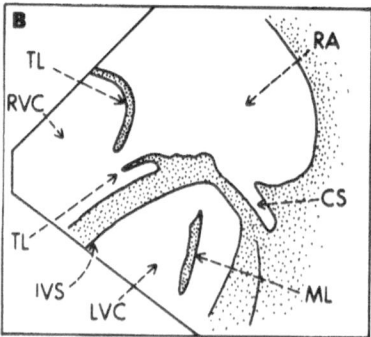

Fig. 2. Panels A and B show an image in the long axis of the tricuspid valve. (Position II). RA = right atriums; RVC = right ventricular chamber; TL = tricuspid leaflet; IVS = interventricular septum; LVC = left ventricular chamber; ML = mitral leaflet; CS = coronary sinus. The chest wall is at the left.

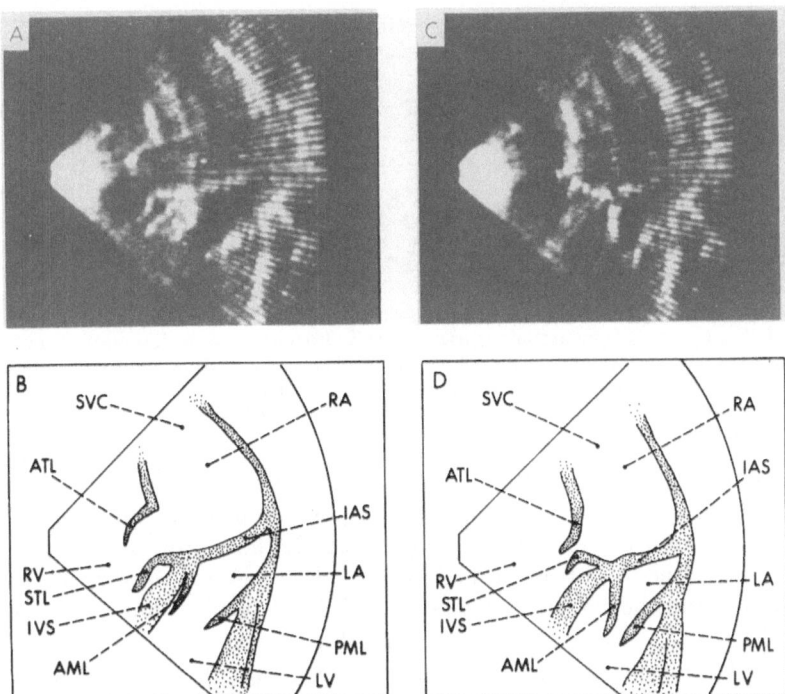

Fig. 3. Stop frames and matched schematic diagrams of two-dimensional scans indicating the structures seen in a normal patient through position II. A and B, open tricuspid valve in diastole. AML = anterior mitral leaflet; ATL = anterior tricuspid leaflet; IAS = interatrial septum; LA = left atrium; LV = left ventricle; PML = posterior mitral leaflet; STL = septal tricuspid leaflet; SVC = superior vena cava. The chest wall is at the left.

cross-sectional images of cardiac structures are presented in a circular sector format at varying azimuth angles to 90 degrees. Much detail is lost from the original real-time recording with still-frame illustrations for two reasons. First, visual integration of motion that normally accompanies real-time playback is lost when still frames are displayed. Second, a single video frame represents only one half of the information provided in real-time due to the 2:1 interlace of the scan into the video format.

CLINICAL EXAMPLES

Echocardiographic examination of the right side of the heart is occasionally best facilitated by contrast techniques. In our laboratory 8–10 ml of normal saline is injected rapidly into an antecubital vein. A resultant bolus of microcavitations produced by the rapid injection is seen to transmit the right heart (Fig. 4).

This technique has been shown to be useful for the detection of tricuspid insufficiency, by two-dimensional echocardiography, by observing the to and fro motion of the microcavitations across the tricuspid valve (5).

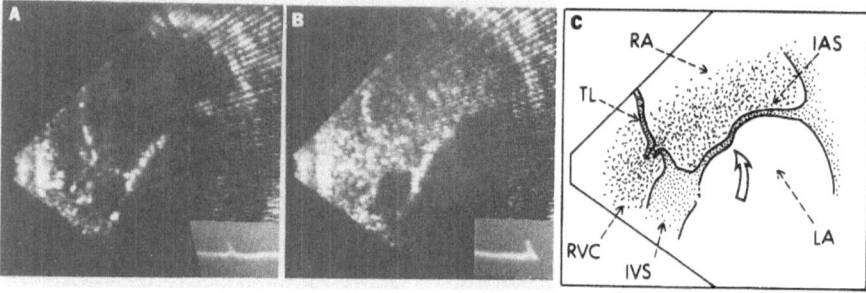

Fig. 4. Frames in the long axis of the tricuspid valve from a patient with tricuspid regurgitation. Panel A is a diastolic frame before the bolus injection of saline. Panel B is an early systolic frame after the saline injection and shows microcavitations in both the right atrium and right ventricle. Panel C is a schematic of panel B. The open arrow in panel C shows the region of the foramen ovale. The chest wall is at the left.

Occasionally, swirling of the microcavitations in the right atrium in patients with normal tricuspid valves make it impossible to differentiate from small degrees of tricuspid insufficiency and, therefore, limits this approach.

To overcome this problem the long axis of the inferior vena cava should be examined and the systolic appearance of the microcavitations noted within it when tricuspid insufficiency is present (Fig. 5). The inferior vena cava is located by placing the transducer in the subxyphoid area, parallel to the long axis of the patients torso and just to the right of the midline. This approach significantly increases the sensitivity and specificity of two-dimensional echocardiography for the detection of tricuspid insufficiency. Because no cathether is across the tricuspid valve this may be the most useful clinical method for the detection of tricuspid insufficiency available.

M-mode echocardiography may also be used for the detection of tricuspid insufficiency (6). Using a similar subxyphoid transducer location as with the two-dimensional approach, the inferior vena cava appears on M-mode as a tubular structure, 8 to 10 cm in depth and approximately 2 cm in diameter.

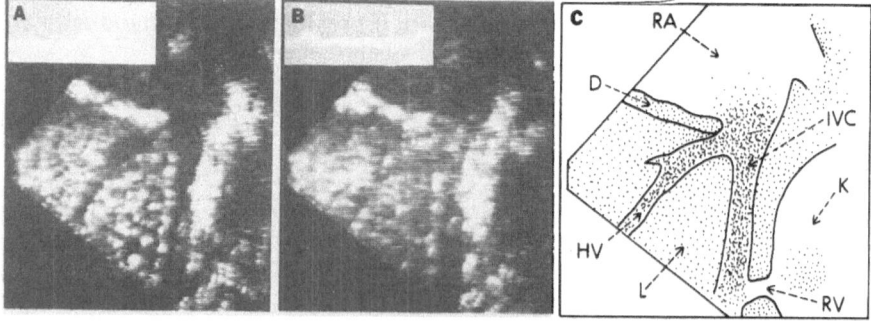

Fig. 5. Frames in the plane of the right atrium and inferior vena cava, from a patient with tricuspid regurgitation. Panel A is a diastolic frame, before the injection of saline into an antecubital vein. Panel B is a systolic frame after the saline injection and demonstrates the appearance of microcavitations in the inferior vena cava and hepatic vein. D = diaphragm; K = kidney; RV = renal vein; L = liver; HV = hepatic vein. The abdominal wall is at the left.

Rapid inspiration by the patient collapses the inferior vena cava and serves to differentiate it from abdominal aorta (Fig. 6). Tricuspid insufficiency is again documented by the systolic appearance of microcavitations in the inferior vena cava. This approach appears superior to two-dimensional echocardiography because it allows for easy correlation of the microcavitations to the electrocardiogram. The importance of this ability is demonstrated in the bottom panel of Figure 6 where microcavitations appear, prior to the QRS of the electrocardiogram, in presystole. This indicates a false positive for tricuspid insufficiency as this patient had impaired right ventricular filling due to uremic pericarditis and cardiac tamponade.

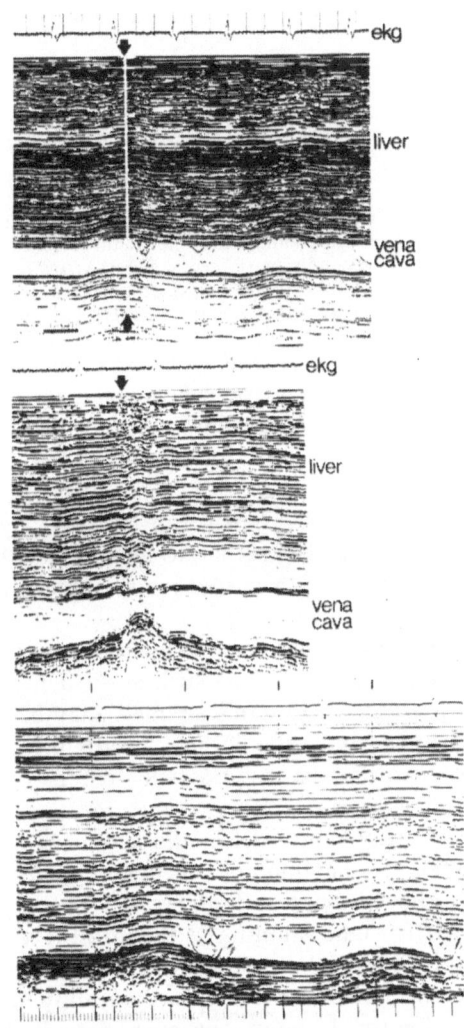

Fig. 6. M-mode echovenacavagrams. Top: Systolic appearance of micro-cavitations indicating tricuspid insufficiency. Middle: Inspiration causes collapse of inferior vena cava. Bottom: Presystolic appearance of microcavitations in a patient with pericardial tamponade.

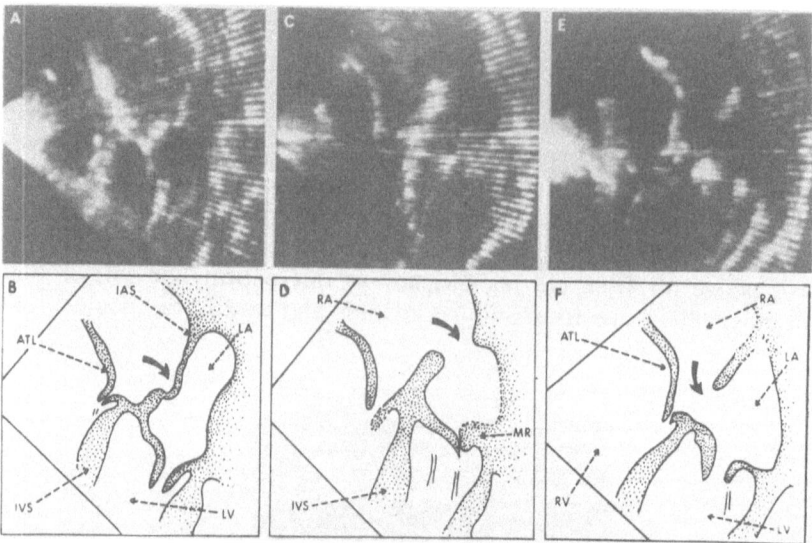

Fig. 7. Systolic frames in the long axis of the tricuspid valve and interatrial septum. Panels A and B are from a normal subject. Arrow in B indicates the area of the foramen ovale. Panels C and D are from a patient with an ostium secundum atrial septal defect. Arrow in D indicates the area of the septal defect. Panels E and F are from a patient with an ostium primum atrial septal defect. Arrow in F indicates the area of the septal defect. MR = mitral ring. The chest wall is at the left.

Although little data is yet available, tricuspid prolapse usually appears as a billowing of one or more of the valve leaflets above the level of the valve ring. Since normal tricuspid valve coaptation is at, or slightly above, the level of the ring this diagnosis should be cautiously made.

Valve thickening with tethering of the leaflet tips seen by two-dimensional echocardiography indicates the presence of tricuspid stenosis. Reduction in the tricuspid EF slope is also seen. No data currently exists for direct measurement of the stenotic tricuspid valve orifice by two-dimensional echocardiography.

Two-dimensional echocardiography extends the use of M-mode for the detection of certain congenital lesions such as Ebstein's anomaly and atrial septal defect. The presence of Ebsten's anomaly may be confirmed by noting displacement of the tricuspid valve leaflets distally into the right ventricular cavity (7). Use of contrast techniques will demonstrate the tricuspid insufficiency if present.

In some cases of atrial septal defect the actual anatomic defect may be visualized (Fig. 7) (8). More commonly, the combined use of two-dimensional echocardiography and contrast techniques will reveal a negative contrast effect due to the left to right shunting at the atrial level (Fig. 8) (9).

Since all patients with atrial septal defect have some degree of right-to-left shunting, contrast two-dimensional echocardiography may be used to detect this phenomenon. Figure 9 shows one such patient. Using this criterion provides the most sensitive indicator for the presence of an atrial septal defect that is currently available.

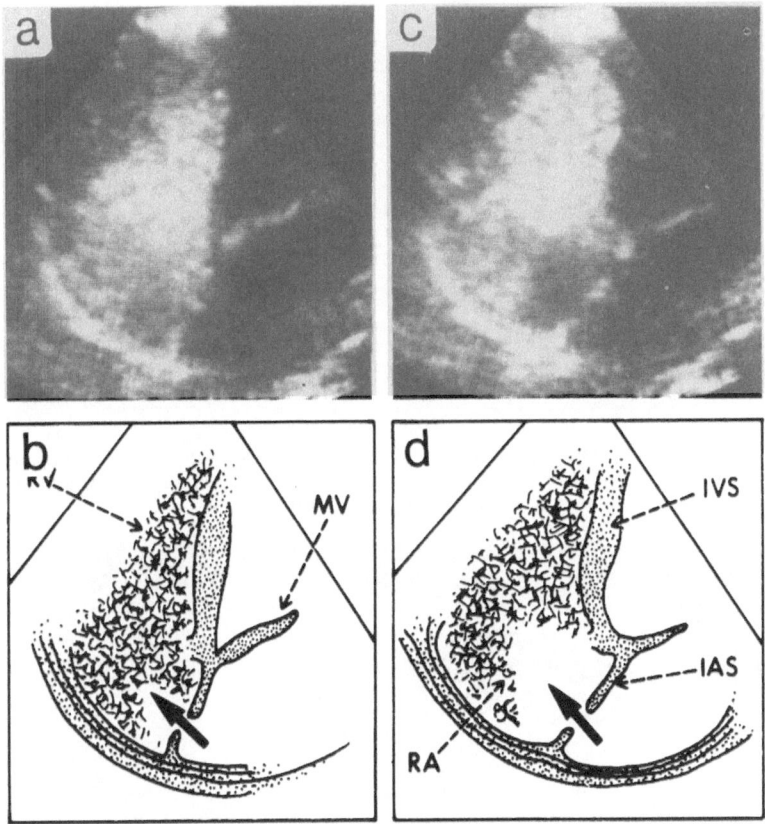

Fig. 8. Sequential late diastolic stop-frame videotape images in the apical four-chamber view (Position Ib) with accompanying schematic diagrams from a patient who had an ostium secundum atrial septal defect. Blood without microcavitations (negative contrast) is seen to enter the right atrium (panels a and b) and partially fill it (panels c and d). The chest wall is at the top.

Rare congenital lesions such as persistent left superior vena cava may also be detected by contrast two-dimensional echocardiography. Although this lesion is usually benign it has important implications in patients undergoing cardiovascular bypass for correction of other cardiac defects. Injection of contrast should routinely be made into a left antecubital vein or this lesion may be easily missed (Fig. 10).

As with M-mode echocardiography, two-dimensional echocardiography is advantageous for detection of right sided mass lesions such as those noted as a result of vegetative endocarditis or tumor (11, 12). Two-dimensional echocardiography has the advantage over M-mode because localization of the mass, measurement of its size and assessment of other characteristics are possible.

Figure 11 demonstrates a mass lesion due to *Proteus mirabilis* attached to the posterior tricuspid leaflet in a drug addict. In real-time the vegetative lesion appeared to "roll" down the leaflet in diastole. Several days after this

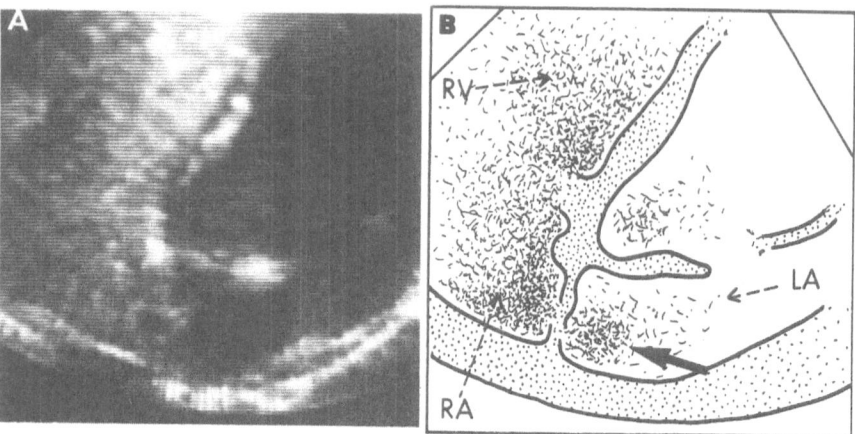

Fig. 9. A moderate right-to-left atrial level shunt using the apical four-chamber view (Position Ib) in a patient with atrial septal defect. The arrow indicates a small, dense cloud of microcavitations just as they appear in the left atrium. The chest wall is at the top.

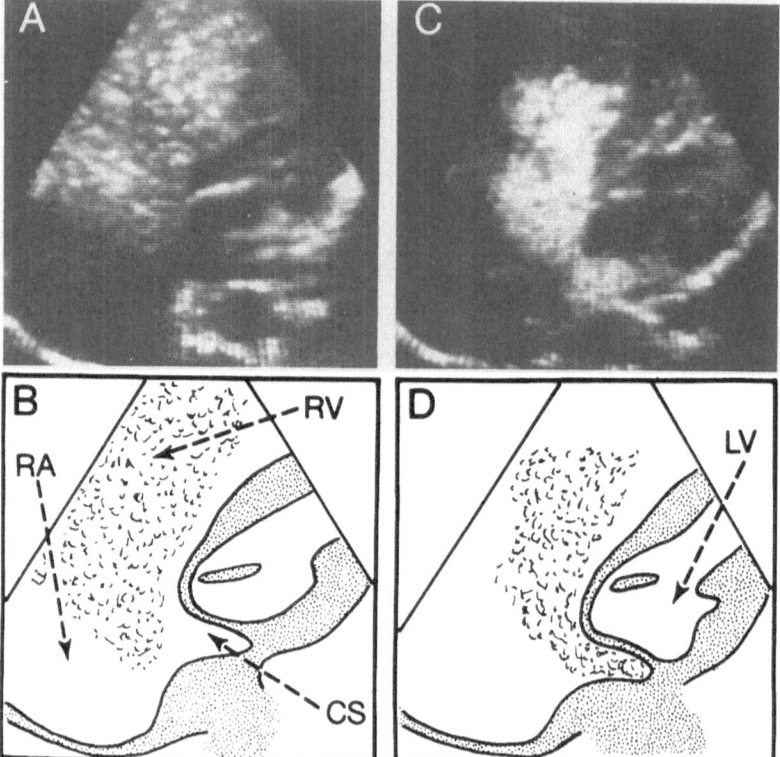

Fig. 10. Tangential apical four-chamber views following injection of echocardiographic contrast. Panel A shows the contrast distribution following injection from a peripheral right arm vein. The right atrium and right ventricle opacify normally. Note the absence of contrast in the area of the coronary sinus. Panel C illustrates the distribution following injection of contrast from a peripheral left arm vein. Note the complete opacification in the area of the coronary sinus.

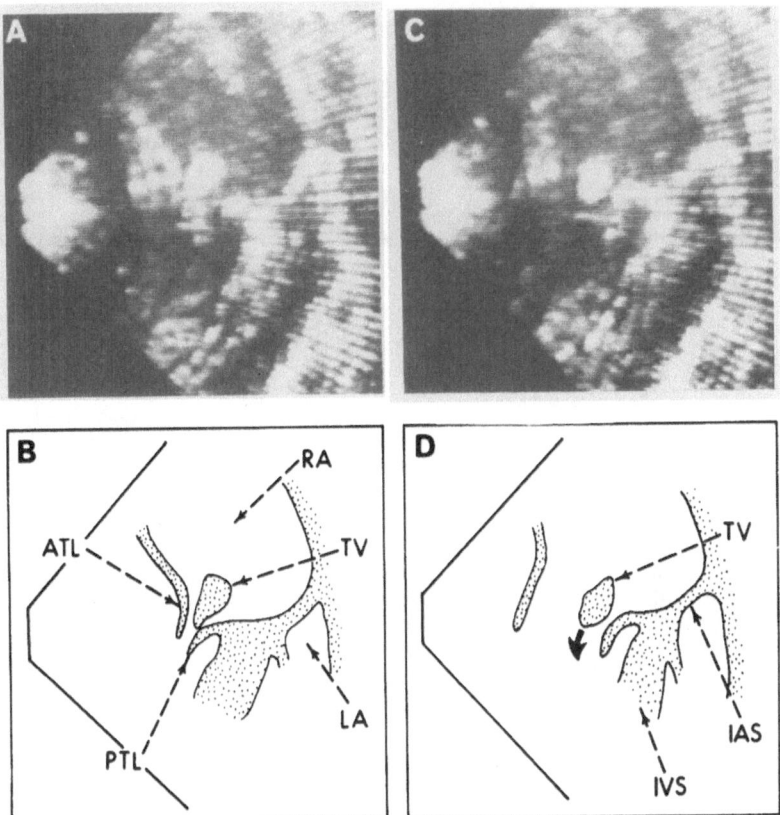

Fig. 11. Serial stop-frame photos and schematic diagrams of the anterior and inferior tricuspid valve leaflets of a patient with tricuspid endocarditis. Panel A and B – vegetation seen in systole on the atrial surface of the tricuspid valve. Panel C and D – vegetation seen moving through tricuspid orifice in early diastole TV = tricuspid vegetation. The chest wall is at the left.

scan was performed the patient experienced sudden onset of chest pain that accompanied disappearance of the lesion on repeat echocardiographic study.

Figure 12 shows a flail anterior tricuspid valve leaflet in a patient due to leaflet destruction from bacterial endocarditis. Prior scans documented a series of events from detection of presence of a mass lesion at first, followed by development of severe leaflet prolapse within several weeks and then eventually progressing to the flail leaflet shown.

Mass lesions due to tumor, particularly those in the right atrium, are often difficult to detect by M-mode. Altered reflectance characteristics of certain tumors may rarely render some acoustically undetectable. Contrast two-dimensional echocardiography should always be employed when such tumors are suspected. Figure 13 shows a barely perceptable tumor that was readily outlined by the use of contrast techniques.

Lesions of the right ventricular outflow tract such as aneurysm of the interventricular septum, pulmonic insufficiency and compression at the main

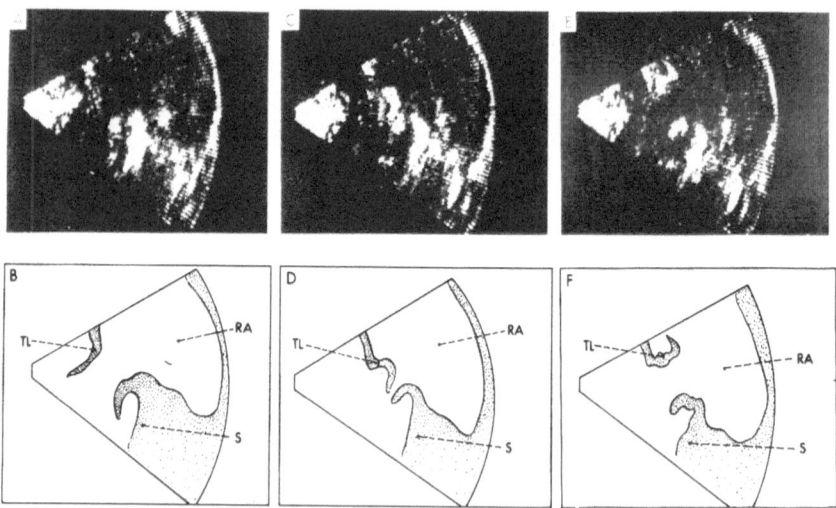

Fig. 12. Single frame photos and matched schematic diagrams from the two-dimensional scan through position II in a patient with flail tricuspid leaflet due to vegetative endocarditis. Panels A and B: The tricuspid valve leaflets open in diastole. Panels C and D: Early systolic prolapse of the anterior tricuspid leaflet. Panels E and F: Mid to late systolic flail of the anterior tricuspid leaflet. The chest wall is at the left.

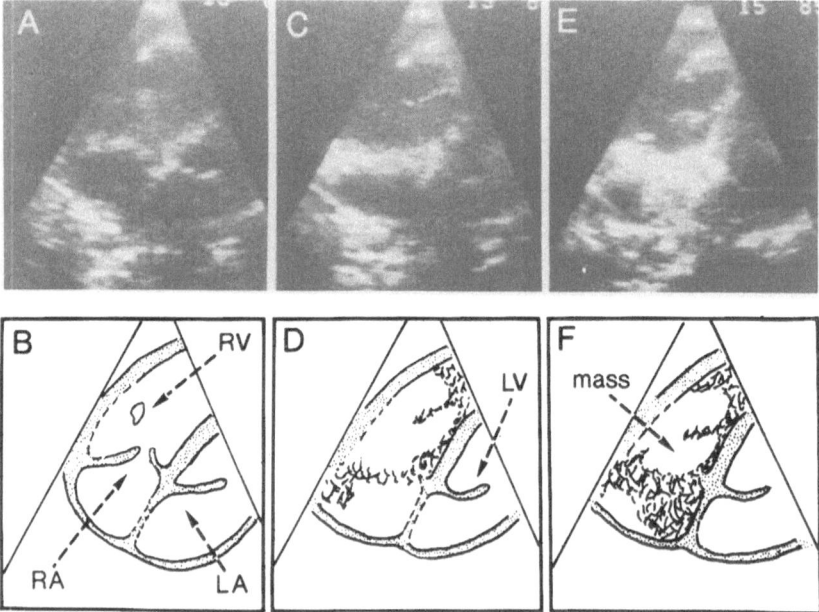

Fig. 13. Apical four-chamber views of patient with right ventricular tumor. Panel A: No contrast. Panels C and E show contrast outlining lobulated tumor. The chest wall is at the top.

stem pulmonary arteries are also possible. Use of contrast two-dimensional echocardiographic approaches is, usually, necessary (13).

CONCLUSIONS

The echocardiographer must be aware that maximum use of echocardiographic techniques for the delineation of right-sided cardiac lesions is not always easily accomplished. Physical or historical evidence indicating suspicion of right-sided lesions is often minimal. Casual echocardiographic examination of the right side of the heart may then fail to reveal important diagnostic information.

Proper interaction with the clinical data concerning history, physical examination and results of other tests such as chest X-ray may frequently direct the echocardiographer to perform a more careful examination of right-sided structures. Judgment concerning when to employ contrast techniques or when to examine the inferior vena cava may then be properly implemented. In time, it is likely that these approaches will be extended to the evaluation of a wider variety of other right-sided cardiac abnormalities.

REFERENCES

1. Feigenbaum H: Echocardiography. Philadelphia. Pa., Lea and Febiger, 1976.
2. Silverman NH, NB Schiller: Apex cardiography: a two-dimensional technique for evaluating congenital heart disease. Circulation 57:503, 1978.
3. von Ramm OT, FL Thurstone: Cardiac imaging using a phased-array ultrasound system. I. System design. Circulation 53:258, 1976.
4. Kisslo J, OT von Ramm, FL Thurstone: Cardiac imaging using a phased-array ultrasound system. II. Clinical technique and application. Circulation 53:62, 1976.
5. Lieppe W, VS Behar, R Scallion, JA Kisslo: Detection of tricuspid regurgitation with two-dimensional echocardiography and peripheral vein injections. Circulation 57:128, 1978.
6. Myers S, JA Kisslo, TD Fraker: Practical M-mode venacavography. (Abstr) Proceedings of the American Institute of Ultrasound in Medicine 1:16, 1978.
7. Ports TA, NH Silverman, NB Schiller: Two-dimensional echocardiographic assessment of Ebstein's Anomaly. Circulation 58:336, 1978.
8. Lieppe W, R Scallion, VS Behar, JA Kisslo: Two-dimensional echocardiographic findings in atrial septal defect. Circulation 56:447, 1977.
9. Fraker TD, PJ Harris, VS Behar, JA Kisslo: Detection and exclusion of interatrial shunts by two-dimensional echocardiography and peripheral venous injection. Circulation 59:379, 1979.
10. Stewart JA, TD Fraker, DA Solsky, NK Wise, JA Kisslo: Detection of persistent left superior vena cava by two-dimensional contrast echocardiography J Clin U 1979 (in press).
11. Kisslo J, OT von Ramm, R Haney, R Jones, SS Juk, VS Behar: Echocardiographic evaluation of tricuspid valve endocarditis. An M-mode and two-dimensional study. Am J Cardiol 38:502, 1976.
12. Crawford F, AS Wechsler, JA Kisslo: Tricuspid endocarditis in a drug addict: Detection of tricuspid vegetations by two-dimensional echocardiography. Chest 74:473, 1978.
13. Klicpera M, TD Fraker, J Kisslo: Clinical utility of identification of the right ventricular outflow tract, pulmonary artery and its bifurcation by contrast two-dimensional echocardiography. (Abstr) Am J Cardiol 41:391, 1978.

DETERMINATION AND CONSEQUENCES OF BIAS AND RANDOM ERROR IN ECHOCARDIOGRAPHIC MEASUREMENTS

J. LUBSEN

Echocardiography is an accepted, non-invasive tool used to measure dimensions of cardiac structures and to assess cardiac function. The technique is not a simple one and requires skill and practice from the examiner. The resolution is limited by physical principles. It is therefore of interest to determine the extent to which echocardiographic measurements are subject to error.

BIAS AND RANDOM ERROR IN BIOLOGIC MEASUREMENTS

Like any other measurement, an echocardiographic measurement M can be described as $M = T + E$; where "T" represents the true dimension or parameter value and "E" the deviation of the measurement from the true value. If the measurement is repeated at a certain level of T, E will vary from measurement to measurement. The average of E may be thought of as a constant systematic error or bias which is present in every measurement. Furthermore, a random component is present in E which varies from measurement to measurement. Thus, we may rewrite $M = T + E$ as $M = T + B + e$, where "B" represents the bias component of E and "e" the random component of E. B is a constant, which may depend on T. The random component e has a mean of zero and a variance denoted by "var(e)", which also may depend on T. The term "accuracy" is often used to denote the bias component and the term "precision" to denote the random component. The reliability of a measuring device is reflected in the magnitudes of B and var(e).

Bias in itself is not a serious problem as long as it can be kept constant over time and its magnitude is known. However, the random error cannot be taken into account in individual measurements and must therefore be kept as small as possible.

HOW CAN WE DETERMINE THE BIAS AND RANDOM ERROR OF A MEASUREMENT?

It is simple if one can obtain a series of measurements at a constant and known level of T. It follows from $M = T + B + e$ that the mean of M, denoted by $\bar{M}$, equals $T + B$ since B is a constant and $\bar{e} = 0$ by definition. Thus, if T is known, B may be estimated as $\bar{M} - T$. Also, it follows directly from the definitions that var(e) is estimated by the variance of M as determined from the series. By repeating the experiment at different levels of T, we may determine whether B and/or var(e) depend in any way on T itself. If T is unknown, it is impossible to estimate B but var(e) may still be estimated by var(M) as long as T can, although unknown, be kept constant for a series of measurements. Most investigators do not know that var(e) may also be determined from a series of pairs of duplicate measurements made with two measuring devices M_1 and M_2. We then have $M_1 = T_1 + B_1 + e_1$ and $M_2 = T_2 + B_2 + e_2$. If we assume that e_1 and e_2 are independent of each other and of T (which is reasonable when measurements are made independently, and the range of potential values of T is small) and that each measurement pair is a true duplicate from the same subject (i.e. $T_1 = T_2 = T$) we can write the following equations: $\bar{M}_1 = \bar{T} + B_1$, $\bar{M}_2 = \bar{T} + B_2$, var($M_1$) = var($T$) + var($e_1$), var($M_2$) = var($T$) + var($e_2$). These relationships follow immediately from the definitions of B and e and the above assumptions.

It can further be shown that var(T) is estimated by the covariance of the duplicate measurements, denoted by cov(M_1, M_2). It appears therefore that $[B_1 - B_2]$ is estimated by $[\bar{M}_1 - \bar{M}_2]$, var(e_1) by $[\text{var}(M_1) - \text{cov}(M_1, M_2)]$, and var($e_2$) by $[\text{var}(M_2) - \text{cov}(M_1, M_2)]$. It is obvious that there are many potential applications for these estimations, which were first derived by Grubbs (1) in 1948. An estimate of $[B_1 - B_2]$ allows us to compare measurements which were made with the two measuring devices on the same subject. The magnitude of var(e_1) and var(e_2) give an idea of the relative precision of the two devices. It should be noted that the correlation coefficient between M_1 and M_2, which is often reported in the literature when two alternative measurements are compared, depends both on var(e_1) and var(e_2) and is unaffected by the magnitude of $[B_1 - B_2]$. Therefore, correlation coefficients do not give any insight into the relative accuracy and precision of different methods.

WHAT ARE THE CONSEQUENCES OF THE PRESENCE OF BIAS AND RANDOM ERROR IN ECHOCARDIOGRAPHIC MEASUREMENTS?

Even in experimental situations, it will often be impossible to obtain the true value of the dimension or functional parameter which is measured. Therefore, the absolute magnitude of B is usually unknown. This is not particularly important so long as it can be assumed that B remains constant. Therefore, meticulous care should be taken to achieve this in the echocardiographic laboratory. If this cannot be guaranteed, "normal" ranges used as reference values lose their applicability completely. Also, when following a patient's cardiac condition over time, it is a "conditio sine qua non" that any change found should not be ascribable to a change in B, due, for instance, to a drift in the calibration of the echocardiograph, measurement device, etc.

Assuming that B can be kept constant, random error is then of greater concern. It follows from var(M) = var(T) + var(e) that random error leads to a higher measurement variability than the biological variability represented by var(T) and therefore to wider "normal" ranges and less distinction between health and disease. In follow-up studies on the same patient, random error leads to greater instability of the measurement and therefore hampers the detection of a trend or leads to "regression-to-the-mean" problems. Finally, random error leads to a less apparent relationship between parameters which are in fact related. For instance, there should be a marked relationship between body surface area and various left ventricular dimensions. If any of the measurements used to derive these parameters are subject to considerable random error, the relationship may become undetectable in practice.

It is concluded that bias and random error should be a matter of great concern and study in the echocardiographic laboratory. The examiner should be aware of the implications they have for the interpretation of echocardiographic measurements.

REFERENCE

1. Grubbs FE: On estimating precision of measuring instruments and product variability. J Am Stat Assn 43:243, 1948.

DIFFERENCES IN THE ECHOCARDIOGRAPHIC DIMENSIONS OF THE HEART BETWEEN FEMALES AND MALES

R.S. RENEMAN, J.J.F. SCHMITZ, L.H.E.H. SNOECKX, and J.A.C. LAMBREGTS

Abstract. The echocardiographic dimensions of the aorta and the heart were determined in healthy adults, who were not regularly participating in athletic activities. The volunteers were grouped according to age and sex. The aortic and cardiac dimensions were larger in males than in females, especially in the older age group (30–42 years). Most of these differences disappeared when the dimensions were adjusted for body surface area or body weight. It is questionable, however, whether this adjustment is permissible, since no clear relation could be found between the dimensions on the one hand and body surface area and body weight on the other. In our opinion, echocardiographic studies of the dimensions of the aorta and the heart should take differences between females and males into account.

INTRODUCTION

In the absence of cardiac disease, the echocardiographic dimensions of the heart depend among other things on the arterial blood pressure level (2, 11) and the amount of physical exercise performed (1, 8, 9, 13). Moreover, there are indications that these dimensions vary with age (5, 6, 12). Therefore, proper information about the echocardiographic dimensions of the heart in normal subjects can only be obtained when those taking part in the study do not participate regularly in athletic activities and have normal blood pressure levels and when their ages are taken into consideration. In general, little or no attention is paid to possible differences between the sexes in the echocardiographic dimensions of the aorta and the heart. In most studies the data obtained in females and males are grouped together, while, occasionally, the dimensions are adjusted for body surface area or body weight in order to remove the differences between the sexes (12). This adjustment assumes that a particular relation exists between the echocardiographic dimensions on the one hand and body surface area and body weight on the other. Although certain relations between cardiac dimensions and body surface area have been described in children and adolescents (4, 7, 10), when cardiac structures are still growing, no information could be found about this relation in adults.

The present study was conducted in order to investigate, in adults, whether or not differences in aortic and cardiac dimensions between females and males do exist and whether there is a relation between these dimensions on the one hand and body surface area and body weight on the other.

METHODS

The dimensions of the aorta and the heart were determined echocardiographically in 108 volunteers, who were randomly selected from the population registers. Volunteers were excluded from the study if they were physically or mentally disabled or were rejected for any form of sport or were involved in athletic activities more than once a week.

The subjects were divided into four groups. Group I consisted of males, aged 18–30; Group II consisted of females, aged 18–30; Group III consisted of males, aged 30–42 and Group IV consisted of females, aged 30–42. These age-groups were selected because the volunteers had to serve as controls for comparison with athletes.

To eliminate abnormalities, all volunteers had a physical examination of heart and lungs, an antero-posterior chest X-ray and a standard 12-lead ECG. Cuff blood pressure measurements were obtained three times. The last value, usually determined following the echocardiographic examination, was taken as the subject's reading. The echocardiograms of volunteers with raised blood pressure readings, i.e. higher than 140/95 mm Hg in females and higher than 140/90 mm Hg in males, were not used for further analysis. Heart rate was calculated from the ECG. Height and body weight were measured in all volunteers and body surface area was calculated from these parameters according to the method of Engström and Herzog (3).

The echocardiograms were made with the subject in a recumbent, left lateral position, using a Cardiovisor (Organon Teknika). A 2.25 MHz transducer, which focusses at 7.5 cm, or a 4.5 MHz transducer was positioned in an appropriate intercostal space so that the thickness of the interventricular septum (IVS), the left ventricular internal diameter (LVID) and the thickness of the posterior wall of the left ventricle (LVPW) could be determined simultaneously. In these recordings, the tip of the anterior leaflet of the mitral valve could just be detected. The internal diameters of the right ventricle (RVID), the aorta (A_OID) and the left atrium (LAID) were also determined. The end-diastolic dimensions of the IVS and of the left and right ventricles were assessed just before the start of isovolumic contraction. Those of the aorta and the left atrium were determined at the beginning of the upstroke of the R wave of the ECG. The end-systolic dimensions of the IVS and of the left and right ventricles were assessed at the moment that the IVS and the LVPW were moving in the same direction. The aortic and left atrial dimensions in systole were determined at the moment of aortic valve closure. In general, the values shown represent an average of the measurements made during three successive heart beats. Only echocardiograms of sufficiently high quality, i.e. unambiguous recognition of the structures, were used for the measurements.

Differences between the data in the various groups were evaluated for statistical significance by applying Students's t-test ($P < 0.05$). Comparison of the aortic and cardiac dimensions was not only made for the absolute values, but also for the dimensions adjusted for body surface area or body weight. In

addition the relation between the absolute dimensions and the latter parameters was determined, using Pearson's correlation coefficient.

RESULTS

After exclusion of the echocardiograms of mediocre or poor quality ($n = 25$)
and of the volunteers with raised blood pressure ($n = 7$), the distribution of
the subjects over the four groups was as follows. Group I: $n = 17$, age:
23.7 $\pm$ 3.6 ($\bar{x} \pm$ sd); Group II: $n = 21$, age: 23.1 $\pm$ 3.1 ($\bar{x} \pm$ sd); Group III: $n = 19$,
age: 34.5 $\pm$ 3.4 ($\bar{x} \pm$ sd) and Group IV: $n = 19$, age: 35.6 $\pm$ 4.0 ($\bar{x} \pm$ sd). In these
subjects the chest X-ray and the ECG showed no evidence of abnormality.

The mean absolute values and the standard deviations of the measured
end-diastolic and end-systolic dimensions of the aorta and the heart as well
as the heart rate, blood pressure, body weight, height and body surface area
values in the four groups are presented in Table 1. Comparison of Group I
and II revealed that body surface area, height and end-diastolic and end-
systolic RVID were smaller and body weight was lower in females than in
males. In the older age-group, the differences between the sexes were more
pronounced (cf. Group III and IV). In this group, body surface area, height,
end-diastolic A_0ID and LVID and end-systolic A_0ID and LVID were
smaller and body weight was lower in females than in males. Besides, the IVS
and LVPW were thinner in females than in males, both at the end of diastole
and at the end of systole. In the younger, as well as in the older-age group, no
significant differences in blood pressure and heart rate could be detected
between females and males.

When aortic and cardiac dimensions were adjusted for body surface area
or body weight (Table 2), all differences between females and males disappeared in the older-age group (cf. Group III and IV). In the younger age-
group, end-diastolic and end-systolic RVID remained larger in males than in
females.

Both in females and in males, the absolute aortic and cardiac dimensions
tended to be larger in the older age-group (Table 1). However, in men only,
significant differences were found in end-diastolic LVID and end-systolic IVS
and LVPW thickness (cf. Group I and III). In women only the differences in
end-diastolic RVID and end-systolic IVS thickness were significant (cf.
Group II and IV).

The correlation coefficients for the dimensions of the aorta and the heart,
related to body surface area or body weight are listed in Table 3. These data
show that, in general, poor correlations were found.

DISCUSSION

This study indicates that in healthy adults, who are not regularly participating in athletic activities, the dimensions of the aorta and the heart are larger

Table 1. The mean absolute values and standard deviations of the determined variables and parameters. Comparison between the various groups.

Variables-Parameters		Group I	Group II	Group III	Group IV
A_oID (mm)	ED	29.8 ± 4.2	28.3 ± 6.4	32.3 ± 4.2	26.8 ± 5.4°
	ES	32.9 ± 4.2	30.0 ± 5.4	34.8 ± 4.5	30.4 ± 5.2°
LAID (mm)	ED	25.9 ± 6.7	21.5 ± 6.1	25.6 ± 6.7	23.9 ± 5.8
	ES	34.4 ± 6.1	31.3 ± 5.5	36.4 ± 6.5	32.8 ± 6.6
RVID (mm)	ED	28.5 ± 7.7	20.1 ± 5.3+	26.0 ± 6.6	25.0 ± 5.9*
	ES	25.6 ± 5.4	18.9 ± 4.9+	24.6 ± 5.6	21.8 ± 5.1
IVS thickness (mm)	ED	8.5 ± 2.4	7.2 ± 1.6	9.4 ± 1.9	8.0 ± 2.1°
	ES	11.3 ± 2.8	10.2 ± 1.7	13.9 ± 2.6†	12.1 ± 2.6°*
LVID (mm)	ED	50.4 ± 5.5	49.2 ± 4.4	54.5 ± 5.6†	48.9 ± 4.7°
	ES	37.4 ± 6.2	34.7 ± 3.6	37.1 ± 4.2	32.7 ± 4.0°
LVPW thickness (mm)	ED	8.2 ± 1.5	7.5 ± 1.2	8.9 ± 1.4	7.5 ± 1.8°
	ES	12.8 ± 1.8	12.2 ± 2.1	14.5 ± 2.5†	12.7 ± 2.3°
Heart rate (beats/min)		65.8 ± 10	68.8 ± 12	63.6 ± 7.5	67.8 ± 13.7
Blood pressure (mm Hg)	Syst.	125.4 ± 11	122.6 ± 11.4	126.5 ± 10.2	125.7 ± 9.1
	Diast.	82.1 ± 7.2	79.9 ± 8.7+	84.6 ± 6.4	80.2 ± 9.3
Weight (kg)		67.9 ± 7.4	61.2 ± 8.7+	73.5 ± 8.0†	62.9 ± 7.2°
Height (m)		1.763 ± 0.086	1.687 ± 0.067+	1.755 ± 0.057	1.633 ± 0.056°*
Body surface area (m²)		1.86 ± 0.13	1.72 ± 0.13+	1.92 ± 0.12	1.70 ± 0.11°

Group I = males, aged 18–30 (n=17)
Group II = females, aged 18–30 (n=21)
Group III = males, aged 30–42 (n=19)
Group IV = females, aged 30–42 (n=19)

° = significantly different from Group III

+ † = significantly different from Group I
* = significantly different from Group II

significant: $p < 0.05$.

Table 2. The mean values and standard deviations of the aortic and cardiac dimensions, adjusted for body surface area (BSA) or body weight (BW). Comparison between males and females.

Variables		Group I		Group II		Group III		Group IV	
		BSA[1]	BW[2]	BSA	BW	BSA	BW	BSA	BW
A_oID	ED	16.2±2.4	44.5± 7.8	16.1±3.3	45.9± 9.5	16.7±2.3	43.9± 7.1	16.2±2.1	43.3± 9.6
	ES	17.7±2.5	49.0± 8.7	17.0±2.7	48.5± 8.2	18.1±2.5	47.5± 7.9	17.4±3.3	49.3± 9.5
LAID	ED	13.9±3.4	38.2± 9.5	12.5±3.5	33.8± 9.5	13.9±3.2	36.5± 8.5	13.7±3.3	38.8± 8.8
	ES	18.5±3.1	50.8± 8.2	17.6±3.0	50.8± 8.3	19.7±3.3	51.5± 9.5	18.4±3.8	53.2± 9.3
RVID	ED	15.2±4.4	41.9±11.6	11.9±3.7*	32.7± 9.6+	13.8±3.1	37.9± 7.6	14.0±4.1	38.7± 9.7
	ES	13.7±3.0	37.6± 8.7	11.1±3.1*	31.1± 8.2+	13.0±2.4	34.4± 6.3	12.2±3.5	33.7± 8.6
IVS thickness	ED	4.5±1.3	12.5± 3.3	4.2±0.8	11.9± 2.7	4.9±1.0	12.9± 3.0	4.7±1.5	13.0± 4.3
	ES	6.1±1.5	16.6± 4.0	5.9±1.0	16.8± 2.7	7.3±1.6	19.1± 4.7	7.0±1.8	19.6± 5.4
LVID	ED	27.2±3.4	74.9±10.6	28.7±2.8	81.6±11.4	28.4±3.2	74.6±10.5	28.3±3.4	78.3±10.0
	ES	21.3±3.0	55.5±10.1	20.2±2.1	57.6± 8.4	19.4±2.3	50.9± 7.3	18.8±2.5	52.4± 6.5
LVPW thickness	ED	4.4±0.8	12.0± 2.2	4.4±0.7	12.5± 2.5	4.6±0.8	12.2± 2.3	4.4±1.2	12.5± 3.1
	ES	6.9±1.1	18.9± 3.3	7.1±1.2	20.1± 4.0	7.6±1.1	19.6± 2.9	7.4±1.7	20.7± 4.8

1) $\dfrac{\text{dimensions in mm}}{\text{body surface area in m}^2}$ 2) $\dfrac{\text{dimensions in mm}}{\text{body weight in kg}} \times 100$

*, + = significantly smaller than in Group I ($p<0.05$). See Table 1 for group composition.

Table 3. The correlation coefficients for the aortic and cardiac dimensions, related to body surface area (BSA) or body weight (BW).

Variables		Group I		Group II		Group III		Group IV	
		BSA	BW	BSA	BW	BSA	BW	BSA	BW
AoID	ED	0.22	0.15	0.54	0.43	0.13	0.17	0.23	0.31
	ES	0.11	-0.35	0.56	0.40	0.15	0.13	0.23	-0.06
LAID	ED	0.15	0.31	0.02	0.37	0.22	0.31	0.26	0.37
	ES	0.28	0.40	0.24	-0.21	0.17	0.26	0.45	0.53
RVID	ED	-0.04	0.15	0.12	0.15	0.30	0.34	-0.15	0.14
	ES	0.05	0.06	0.06	0.23	0.55	0.48	0.13	0.08
IVS thickness	ED	0.21	0.34	0.36	0.36	0.13	0.09	0.33	-0.40
	ES	0.23	0.36	0.04	0.35	0.09	-0.21	0.30	0.38
LVID	ED	0.06	0.07	0.31	0.32	0.24	0.29	0.29	0.35
	ES	0.12	0.30	0.36	0.28	0.27	0.28	0.07	0.47
LVPW thickness	ED	0.28	0.33	0.21	0.08	0.04	-0.01	-0.27	-0.20
	ES	0.05	0.03	0.57	0.67	0.57	0.70	0.17	-0.03

See Table 1 for group composition.

in males than in females, especially in the older age-group (30–42 years). Most of the differences between females and males disappear when the dimensions are adjusted for either body surface area or body weight, which is in agreement with the findings of Valdez and co-investigators (12). It is questionable, however, whether this adjustment is permissible, because the correlation coefficients for the aortic and cardiac dimensions related to body surface area or body weight are generally poor, suggesting that, in these age-groups, the dimensions are not really dependent on body surface area or body weight.

The disappearance of most of the differences in dimensions between females and males after adjustment for body surface area or body weight probably results from the significant differences between the latter parameters in both sexes. The present findings indicate that, in adults, differences in the dimensions of the aorta and the heart between females and males should be taken into account.

In the age-groups investigated in the present study, the dependency of the aortic and cardiac dimensions on age is limited. For some of the dimensions this dependency might increase with age, as indicated by the increasing left ventricular wall thickness and aortic root diameter with age (6).

The IVS and LVPW thickness values found in this study are in accordance with those reported in the literature. However, the end-diastolic and end-systolic LVID values found in these studies are smaller than those obtained in our study. The slightly higher LVID readings probably result from an oblique orientation of the sound beam, due to tilting of the transducer when searching for the largest diameter.

In conclusion, the present findings indicate that, in echocardiographic studies of the dimensions of the aorta and the heart, differences between females and males must be taken into account and that these differences should be considered when control groups are compared with patients or athletes.

ACKNOWLEDGEMENTS

The authors are greatly indebted to Drs. Leo Strijbosch for his assistance in the statistical evaluation of the data and to Mrs. Mariet de Groot and Mrs. Joke Hoozemans for their help in preparing the manuscript.

REFERENCES

1. Allen HD, SJ Goldberg, DJ Sahn, N Schy, R Wojcik: A quantitative echocardiographic study of champion childhood swimmers. Circulation 55 (1): 142, 1977.
2. Dunn FG, P Chandraratna, JGR de Carvalho, LL Basta, ED Frohlich: Pathophysiologic assessment of hypertensive heart disease with echocardiography. Am J Cardiol 39:789, 1977.
3. Engström CG, P Herzog: Ventilation nomogram for practical use with the Engström respirator. Acta Chir Scand, suppl. 245, 37, 1959.
4. Feigenbaum H: Echocardiography, 2nd edition, Philadelphia, Pa., Lea & Febiger, 1976.

5. Gardin JM, WL Henry, DD Savage, SE Epstein: Echocardiographic evaluation of an older population without clinically apparent heart disease. Am J Cardiol 39:277, 1977 (abstract).
6. Gerstenblith G, JW Frederiksen, ML Weisfeldt, NW Shock, NJ Fortuin: Echocardiographic changes in a normal adult aging population. Circulation 52 (4), suppl. II, 135, 1975 (abstract).
7. Henry WL, J Ware, JM Gardin, SI Hepner, J McKay, M Weiner: Echocardiographic measurements in normal subjects. Circulation 57 (2): 278, 1978.
8. Morganroth J, BJ Maron, WL Henry, SE Epstein: Comparative left ventricular dimensions in trained athletes. Ann Intern Med 82:521, 1975.
9. Roeske WR, RA O'Rourke, A Klein, G Leopold, JS Karliner: Noninvasive evaluation of ventricular hypertrophy in professional athletes. Circulation 53 (2): 286, 1976.
10. Rogé CLL, NH Silverman, PA Hart, RM Ray: Cardiac structure growth pattern determined by echocardiography. Circulation 57 (2): 285–290, 1978.
11. Schlant RC, S Heymsfield, JM Felner, C Gilbert, J Perkins, N Shulman, B Blumenstein: Echocardiographic studies of left ventricular function and anatomy in uncomplicated essential hypertension. Am J Cardiol 37:170, 1976 (abstract).
12. Valdez R, J Motta, R Martin, E London, W Haskell, R Popp, L Horlick: Survey of a normal population with the echocardiogram. Am J Cardiol 39:277, 1977 (abstract).
13. Zeldis SM, J Morganroth, S Rubler: Cardiac hypertrophy in response to dynamic conditioning in female atheletes. J Appl Physiol 44 (6):849, 1978.

ASSESSMENT OF ATRIAL SEPTAL DEFECTS BY CROSS-SECTIONAL ECHOCARDIOGRAPHY

P.D.V. BOURDILLON, R.A. FOALE, and A.F. RICKARDS

INTRODUCTION

In the investigation of atrial septal defects by M-mode echocardiography the features described have included dilatation of the right ventricle, reversed motion of the interventricular septum, and increased amplitude of opening motion of the tricuspid relative to the mitral valve. These criteria have been found to be lacking in sensitivity and specificity. In general it is not possible to visualize the interatrial septum directly by M-mode echocardiography although this can be done using cross-sectional echocardiography (1). With the additional use of injections of contrast the presence or absence of interatrial shunts can also be assessed (2). The purpose of this study was to evaluate the use of cross-sectional echocardiography combined with contrast injections into peripheral arm veins in the investigation of patients with atrial septal defects.

PATIENTS AND METHODS

Fifteen patients with atrial septal defects, age range 6 to 42 years, were studied. Eleven patients had a dominant left-to-right shunt demonstrated by oxygen saturation estimations at cardiac catheterization, with no detectable right-to-left shunt. Nine of these patients had an ostium secundum atrial septal defect, one a sinus venosus atrial septal defect, and one had Lutembacher's syndrome of an ostium secundum atrial septal defect and mitral stenosis. Four patients who were clinically cyanosed had a dominant right-to-left shunt, 2 with total anomalous pumonary venous drainage, 1 with a secundum atrial septal defect and pulmonary hypertension at systemic level (Eisenmenger syndrome), and 1 with complex congenital heart disease including dextrocardia and double outlet right ventricle with free mixing across an atrial septal defect. All patients except one were also investigated by cardiac catheterization, the one exception being the patient with Eisenmenger's syndrome in whom the diagnosis was subsequently confirmed at postmortem examination.

The patients were studied by M-mode and cross-sectional echocardiography using a mechanical 30° sector scanner.* The interatrial septum was

* Smith-Kline Instrument Company Limited.

Charles T. Lancée (ed.), Echocardiology, 61–65. All rights reserved
Copyright © 1979 by Martinus Nijhoff Publishers bv, The Hague/Boston/London

visualized using a conventional short axis view, with the transducer held at
the third or fourth interspace at the left sternal edge. Indocyanine green dye,
5% dextrose or normal saline were injected as contrast into a peripheral arm
vein. In addition to the 15 patients with atrial septal defects 10 patients with
an intact interatrial septum were also studied using peripheral contrast
injections.

The images were initially viewed on an oscilloscope and stored on magnetic tape. They were subsequently recorded on 35 mm film using a cine
camera synchronized with the sweep of the scanning ultrasound beam to
produce moving cine film at 15 frames per second.

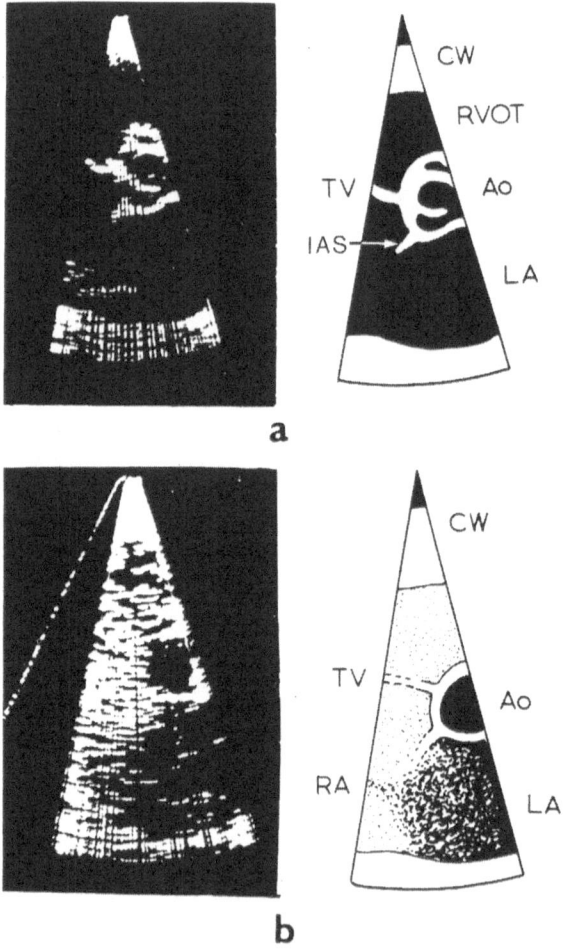

Fig. 1. Atrial septal defect, left-to-right shunt. a) before, b) after contrast injection, Cw = chest
wall, RVOT = right ventricular outflow tract, AO = aorta, TV = tricuspid valve, LA = left atrium,
IAS = interatrial septum.

RESULTS

The interatrial septum was visualized in all patients studied. In the 11 patients with an atrial septal defect and a left-to-right shunt the defect was seen in the septal image with a free "edge" moving with a fixed relationship to the aortic root (Fig. 1). In 3 of the patients with a right-to-left shunt a similar appearance was seen (Fig. 3), but in the patient with complex congenital heart disease the septal defect was not consistently seen. The appearance of the interatrial septum in patients with a septal defect differs from that in patients with an intact septum in that, although there is often variable loss of echoes in the image of an intact septum as the septum moves across the plane of ultrasound during the cardiac cycle, there is no position of

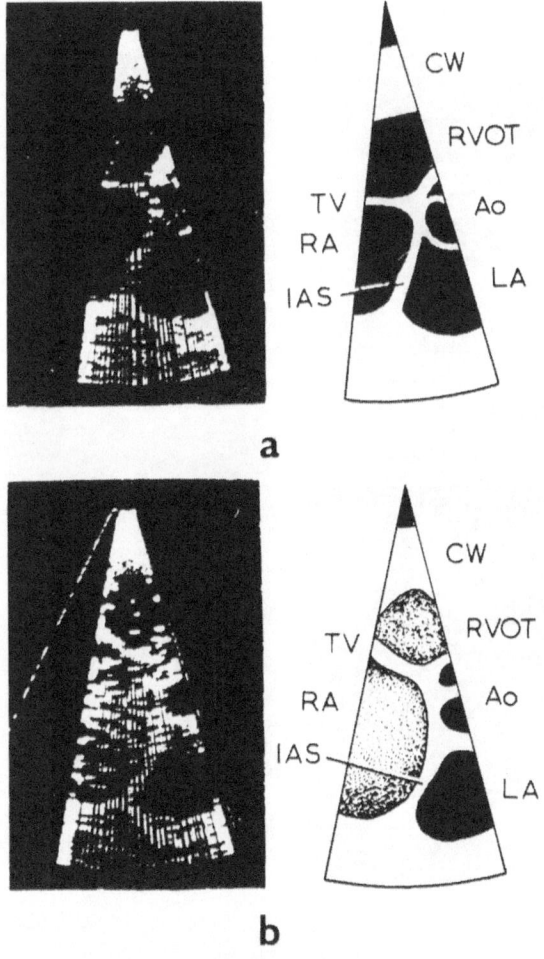

Fig. 2. Intact interatrial septum. Abbreviations as for figure 1.

the ultrasound plane in which a fixed edge is seen moving with a constant relationship to the aortic root.

Following injection of contrast into a peripheral arm vein in patients with an intact interatrial septum, contrast is seen initially in the right atrium and subsequently in the right ventricular outflow tract (Fig. 2). No contrast is observed in the left atrium and the interatrial septum is outlined by the contrast in the right atrium. In the patients with a dominant right-to-left shunt free transfer of contrast from right atrium to left atrium was observed (Fig. 3), with contrast subsequently appearing in the aortic root. In 8 of the patients with a dominant left-to-right shunt some degree of transfer of contrast from right atrium to left atrium was observed (Fig. 1). The 3 patients with a left-to-right shunt in whom contrast was not observed to enter the left atrium were the patient with Lutembacher's syndrome in whom there was a 5

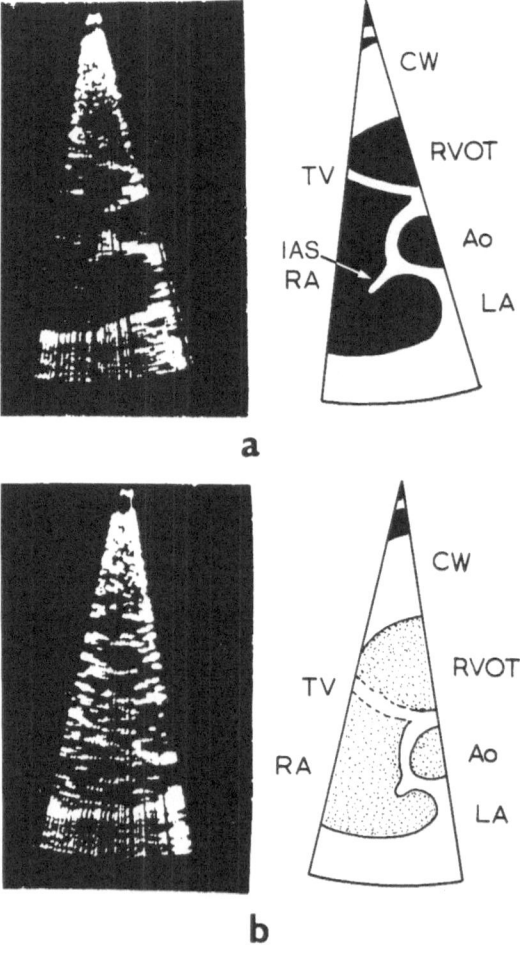

Fig. 3. Atrial septal defect, right-to-left shunt.

mm Hg pressure difference between left atrium and right atrium due to the presence of mitral stenosis in addition to the secundum atrial septal defect; one patient with a secundum atrial septal defect and a very small left-to-right shunt with a pulmonary to systemic flow ratio of 1.3:1; and a patient in whom it was considered that an inadequate injection of contrast was made.

DISCUSSION

The interatrial septum can be consistently visualized using cross-sectional echocardiography. We have confirmed the findings of Dillon et al. (1) that an atrial septal defect can be seen with this technique and that the appearance of a true defect differs from the apparent defect in the septal image that may be seen in patients with an intact interatrial septum. This relatively specific appearance is observed if the defect is within the plane of the ultrasound sector scan which has to be varied during the course of the examination in order to obtain an optimum image.

The use of contrast injections into peripheral veins enhances the practical value of the technique. The appearance of a defect in the septal image is a negative and, to some extent, subjective finding, but the transfer of contrast echoes from right atrium to left atrium is a positive feature which confirms the presence of a defect. The results we have obtained using this technique are similar to those of Fraker et al. (2) in that most patients with an atrial septal defect and a left-to-right shunt show some degree of transfer of contrast echoes from right atrium to left atrium after injection into a peripheral arm vein.

SUMMARY AND CONCLUSIONS

Cross-sectional contrast echocardiography has been used to study 15 patients with atrial septal defects and 10 patients with an intact interatrial septum. The septum can be consistently visualized by this technique and a relatively specific appearance of the interatrial septum is observed in patients with an atrial septal defect. Injection of contrast into a peripheral arm vein helps to confirm the presence or absence of an atrial septal defect.

REFERENCES

1. Dillon JC, AE Weyman, H Feigenbaum, R Eggleton, K Johnston: Cross-sectional echocardiography examination of the interatrial septum. Circulation 55:115, 1977.
2. Fraker TD, S Myers, JA Kisslo: Detection and exclusion of interatrial shunts by contrast two-dimensional echo. Circulation 58:187 (Abstr), 1978.

A COMBINED ECHOCARDIOGRAPHIC AND PHONOCARDIOGRAPHIC STUDY ON THE GENESIS OF DIASTOLIC HEART SOUNDS

B. DENEF, F. VAN DE WERF, H. DE GEEST, and H. KESTELOOT

INTRODUCTION

The combination of phono- and echocardiography has a diagnostic value that may be lacking when these two techniques are employed either separately or serially.

Recently, interesting clinical investigations on the origin of heart sounds have been performed using this combined technique (1–7). On the basis of a large number of simultaneous recordings of phono- and echocardiograms, Craige et al. offered new evidence concerning the genesis of heart sounds, considering the origin of the high frequency sounds as "valvular" and of the low frequency sounds as "ventricular" (8).

The "valvular" concept of the origin of high-frequency heart sounds, however, has been contradicted by other investigators (9).

Most of these studies investigate the genesis of first and second heart sound, ejection sounds and opening snaps, whereas echocardiographic studies on the genesis of other diastolic heart sounds are rare.

In this paper, we shall present some unusual phono-echocardiographic findings which will provide some additional insights into the genesis of diastolic heart sounds.

METHODOLOGY

Standard methods were used for the registration of the echo- and phonocardiogram. The recordings were made with a 2.25 MHz Irex ultrasound transducer (med. int. focus), using an Irex I ultrasonoscope and recorder and a microphone that can be fixed to the chest wall by a suction device. The phonocardiograms were also recorded on a 6-channel, ink-jet, direct-writing recorder (Siemens-Elema).

RESULTS

1. Figure 1 illustrates a combined phono-echocardiogram in a patient with a calcified mitral valve, without a pressure gradient between left atrium and left ventricle at catheterization.

During clinical examination, and on the phonocardiogram, a pre-systolic

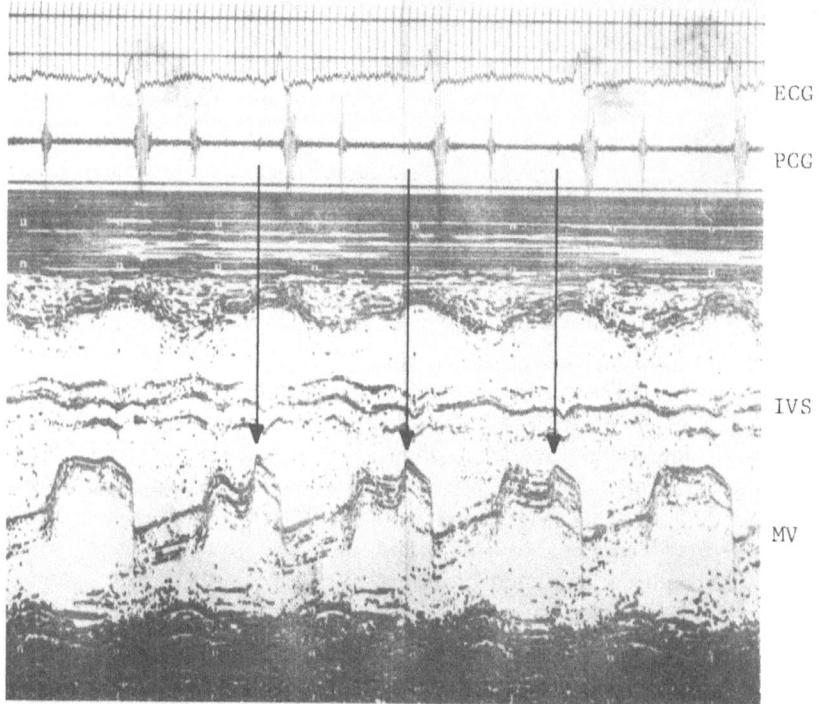

Fig. 1.

click was found, but only as an intermittent phenomenon despite a constant sinus rhythm without changing R-R or P-Q intervals.

The simultaneously recorded echocardiogram indicates that this high-frequency sound has a valvular origin, as it exactly coincides with the time of the abrupt maximal opening of the mitral valve during atrial contraction. The pre-systolic click is absent whenever this abrupt reopening of the mitral valve during atrial contraction does not occur. This unusual case, which has not been described previously, strengthens the "valvular" theory on the genesis of high-frequency heart sounds.

2. Figure 2a, b shows a phonocardiogram and an echocardiogram recorded in a patient with atrial flutter and a high degree of atrioventricular block.

Regular undulations of equal amplitude on the mitral valve leaflets are seen during diastole, corresponding precisely to the atrial flutter waves in the ECG. On the phonocardiogram, low-frequency diastolic sounds following each flutter wave are seen, but only in the late part of a prolonged diastole.

These findings indicate that these low-frequency diastolic heart sounds are not of valvular origin. They are more likely to originate from vibrations within the heart walls. Regular undulations are indeed seen on the interventricular septum and the left ventricular posterior wall. The fact that the atrial sounds are only visible during end-diastole indicates an interaction between left atrial contraction and the left ventricular wall during diastole in the genesis of these low-frequency diastolic heart sounds. These sounds only become apparent above a certain degree of left ventricular filling and wall tension.

3. Figures 3 to 5 illustrate combined phono-echocardiograms recorded in a patient with a Björk-Shiley mitral valve prosthesis during episodes of atrial flutter.

The genesis of the multiple diastolic clicks on the phonocardiogram can only be clarified by studying the simultaneously recorded mitral valve echo. The diastolic clicks originate from the abrupt opening and closure of the

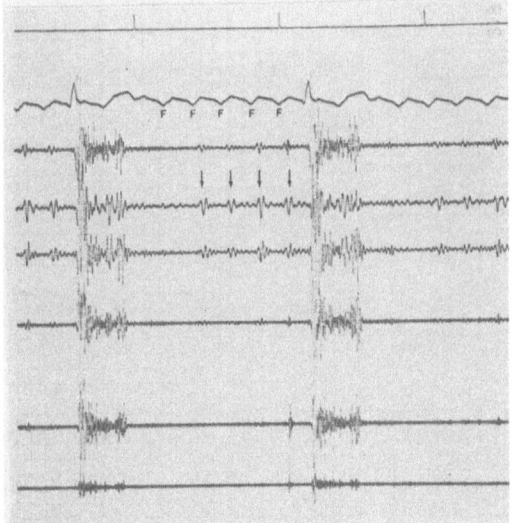

Fig. 2a.

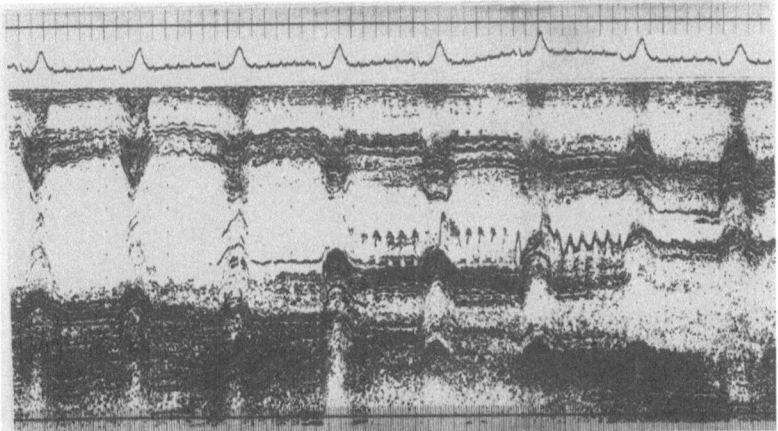

Fig. 2b.

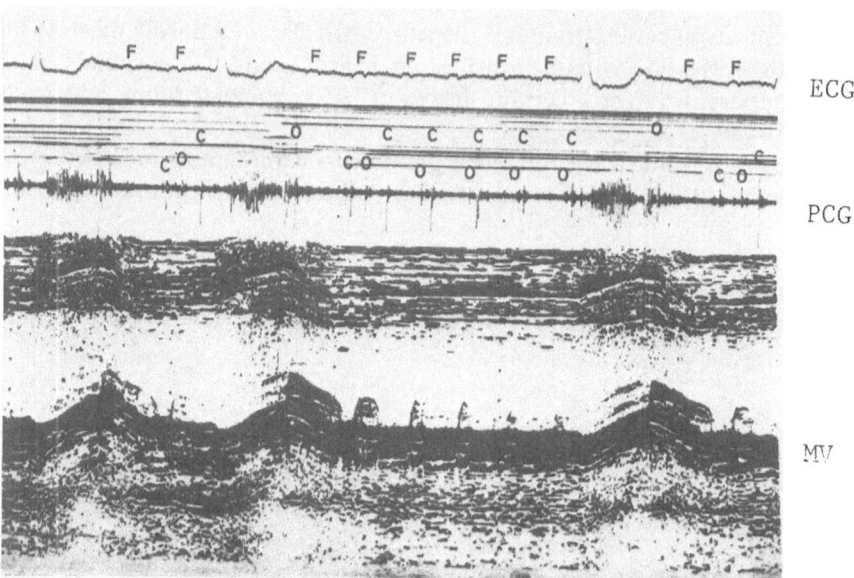

Fig. 3.

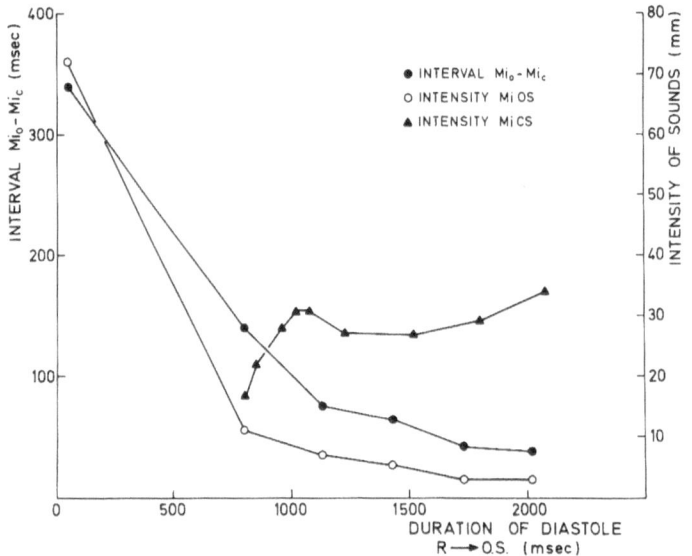

Fig. 4.

prosthetic valve as a result of the mechanical activity of the atrial flutter
waves. The variable intensity and timing of these clicks are functions of the
duration of diastole and the degree of left ventricular filling. The intensity of
the opening sound (MiOS) decreases, of the closure sound (MiCS) increases
and the duration of the valve opening (interval Mi_O-Mi_C) decreases

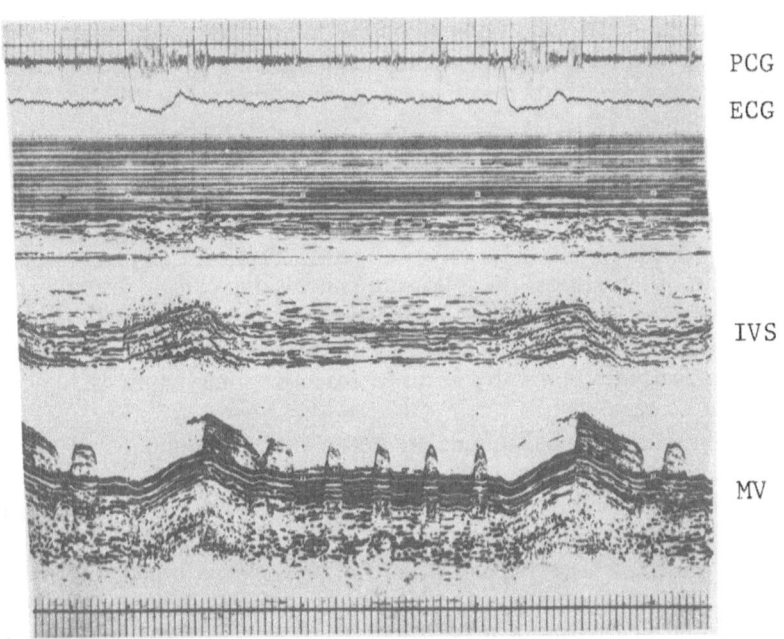

Fig. 5.

progressively as LV filling progresses (Figs. 3 and 4). The total excursion of the valve disk, however, does not change significantly (Fig. 5).

These findings can be explained by an interaction between the mechanical activity of the left atrium and LV wall tension: the increase in wall tension occurring during LV filling shortens the time that the left atrial contraction can keep the valve in open position, decreases the opening – and increases the closing – velocity of the valve and consequently influences the relative intensity and timing of the related sounds.

DISCUSSION

The origin of heart sounds occurring during ventricular systole is always complex. Valvular sounds, whether opening or closing sounds, are always accompanied by acceleration or deceleration of blood mass. Deceleration of mass may generate oscillations by transforming kinetic into vibratory energy. As a result, the tension in the valve structures cannot be isolated from other physical phenomena. During diastole, however, the kinetic energy of any moving blood mass is certainly markedly lower than during systole. High-frequency heart sounds coinciding with the end of rapid valvular movements during diastole are thus further proof of the fact that a valvular component exists in these sounds. The initial vibrations of these sounds should coincide with the end of rapid valvular movements determined by echocardiography, as has been beautifully demonstrated by Craige and co-workers. The presence of low-frequency vibrations in the ventricular wall coinciding with low frequency precordial vibrations is highly interesting. One might speculate whether or not the kinetic energy present in the wall during movement could also be transformed into low frequency vibrations when this movement is abruptly halted.

CONCLUSIONS

From these observations, the following conclusions can be drawn:
1. High-frequency diastolic heart sounds (opening snaps, pre-systolic clicks) are of valvular origin. They only originate at the moment when the atrioventricular valve abruptly reaches its maximum excursion (case 1).
2. Low frequency atrial sounds are not of valvular origin. Most likely they originate from heart wall vibrations as the result of an interaction between the mechanical activity of the left atrium and left ventricular diastolic wall tension (case 2).
3. The mechanical activity of atrial flutter waves is important since they are able to open and close prosthetic heart valves and to generate diastolic heart sounds (case 2 and 3).
4. Combined echo-phonocardiography is of great value for clarifying some unusual auscultatory and phonocardiographic phenomena and can provide new insights in the genesis of heart sounds.

REFERENCES

1. Craige E.: Echocardiography in studies of the genesis of heart sounds and murmurs. In: Progress in Cardiology, Yu PN, Goodwin JF (eds), Philadelphia, Lea and Febiger, 1975.
2. Craige E.: On the genesis of heart sounds: Contributions made by echocardiographic studies. Circulation 53:207, 1976.
3. Waider W, E Craige: First heart sound and ejection sounds: Echocardiographic and phonocardiographic correlation with valvular events. Am J Cardiol 35:346, 1975.
4. Leatham A, GL Leech: Observations on the relation between heart sounds and valve movements by simultaneous echo and phonocardiography. Brit Heart J 37:557, 1975, (abstract).
5. Mills P, R Chamusco, S Moos et al.: Echophonocardiographic studies of the contribution of the atrioventricular valves to the first heart sound. Circulation 54:944, 1976.
6. Chandraratna PAN, JM Lopez, LS Cohen: Echocardiographic observations on the mechanism of production of the second heart sound. Circulation 51:292, 1975.
7. Anastassiades PC, MA Quinones, W. Gaasch et al.: Aortic valve closure: Echocardiographic, phonocardiographic and hemodynamic assessment. Am Heart J 91:228, 1976.
8. Mills P, E Craige: Echophonocardiography. Progr Cardiovascul Dis 20:337, 1978.
9. Luisada AA, DM MacCanon, S Kumar et al.: Changing views on the mechanism of the first and second heart sounds. Am Heart J 88:503, 1974.

SUBXIPHOID VERSUS STANDARD
M-MODE ECHOCARDIOGRAPY

G. GULLACE

The use of subxiphoid (SUBX) M-mode echocardiography has been rather limited, as can be seen from the few studies published; these concern more bronchopneumopathics than cardiopathics (1, 3, 4, 5). Probably this limited use can be attributed to the presumed unreliability of the spatial parameters and to the subxiphoid echocardiographic anatomy not being well established.

This paper compares the morphologic, topographic and technical aspects together with the parameters of space, time and velocity, obtained from the SUBX with the ones obtained by the standard techniques (ST).

METHODS

Two echocardiographic tracings were obtained, using both ST and SUBX, in 60 patients (15 normal and 45 cardiopathic).

SUBX was set up as follows: the transducer was positioned at the costalxiphoid arch and depressed slightly on the abdominal wall; the ultrasonic beam was directed upwards and towards the back until the tricuspid valve (TV) was visualized. The visualization was obtained when the beam was directed medially, almost parallel to the left sternal edge, and towards the back.

Position A. The beam was directed towards the back until the aortic root was visualized. In this position, therefore, the beam was medial on the frontal plane and directed towards the back on the sagittal plane (Fig. 1).

Position C. The beam was directed laterally from position A to the left shoulder on the frontal plane, and more inclined to the back on the sagittal plane than the beam in position A. (Fig. 1).

Position B. The beam was directed a little laterally on the frontal plane and forwards on the sagittal plane as compared with position A (Fig. 1).

All the patients were in a supine position, in some cases they were invited to bend their legs or to arch their backs by placing a cushion in the small of the back.

A recording was defined as "good" when the most of the points of the structures necessary for space and time measurements were sufficiently clear, and as "complete" when a "good" visualization of all the structures was obtained. "Anterior" was considered to be the area nearest the transducer and "posterior" the area farthest away.

74

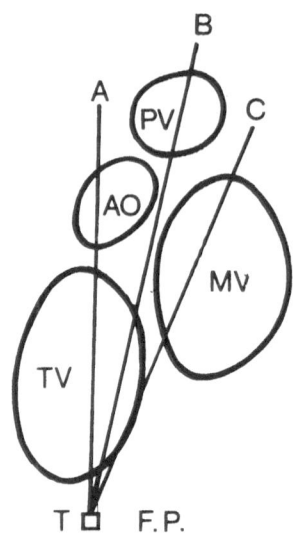
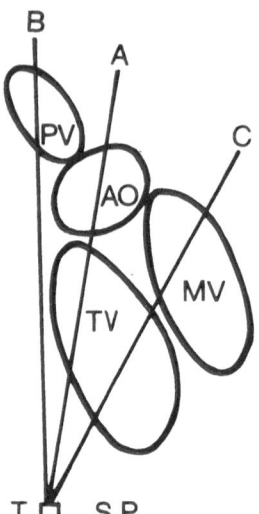

Fig. 1. F.P. = frontal plane; S.P. = sagittal plane; T = transducer; AO = aorta; PV = pulmonary valve; MV = mitral valve; TV = tricuspid valve; A = position A; B = position B; C = position C.
The transducer is positioned at the costal-xiphoid arch and directed upwards (A), laterally and forwards (B), more laterally and backwards (C).

The most important parameters of space, time and velocity were obtained from all tracing. The mean values obtained by SUBX were compared to the ones obtained by ST.

RESULTS

Taken in order from the transducer, position A provided a visualization of the anterior (near) wall of the right ventricle (RV), the TV, the interventricular septum (IVS), the anterior (near) wall, cusps and posterior (far) wall of the aorta (AO), and the cavity and posterior (far) wall of the left atrium (LA) (Fig. 2A).

Position C provided a visualization of the anterior wall and cavity of RV, sometimes the TV, the IVS, the mitral valve (MV) and the cavity and posterior (far) wall of the left ventricle (LV) (Fig. 2C).

Position B provided a visualization of the diastolic phase of TV, the outflow tract of RV, echoes presumably reflected by the crista supraventricularis, the pulmonary valve (PV) and no cavity or echo-free space behind it (Fig. 2B).

The following statements are based on scans from position B through A and C (Fig. 2).

(a) There is a continuity between the near wall of AO and IVS, between the far wall of AO and MV and between the far wall of LA and PW;

b) The PV is the farthest valve from the transducer and, therefore, farther away than AO;

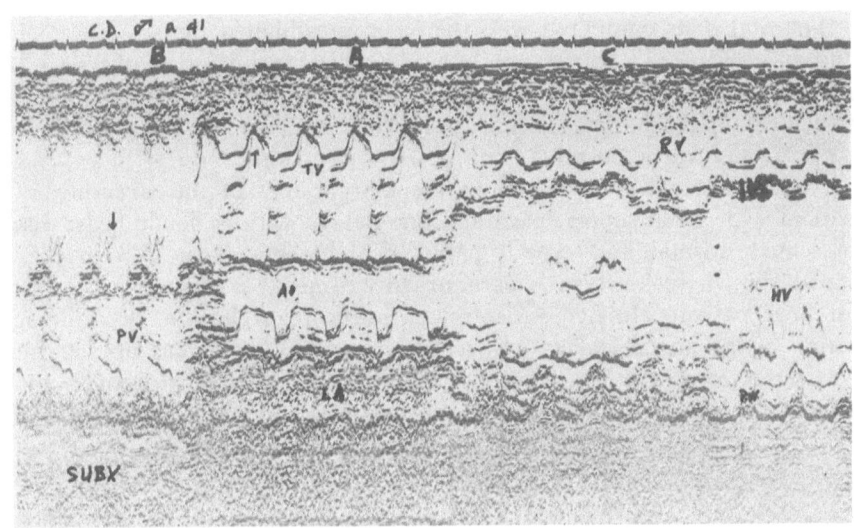

Fig. 2. A scan made from the B to the A to the C position by the subxiphoid echocardiographic technique (SUBX). It is possible to identify the pulmonary (PV), aortic (AO) mitral (MV) and tricuspid (TV) valve, the right ventricle (RV), the interventricular septem (IVS), the left atrium (LA) and the cavity and posterior wall (PW) of the left ventricle. The arrows indicate the anterior and posteror leaflets of TV.

c) There is no cavity behind the PV, whereas a cavity (the LA) is always present behind AO.

The recording was good:

		ST	SUBX	
for MV	in	59 (98%)	42 (70%)	patients
for AO	in	58 (97%)	54 (90%)	patients
for PV	in	48 (80%)	54 (90%)	patients
for TV	in	39 (65%)	54 (90%)	patients
for LV+RV	in	57 (95%)	48 (80%)	patients
and "complete"	in	39 (65%)	42 (70%)	patients

The ST and SUBX, when considered as one method only, provided a "complete" recording in 54 (90%) patients.

Patients with obesity, pulmonary emphysema and thoracic malformations in the case of ST and stiffness of the abdominal wall and pectus excavatum in that of SUBX, did not provide a "good" or "complete" visualization of the structures.

The systolic time intervals of the right and left ventricle did not show significant differences when the ST was compared to the SUBX. However, either the difference between the right and left ejection time or the electro-mechanically derived duration of systole, provided a useful means of identifying the semilunar valve, whether AO or PV.

The SUBX as compared with the ST, overestimated the systolic ($+10\%$) and diastolic ($+11\%$) dimension of LV ($p<0.1$), the dimension of RV ($+18\%$; $p<0.05$), of AO ($+14\%$; $p<0.05$) and thickness of IVS ($+7\%$; $p<0.1$) and underestimated the dimension of LA (-20%; $p<0.01$) and the septal (-30%; $p<0.01$) and aortic cusp (-20%; $p<0.01$) excursions.

No difference was observed in the morphology of the structures. One patient with atrial septal defect and one patient with ischemic heart disease presented normal and type-B paradoxical movement of IVS in ST, respectively; whereas a type-A paradoxical movement was observed in SUBX for both patients. In five patients with aortic regurgitation, diastolic separation of the aortic leaflets was recorded in SUBX; whereas no separation was observed in the ST recordings of the same patients. Moreover, such a separation was not recorded in the other patients, whether with ST or SUBX.

CONCLUSION

As this study shows, subxiphoid echocardiography supplements the standard techniques by providing a good visualization of cardiac structures.

Previous papers, (3) and (5) have discussed problems of topography and of identification of the pulmonary and aortic valve by this technique. The underestimation of the left atrial dimension agrees with the data previously reported (1, 2), whereas the estimates of the other dimensions and excursional amplitudes disagree with these reports. The overestimation and underestimation shown by SUBX can be explained by the fact that the beam intersects the structures almost perpendicularly in ST; whereas, in SUBX, the beam is at an angle and intersects the structures along a plane more closely parallel to the structures themselves.

In this study, the SUBX provided a better visualization of TV and PV than did the ST. This is particularly important and useful in the evaluation of right ventricular performances.

At present, any explanation of the different morphological aspects observed in some cases is hazardous since patients were selected at random for the study and there was limited experience with SUBX.

In conclusion, the SUBX should be considered as a useful tool for the visualization of the right cardiac structures and, therefore, for the study of a variety of cardiopathies.

REFERENCES

1. Chang S, H Feigenbaum: Subxiphoyd echocardiography. J Clin Ultrasound 1:14, 1973.
2. Chang S, H Feigenbaum: Subxiphoyd echocardiography. Chest 68:2, 1975.
3. Gullace G: Ecocardiografia subxifoidea: aspetti morfologici e topografici. Atti 39° Congresso Nazionale della S.I.C., Milano, 1978 (in press).
4. Ravault MC, C Pernot: Abord sous-xiphoidien en echocardiographie pediatrique. Coeur 8:871, 1977.
5. Rusconi C, G Orlando, C Spedini, G Grati: Ecocardiografia subxifoidea: arteria polmonare o aorta? Giorn It Cardiol 7:870, 1977.

ABSOLUTE INTRACARDIAC BLOOD VELOCITIES MEASURED WITH CONTINUOUS WAVE DOPPLER AND A NEW REAL-TIME SPECTRAL DISPLAY

D.S. TUNSTALL PEDOE, P.C. MACPHERSON, and S.J. MELDRUM

INTRODUCTION

To realize the full potential of the diagnostic information carried by intracardiac blood velocity patterns requires measurement of their absolute velocities, direction and timing. The severity of a valve stenosis may be judged by its peak jet velocity. The importance of a regurgitant jet may be assessed by its size and duration, its absolute velocity depending on the transvalvar gradient. In order to explore the diagnostic and haemodynamic information carried by the absolute blood velocities, these have been measured transcutaneously using continuous wave 2 MHz Doppler ultrasound.

Pulsed Doppler cannot be used for these high jet velocities, which give rise to Doppler shifts in excess of those measurable by currently available equipment. Typical pulsed Doppler equipment has a pulse repetition frequency (PRF) of 10 kHz for depths of up to 7.5 cm which for a 2 MHz carrier restricts the maximum velocity that can be measured to 1.9 m/sec, and to even lower velocities at greater depths or for higher carrier frequency.

A directional, real-time, spectral display of the Doppler signal is favoured, since this gives all the information retrieved by the beam of ultrasound, giving unambiguous measurement of the peak velocity; unlike mean or maximum velocity estimators, that give a unique value for a complex, often bidirectional, wide band of velocities and are often sensitive to gain adjustment.

THE INVESTIGATION SYSTEM

This consists of an ultrasonic Doppler velocimeter*, spectrum analyser, display and fibre-optic recorder as shown in Figure 1.

Blood velocities are translated by the velocimeter to frequencies in the audio range and presented as two outputs, both of which give the magnitude of frequency shift, with direction information being contained in their relative phase. A phase to frequency converter combines these to produce signals above or below 4 kHz, depending on the direction of flow.

The ECG is displayed on the record and is used to indicate the onset of

---

* Pedof, SINTEF, Trondheim, Norway.

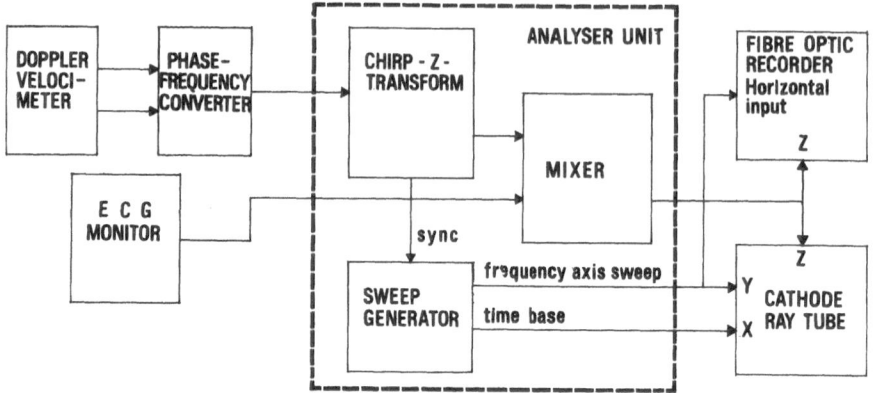

Fig. 1. The investigation system.

each cardiac cycle. This is necessary to interpret the spectra in cases of complex flow dynamics.

SPECTRUM ANALYSER

The analyser calculates spectral intensities using a chirp-Z-transform (CZT), modified to obtain continuous, real-time operation. This technique is parti- cularly suited to the capabilities of transversal filters using charge coupled device (CCD) technology. In its simplest terms, the analyser performs the transform by numerous multiplications and additions of discrete Doppler time samples with frequency sweeps called "chirps." Most of this is achieved by the transversal filter. At any one time, 512 samples are delayed in the analyser and transformed to produce a single discrete sample of the fre- quency spectrum. For continuous operation, a spectral component is calcu- lated every time the input is sampled, following a 512 step sequence. This goes from the maximum frequency to zero, then back to the maximum again, each spectrum consisting of 256 steps, the maximum frequency being limited to half the sample rate, by Nyquist's theorem.

In this application a 40 kHz clock was used, giving a range of 20 kHz in 78 Hz steps. Spectra are produced in 6 msec corresponding to a rate of 156 per second. Frequency resolution is limited to about 3 steps (234 Hz) by finite sampling in the time domain, since time limited samples contain slightly different spectral components from those of a continuous waveform. This should have little effect, however, on the wide band spectrum of Doppler signals.

DISPLAY

The usual sonogram display format is used where spectral intensity is achieved by Z-modulation of a cathode ray tube with X and Y sweeps, producing time and frequency axes, respectively. A fibre-optic recorder provides hard copy, with the paper movement producing the time axis.

BLOOD VELOCITY MEASUREMENTS

Measurements are made using this system by exploring the precordium with a beam of ultrasound, and then aligning the probe with any high velocity jet detected. For accurate measurement of velocity, alignment of the probe with the jet is essential. Figure 2 illustrates how this is done for mitral valve disease.

The probe's alignment with the jet can be checked by using the range-gated facility of the equipment. When correctly aligned, the jet can be sampled over a considerable depth, and will also give the highest velocity reading when the apparatus is switched to continuous wave operation.

PATIENTS STUDIED

Although a variety of cardiological conditions, including pulmonary and tricuspid valve disease have been studied, the principal use has been for the study of mitral valve disease and the effects of arrhythmias.

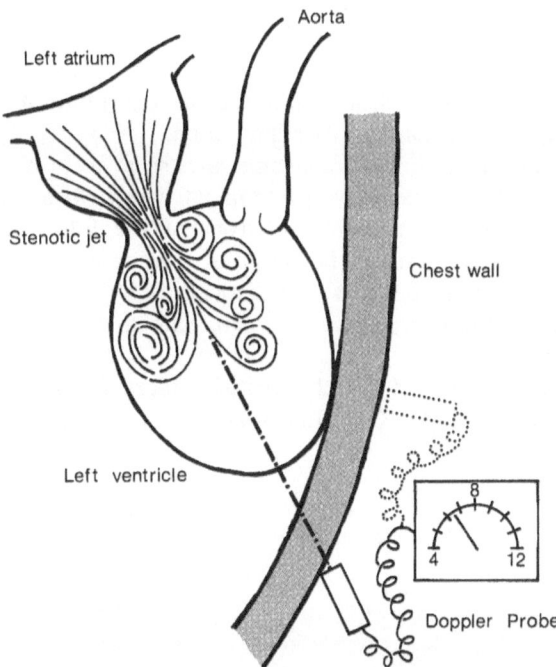

Fig. 2. Transcutaneous measurement of blood velocity through the mitral valve.

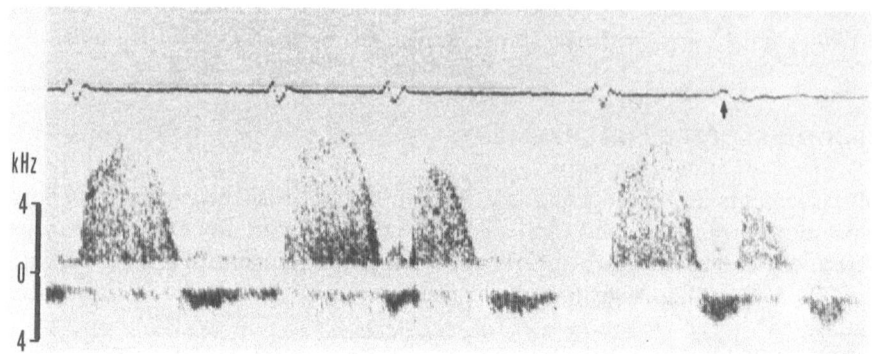

Fig. 3. A real time direction spectral display of transmitral blood velocity in mitral regurgitation.

Twenty patients with mitral valve disease have been studied. In 15 a high velocity regurgitant jet was detected passing back into the left atrium. Velocities as high as 5 m/sec have been measured. An example is shown in Figure 3.

This patient has mitral regurgitation, and was in atrial fibrillation with occasional ventricular ectopic beats. The arrow indicates a ventricular ectopic beat, which does not generate as high a regurgitant jet velocity as the normally conducted beat with the same antecedent cycle length. The regurgitant jet velocity is shown as a positive Doppler shift above the zero calibration, and the inflow to the left ventricle is shown as the negative velocity in diastole.

In two patients with pansystolic murmurs, a high velocity jet was detected passing from the left ventricle into the right, with an orientation suggesting ventricular septal defect rather than mitral regurgitation. This was subsequently confirmed at cardiac catheterization.

Although anatomical limitations sometimes seem to prevent measurement of the absolute blood velocity, preliminary work with this new display technique, suggests that real-time analysis of the full spectrum of blood velocities will greatly increase the range of cardiac conditions in which the Doppler technique may be used diagnostically. The technique appears to be of considerable value in many cases where echocardiography is unhelpful.

This work was supported by the British Heart Foundation. Fibre-optic recorder loaned by Smith Kline Instruments.

B. APPLICATIONS IN ISCHEMIC DISEASE

SENSITIVITY AND SPECIFICITY OF M-MODE AND CROSS-SECTIONAL ECHOCARDIOGRAPHIC FINDINGS IN PATIENTS WITH CORONARY ARTERY DISEASE

H. FEIGENBAUM, A.E. WEYMAN, B. CORYA, S. RASMUSSEN,
L. SAM WANN, E. ROGERS, R. GODLEY, and J.C. DILLON

ASSESSMENT OF OVERALL PERFORMANCE OF THE ISCHEMIC LEFT VENTRICLE

The most common echocardiographic technique for evaluating the left ventricle utilizes dimensions between the interventricular septum and the posterior left ventricular wall. By obtaining diastolic and systolic dimensions one can gain knowledge concerning the size of the left ventricle and the manner in which it is functioning. Investigators have used these dimensions to estimate ventricular volumes and measure fractional shortening and circumferential shortening. Unfortunately, there are well-recognized limitations to this echocardiographic technique (1, 2, 3). These limitations are extremely important in the setting of ischemic heart disease.

Figure 1 is an M-mode scan from a patient with coronary artery disease.

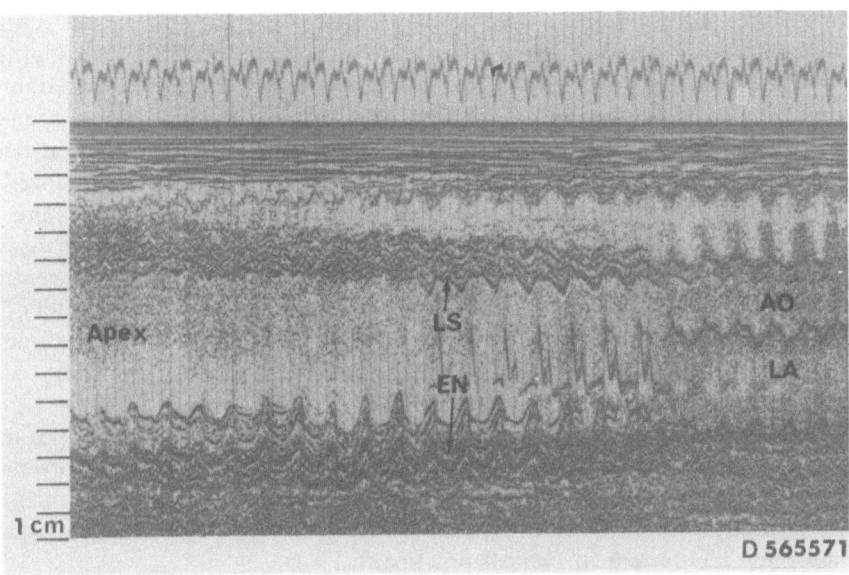

Fig. 1. M-mode scan from the left ventricular apex to the base of the heart in a patient with an anterior septal infarction and aneurysm involving the anterior wall. The septal (LS) and posterior endocardial (EN) echoes move normally near the base of the heart at the level of the mitral valve; however, there is an abrupt cessation of septal motion as the ultrasonic beam approaches the apex. (From Dillon JC, H Feigenbaum, BC Corya, S Peskoe, S Chang: M-mode echocardiography in the evaluation of patients for aneurysmectomy. Circulation 53:657, 1976.)

The distance between the left side of the septum (LS) and the posterior left ventricular endocardium (EN) is 5.8 cm, which is slightly above normal; however, the septal and posterior walls move fairly well at the level of the mitral valve apparatus. If the echocardiographic recording were limited to the area just beyond the level of the mitral valve, where the LS and EN labels are indicated, one would assume that other than slight dilatation, overall left ventricular performance is satisfactory. As this scan demonstrates, however, the apical portion of the septum does not move. As one might anticipate, the angiographic left ventricular assessment of ventricular function was significantly depressed. In fact, on the angiogram the apical half of the ventricle was aneurysmal, and the overall angiographic ejection fraction was quite poor. Thus, it should be perfectly obvious that there are very important limitations to using echocardiographic dimensions of the basal half of the ventricle to predict global ventricular performance, especially ejection fraction.

Despite these limitations it is still possible to use echocardiography to gain some information concerning overall left ventricular performance. Although the usual echocardiographic dimension used to estimate left ventricular diastolic volume is inaccurate in patients with segmental disease, there is still some value in this dimension even in such patients. The diastolic measurement may still provide a rough estimate of the overall size of the left ventricle (4). There is evidence to suggest that this standard echocardiographic measurement may be helpful in judging the extent of ventricular damage, since the basal portion of the left ventricle is usually the last area of the heart to be involved with coronary artery disease (5, 6, 6a). Left ventricular dilatation at the level of the mitral valve is frequently a sign of advanced left ventricular disease. Thus, if one uses the standard echocardiographic left ventricular measurement as a simple dimension and does not try to measure volumes, it may still be useful in assessing the status of the ischemic ventricle, particularly when the chamber is severely damaged. Unfortunately, this measurement is not a very sensitive indicator of left ventricular dysfunction and left ventricular dilatation is obviously not specific for coronary artery disease.

There have been several efforts to measure left ventricular volumes using cross-sectional echocardiography (7–10). Many of these studies are promising and attractive. Unfortunately, there are still many technical difficulties and confirmation by other investigators will be necessary before we can begin to use these techniques in clinical practice.

The mitral valve may be helpful in reflecting haemodynamic changes in patients with coronary artery disease. It has been noted that patients with coronary artery disease and elevated left ventricular diastolic pressures frequently exhibit abnormal closure of the mitral valve with prolongation of the A-C interval and a notch or plateau between these two points (5, 6, 11). Although this measurement does not correlate well with left ventricular diastolic pressure (12, 13), this finding appears to be abnormal and can have some prognostic value (5, 6).

There are several techniques described which use the mitral valve for estimating mitral valve flow or left ventricular stroke volume in patients with coronary artery disease. One technique utilizes a measurement of the cross-sectional area of the aorta together with the rate of systolic closure of the mitral valve (14). These two measurements, combined with left ventricular ejection time measured from the aortic valve echogram, provide a formula for measuring cardiac output. Another technique utilizes the mitral valve echogram together with the electrocardiogram to arrive at a formula for assessing mitral valve flow (15). The echocardiographic measurements include the separation between the anterior and posterior mitral leaflets at the E point and the D-E slope. The electrocardiographic measurements included heart rate and PR interval. The formula derived is:

$$\text{Stroke Volume} = \left(\frac{\text{EE}}{\text{HR}} + \text{PR} \right) \times 100 + \frac{2 \times \text{DE}}{\text{HR}}.$$

Both of these techniques obviously need further confirmation. The latter study recently has been reproduced by an independent group of investigators (16), so hopefully, this technique may prove to be useful in estimating mitral valve flow or cardiac output in patients with coronary artery disease.

One group of investigators has noted that the separation between the mitral valve E point and the most downward portion of the left ventricular septum can provide an estimate of overall ventricular performance (17). This technique probably utilizes the fact that when the ventricle is severely damaged, it dilates and mitral valve flow decreases. In a group of patients with coronary artery disease, this E point-septal separation correlated with angiographic ejection fraction (17). Unfortunately, as with any technique which utilizes left ventricular dimensions, this measurement again is not very sensitive. For example, there could be significant apical disease and the E point-septal separation could be normal.

Another group of investigators has correlated the timing of mitral valve opening and the dimensional changes of the left ventricular cavity to judge left ventricular performance (18, 19). Normally, the mitral valve begins to open at about the same time as the left ventricular dimension begins to widen in early diastole. With the use of a computer the authors demonstrated that in patients with coronary artery disease there was an outward motion of the left ventricle prior to mitral valve opening. Thus, there appeared to be a distortion of the shape of the ventricle during isovolumic relaxation (20). The sensitivity and specificity of this technique has not been evaluated.

In summary, although there are significant limitations to echocardiography's ability to assess overall left ventricular performance in patients with coronary artery disease, there are several techniques which have been described, many of which are very promising. Unfortunately, it is difficult to assess specificity and sensitivity because the gold standard is primarily angiography and the differences between echocardiography and angiography are significant. Thus, one can anticipate considerable future work using animal models to hopefully eliminate the inherent differences between angiography and echocardiography.

DETECTION OF ISCHEMIC MUSCLE

The ischemic muscle can be detected echocardiographically with a fairly high degree of sensitivity. Both animal (21, 22) and clinical studies (5, 23, 24) have documented that when the muscle becomes ischemic, its motion is altered almost immediately. With the high sampling rate inherent in M-mode echocardiography, wall motion is recorded very well. Figure 2 demonstrates serial echograms of a patient who was in the hospital with suspected coronary artery disease. On December 9, 1974, the left septum (LS) and posterior left ventricular endocardium (EN) were moving reasonably well, even though the echocardiographic study was not technically excellent. The following morning, the patient developed chest pain, and one notes a dramatic change in the posterior left ventricular wall motion.

Figure 3 demonstrates possibly an even more specific finding with acute myocardial ischemia. In this patient, the interventricular septum not only is moving paradoxically, or upward, during ventricular systole, but the septal

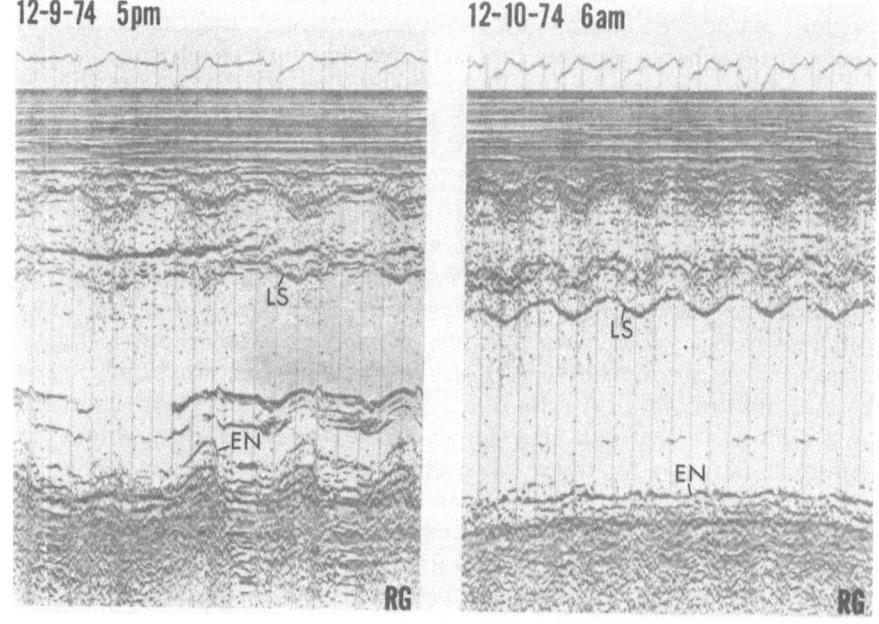

Fig. 2. Serial echograms from a patient with chest pain who eventually developed an inferior myocardial infarction. On 12/09/74, the echogram demonstrates reasonably good septal (LS) and endocardial (EN) motion. At 6 A.M. on 12/10/74, the patient had severe chest pain and the posterior endocardial echo stopped moving. (From Feigenbaum H: *Echocardiography* (2nd edition), Philadelphia, Pa., Lea & Febiger, 1976.)

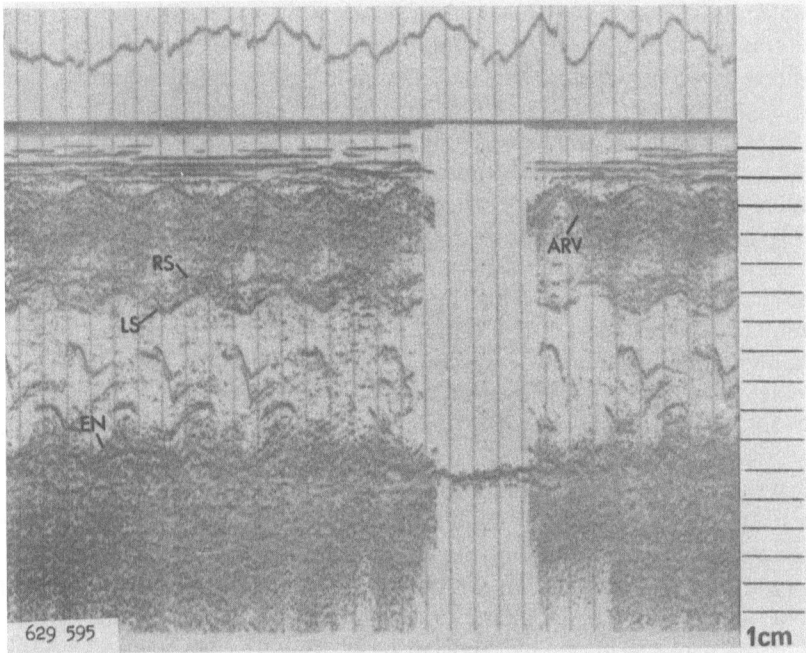

Fig. 3. Left ventricular echogram from a patient with an acute myocardial infarction. The septal echoes move anteriorly during ventricular systole. The distance between the right (RS) and left (LS) septal echoes is greater at end-diastole than at end-systole. Thus, there is thinning of the interventricular septum with ventricular contraction. ARV = anterior right ventricular wall, EN = posterior left ventricular endocardium. (From Feigenbaum H: *Echocardiography* (2nd edition), Philadelphia, Pa., Lea & Febiger, 1976.)

thickness is actually less during systole than during diastole, which is the opposite of normal. There is good laboratory (25, 26) and clinical evidence (27, 28) that ventricular wall thinning may be fairly specific for acute ischemia. Thus, M-mode echocardiography not only is able to record segmental ventricular wall motion with a high degree of sensitivity, but the technique has the capability of recording ventricular wall thickening or thinning, which may be more specific for ischemia than is abnormal wall motion.

There have been attempts to predict anatomy of the coronary arteries by segmental wall motion abnormalities on the echocardiogram (29, 30, 31). There is conflicting evidence in the literature as to just how well echocardiography can predict the coronary anatomy (32). Most investigators agree that if the interventricular septal motion is abnormal, there is a high probability that there is a proximal left anterior descending or a left main coronary artery obstruction. However, normal septal motion in no way precludes the possibility of obstruction in these arteries (32). One study shows that septal motion correlates better with myocardial perfusion of the septum, rather than with anatomic obstructions of the coronary arteries (33). For example, a tight proximal LAD obstruction with good collateral fill of the vessel may result in normal septal motion. However, if perfusion of the septum is poor or absent, then the likelihood of abnormal septal motion is quite high. The use of the posterior ventricular wall motion to predict coronary anatomy is even less reliable.

One need not restrict the echocardiographic examination to merely the proximal portion of the interventricular septum and the posterior ventricular wall. It has been demonstrated that one can also record echoes from the anterior left ventricular wall (34) and from multiple other areas of the ventricle (35). However, despite these multiple examinations, the M-mode technique still does not examine all of the ventricle. Cross-sectional echocardiography adds significantly to the ability to examine areas of the left ventricle not commonly seen with M-mode echocardiography. An important area which is not easily recorded with the M-mode technique is the cardiac apex. Figure 4 demonstrates a cross-sectional, long-axis echogram of the apex (AP). During diastole, the posterior wall of the apex (AP) is in a straight line with the body of the left ventricle (LV). However, during systole, one can appreciate an outward bulge of the posterior apical portion of the ventricle (arrow). Thus, this patient has dyskinesis of the left ventricular apex. This type of abnormality is common and is difficult to record with M-mode echocardiography. The medial and lateral walls of the left ventricle are also

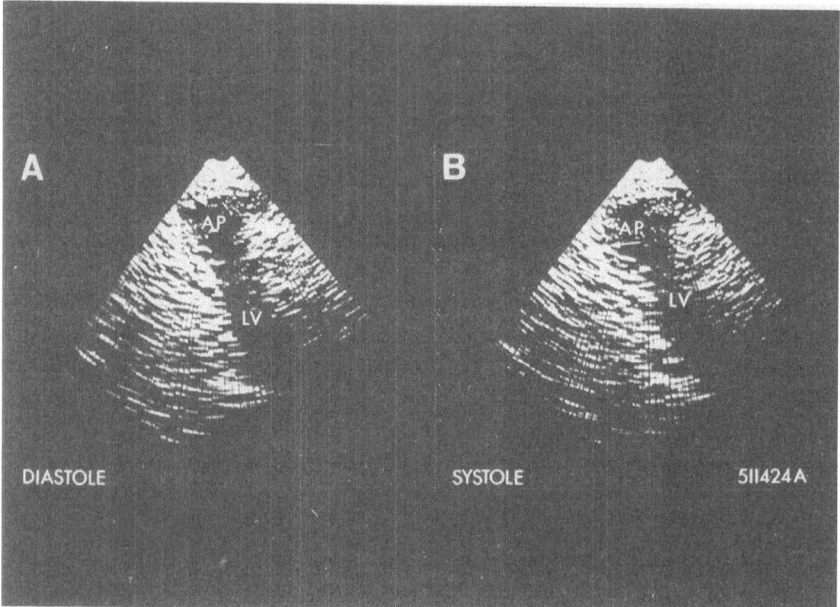

Fig. 4. Cross-sectional echocardiographic examination of the left ventricular apex in a patient with a dyskinetic apex (AP). During diastole the posterior border of the apex is in line with the posterior wall of the left ventricle (LV). During systole there is an outward bulging (arrow) of the apex.

areas which are difficult to record with M-mode echocardiography and now are accessible to the examiner using the cross-sectional technique.

There have been several attempts at correlating the cross-sectional examination with angiocardiograms looking at ischemic segments (36, 37). One study which looked only at the ventricular apex showed an excellent correlation between the two examinations (36). However, if one examines multiple areas of the left ventricle and correlates the echocardiographic findings with the angiogram, there will be greater disparity. In one fairly large study which correlated the echocardiographic and angiographic findings, the overall correlation was good; however, there were significant differences (37). Retrospective analysis of the differences found that there were interpretation and technical errors of both the angiograms and the echograms. In addition, the authors emphasized the inherent differences in echocardiography and angiography. Echocardiography utilizes reflected ultrasound to obtain a cross-section or tomogram of the heart. Angiography records the shadow of the angiographic dye. Theoretically, one would see areas on the echocardiogram which would be hidden from view on the angiogram. The most common problem is that the common angiographic and echocardiographic views are looking at different areas. The diagram of the RAO angiogram in Figure 5 shows an akinetic anterior wall, whereas the echogram (Fig. 5B) shows a dyskinetic septum not seen on the RAO angiogram.

Since echocardiography can detect ischemic muscle, investigators have recently been doing echocardiographic studies during stress (24, 38–41). As one might anticipate, there are significant technical difficulties in examining

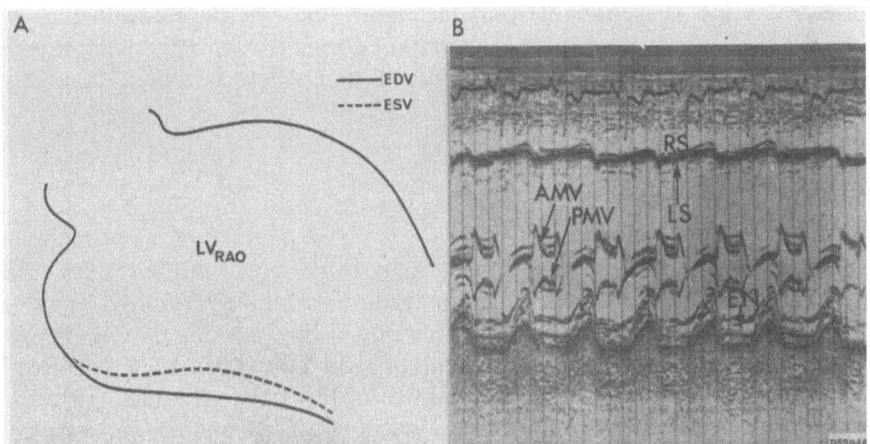

Fig. 5. Drawing of a left ventricular angiogram in the right anterior oblique projection and a left ventricular echogram in a patient with coronary artery disease and a scarred anterior wall and interventricular septum. The angiogram shows an akinetic anterior left ventricular wall. The echocardiogram demonstrates an interventricular septum which moves paradoxically and is thinner and more echo-producing than normal. RS = right side of the septum, LS = left side of the septum, AMV = anterior mitral valve leaflet, PMV = posterior mitral valve leaflet, EN = posterior left ventricular endocardium. (From Jacobs JJ, H Feigenbaum, BC Corya, JF Phillips: Detection of left ventricular asynergy by echocardiography. Circulation 48:263, 1973.)

the left ventricle echocardiographically during exercise. Originally, hand-grip stress was attempted (24). Although one could obtain satisfactory echocardiograms, this form of stress did not routinely produce angina. More recently, individuals have been using supine leg exercise (38–41). Preliminary data are encouraging, and one may find increased use of supine leg exercise to bring out latent ventricular wall motion abnormalities in patients with coronary artery disease.

With the advent of cross-sectional echocardiography, another application which may prove to be extremely important is the estimation of functional infarct size as judged by the amount of muscle moving abnormally (42–48). Although the echocardiographic findings overestimate the amount of infarction found pathologically, the abnormal wall motion may still be the prime factor in determining pump function of the ischemic ventricle. Since the cross-sectional approach can now usually examine the entire ventricle, it is possible to derive formulae which quantitate the amount of muscle which is moving abnormally. Several different approaches have been suggested. Further experience and confirmation from multiple investigators will be necessary to determine the accuracy and reliability of these techniques. The experience to date has been encouraging.

Thus, echocardiography is proving to be sensitive and reliable in judging wall motion in patients with coronary artery disease. With the advent of cross-sectional echocardiography, the entire ventricle is now accessible to the echocardiographer for examination, and attempts at quantitating the amount of abnormally moving muscle are now being made. Such parameters as wall thickening may be more specific for ischemia than are wall motion abnormalities. It is possible that techniques may be developed which will permit the echocardiographic examination during ischemia-inducing exercise. Unfortunately, most of these techniques are too new to be able to assess their true specificity or sensitivity.

COMPLICATIONS OF MYOCARDIAL INFARCTION

Another major role for echocardiography in patients with coronary artery disease is in the detection of complications secondary to myocardial infarction. Among the acute complications, one would include the development of pericardial effusion. Echocardiography, of course, is very sensitive in detecting pericardial effusion, irrespective of the cause. Another fairly early complication would be rupture of the interventricular septum. In one report, investigators noted dilatation of the right ventricle when the interventricular septum ruptured (49). Another group noted a peculiar pattern of mitral valve motion with this complication (50). More recently, a cross-sectional echocardiographic study noted a bulging of the interventricular septum into the right ventricle in patients with a ruptured septum (43). There was aneurysmal dilatation of the interventricular septum at the site of ventricular rupture.

Papillary muscle rupture has been noted echocardiographically (51). All of the signs of a flail mitral valve with acute left ventricular volume overload may be noted with this sometimes catastrophic complication. A somewhat later complication would include development of left ventricular clots. These clots frequently occur at the site of severe left ventricular dyskinesis or even aneurysm formation. An increasing number of reports are now in the literature concerning the detection of left ventricular clots using cross-sectional echocardiography (52, 53). These clots are almost invariably located in the left ventricular apex, and the four-chamber, cross-sectional view seems to be the best in making this diagnosis.

Among the complications of chronic coronary artery disease, the most important is aneurysm formation. Echocardiography, particularly cross-sectional echocardiography, is proving to be extremely sensitive and specific for the detection of ventricular aneurysms (54, 55). Figure 6 shows an echocardiogram and a diagram of a commonly seen apical ventricular aneurysm. This type of aneurysm is a frequent complication of coronary artery disease and is detected echocardiographically in a high percentage of patients. In a study correlating the echocardiographic detection of apical aneurysms with those seen angiographically, the correlation was extremely good with very few, if any, aneurysms missed on the echocardiogram (54). A technical point to be noted is that the illustration in Figure 6 is actually made from two different echocardiographic recordings. An echogram of the aneurysm was superimposed on another echogram of the body of the left ventricle. The reason for making this composite photograph is to emphasize

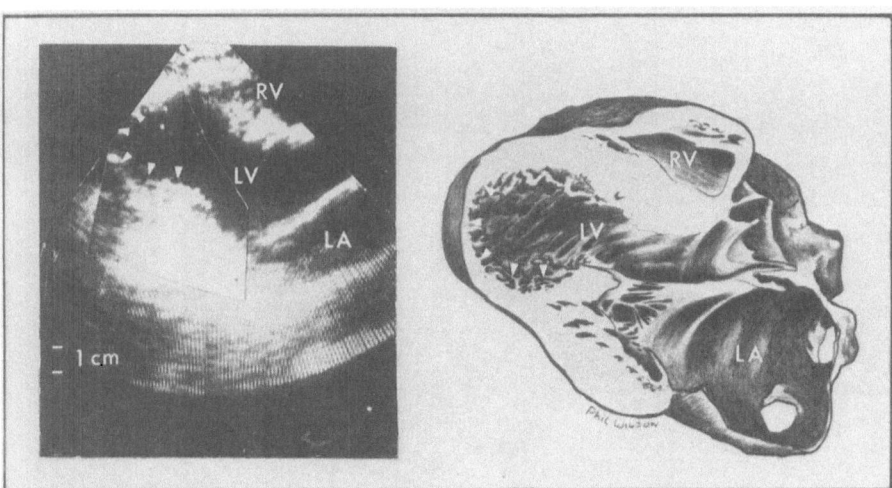

Fig. 6. Cross-sectional echocardiogram and diagram of a large apical aneurysm. The aneurysm is denoted by the arrowheads both on the echogram and the diagram. The echogram is a composite of two recordings, since the apex and the left ventricular outflow tract do not lie in the same plane. (From Rogers EW, H Feigenbaum, AE Weyman: Echocardiography for quantitation of cardiac chambers. In: Progress in cardiology, VIII, Yu P, Goodwin J (eds), Philadelphia, Pa. Lea & Febiger, (in press).

the fact that the left ventricular apex, as seen in Figure 4, is not in the same plane as the body and outflow tract of the left ventricle. Thus, one cannot obtain a single echogram looking exactly like Figure 6. The composite photograph also was made to help in the orientation of the reader.

Another important echocardiographic view for the detection of aneurysms is the four-chamber view. Figure 7 shows an echogram and a diagram of a normal four-chamber examination while Figure 8 demonstrates the findings with aneurysmal dilatation of the apical half of the left ventricle. The septal distortion and dilatation seen in Figure 8 is proving to be common in patients with coronary artery disease and appears to be a fairly reliable sign of aneurysmal dilatation of the apical half of the ventricle.

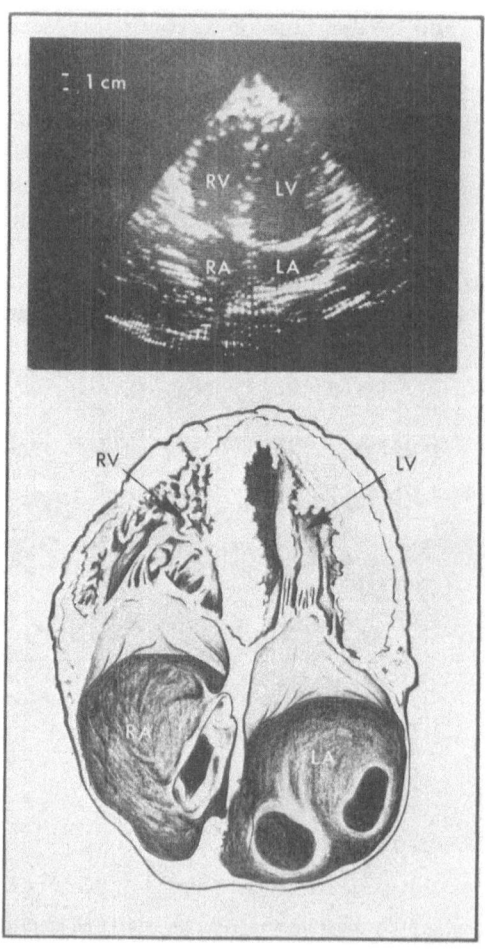

Fig. 7. Four-chamber echogram and diagram of a normal heart. RV = right ventricle, LV = left ventricle, RA = right atrium, LA = left atrium. (From Rogers EW, H Feigenbaum, AE Weyman: Echocardiography for quantitation of cardiac chambers. In: Progress in cardiology. VIII, Yu P, Goodwin J (eds), Philadelphia, Pa., Lea & Febiger, (in press).

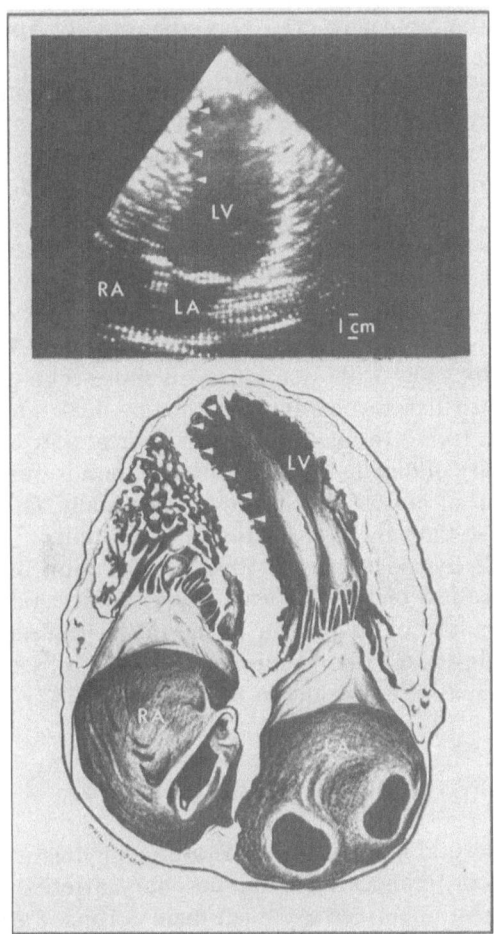

Fig. 8. Four-chamber echogram and diagram of a patient with an apical left ventricular aneurysm (arrowheads). LV = left ventricle, RA = right atrium, LA = left atrium. (From Rogers EW, H Feigenbaum, AE Weyman: Echocardiography for quantitation of cardiac chambers. In: Progress in cardiology, VIII, Yu P, Goodwin J (eds), Philadelphia, Pa., Lea & Febiger, (in press).

Success of surgical removal of an aneurysm is in large part dependent upon the amount of myocardium remaining after aneurysmectomy, and echocardiography may be valuable in assessing that part of the ventricle not involved in the aneurysm. The M-mode examination can be useful in assessing the status of the noninfarcted muscle (6). If the base of the ventricle remains normal in size and there is good motion of both the septal and posterior ventricular walls (Fig. 1), then the prospect of successful aneurysmectomy is very high. One can make a similar assessment using cross-sectional techniques to quantitate the amount of muscle which continues to move normally (55, 56). Thus, echocardiography is proving to be very helpful in the management of patients with known or suspected ventricular aneurysms.

Although less common, false aneurysms of the left ventricle have also been detected echocardiographically (57). This abnormality appears as a large, relatively echo-free space, usually behind the posterior left ventricular wall. This complication resembles loculated pericardial effusion. Both M-mode and cross-sectional techniques have detected this abnormality.

Another common complication of myocardial infarction is scar formation. The necessity of identifying scar is enhanced by increasing use of coronary revascularization. It is obvious that scarred myocardium will not resume normal contraction when revascularized. There is a clinical study showing how one can make the diagnosis of scar using M-mode echocardiography (58). Figure 4 shows a diagram of an angiogram and an echogram from a patient with chronic coronary artery disease. In Figure 4B, the septum is thin, moves paradoxically with systole, and is more echo-producing than is the posterior ventricular myocardium. Although there are many technical details involved in trying to make the assessment of scar echocardiographically, the probability of having a scarred myocardium is quite high if one can find a thin segment of muscle which moves abnormally, fails to thicken, and is more echointense than the surrounding myocardium.

Papillary muscle dysfunction is another complication of coronary artery disease. A recent study of such patients using cross-sectional echocardiography noted the failure of coaptation of the mitral leaflets and evidence of infarction involving the papillary muscles (59). This observation obviously must await confirmation before it can be used clinically.

EXAMINATION OF THE CORONARY ARTERIES

There have been several reports in the literature demonstrating that echocardiography can record echoes from the coronary arteries (60, 61, 62). The coronary artery most often seen is the left main coronary artery. Most of the studies to date have used cross-sectional echocardiography to examine the coronary arteries. Obstructions in the left main coronary artery have been noted; however, there has been no study demonstrating sensitivity or specificity using this examination. As one would anticipate, there are many technical difficulties. One is attempting to examine a relatively small structure which is moving in three-dimensional space, thus one can cut across the artery in various unpredictable ways, many of which could simulate the appearance of obstructions. Thus, further investigation is obviously necessary before one can use this technique clinically to detect or exclude obstructions of the left main coronary artery.

A recent report demonstrated that one could detect high-intensity echoes, presumably from atherosclerotic plaques in the vicinity of the left coronary artery (63), by utilizing computer processing of the echocardiographic data to enhance the strong specular echoes. These high-intensity echoes were noted in a high percentage of patients with disease of the left coronary artery. This same study indicated that one could record these abnormal echoes from the proximal portion of the left anterior descending coronary artery as well as from the left main coronary artery. Although the location of these high-intensity echoes did not correlate well with the site of obstructing lesions, the correlation between the presence of these abnormal echoes and the presence of diseased coronary arteries was very high. It will be interesting to see if this technique proves to be a practical application for echocardiography.

SUMMARY

How echocardiography is used in the management of patients with coronary artery disease depends to a large degree upon one's approach to these patients. If one feels that all patients with known or suspected coronary artery disease warrant angiographic study and that the angiography is the gold standard by which to manage patients, then one could argue that echocardiography is superfluous and that few individuals with coronary artery disease warrant echocardiographic study. However, if one recognizes that there are inherent differences in the echocardiographic and angiographic examinations and that there are some areas seen on the echocardiogram which are hidden from view on the angiogram, then echocardiography should be useful, especially in the markedly diseased ventricle. There may be areas of well contracting left ventricle missed on the angiogram. If the clinician is willing to exclude the possibility of surgery if the ventricle is severely diseased, then an echocardiogram can make this assessment prior to angiographic study and these individuals can be saved from an unnecessary catheterization. On the other hand, if surgery will be seriously considered, irrespective of how bad the ventricular function might be, then echocardiography may represent a redundant examination.

If the primary indication for consideration of surgery is the possibility of an aneurysm, then echocardiography can be a definitive examination. The data thus far indicate that echocardiography should be able to find or exclude an aneurysm reliably and should be able to assess the function of the remaining ventricle.

Possibly the most useful application of echocardiography will be in the setting of acute myocardial infarction. If one desires an assessment of ventricular performance and infarct size, then echocardiography could be the diagnostic tool of choice. Serial examinations are quite feasible and practical, and should be useful in detecting complications such as clots, pericardial effusion, aneurysm formation, and disruption of the mitral valve apparatus.

The echocardiographic examination of the coronary arteries is interesting and exciting but is far too preliminary to use in managing patients with coronary artery disease.

REFERENCES

1. Feigenbaum H: Echocardiographic examination of the left ventricle. Circulation 51:1, 1975.
2. Popp RL, EL Alderman, OR Brown, DC Harrison: Sources of error in calculation of left ventricular volumes by echography. Am J Card 31:152, 1973.

96

H. FEIGENBAUM ET AL.

3. Teichholz LE, T Kreulen, MV Herman, R Gorlin: Problems in echocardiographic volume determinations: Echocardiographic-angiographic correlations in the presence or absence of asynergy. Am J Card 37:7, 1976.
4. Sweet RL, RE Moraski, RO Russel, Jr, and CE Rackley: Relationship between echocardiography, cardiac output, and abnormally contracting segments in patients with ischemic heart disease. Circulation 52:634, 1975.
5. Corya BC, S Rasmussen, SB Knoebel, H Feigenbaum: Echocardiography in acute myocardial infarction. Am J Card 36:1, 1975.
6. Dillon, JC, H Feigenbaum, AE Weyman, BC Corya, S Peskoe, S Chang: M-mode echocardiography in the evluation of patients for aneurysmectomy. Circulation 53:657, 1976.
6a. Nieminen M, J Heikkila: Echoventriculography in acute myocardial infarction II: Monitoring of left ventricular performance. Brit Heart J 38:271, 1976.
7. Schiller N, D Drew, H Acquatella, R Boswell, E Botvinick, B Greenberg, E Carlsson: Noninvasive, biplane quantitation of left ventricular volume and ejection fraction with a real-time two-dimensional echocardiography system. Circulation 54:II–23, 1976 (abstract).
8. Wyatt HL, M Heng, S Meerbaum, R Davidson, S Lee, E. Corday: Quantitative left ventricular analysis in dogs with the phased array sector scan. Circulation 56:III–152, 1977 (abstract).
9. Chaudry KR, S Ogawa, FJ Pauletto, FE Hubbard, LS Dreifus: Biplane measurements of left and right ventricular volumes using wide angle cross-sectional echocardiography. Am J Card 41:391, 1978 (abstract).
10. Maughan WL, LW Eaton, JB Garrison, AA Shoukas, JL Weiss: Accurate volume determination in the isolated ejecting canine left ventricle by two-dimensional echocardiography. Circulation 58:910, 1978 (abstract).
11. Konecke LL, H Feigenbaum, S Chang, BC Corya, JC Fischer: Abnormal mitral valve motion in patients with elevated left ventricular diastolic pressures. Circulation 47:989, 1973.
12. Talner NS, AG Campbell: Recognition and management of cardiologic problems in the newborn infant. Prog Cardiovasc Dis 15:159, 1972.
13. Lewis JR, JO Parker, GW Burggraf: Mitral valve motion and changes in left ventricular enddiastolic pressure: A correlative study of the PR-AC interval. Am J Card 42:383, 1978.
14. Lalani AV, SJK Lee: Echocardiographic measurement of cardiac output using the mitral valve and aortic root echo. Circulation 54:738, 1976.
15. Rasmussen S, BC Corya, H Feigenbaum, MJ Black, DE Lovelace, JF Phillips, RJ Noble, SB Knoebel: Stroke volume calculated from the mitral valve echogram, in patients with and without ventricular dyssynergy. Circulation 58:125, 1978.
16. Scheele W, R Kraus, HN Allen, SW Halpem: Use of M-mode echocardiography to determine stroke volume. Am J Card 43:411, 1979 (abstract).
17. Massie BM, NB Schiller, RA Ratshin, WW Parmley: Mitral-septal separation: New echocardiographic index of left ventricular function. Am J Card 39:1008, 1977.
18. Upton M, D Gibson, D Brown: Echocardiographic assessment of abnormal left ventricular relaxation in man. Circulation 52:II–134, 1975 (abstract).
19. Doran JH, TA Traill, DJ Brown, DG Gibson: Detection of abnormal left ventricular wall movement during isovolumic contraction and early relaxation. Comparison of echo- and angiocardiography. Brit Ht J 40:367, 1978.
20. Upton MT, DG Gibson, DJ Brown: Echocardiographic assessment of abnormal left ventricular relaxation in man. Brit Heart J 38:1001, 1976.
21. Kerber RE, ML Marcus, J Ehrhard, R Wilson, FM Abboud: Correlation between echocardiographically demonstrated segmental dyskinesis and regional myocardial perfusion. Circulation 52:1097, 1975.
22. Kerber RE, FM Abboud: Echocardiographic detection of regional myocardial infarction. Circulation 47:997, 1973.
23. Jacobs JJ, H. Feigenbaum, BC Corya, JF Phillips: Detection of left ventricular asynergy by echocardiography. Circulation 48:263, 1973.
24. Widlansky S, PL McHenry, BC Corya, JF Phillips: Coronary angiography, echocardiographic and electrocardiographic studies on a patient with variant angina due to coronary artery spasm. Am Heart J 90:631, 1975.
25. Sasayama S, D Franklin, J Ross, WS Kemper, D McKown: Dynamic changes in left ventricular wall thickness and their use in analyzing cardiac function in the conscious dog. A study based on a modified ultrasonic technique. Am J Card 38:870, 1976.
26. Kerber RE, ML Marcus, R Wilson, J Ehrhardt, FM Abboud: Effects of acute coronary

occlusion on the motion and perfusion of the normal and ischemic interventricular septum. Circulation 54:928, 1976.

27. Dumesnil JG, JL Laurenceau, A Labatut, S Gagne: Echocardiographic study of changes in regional ventricular function following nitroglycerine and surgical correlation. Circulation 52:II-134, 1975 (abstract).

28. Corya BC, S. Rasmussen, H Feigenbaum, SB Knoebel, MJ Black: Systolic thickening and thinning of the septum and posterior wall in patients with coronary artery disease, congestive cardiomyopathy, and atrial septal defect. Circulation 55:109, 1977.

29. Brown OR, RL Popp, DC Harrison: Abnormal interventricular septal motion in patients with significant disease of the left anterior descending coronary artery or other conditions of septal failure. Am J Card 31:123, 1973.

30. Joffe CD, H Brik, LE Teichholz, MV Herman, R Gorlin: Echocardiographic diagnosis of left anterior descending coronary disease. Am J Card 40:11, 1977.

31. Dortimer AC, RL DeJoseph, RA Shiroff, AJ Liedtke, R Zelis: Distribution of coronary artery disease. Prediction by echocardiography. Circulation 54:724, 1976.

32. Gordon, MJ, RE Kerber: Interventricular septal motion in patients with proximal and distal left anterior descending coronary artery lesions. Circulation 55:338, 1977.

33. Kolibash AJ, BM Beaver, PK Fulkerson, S Khullar, RF Leighton: The relationship between abnormal echocardiographic septal motion and myocardial perfusion in patients with significant obstruction of the left anterior descending artery. Circulation 56:780, 1977.

34. Corya BC, H Feigenbaum, S Rasmussen, MJ Black: Anterior left ventricular wall echoes in coronary artery disease. Linear scanning with a single element transducer. Am J Card 34:652, 1974.

35. Heikkila J, M Nieminen: Echoventriculographic detection, localization, and quantification of left ventricular asynergy in acute myocardial infarction. A correlative echo and electro-cardiographic study. Brit Heart J 37:46, 1975.

36. Hickman HO, AE Weyman, LS Wann, JF Phillips, JC Dillon, H Feigenbaum, J Marshall: Cross-sectional echocardiography of the cardiac apex. Circulation 56:III-153, 1977 (abstract).

37. Kisslo JA, D Robertson, BW Gilbert, O vonRamm, VS Behar: A comparison of real-time, two-dimensional echocardiography and cineangiography in detecting left ventricular asynergy. Circulation 55:134, 1977.

38. Strom J, W Frishman, U Elkayam, T LeJemtel, H Ribner, J Strobeck, J Stein, E Sonnenblick: Pre and post exercise echocardiography in evaluating ischemic ECG changes in patients without chest pain. Circulation 56:III-198, 1977 (abstract).

39. Mason SJ, JL Weiss, ML Weisfeldt, JB Garrison, NJ Fortuin: Exercise echocardiography: Detection of wall motion abnormalities during ischemia. Circulation 56:III-6, 1977 (abstract).

40. Crawford MH and W Amon: Echocardiographic evaluation of left ventricular performance during supine and upright bicycle exercise. Am J Card 41:405, 1978 (abstract).

41. Wann LS, JC Dillon, CC Hallman, JV Faris, AE Weyman, H Feigenbaum: Exercise cross-sectional echocardiography: Technical feasibility and comparison to cardiac catheterization and ECG/Thallium-201 treadmill exercise. Circulation 58:158, 1978 (abstract).

42. Weyman AE, TD Franklin, KM Egenes, D Green: Correlation between extent of abnormal regional wall motion and myocardial infarct size in chronically infarcted dogs. Circulation 56:III-72, 1977 (abstract).

43. Heger J, AE Weyman, RJ Noble, JC Dillon, H Feigenbaum: An analysis of the site, extent, and hemodynamic consequences of acute myocardial infarction by cross-sectional echo-cardiography. Circulation 56:III-152, 1977 (abstract).

44. Heng MK, T-W Lang, T Toshimitsu, S Meerbaum, HL Wyatt, S-S Lee, R Davidson, E Corday: Quantification of myocardial ischemic damage by 2-dimensional echocardiography. Circulation 56: III-125, 1977 (abstract).

45. Hestenes JD, MK Heng, HL Wyatt, S Meerbaum, E Corday, R Nathan: Circumferential segmental wall motion of the left ventricle estimated from phased array sector scan ultrasound image. Am J Card 41:437, 1978 (abstract).

46. Rogers EW, AE Weyman, H Feigenbaum, JJ Heger, JC Dillon: Predicting survival after myocardial infarction by cross-sectional echo. Circulation 58:907, 1978 (abstract).

47. Meltzer RS, JN Woythaler, AJ Buda, JC Griffin, R Kernoff, RL Popp, RP Martin: Non-invasive quantification of infarct size by two-dimensional echocardiography. Circulation 58:723, 1978 (abstract).

48. Weiss JL, BH Bulkley, SJ Mason: Two-dimensional echocardiographic quantification of

myocardial injury in man: Comparison with post mortem studies. Circulation 58:595, 1978 (abstract).

49. DeJoseph RL, SF Seides, A Lindner, AN Demato: Echocardiographic findings of ventricular septal rupture in acute myocardial infarction. Am J Card 36:346, 1975.

50. Chandraratna PAN, PK Balashandran, PM Shah, M Hodges: Echocardiographic observations on ventricular septal rupture complicating acute myocardial infarction. Circulation 51:506, 1975.

51. Jamal N, W Winters, J Nelson: Echocardiographic features of flail mitral valve leaflets: Ruptured chordae tendineae versus ruptured papillary muscle. Circulation 58:157, 1978 (abstract).

52. Neumann A, W Bommer, L Weinert, T Grehl, DT Mason, EA Amsterdam, AN DeMaria, Identification of left ventricular thrombi by cross-sectional echocardiography. Am J Card 41:392, 1978 (abstract).

53. Seward JB, GM Gura, DJ Hagler, AJ Tajik: Evaluation of M-mode echocardiography and wide-angle two-dimensional sector echocardiography in the diagnosis of intracardiac masses. Circulation 58:909, 1978 (abstract).

54. Weyman AE, SM Peskoe, ES Williams, JC Dillon, H Feigenbaum: Detection of left ventricular aneurysms by cross-sectional echocardiography. Circulation 54:936, 1976.

55. Rakowski H, RP Martin, JN Schapira, L Wexler, JF Silverman, PR Cipriano, DF Guthaner, RL Popp: Left ventricular aneurysm: Detection and determination of resectability by two-dimensional ultrasound. Circulation 56:III–153, 1977 (abstract).

56. Barrett M, Y Charuzi, R Davidson, N Buchbinder, HL Wyatt, HJC Swan, E Corday: Assessment of left ventricular function in the presence of aneurysm by cross-sectional echocardiography. Circulation 58:733, 1978 (abstract).

57. Roelandt J, M Van Den Brand, WB Vletter, J Nauta, and PG Hugenholtz: Echocardiographic diagnosis of pseudoaneurysm of the left ventricle. Circulation 52:466, 1975.

58. Rasmussen S, BC Corya, H Feigenbaum, SB Knoebel: Detection of myocardial scar tissue by M-mode echocardiography. Circulation 57:230, 1978.

59. Godley RW, AE Weyman, H Feigenbaum, EW Rogers, D Green: Patterns of mitral leaflet motion in patients with probable papillary muscle dysfunction. Am J Card 43:411, 1979 (abstract).

60. Weyman AE, H Feigenbaum, JC Dillon, KW Johnston, RC Eggleton: Non-invasive visualization of the left main coronary artery by cross-sectional echocardiography. Circulation 54:169, 1976.

61. Inoue K, K Kuwaki, K Ueda, T Shirai, T Utsunomiya: M-mode echocardiogram of the coronary artery. Am J Card 41:391, 1978 (abstract).

62. Ogawa S, FE Hubbard, FJ Pauletto, KR Chaudry, CC Chen, AN Moghadam, LS Dreifus: A new approach to non-invasive left coronary artery visualization using phased array cross-sectional echocardiography. Circulation 58:729, 1978 (abstract).

63. Rogers EW, H Feigenbaum, AE Weyman, JC Dillon, LS Wann, RC Eggleton, KW Johnston: Possible detection of coronary atherosclerosis by cross-sectional echocardiography. Circulation 58:209, 1978 (abstract).

ULTRASONIC IMAGING OF EXPERIMENTAL MYOCARDIAL INFARCTS*

R. GRAMIAK, R.C. WAAG, E.A. SCHENK, P.P.K. LEE,
K. THOMSON, and P. MACINTOSH

The detection of early myocardial infarction by direct inspection of the reflection characteristics of normal and infarcted myocardium represents an important clinical goal in the evaluation of patients with coronary artery disease. Little has been published about this important topic, probably because routine clinical examinations have provided no indication that the muscle change produced by infarction can be detected by reflected ultrasound. The success of computerized axial tomography in demonstrating experimental infarcts (1) prompted us to examine the possibility that ultrasound could be used in a similar manner to detect and image the changes produced by myocardial infarction. To accomplish our goals, we elected to circumvent the signal processing inherent in commercial systems in order to quantitate signal amplitudes directly and to select an image processing mode considered best for differentiating normal from abnormal cardiac muscle by using a computer-based data acquisition and image processing system (2). The purpose of this report is to present our experience from an experimental study dealing with infarcts of various durations.

MATERIAL AND METHODS

The left anterior descending coronary artery was occluded by catheter placement of plastic plugs (3) in nine mongrel dogs to produce infarcts ranging in age from 30 min to 8 days. Prior to sacrifice, each animal was injected intravenously with Thioflavin S which demonstrates perfusion by its fluorescence under ultraviolet light (4). The heart was excised, flushed with saline, and the chambers were distended prior to placement in a water bath for ultrasonic study. A commercially available B-scanner was used to obtain 3 equally spaced short axis views of the left ventricle from apex to base. The ultrasonic signals were digitized in 8-bit samples (256 amplitudes) and placed in a matrix of 256 × 256 points for analysis of the reflectance characteristics of normal and abnormal muscle. Histograms of echo amplitude distribution were calculated throughout the image and used to separate the image into individual bands of amplitude range to describe the amplitude characteristics of the myocardium by noting the specific bands in which it appeared.

* This work was supported in part by the National Institutes of Health, Grant 5 RO1 HL 15016.

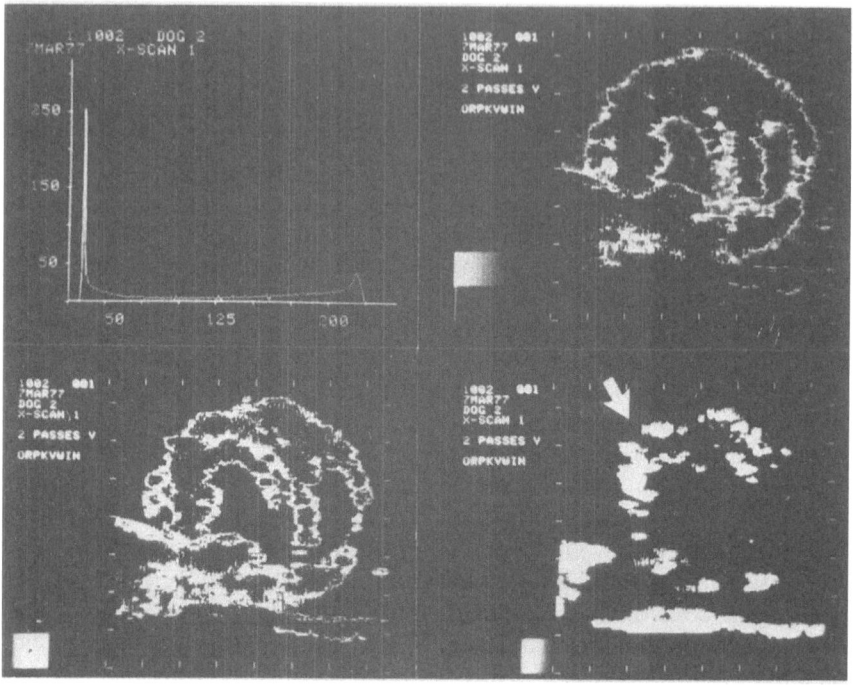

Fig. 1. Amplitude band imaging. A histogram of the signal amplitudes contained in a B-scan image is shown in the upper left and was used to divide the available signals into bands for selective imaging. In the upper right, amplitudes of 60–130 are illustrated while the lower panels demonstrate levels of 131–160 (left) and 213–225 (right). The arrow indicates a region of high amplitude returns from the myocardium.

From these images, the minimal, mean, and maximal reflection amplitudes were derived for normal and infarcted myocardium. In addition, 32×32 matrix element windows were placed over portions of the myocardium to provide histograms of amplitude distribution in selected regions from which the minimal, mean, and maximal signal amplitudes, as well as the standard deviation, were derived (Fig. 2).

Muscle damage was described by establishing a ratio of signal amplitude in a known infarct to normal myocardium, a technique which tended to minimize differences in signal amplitude related to the scanning technique.

Following ultrasonic study, the hearts were sectioned in planes which duplicated those used in the ultrasonic scans and the extent of muscle involvement was determined by combining the perfusion deficit and the distribution of microscopic changes which included dehydrogenase enzyme activity, myofiber structure, cellular infiltration, connective tissue proliferation and changes in myofiber elasticity, which appeared as a wavy pattern of the myofibers.

The ultrasonic images were processed to show abnormal amplitude areas as white and normal myocardium as gray against a black background. Correlation of the ultrasonic findings with the perfusion-histology studies was considered good when the ultrasonic study identfied abnormal muscle in

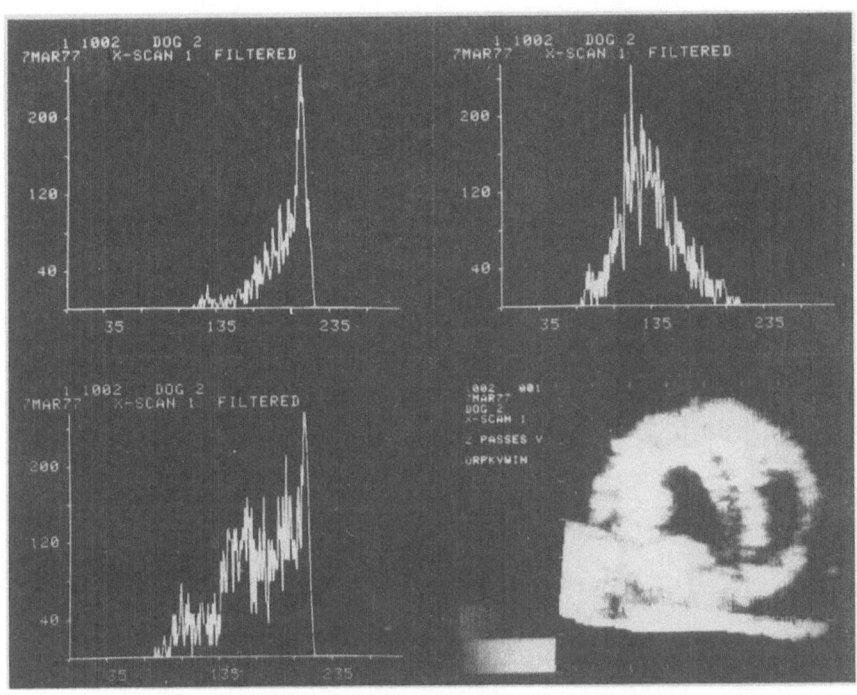

Fig. 2. Limited area histogram analysis. Original B-scan data, presented in 16 shades of gray, with 32 × 32 matrix point windows, is shown in the lower right. Amplitude histograms obtained from the individual windows are arranged to correspond to their anatomic location in the heart. The upper right is from normal myocardium, the upper left is from an area of proved infarction, while the lower left is from a region which proved to represent a false positive.

the correct position and demonstrated more than 50% of its size. When 50% or less of the real size was imaged, the study was designated as underestimated, while others were classified as false positive or false negative when the ultrasonic findings were not in the correct location.

RESULTS

Twenty-one of the 27 planes obtained in the study were technically adequate and revealed that areas of myocardial damage were characterized as regions of high signal amplitude as compared with normal myocardium (Fig. 3).

Good correlation was obtained in 10 of the 21 planes, 6 planes represented underestimation and there were 5 false positive or false negative findings. Infarcts of 24 hours or less were present in 5 animals and, in this group, a good correlation was found in 8 of 11 planes and underestimation occurred in 2 additional planes. There was a single false positive in this group. When older occlusions of 2–8 days duration were examined separately, a good correlation was present in only 2 of 10 planes, 4 were underestimated and there were 2 false positives and 2 false negatives.

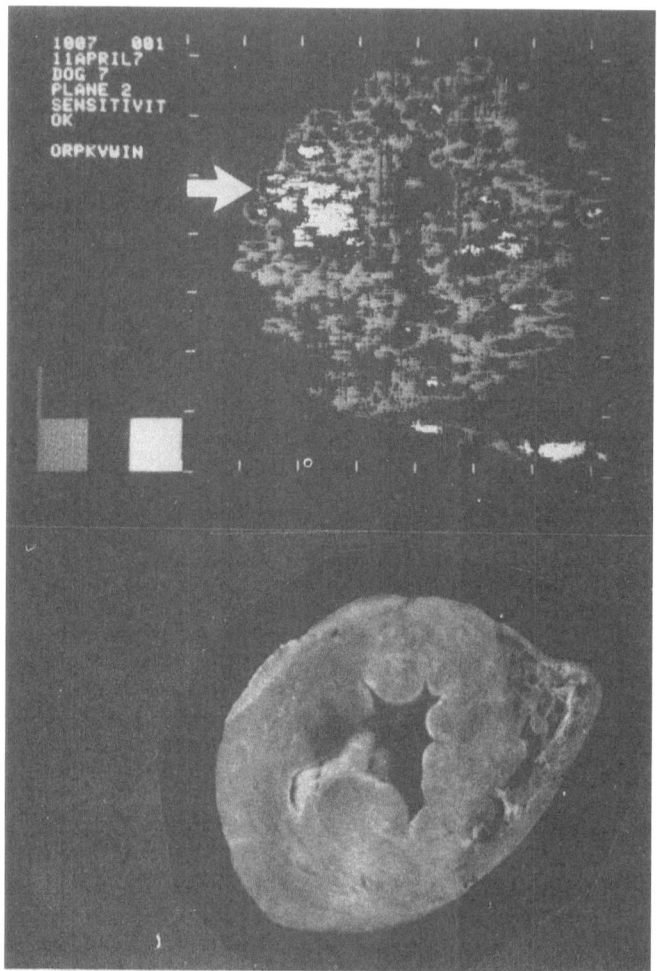

Fig. 3. Thirty-minute infarct. A tri-stable image (upper) shows normal myocardium as gray and an area of early infarction (arrow) as white. The lower panel represents a corresponding Thioflavin S fluorescence image in which the perfusion deficit appears black with some adjacent mottling.

Table 1. Correlations.

	Animals	Planes	Occl duration	Good agree	Under estimate	False pos or neg
Overall	9	21	30 min–8 days	10	6	5
Early infarcts	5	11	30 min–24 hrs	8	2	1
Older infarcts	4	10	2–8 days	2	4	4

Quantitative analysis of signal amplitude was carried out in all cases, showing good correlation using the technique of amplitude band imaging. Normal myocardium was characterized by an average lower limit of 60 (of 256 amplitudes), a mean of 122, and a maximum of 156. Infarcts were consistently higher with a minimum of 156, mean of 193, and a maximum of 219. The ratio of infarct/normal ranged from 1.4 to 2.6. Similar findings were obtained by small window histogram analysis.

Table 2. Amplitude analysis of normal myocardium and infarcts with good correlation*.

| | Amplitude Band Imaging | | |
	Mini	Mean	Maxi
Normal myocardium	60	122	156
Infarct	156	193	219
Infarct/Normal	2.6	1.6	1.4
	Histograms			
	Mini	Mean	Maxi	S.D.
Normal myocardium	41	84	133	20
Infarct	73	148	196	26
Infarct/Normal	1.8	1.8	1.5	

*all data represent group averages

Three false positives could not be distinguished from true infarcts based on quantitative data (Fig. 4).

In a case of underestimation, the "missed" portion of the infarct showed an infarct/normal ratio in the range of true infarcts but it was lower than the adjacent area of recognized infarction which contained higher amplitude signals.

A large 4-hour infarct showed good correlation with the microscopic distribution of abnormality, though about 50% of the infarct had undergone reperfusion. It is interesting that the reperfused portion contained slightly higher signal amplitudes than the non-perfused (Fig. 5).

In another specimen, normal muscle was evaluated in an anterior and posterior position in the heart and showed that a sizeable decrease in amplitude was present in the posterior sample (mean anterior 133 posterior 86). However, this did not result in any confusion since the infarct was clearly imaged.

DISCUSSION

Amplitude characterization of normal and infarcted myocardium was first attempted by Wild et al. (5) in 1956 when they demonstrated an infarct of unspecified age as an area of decreased reflection as compared with normal muscle. More recently, Joynt et al. (6) referred to studies similar to ours in which the infarcted area also produced higher amplitudes than normal

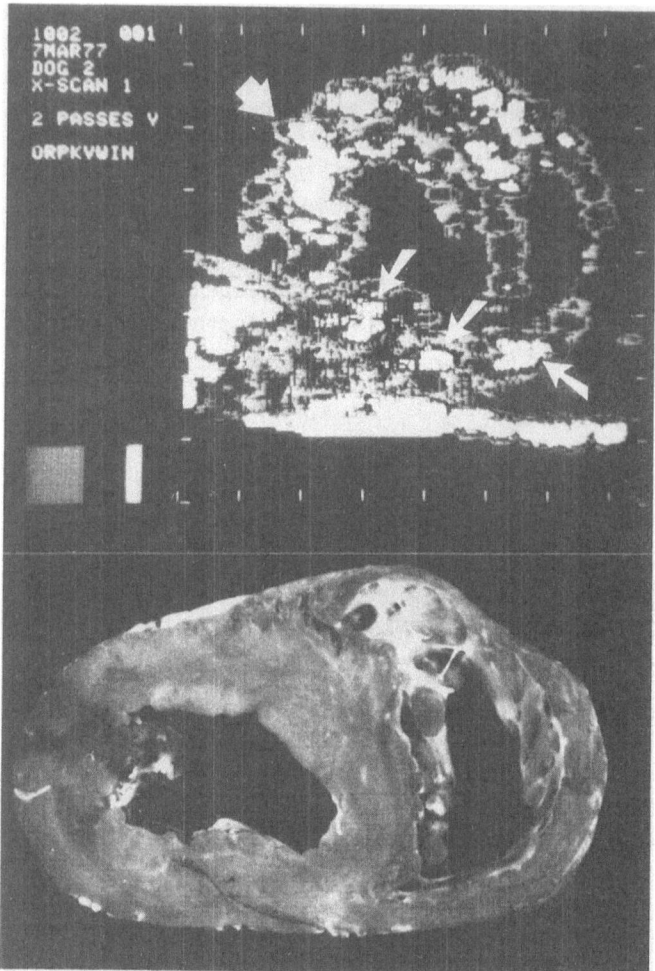

Fig. 4. False positive findings in the presence of myocardial infarction. The infarction (upper arrow) appears as a region of high signal amplitude. Similar appearing false positive zones (lower arrows) are shown. The high amplitude echoes obtained in the upper portion of the right ventricle probably arise from fibrous elements which are part of the tricuspid valve apparatus. The lower image is a Thioflavin S perfusion study.

muscle. Myocardial scarring has been described by Rasmussen (7) as a pattern of wall thinning and increased echo amplitude. Clearly, the detection of myocardial change appears feasible but is currently at its earliest stage of development.

We have not been able to identify a specific tissue change which is responsible for the increased reflectivity seen in our experimental study. To be considered as possible sources, working alone or in combination, are diminished blood content of the myocardium, lactate accumulation, ion and water shifts, and changes in the elasticity of myofibers. We are also at a loss to explain the mechanism of false positives and false negatives. The latter

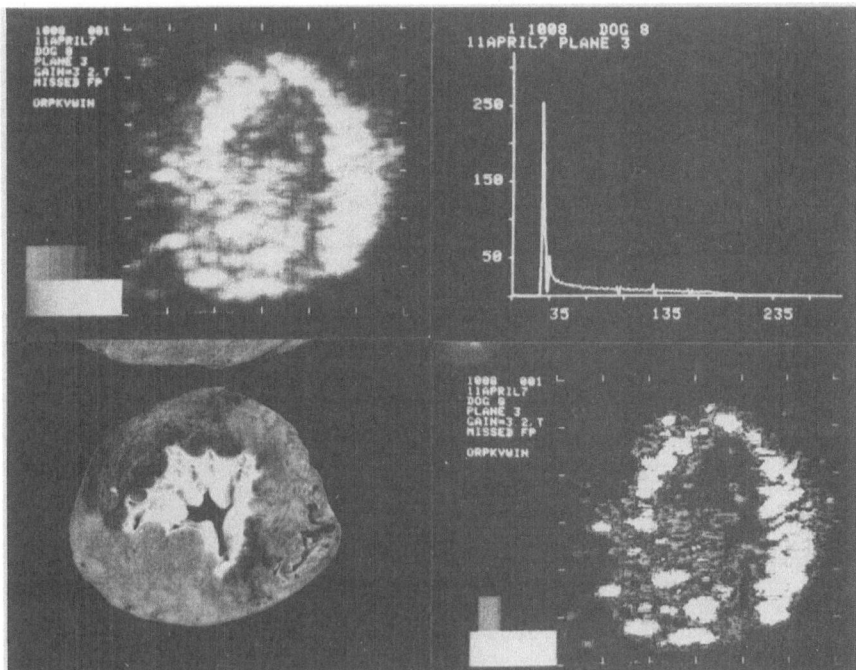

Fig. 5. Four-hour infarct. Original ultrasound data in 16 shades of gray is shown in the left upper panel, total image histogram in the right upper, and the Thioflavin S perfusion distribution in the lower left. The tri-stable image (lower right) demonstrates an ultrasonically typical, large infarct which closely matches the distribution of tissue changes observed microscopically. The right side of the infarct, involving the septum, shows mostly good perfusion with spotty zones of poor perfusion. The posterior left ventricular wall demonstrated focal evidence of infarction, represented as isolated regions of high amplitude in the tri-stable image.

could well be related to instrument sensitivity setting since unduly high gain was accompanied by infarct/normal ratios of 1 for maximum histogram values and probably indicates receiver saturation. In addition, uneven scanning, drop outs and shadowing could play a role in the production of false negatives. Low amplifier gain, on the other hand, tends to under-represent normal myocardium so that infarct/normal ratios may be as high as 4.0.

We have not, as yet, extended our studies to living patients since we do not have the capability to digitize and store the ultrasonic signals at the rate they are generated in real-time studies nor in the volumes necessary in clinical examination. However, we are hopeful that digital storage of single frames and proper post-processing will allow sufficient flexibility to permit signal amplitude evaluation as well as histogram-based image processing to search for similar changes in living hearts.

The development of an ultrasonic capability to detect and map early infarcts with real-time systems, especially when the electro-cardiographic pattern and blood enzyme changes have not yet stabilized, would represent a significant advance in the diagnostic workup of patients with suspected myocardial infarction.

ACKNOWLEDGEMENT

Figures 2, 3, 6, 7 and 8 first appeared in 'Ultrasonic Detection of Myocardial Infarction by Amplitude Analysis', Radiology 130:713–720, 1979. The permission by the authors of the article and The Radiological Society of North America Inc. to include these figures in the present paper is gratefully acknowledged.

REFERENCES

1. Adams DF, SJ Hessel, PF Judy, JA Stein, HL Abrams: Differing attenuation coefficients of normal and infarcted myocardium. Science 192:467, 1976.
2. Gramiak R, RC Waag: Cardiac reconstruction imaging in relation to other ultrasound systems and computed tomography. Am J Roentgenol 127:91, 1976.
3. Lappin HA, EH Botvinick, WW Parmley, JV Tyberg: Special Communications: Myocardial infarction in closed-chest dogs: a simplified method for production. J of Applied Physiology 5:831, 1975.
4. Kloner RA, CE Ganote, KA Reimer, RB Jennings: Coronary flow during acute myocardial ischemia. Fed Proc 33:592, 1974 (abstract).
5. Wild JJ, HD Crawford, JM Reid: Visualization of the excised human heart by means of reflected ultrasound or echography. Am Heart J 54:903, 1957.
6. Joynt L, A Macovski, D Boyle: Techniques for in vivo tissue characterization. Program & Abstracts, 3rd International Symposium on Ultrasonic Imaging and Tissue Characterization, 5–7 June 1978, National Bureau of Standards, Gaithersburg, Md., 1978, p. 59.
7. Rasmussen S, BC Corya, H Feigenbaum, SB Knoebel: Detection of myocardial scar tissue by M-mode echocardiography. Circulation 57:230, 1978.

CROSS-SECTIONAL ECHOCARDIOGRAPHY IN ACUTE MYOCARDIAL INFARCTION

A. BLOCH, J.-D. MORARD, CH. MAYOR, and J.J. PERRENOUD

The present investigation was designed in order to study echocardiographic variations in patients admitted with acute myocardial infarction. Another purpose was to better define the role of echocardiography in the coronary care unit (CCU). Forty-three patients were initially studied, but 8 had to be excluded because their echocardiograms were of inadequate technical quality. Complete M-mode and real-time cross-sectional echocardiograms were recorded serially in 35 patients. There were 27 males and 8 females. Ages ranged from 34 to 72 years (mean: 54 years). M-mode tracings were obtained with an Ekoline 21 A. Cross-sectional echocardiogram studies were performed using a mechanical sector scanner (Ekosektor I) with a 30° wide angle. The first echocardiogram was recorded in the CCU on day 1, 2 to 15 hours after the beginning of chest pain. The following recordings were performed on day 2 and 3 and once more before hospital discharge.

Localization of the myocardial infarction on sector-scan and ECG showed excellent correlation in 29/35 patients. Discrepancy between the two methods in localizing the myocardial infarction was present in 1 patient. In 3 other patients the myocardial infarction could be localized on sector-scan but not on ECG; one of them had an inferior infarction which was not apparent on ECG; two others had an anterior myocardial infarction with left bundle branch block. Two patients out of 3 with a subendocardial myocardial infarction on ECG had a normal crosssectional study.

Moreover, the cross-sectional echocardiograms were very useful for assessing the regional movements of areas difficult to study on ECG such as the interventricular septum and the left ventricular apex.

Contraction of the infarcted area was studied serially with combined use of M-mode and cross-sectional echocardiography. Regional contraction improved progressively (Figs. 1–2) in 20 of the 35 patients; the improvement usually started on day 2.

Regional contraction worsened in 4 patients, of whom 2 progressively developed a left ventricular aneurysm. Regional contraction of the infarcted area in 11 patients remained unchanged during the whole hospital stay.

The thickness and optical density of the infarcted segments were studied on M-mode recordings when these segments could be adequately visualized. The infarcted areas appeared optically denser and/or thinner on discharge echocardiograms than on the first recording in 11 patients.

The size of the myocardial infarction was assessed semi-quantitatively on the first cross-sectional recording. This assessment (small, medium or large

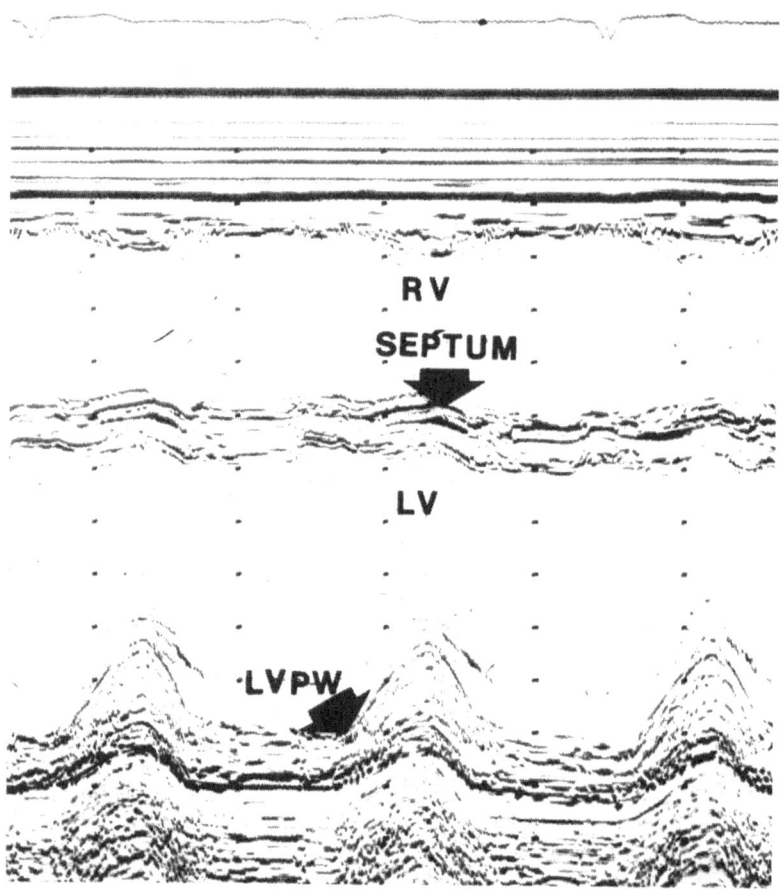

Fig. 1. 50 year-old man admitted with an anterior myocardial infarction. M-mode echocardio-gram recorded 6 hours after the onset of chest pain showing abnormal motion of the interventricular septum.

myocardial infarction) was later correlated with the peak level of the total seric creatine phosphokinase (100–400, 400–900, 900–1500 U). Patients with past history of myocardial infarction and patients whose infarction could not be detected on sector scan were excluded from this evaluation. Excellent correlation between CPK-level and sector-scan was found in 26/30 patients when assessing myocardial infarction size semi-quantitatively.

In conclusion, serial echocardiograms appear very useful in the non-invasive assessment of acute myocardial infarction. 1) Cross-sectional recordings improve ECG's ability to localize acute myocardial infarction. 2) Cross-sectional recordings help in assessing the regional movements of ventricular segments which are difficult to study on ECG. 3) Cross-sectional and M-mode recordings allow demonstration of progressive modifications of left ventricular contraction after acute myocardial infarction. Regional contraction improves progressively in most patients; it appears to worsen in

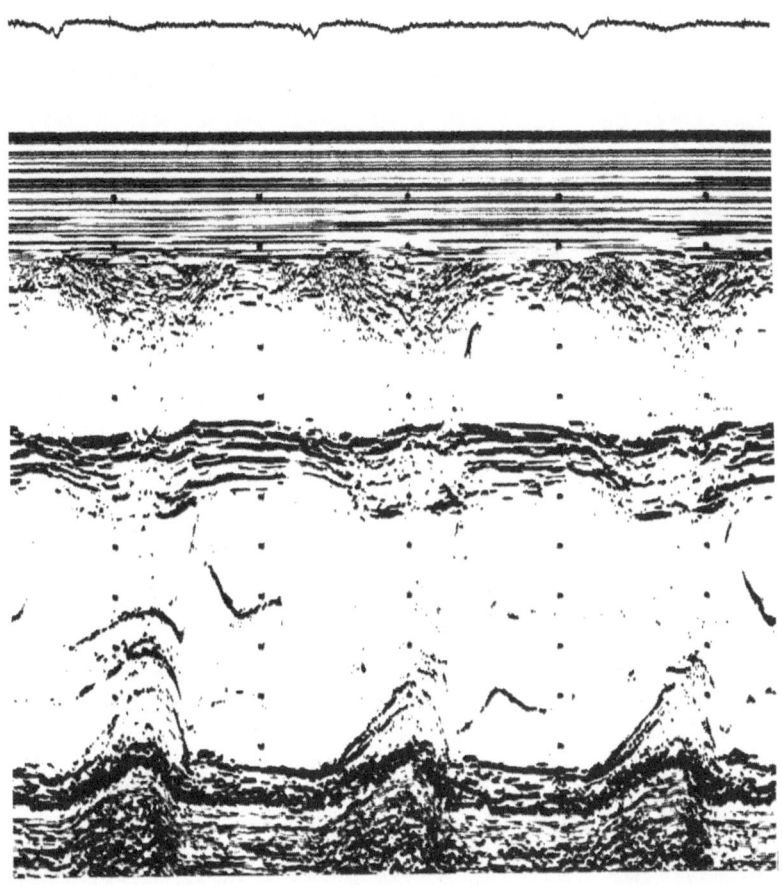

Fig. 2. Same patient. M-mode echocardiogram recorded 13 days after acute myocardial infarction.

some, with occasional development of a left ventricular aneurysm. 4) Echocardiographic studies may show progressive changes in optical density and thickness of infarcted ventricular segments. 5) Cross-sectional recordings enable very early semi-quantitative assessment of the size of an acute myocardial infarction. Echocardiography may therefore prove useful for assessing the effect of pharmacologic interventions on infarct size.

EFFECT OF CORONARY ARTERY OCCLUSION AND REPERFUSION ON THE TIME COURSE OF MYOCARDIAL WALL THICKNESS

F.J. TEN CATE, P.D. VERDOUW, A.H. BOM, and J.R. ROELANDT

INTRODUCTION

Measurement of changes in segment length has provided valuable information about the contractile state of normal and ischemic areas of the myocardium (1–3). It has also been shown that changes in segment length are inversely related to those of wall thickness (3). Until recently, the determination of wall thickness encountered numerous technical problems. The introduction of small transducers (ultrasound principle) which can be sutured on the epicardium has stimulated the study of changes in wall thickness (4, 5), but analysis of the tracings has been restricted to the measurement of wall thickness at end-diastole and end-systole only. So far, no attention has been paid to the time course of wall thickness throughout the cardiac cycle. This study describes these events as they occur throughout two minutes of coronary artery occlusion, followed by ten minutes of reperfusion, paying particular attention to the diastolic phases.

MATERIALS AND METHODS

Studies were performed on young pigs (20–28 kg) which were anesthetized and catheterized as described earlier (6). Left ventricular and ascending aortic pressures were obtained from 7F Millar catheters. The heart was exposed via a midsternal split, and the left anterior descending coronary artery (LAD) was dissected free.

A Krautkramer-Branson 5 MHz Aerotech transducer was sutured on the epicardium in the area perfused by the LAD (Fig. 1).

REGISTRATION AND ANALYSIS OF DATA

The echocardiogram was displayed continuously on a modified Smith-Kline Ekoline 20A ultrasonoscope. At the time of the measurements the echocardiogram, left ventricular pressure (LVP), its first derivative (LVdP/dt), and the pressure in the root of the aorta (AP) were simultaneously written at a paper speed of 50 mm/sec on linagraph direct print photographic paper (Eastman Kodak) via a Honeywell fiberoptic recorder (LS 6). Before control measurements were taken, a bolus of saline (1–2 ml) was injected into the left

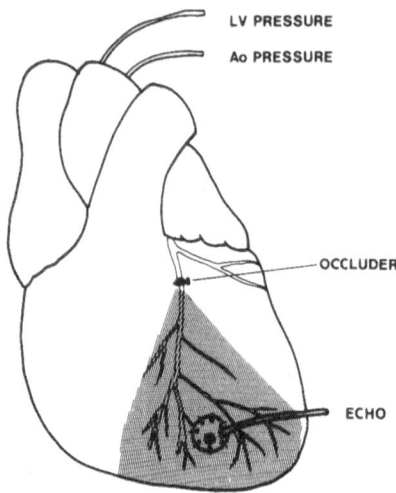

Fig. 1. Illustration of the heart with the site of the ultrasound crystal. Aortic pressure is measured in the root of the aorta.

ventricular cavity, thus providing clearer registration of the blood-endocardium interface. The echocardiograms were analyzed on a digitizing tablet which was connected to a PDP-11/10 computer (7). The following values were determined: end-diastolic (EDT), end-systolic (EST) and maximal (max T) wall thickness. End-diastole was defined as the occurrence of the onset of the upstroke of LVdP/dt, while end-systole was taken as the occurrence of the incisura of the central aortic pressure. Furthermore, the time interval from end-systole to maximal wall thickness ($t_{\text{max } T}$) was measured (Fig. 2). Differentiation of the wall thickness tracings (with the aid of the PDP-11) gave maximum velocity of thickening (max dT/dt/T) and thinning (min dT/dt/T). Each value was determined as the average of five consecutive beats, all traced in duplicate.

RESULTS

Global haemodynamics during occlusion and reperfusion

There were no appreciable changes in heart rate during the course of the experiments (Table 1). Mean arterial pressure decreased by 20% during occlusion, but returned to control values within 2 minutes after reperfusion. The most striking changes were found in left ventricular end-diastolic pressure (LVEDP), which doubled within 30 sec after occlusion was started. LVEDP returned to control within seconds after reperfusion.

The maximum rates of rise (max LVdP/dt) and fall (min LVdP/dt) of the left ventricular pressure decreased respectively increased during occlusion (25% and 45% respectively). Immediately after reperfusion max LVdP/dt increased to

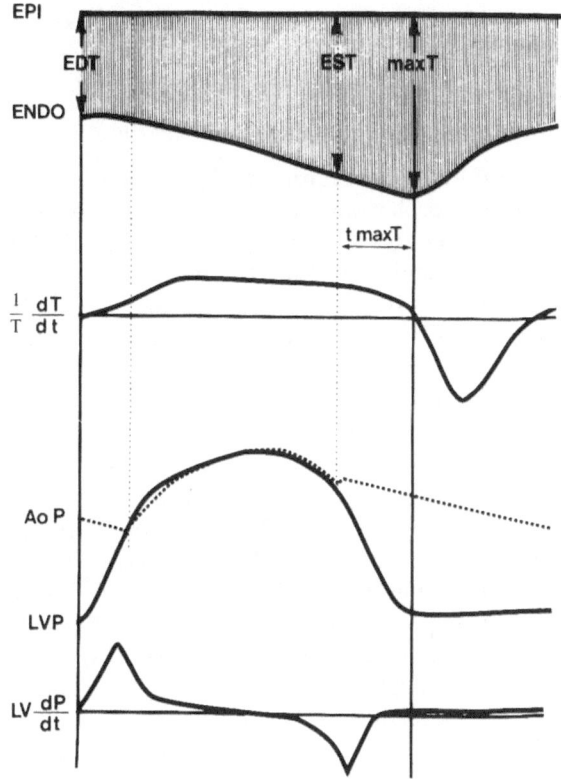

Fig. 2. Definition of wall thickness parameters. The endocardium and the velocity of wall thickness changes ($dT/dt/T$) are redrawn from an original tracing obtained during control. Notice that maximal wall thickness (max T) is reached after closure of the aortic valve.

Table 1. Hemodynamic parameters during control, 2min of LAD occlusion and reperfusion in pigs.

	Control	LAD occlusion		Reperfusion	
		30 sec	90 sec	2 min	10 min
HR (beats/min)	96 ± 7	100 ± 6	108 ± 6	97 ± 6	96 ± 6
MAP (mmHg)	81 ± 8	69 ± 6*	64 ± 7*	85 ± 1.5	82 ±7
LVEDP (mm Hg)	7.8 ± 1.2	13.5±2.2*	17.2±2.5*	8.8±1.5	8.2 ±1.2
Min LVdP/dt (mmHg/sec)	2030 ±370	1500 ±290*	1510 ±290*	2390 ±440	2010 ±310
Min LVdP/dt (mmHg/sec)	−1460 ±250	−820 ±100*	−1010 ±220*	−1540 ±320	−1380 210

LAD = left anterior descending coronary artery;
HR = heart rate;
MAP = mean arterial pressure;
LVEDP = left ventricular end-diastolic pressure;
Max LVdP/dt = maximal rate of rise of left ventricular pressure;
Min LVdP/dt = maximal rate of fall of left ventricular pressure;
*Values significantly different vs control ($p < 0.05$).

values above control of 20% ($p < 0.05$). Min LVdP/dt returned to control values without a significant overshoot.

Myocardial wall thickness during occlusion and reperfusion

An example of a continuous echocardiographic tracing of myocardial wall thickness during control, occlusion and reperfusion is shown in Figure 3.

During control, a percentage thickening ($100 \times$ (max T-EDT)/EDT)% of $62\% \pm 13\%$ ($\bar{x} \pm$ SE) was found. A striking feature is that max T was reached after closure of the aortic valve ($t_{\max T} = 52 \pm 10$ msec, $p < 0.001$). Although most of the thickening (87%, Fig. 4) occurred during ventricular ejection, there was still a significant increase (13%) in wall thickness in early diastole, when the ventricular pressure fell sharply. The velocity of wall thickening was nearly constant, in contrast to the velocity of wall thinning which had a sharply defined maximum. Consequently the maximum velocity of thinning (min dT/dt/T) was consistently larger than the maximum velocity of thickening (60 ± 20 sec^{-1} vs 30 ± 4 sec^{-1}). EDT started to decrease immediately after the LAD was occluded and was only $81\% \pm 5\%$ (p < 0.005) of control after 90 sec of occlusion, but returned towards control within 30 sec of reperfusion (Fig. 3). After 30 sec of occlusion no systolic thickening of the myocardial wall was observed and, in fact, after 90 sec a systolic thinning had even occurred. However, diastolic wall thickening was much larger than during control (Fig. 3). Nevertheless total thickening had decreased to 17% $\pm 1\%$ of EDT after 90 sec of occlusion. The increase in early diastolic thickening was associated with a dramatic prolongation of $t_{\max T}$ from 52 ± 10 msec to (134 ± 16 msec, p < 0.001). Min dT/dt/T was reduced in five of the six animals but slightly elevated in the other. Max dT/dt/T becomes meaningless because it was absent during systole and the irregular pattern of thickening

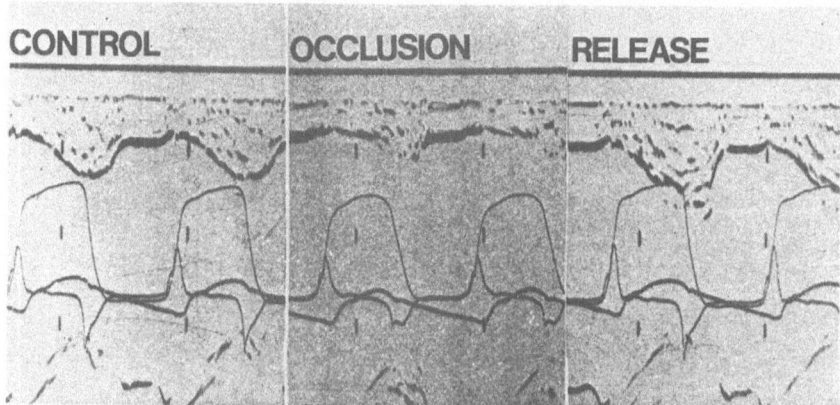

Fig. 3. Echocardiograms obtained during control, after 90 sec of coronary artery occlusion and reperfusion. The motion of the endocardial wall is traced and processed with the aid of digitizing tablet and PDP-11 computer.

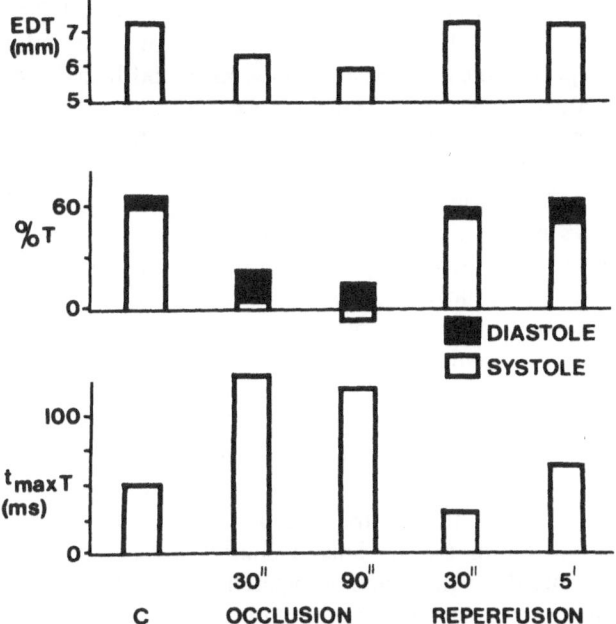

Fig. 4. From top to bottom: myocardial wall thickness at the end of left ventricular end-diastole, percentage of wall thickening and the time at which wall thickness reaches its maximum value. Notice that, during ischemia, nearly all wall thickening occurs during early diastole and that the increased diastolic thickening is associated with a prolongation of $t_{\max T}$.

during diastole did not allow a reliable determination of $dT/dt/T$ during that phase. A small but significant overshoot ($p < 0.05$) was seen in EST and max T in the early reperfusion period. The other wall thickness parameters resumed control values within the first minutes of reperfusion.

DISCUSSION

Considerable attention has been focussed on the study of the regional function of the myocardium. Measurement of changes in segment length is accepted as a reliable indicator for demonstrating the absence or presence of ischemia (1–3, 8, 9). Sasayama et al. (3) have demonstrated that changes in segment length and wall thickness are inversely related. This hypothesis certainly holds for the normally contracting myocardium, but probably does not hold when endocardial ischemia occurs. Myocardial wall thickness determinations (which are transmural measurements) might reveal abnormalities when segment length changes (which are measured along the epicardium) are normal.

Wall thickness has been studied in the past, but has only started to receive considerable attention since the introduction of ultrasound transducers which can be sutured on the epicardium.

Wall thickness increased during systole by about 55% of the EDT value. Other investigators (3, 4, 10) have reported somewhat lower values (30–50%). Differences in species, sites of measurements, EDT and heart rate are possible explanations for this disparity. During occlusion, systolic thickening decreased to akinesis (no systolic thickening) within 30 sec. In the following minute, the wall became dyskinetic (systolic thinning). These observations are in agreement with the findings of other investigators (5, 8, 9). Most striking are the increases in the diastolic thickening and $t_{max\ T}$ during ischemia. This may be related to the observation that the relative changes in min LVdP/dt are larger than the relative changes in max LVdP/dt. Thus, while the ischemic myocardium does not contribute to the overall contractile state of the heart, it opposes diastolic relaxation by its enhanced diastolic thickening. The mechanism of this increased diastolic thickening is not known.

Our earliest measurements in the reperfusion period were taken after 30 sec and repeated 90 sec later. EDT was, at that time slightly, but not significantly, larger than during control. Other authors have reported significantly increased EDT values in the early reperfusion period after occlusions varying from 5–15 min (4, 5). This overshoot over the control value is thought to be caused by the reactive hyperemic flow. The occlusion periods in our study were much shorter (2 min) and it is possible that the hyperemic flow (which was not measured in our study) had subsided and was not large enough at the time of our first measurements during reperfusion to give increased EDT values.

Since Gaasch and Bernhard (4) showed that an increased coronary flow, is associated with an increased end-diastolic wall thickness, it is attractive to speculate that the prolonged myocardial wall thickening during early diastole is related to the particular coronary flow pattern (90% of the flow occurs during diastole). However, such a concept is not supported by the increased diastolic wall thickening during coronary artery occlusion.

Velocities of wall thickening (dT/dt) have only been determined in studies in which wall thickness was determined by röntgen videometry (11, 12). This method, which can be used in patients, is cumbersome and the results are debatable. The authors describe systolic wall thickening of up to 160%. Consequently dT/dt was much larger than in our study. We also found that dT/dt/T was fairly constant during ejection (Fig. 2) in contrast to min dT/dt/T which was sharply defined.

These observations on myocardial wall thickness changes may prove to be helpful in the evaluation of therapeutic interventions in patients with ischemic heart disease. Such measurements might be used to determine whether or not these interventions affect ischemic areas, non-ischemic areas or both.

ACKNOWLEDGEMENT

We would like to thank the Interuniversitair Cardiologisch Instituut (ICI) for the use of the PDP-11/10 computer.

REFERENCES

1. Theroux P, D Franklin, J Ross, WS Kemper: Regional myocardial function during acute coronary artery occlusion and its modification by pharmacoligic agents in the dog. Circ Res 35:986, 1974.
2. Banka VS, RH Helfant: Temporal sequence of dynamic contractile characteristics in ischemic and nonischemic myocardium after acute ligation. Am J Cardiol 34:158, 1974.
3. Sasayama S, D Franklin, J Ross, WS Kemper, and D McKown: Dynamic changes in left ventricular wall thickness and their use in analyzing cardiac function in the conscious dog. Am J Cardiol 38:870, 1976.
4. Gaasch WH, SA Bernhard: The effect of acute changes in coronary blood flow on left ventricular end-diastolic wall thickness – An echocardiographic study. Circulation 593:598, 1977.
5. Heyndrickx GR, H Baig, P Nellens, I Leusen, MC Fishbein, SF Vatner: Depression of regional blood flow and wall thickening after brief coronary occlusions. Am J Physiol 234:H653, 1978.
6. Verdouw PD, WJ Remme, PG Hugenholtz: Cardiovascular and antiarrhythmic effects of aprindine (AC 1802) during partial occlusion of a coronary artery in the pig. Cardiovasc Res 11:317, 1977.
7. Vogel JA, G van Zwieten, N Bom, WJ Gussenhoven: Echocardiology with Doppler applications and real time imaging, Bom N (ed), The Hague, Martinus Nijhoff Medical Division, 1977.
8. Tomoike H, D Franklin, J Ross: Detection of myocardial ischemia by regional dysfunction during and after rapid pacing in conscious dogs. Circulation 58:48, 1978.
9. Tomoike H, D Franklin, D McKown, WS Kemper, M Guberek, J Ross: Regional myocardial dysfunction and hemodynamic abnormalities during strenuous exercise in dogs with limited coronary flow. Circ Res 42:487, 1978.
10. Kerber RE, ML Marcus, FM Abboud: Echocardiography in experimentally-induced myocardial ischemia. Amer J Med 63:21, 1977.
11. Dumesnil JG, EL Ritman, RL Frye, GT Gau, BD Rurtherford, GD Davis: Quantitative determination of regional left ventricular wall dynamics by rontgen videometry. Circulation 50:700, 1974.
12. Chesebro JH, EL Ritman, RL Frye, HC Smith, BD Rutherford, RE Fulton, JR Pluth, DA Barnhorst: Regional myocardial wall thickening response to nitroglycerin – A predictor of myocardial response to aortocoronary bypass surgery. Circulation 57:952, 1978.

ECHOCARDIOGRAPHIC CHANGES IN VASOSPASTIC ANGINA*

ALESSANDRO DISTANTE, ANTONIO L'ABBATE, ATTILIO MASERI,
LUIGI LANDINI, and CLAUDIO MICHELASSI

The traditional concept that the only cause of angina pectoris is represented by an inadequate increase in blood supply, when myocardial metabolic demand is augmented, has been challenged by recent studies (1). In fact, continuous hemodynamic monitoring of patients with angina at rest has documented that no increase in blood pressure, contractility or heart rate precedes the onset of an ischemic attack (2–5). Nevertheless, no data are available on the changes in ventricular wall motion and dimensions associated with attacks of angina at rest. The purpose of this study was to explore the sequence of ventricular echocardiographic patterns in patients with angina at rest in order to determine the sequence of events at the onset of the attack.

MATERIALS AND METHODS

From the patients admitted to our coronary care unit, we obtained echocardiographic studies in 10 males with frequent attacks of angina at rest, characterized by transient ST segment changes occurring in anterior electrocardiographic leads and with no evidence of previous myocardial infarction. Ultrasonic data have been obtained with a commercially available apparatus (Echo Cardio Visor 03) with a fiber-optic paper recorder, using a 7.5 or a 10 cm single element, focussed transducer. After accurate searching for the acoustic window, and under continuous ECG monitoring of the lead showing the earliest and the most marked ST segment changes during spontaneous ischemic attacks, the ultrasonic study was performed in one or more of the following situations: a) in patients with very frequent spontaneous attacks – as soon as the patient reported the onset of spontaneous chest pain or as soon as ischemic ECG changes were noted on the monitor (3 patients); b) during a routine test for inducing ischemia by ergonovine maleate which reproduces attacks similar to spontaneous ones (5 patients) (6, 7); c) in patients under continuous hemodynamic monitoring (2 patients).

In 8 patients, the presence of coronary vasospasm had been documented directly with coronary arteriographic observations obtained during pain, as illustrated in Figure 1.

Out of 16 ischemic episodes recorded (6 spontaneous and 10 ergonovine

*This work has been partly supported by a grant from C.N.R. Project Biomedical Technology, Subproject B1014, No. 204121/86/81787.

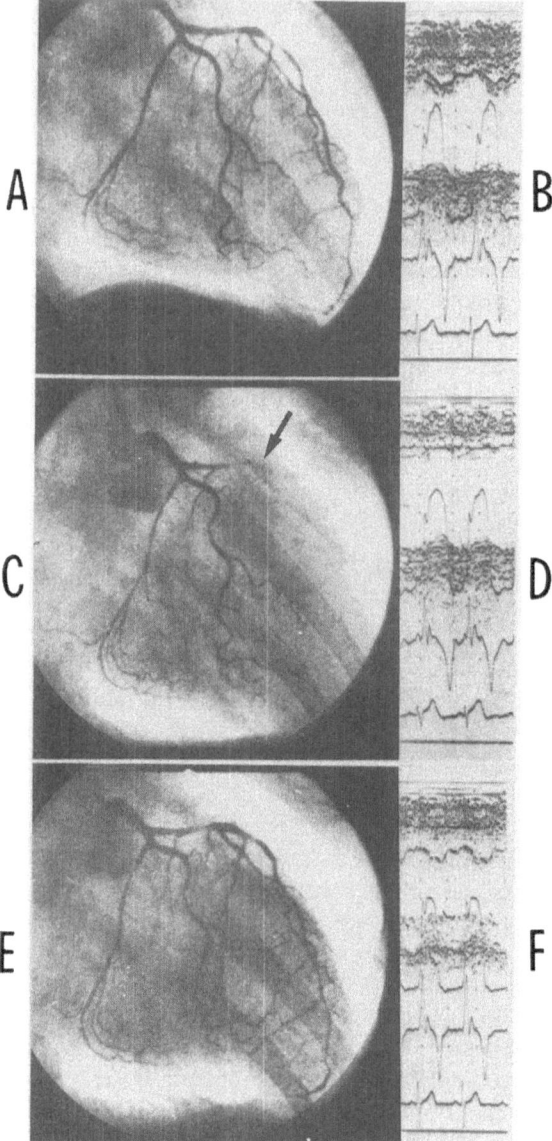

Fig. 1. Selected parts of continuous monitored echocardiogram, LV pressure, d*P*/d*t* and ECG; during an induced ischemic episode, together with selected frames from coronary cineangiography performed during a similar anginal attack. A and B in the absence of pain and ECG changes. C and D during an ischemic attack. Note the absence of visualization of the left anterior descending coronary artery (arrow) and the absence of motion of the inter-ventricular septum, which does not show any systolic thickening. LVEDP is increased, with reduction of LV systolic pressure and peak d*P*/d*t*. In E and F, the reperfusion of LAD artery has occurred, with a return to normal of all the parameters (except for LVSP which is low, because TNG was given to alleviate the attack).

induced), 4 were analyzed with a digitizing apparatus (light-pen on TV monitor, simple computer programs, and printout on a Versatec plotter) both for statistical analysis and in order to compress the large amount of data. The following echocardiographic and, in one case, hemodynamic parameters have been taken into account for the purpose of this study:

A. ECG
B. Contraction (C) and relaxation (R) dP/dt
C. Left ventricular systolic and diastolic pressure (LVSP and LVEDP)
D. Left ventricular systolic (LVSD) and diastolic dimensions
E. Left ventricular percentage fractional shortening (LV%FS)
F. Systolic septal thickness (SEPT. THICK) and percentage thickening
G. Septal and posterior wall motion (SEPT. WALL and POST. WALL).

RESULTS

In 10 patients, 16 episodes of transient myocardial ischemia have been recorded, either characterized by ST segment elevation – 15 – or depression – 1 –. Ten episodes were induced by ergonovine maleate and 6 were spontaneous. Full computerized analysis has been performed in 4 episodes with ST segment elevation, 2 spontaneous and 2 ergonovine induced, in one of which hemodynamic and ultrasound monitoring could be obtained before and during the waxing and waning phases of the attack. The complete time-course of myocardial ischemia could only be studied from the initial onset in the induced episodes, while the time-course of spontaneous episodes could be followed from the onset of pain or of the ischemic changes on the ECG.

Figure 2 shows the time-course of an induced attack. Both ECG changes and pain are very late indicators of ischemia. Reduction of systolic septal thickness (SEPT. THICK) and decrease in contraction (C) and relaxation (R) dP/dt were the first indicators of ischemia. Simultaneously with the decrease in thickening of septal wall there was a reduction in left ventricular fractional shortening (LV%FS) and increase in systolic dimension (LVSD) and diastolic dimension. Left ventricular end-diastolic pressure (LVEDP) changes followed soon after and the product of heart rate and systolic left ventricular pressure (HR × LVSP) did not change until late, when pain appeared and ST changes were already marked. Following the alleviation of the attacks obtained after nitroglycerin s.l., a rebound effect was observed in the septal thickness, left ventricular fractional shortening and contraction dP/dt.

Figure 3 shows the sequence of events during a spontaneous attack in a 29 year old patient with frequent ischemic episodes at rest, most of which were characterized by ST segment elevation or pseudonormalization of a basally negative T wave. The computer printout shows that after a basal recording with normal findings, at the onset of pain as reported by the patient, the septal wall appears akinetic, thin and with a markedly reduced systolic thickening, while the left ventricular dimensions are markedly increased and ECG (lead V$_3$) shows an elevation of the ST segment. Besides absence of

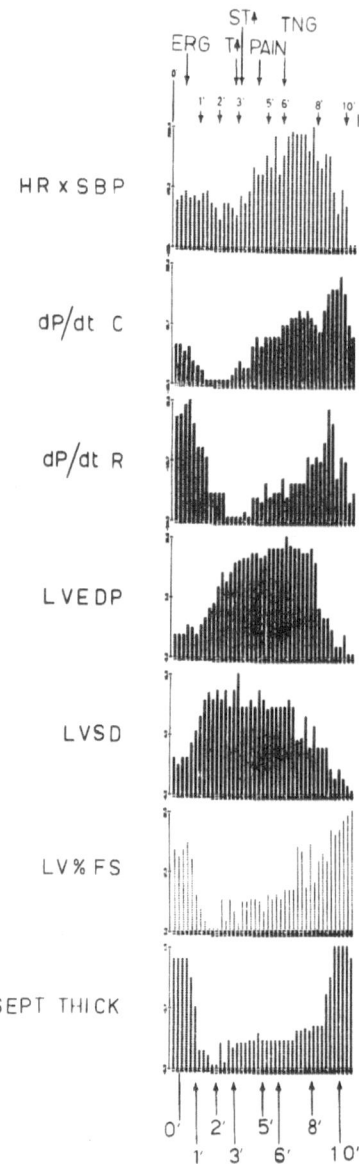

Fig. 2. Complete time-course of an ischemic attack induced by ergonovine maleate. Each vertical bar represents the percentage differences relative to control, averaged over 20 sec: After ergonovine injection the first changes occur in septal thickness (SEPT,THICK.), LV percentage fractional shortening (LV%FS), peak contraction (C) and relaxation (R) dP/dt, and in systolic dimensions (LVSD). Note the prolonged steady state of ischemic changes which are interrupted by TNG s.l., after which a rebound effect in observed in the various parameters.

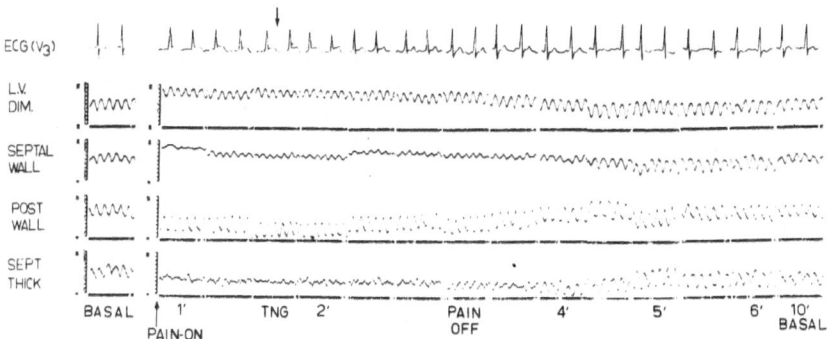

Fig. 3. Echocardiographic monitoring of a spontaneous anginal attack. Basal echocardiogram recorded half an hour before pain. The monitoring started a few seconds after the patient reported the onset of pain. ST segment is elevated, septal wall is already thin and akinetic, LV dimensions are markedly increased. One minute after TNG s.l. pain disappears, while cardiac mechanics return to normal 3 minutes later. Note that 2 minutes after pain-off septum and posterior wall show hyperkinetic motion.

thickening and septal asynergy (paradoxic movement follows akinesis), there is an upward displacement of the septal wall together with a downward displacement of posterior wall, very likely due to the globular shape of the ventricle during ischemia. Nitroglycerin was given when ECG changes showed marked ST segment elevation (arrow).

The qualitative analysis in the other ischemic episodes has consistently shown the same patterns as did the reported examples.

CONCLUSIONS

Previous studies have shown that before an ischemic attack at rest there is no increase in those hemodynamic parameters controlling the myocardial O_2 consumption (2–5), and that the sequence of hemodynamic and electrocardiographic changes observed do resemble those provoked by sudden ligation of a coronary artery in the experimental animal (8–10). Our results show that the increase in ventricular dimensions does not precede the attack but follows a decrease in contraction dP/dt, fractional shortening and systolic thickening of the ischemic region (Fig. 2). Thus, the anginal attacks are neither secondary to an increase in heart rate, systolic or diastolic pressure or dP/dt nor are they preceded by an increase in ventricular dimensions. Therefore, the hypothesis of a "primary" cause of these anginal attacks being coronary vasospasm (1, 3–5, 11–12) is supported by this study. Furthermore, these preliminary results extend our understanding of relationships between transient myocardial ischemia and cardiac mechanics in man, since ultrasonic methods alone or combined with hemodynamic methods provide information (13) otherwise unobtainable on the sequence of the change of dimensions and of wall motion patterns associated with transient ischemic attacks.

REFERENCES

1. Maseri A, S Severi, S Chierchia, O Parodi, A Biagini: Characteristics, incidence and pathogenetic mechanisms of "primary" angina at rest. In: Primary and secondary angina pectoris, Maseri, A, GA Klassen, M Lesch (eds). New York, Grune & Stratton, 1978, p 265.
2. Guazzi M, A Polese, C Fiorentini, F Magrini, MT Olivari, C Bartorelli: Left and right hemodynamics during spontaneous angina pectoris. Comparison between angina with ST segment depression and angina with ST segment elevation. Brit Heart J 37:401, 1975.
3. Maseri A, R Mimmo, S Chierchia, C Marchesi, A Pesola, A L'Abbate: Coronary spasm as a cause of acute myocardial ischemia in man. Chest 68:625, 1975.
4. Chierchia S, C Marchesi, A Maseri: Evidence of angina not caused by increased myocardial metabolic demand and patterns of electrocardiographic and hemodynamic alterations during "primary" angina. In: Primary and secondary angina pectoris, Maseri A, GA Klassen, M Lesch (eds), New York, Grune & Stratton, 1978, p 145.
5. Chierchia S, A Maseri, I Simonetti, C Brunelli: O_2 myocardial extraction in angina at rest. Evidence of a primary reduction of blood supply. Circulation (abstr) 56: (suppl. III) 37, 1977.
6. Schroeder JS, JL Bolen, RA Quint, DA Clark, WG Hayden, CB Higgins, L Wesler: Provocation of coronary spasm with ergonovine maleate. Am J Cardiol 40:487, 1977.
7. Tavazzi L, JA Salerno, M Ray, G Specchia, M Chimenti, L Angoli, S De Servi, A Mussini, P Bobba: Acute myocardial ischemia induced by ergonovine maleate in patients with "primary" angina. In: Primary and secondary angina pectoris, Maseri A, GA Klassen, M Lesch (eds), New York, Grune & Stratton, 1978, p 247.
8. Porter WT: On the results of ligation of the coronary arteries. J Physiol 15:121, 1894.
9. Orias O: The dynamic changes in ventricles following ligation of the ramus descendens anterior. Am J Physiol 100:629, 1932.
10. Tennant R, CJ Wiggers: The effect of coronary occlusion on myocardial contraction. Am J Physiol 112:351, 1935.
11. Hillis LD, E Braunwald: Coronary artery spasm. NEJM 299:695, 1978.
12. Maseri A: Pathogenetic mechanisms of angina pectoris. Expanding views. Thomas Lewis Lecture, London 1977. Brit Heart J (in press).
13. Roelandt J, W Walsh, PG Hugenholtz: Advantages of combined hemodynamic and ultrasonic studies in man. In: Echocardiology Bom N (ed), The Hague, Martinus Nijhoff Medical Division, 1977, p 95.

ASSESSMENT OF REGIONAL WALL MOTION IN CORONARY ARTERY DISEASE BY TWO-DIMENSIONAL ECHOCARDIOGRAPHY

A.F. PARISI, P.F. MOYNIHAN, E.D. FOLLAND, and C.L. FELDMAN

Real-time two-dimensional echocardiography (2 DE) offers a challenging opportunity for physicians interested in identifying the presence of, and quantifying the extent of, regional wall motion abnormalities in coronary artery disease.

In this study, 2 DE was evaluated for its sensitivity to detect and for its ability to determine the size of localized wall motion abnormalities in patients with coronary artery disease. Individuals with and without transmural myocardial infarction were used to conduct a parallel analysis of 2 DE and angiographic techniques.

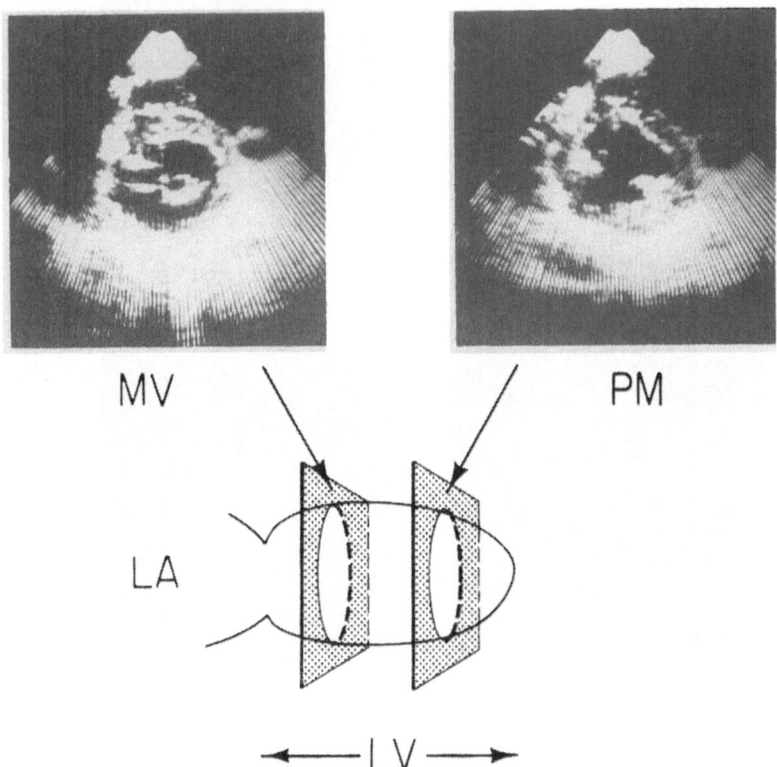

Fig. 1. Schematic of the left ventricle illustrating the orientation of the sections utilized and actual echocardiographic images obtained at each level. MV = mitral valve section, PM = papillary muscle section, LA = left atrium, LV = left ventricle.

Two-dimensional studies were performed with a Varian V-3000 phased array sector scanner. Examinations included cross-sectional (short axis) views at the levels of the mitral valve and papillary muscles in all subjects. Records of all studies were made on a Panasonic NV-3160 videotape recorder with slow-motion stop-action replay capability and displayed on a Conrac SNA-14C monitor. Diastolic and systolic tomographic endocardial outlines were obtained from stop-action frames gated to the electrocardiographic QRS complex and phonocardiographic S_2, respectively. Slow-motion and fast speed playback was used to verify all endocardial outlines. An Electronics for Medicine VVF light pen video digitizer was used for tracing; it was interfaced to a Digital Equipment Corporation PDP-11/05 computer which was specifi-

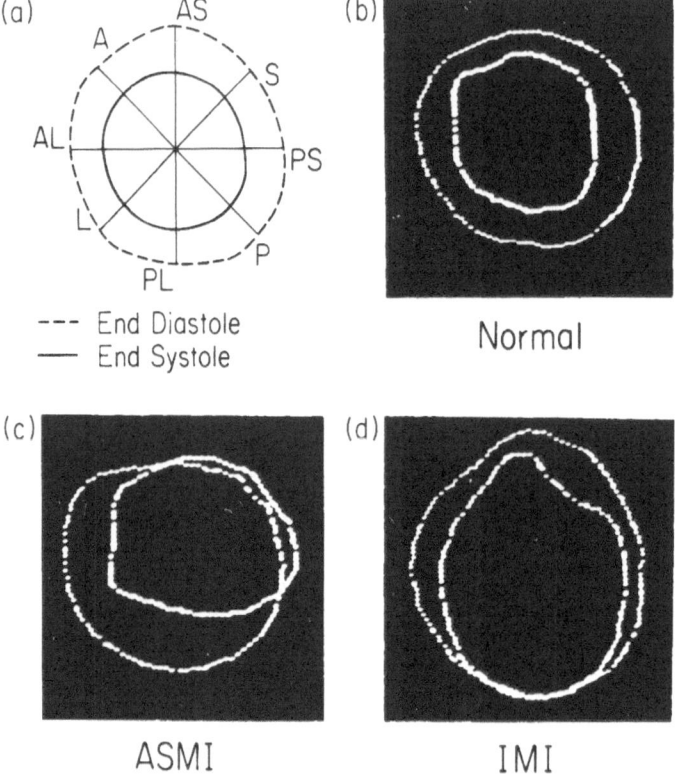

Fig. 2. (a) Schematic demonstration of the axis system imposed on the ventricular outlines for regional analysis. S = septal, PS = postero-septal, P = posterior, PL = postero-lateral, L = lateral, AL = antero-lateral, A = anterior, AS = antero-septal.

(b) Diastolic-systolic pair of mitral valve level outlines of a normal ventricle as displayed by computer after digitizing.

(c) Corresponding diastolic-systolic outlines from a patient with an antero-septal myocardial infarction (ASMI) showing dyskinesis in the antero-septal region.

(d) Corresponding diastolic-systolic outlines from a patient with an inferior myocardial infarction (IMI) showing posterior akinesis.

cally programmed for 2 DE outline storage and analysis. (1) Figure 1 illustrates the 2 DE examination as performed in each subject.

A radial axis system was designed by constructing an initial chord in end-diastole from the mid-septum (S) to the lateral wall (L) in a manner which divided the diastolic area of the cross-section under analysis into anterior and posterior halves of equal area (Fig. 2a). Radii extending from the midpoint of the initial axis were subsequently inserted at 45° angles so as to provide a final framework of 8 hemi-axes and 8 areas corresponding to discrete anatomic locations. In this system papillary muscles were excluded from the drawn outlines; thus a normal ventricle both at the level of the mitral valve and papillary muscles had diastolic and systolic outlines which appeared approximately as two concentric circles (Fig. 2b). The axis system was consistently applied to all ventricles studied; it was also maintained as a fixed

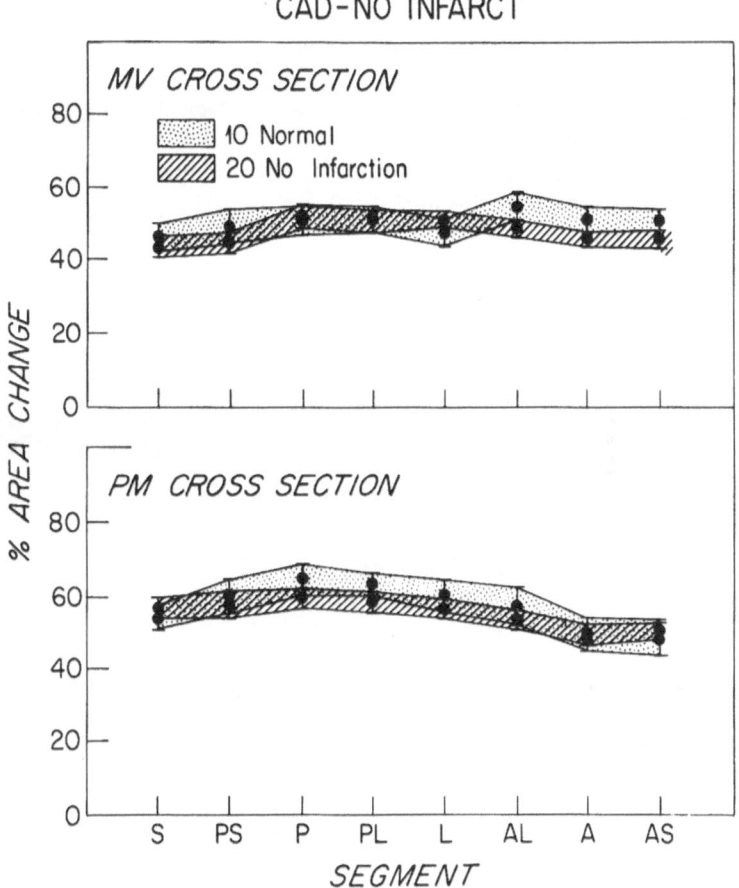

Fig. 3. Regional function plots (mean ±1 standard error) for the group of normal subjects and the group of patients with coronary artery disease (CAD) and no infarction. Segment labeling as in Figure 2.

reference for analysis of all systolic images. Figures 2c and 2d show typical diastolic/systolic outline pairs from patients with antero-septal and inferior myocardial infarction for comparison.

10 normal volunteers and 32 patients being evaluated for coronary artery disease were studied. The patients all had right anterior oblique left ventricular cineangiograms and selective coronary arteriography performed within 72 hours of the 2 DE study. Angiographic outlines were traced by an individual unaware of the 2 DE results. All ventriculographic outlines were also computer analyzed for regional wall motion abnormalities using a Herman-Gorlin axis format. (2). Of the 32 patients, 12 had electrocardiographic evidence of *transmural* myocardial infarction, 6 anterior and 6 inferior. The twenty remaining patients did not have electrocardiographic evidence of transmural infarction.

A normal range of 2 DE regional area shrinkage was established from the group of 10 normal volunteers at both the mitral valve and papillary muscle levels. The subgroup of 20 patients without evidence of transmural infarction failed to differ from normal values at either the mitral valve or papillary muscle level (Fig. 3).

In contrast the patients with transmural myocardial infarctions differed significantly at both levels from established normal values (Fig. 4). The 6 patients with anterior myocardial infarction had depressed area shrinkage in anterior regions both at the mitral valve and at the papillary muscle levels;

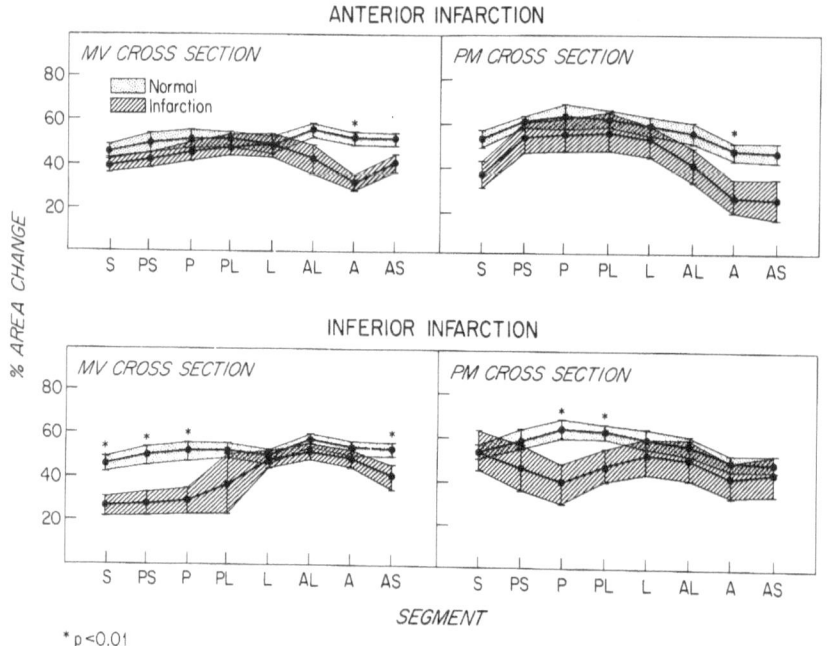

Fig. 4. Regional function plots (mean ±1 standard error) for the group of normal subjects and the groups of patients with anterior myocardial infarction (top) and inferior myocardial infarction (bottom). Segment labeling as in Figure 2.

similarly the 6 patients with inferior infarction had depressed area shrinkage most pronounced in posterior regions at both levels.

When individual patients were considered, 10 of the 12 transmural infarctions were correctly identified and localized by two-dimensional echocardiography when compared to the normal range (mean ± 2 SD for the 10 normal volunteers). In an analogous approach establishing a normal range as two standard deviations from the mean by the computer based ventriculographic analysis system using the Herman-Gorlin axis formulation, 10 of the 12 patients were similarly identified by left ventricular angiography. Thus, the sensitivity of the non-invasive and invasive technique proved to be identical in this small series of patients with transmural infarction. Specificity could not be evaluated similarly since normal regional function is not highly correlated with the absence of electrocardiographic evidence of transmural myocardial infarction.

Multiple regression analysis showed that mitral valve and papillary muscle cross-section area shrinkage contributed equally to total ejection fraction. The average shrinkage from the overall mitral valve and papillary muscle cross-sections correlated directly with angiographic ejection fraction ($r = 0.76$; $p < 0.01$). This indicates that data from two-dimensional echocardiography can be used to determine the extent of regional dysfunction.

We conclude that 2 DE can be utilized profitably to identify and quantify regional wall motion abnormalities by establishing standards of reference derived from normal individuals studied similarly; initial data indicate that in patients with transmural infarction 2 DE has a sensitivity comparable to left ventricular cineangiography for defining regional contraction defects.

REFERENCES

1. Parisi AF, PF Moynihan, ED Folland, DR Jones, CL Feldman: Quantitative Analysis of Left Ventricular Geometry Assessed by Two-Dimensional Echocardiography. Circulation 58:II-10, 1978.
2. Herman MV, R Gorlin: Implications of Left Ventricular Asynergy. Am J Cardiol 23:538, 1969.

ANALYSIS OF VENTRICULAR ASYNERGY IN MYOCARDIAL INFARCTION

A study with real-time cross-sectional echocardiography

YUNG-DAE PARK, HIROSHI SAKAKIBARAT, SEIKI NAGATA, SHINTARO BEPPU, and YASUHARU NIMURA

It is important to know localization and extent of the regional abnormal motion of the left ventricle in the case of myocardial infarction. Many authors have attempted to detect left ventricular asynergy with M-mode echocardiography (1, 2, 3, 5). We have attempted in this study to make a systematic real-time cross-sectional echocardiographic approach to detect the left ventricular asynergy in myocardial infarction and to analyse the cardiac motion in this setting.

SUBJECTS AND METHOD

Fifty-one patients with myocardial infarction underwent M-mode echocardiography, real-time cross-sectional echocardiography, left ventriculography and selective coronary cineangiography. Diagnosis of myocardial infarction was made by classical history, electrocardiographic and enzymological examinations. Their ages ranged from 42 to 68 years.

Commercially available real-time cross-sectional echocardiographs were used which were electronic phased-array sector systems and had wide sector angles (Toshiba SSH-11A and Varian V 3000). Echocardiography was performed with the patients in the supine or left lateral decubitus position. Cross-sectional images were recorded and reviewed with 8 mm cine film and/or videotape.

Echocardiographic cross-sections were set as follows: (1) longitudinal sections along the long axis of the left ventricle from the aorta to the apex, in which the interventricular septum, posterior wall and apex were visualized; (2) a longitudinal section perpendicular to the above sections from the apical approach, in which the interventricular septum and lateral wall were visualized; (3) transverse sections parallel to the short axis at the levels of the mitral leaflet, chordae tendineae, papillary muscle and apex, in which the interventricular septum, posterior wall and lateral wall of each level were visualized; (4) horizontal sections for observation of the right ventricular wall motion (Fig. 1).

RESULTS

Most parts of the left ventricle could be searched by the above-mentioned serial sections. In almost all cases, the wall motion was well visualized in longitudinal sections. However, every section of the left ventricle was not

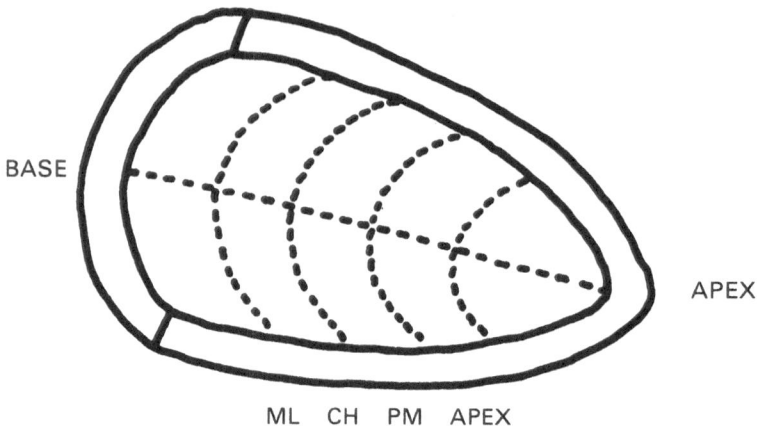

Fig. 1. Schematic illustration of the cross-sections of the left ventricle. Two longitudinal and four short axes were searched. Abbreviations: ML; mitral leaflet, CH; chordae tendineae, PM; papillary muscle.

always clearly visualized; in some cases for example, the transverse section of the apex and the lateral wall of the transverse sections were difficult to assess definitely, because of poor echocardiographic visualization.

The sites of asynergy detected with the above-mentioned serial sections well corresponded to those in left ventriculography. As for the severity of asynergy, which was evaluated as hypokinetic, akinetic and dyskinetic, echocardiographic findings also well corresponded to those in left ventriculography. In some cases, however, the apex was assessed to be more severely asynergic with echocardiography than left ventriculography.

In addition, real-time cross-sectional echocardiography revealed the following characteristic features of the asynergic areas.

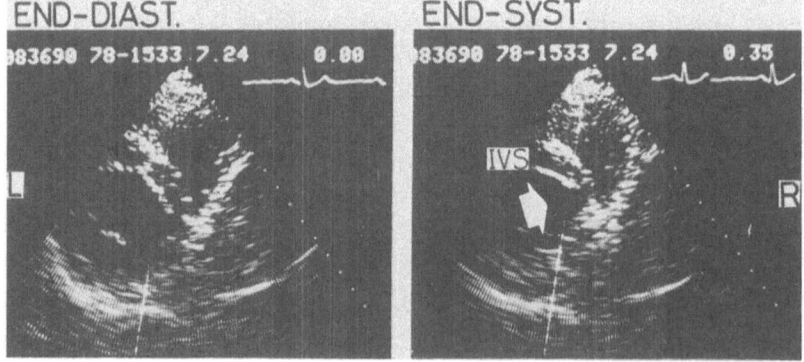

Fig. 2. The transverse section at the level of the chordae tendineae in a case with inferior infarction. Akinesis of the medial half of the posterior wall and systolic anterior movement of the lower part of the interventricular septum were demonstrated. IVS: interventricular septum. R: right side of the patient. L: left side of the patient.

1. *Sliding motion*

The non-contractile area was pulled by the normal contractile area during systole. This motion could be recognized only with real-time observation of echocardiography. On the M-mode echocardiogram, it was manifested as a decrease of systolic excursion and delay of the systolic peak and was difficult to be assessed as akinetic.

2. *Ventricular aneurysm*

In cases with ventricular aneurysm, not only dyskinetic motion, but also the deformed contour of the left ventricular cavity was clearly visualized, especially in the transverse sections.

3. *Inferior infarction*

In cases of inferior infarction, asynergic area was more easily recognized in the transverse sections than in the longitudinal sections, and the asynergic area was observed in the medial half of the posterior wall in almost all cases. Furthermore, the asynergic area extended to the lateral half of the posterior wall and/or the lower part of the interventricular septum, and in some cases even to the right ventricular wall (Fig. 2).

DISCUSSION

In this study, we have attempted to establish a systematic echocardiographic approach to detect left ventricular asynergy. To assess the sites and severity of asynergy, the above-mentioned serial sections were essentially the minimum requirement, although fewer cross sections than in this study might enable one to detect the asynergic area in cases of extensive infarction (4). Though sites of asynergic areas detected with echocardiography well corresponded to those in left ventriculography, echocardiographic evaluation of the severity of asynergy showed some discrepancy with those in left ventriculography. This might be caused by the following two factors: firstly, that both methods assess the wall motion qualitatively, that is, subjectively; and secondly, that the visual field of echocardiography is narrow.

Transverse cross-sections give unique diagnostic information which is denied to other diagnostic procedures. Transverse cross sections demonstrated the end-systolic deformed contour of the left ventricular cavity easily, and in cases of ventricular aneurysm even in diastole. Furthermore, in cases of inferior infarction, the transverse section clearly demonstrated the difference of the motion between the upper and lower parts of the interventricular septum, and between the medial and lateral halves of the posterior wall of the left ventricle. According to our results, studies based on observations using only M-mode echocardiography showed quite surprising correlation between echocardiographic and left ventriculographic findings.

Although care was taken to place the transducer parallel to the line perpendicular to the longitudinal sections at examining the transverse sections, problems remain in the accuracy of the transverse sections at the levels of the papillary muscle and apex.

In conclusion, the above-mentioned serial sections are essentially the minimum requirement to detect the severity and extension of asynergy. It should be emphasized that transverse cross-sections give diagnostic information which is denied by other diagnostic methods.

REFERENCES

1. Jacobs JJ, H Feigenbaum, BC Corya, JF Phillips: Detection of left ventricular asynergy by echocardiography. Circulation 48:263, 1973.
2. Corya BC, H Feigenbaum, S Rasmussen, MJ Black: Anterior left ventricular wall echoes in coronary artery disease, linear scanning with a single element transducer. Am J Cardiol 34:652, 1974.
3. Kerber RE, ML Marcus, J Ehrhardt, R Wilson, FM Abboud: Correlation between echocardiographically demonstrated segmental dyskinesis and regional myocardial perfusion. Circulation 52:1097, 1975.
4. Weyman AE, SM Peskoe, ES Williams, JC Dillon, H Feigenbaum: Detection of left ventricular aneurysms by cross-sectional echocardiography. Circulation 54:936, 1976.
5. Heikkila J, M Nieminen: Echoventriculographic detection, localization, and quantification of left ventricular asynergy in acute myocardial infarction. A correlative echo- and electrocardiographic study. Brit Heart J 37:46, 1975.

C. APPLICATIONS IN LEFT VENTRICULAR FUNCTION ANALYSIS

ABNORMAL LEFT VENTRICULAR RELAXATION AND DIASTOLIC FILLING PATTERNS IN LEFT-SIDED HEART DISEASE

P. HANRATH

In clinical cardiology, until recently, the quantitative description of LV diastolic function was entirely based on left heart catheterization and angiography. With the introduction of computerized techniques for the evaluation of M-mode echograms, a non-invasive, quantitative analysis of left ventricular function became possible. Simultaneous recordings of the left ventricular dimension with the mitral valve echogram and the phonocardiogram or apexcardiogram allow exact determination of the LV isovolumic relaxation time, the LV dimension change during this time period and an analysis of the left ventricular filling pattern in terms of time or dimension changes during the different phases of LV filling.

LEFT VENTRICULAR RELAXATION AND FILLING PATTERN IN NORMAL SUBJECTS

Simultaneous recordings of the left ventricular cavity echogram with the echoes from the mitral valve leaflets, the phonocardiogram or apexcardiogram or even with a left ventricular pressure curve, provide an insight into the time relationship between the opening and closing of both the aortic and mitral valves and the LV dimension changes.

During the LV isovolumic relaxation period – defined as the time interval between aortic valve closure (A_2) and mitral valve opening – only a small dimension change occurs in normal subjects (17).

Several authors – using computerized techniques for the evaluation of LV echograms – have proposed the time interval "minimal LV dimension to mitral valve opening" as an index of the LV isovolumic relaxation time (1, 11, 12, 14). In normal subjects, this time interval does not measure the true isovolumic relaxation time, because aortic valve closure precedes LV minimum dimension. Therefore, the time interval "minimal LV-dimension to mitral valve opening" is only an approximate estimate of LV isovolumic relaxation time. In normal subjects this time-interval is in the range 10 ± 2 ms and is accompanied by a small dimension increase of 0.6 ± 0.5 mm.

The computerized analysis of M-mode echograms has further shown that, in normal subjects during early LV filling, a close time relationship exists between the onset of mitral valve opening, left ventricular wall movement or changes in left ventricular wall thickness (5). With the onset of mitral valve opening, LV dimension increases rapidly and wall thinning starts (9). The peak rate of LV dimension increase and the peak rate of forward movement of the anterior leaflet are synchronous within 2 ± 6 ms. The timing of peak rate of LV wall thinning is always after mitral valve opening and has its peak value within the rapid filling period.

As shown in Figure 1 left ventricular filling can be separated into 3 phases. Rapid filling is observed in early diastole during which the peak filling rate is measured. Then follows a period of slow filling with minimal dimension change. Following the P wave, atrial contraction occurs and results in a late "atrial kick" in the dimension time curve and accordingly in a late second peak of its first derivative.

The duration of the rapid filling phase is defined as the time interval from mitral valve opening to that point were the normalized lengthening rate decreased to 50% of its peak value (3). Similarly, the diameter at the end of the slow filling period just before the "atrial kick" is determined as that point, where the last second lengthening peak has reached half of its maximum. The

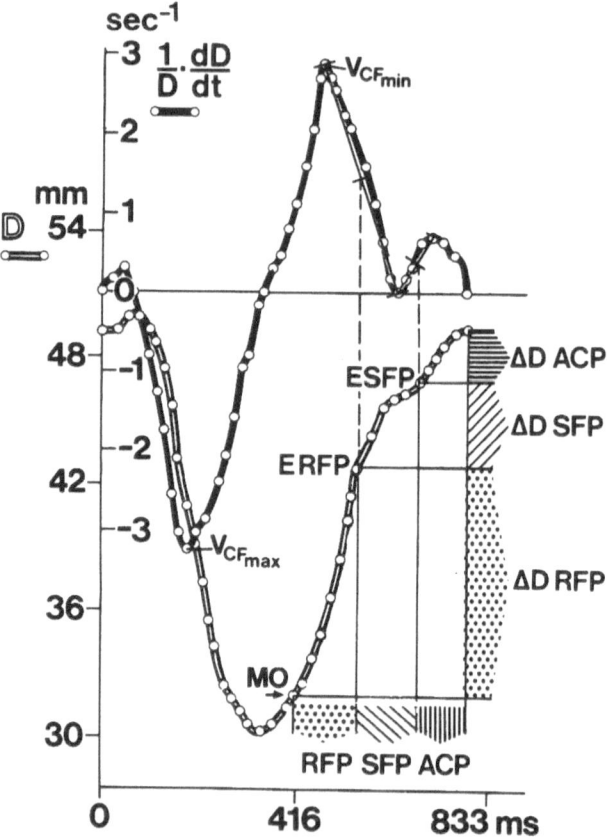

Fig. 1. Dimension-time curve of a normal subject with determination of the rapid (RFP), slow (SFP) and filling period due to atrial contraction (ACP). ΔD = dimension increase, ERFP = end-point of the rapid filling phase, ESFP = end-point of the slow filling period, $V_{CF\,max}$ = peak shortening rate, $V_{CF\,min}$ = peak lengthening rate, MO = mitral valve opening.

dimension increase due to atrial contraction is terminated by the beginning of the following heart cycle.

With this method of break-point determination the contribution of each of three phases of diastole to the total LV filling can be measured in terms of absolute or relative dimension and time changes resp.:

Table 1. Time and relative dimension change during the different phases of LV filling.

Rapid filling time:	$27 \pm 13\%$
Slow filling time:	$52 \pm 16\%$
Time of filling due to atrial contraction:	$20 \pm 18\%$
Dimension increase during rapid filling:	$62 \pm 10\%$
Dimension increase during slow filling:	$22 \pm 9\%$
Dimension increase during atrial contraction:	$16 \pm 10\%$

ABNORMAL LEFT VENTRICULAR RELAXATION

Abnormalities in isovolumic relaxation commonly occurs in patients with coronary heart disease. In patients with normal left ventricular function proven by angiography LV minimal dimension is synchronous with the onset of mitral valve opening. Gibson and co-workers have shown, that in patients with coronary artery disease and LV segmental wall motion abnormalities this close time relation between mitral valve and LV wall movement is lost as is shown in Figure 2 (7, 16). In this echogram of a patient with three-vessel-disease LV function at first sight appears to be good, with a satisfactory posterior wall movement and akinetic septal motion. However, it is apparent, from the mitral valve echo and the LV pressure trace, that virtually all the increase in LV dimension occurs before the onset of mitral valve opening and, therefore, before the onset of left ventricular filling. So the, apparently normal, increase in diastolic left ventricular dimension is no more than a shape change of the left ventricle during isovolumic relaxation. This means that, in this particular case, wall movement is abnormal with disturbed coordination between regional wall movement on one side, and mitral valve opening – as an index of the function of the whole left ventricle – on the other side. This method has proven very sensitive for detecting abnormalities of isovolumic relaxation in patients with coronary artery disease and correlated very closely with the presence of regional reduction in wall motion seen on angiography (4).

Abnormally prolonged left ventricular relaxation, defined as delayed mitral valve opening with regard to minimum left ventricular dimension, has also been reported in patients with severe primary or secondary left ventricular hypertrophy due to cardiomyopathy or chronic pressure overload (12). In comparison with normal subjects the dimension change during this time period was significantly increased (10–14%) and interpreted as an abnormal change of shape of the LV.

However, the onset of mitral valve opening is only one of several ways in

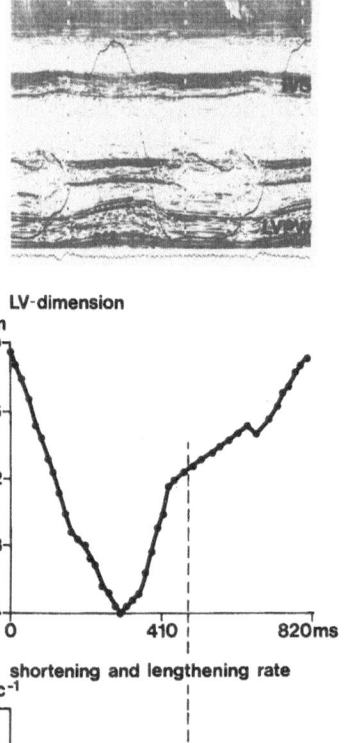

Fig. 2. Echogram of a patient with 3-vessel-disease and prolonged isovolumic relaxation. Delayed mitral valve opening (MO) with regard to end-systolic dimension or aortic valve closure.

which timing of the left ventricular function can be detected. Further evidence of abnormal isovolumic relaxation behaviour can be derived from disturbances in the relation between changes in LV dimension and high-fidelity pressure tracings in the left ventricle and the aorta. In normal subjects the shape of the loop is rectangular (Fig. 3), because, during isovolumic contraction and relaxation, the LV pressure changes at constant LV dimension (16). Similar results can be derived from simultaneous recordings of the left ventricular echo- and apexcardiogram (18). The simultaneous recording of the apexcardiogram is necessary in order to know the timing of aortic valve closure. Like the pressure-dimension loop, the relation between the

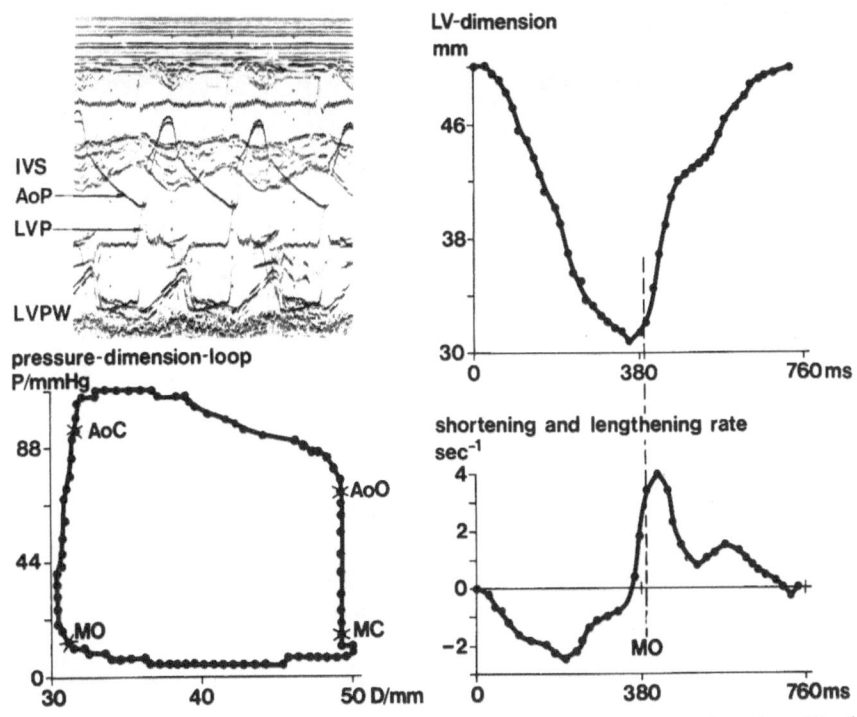

Fig. 3. Simultaneous LV echogram and pressure measurement in a normal subject. Nearly rectangular pressure – dimension – loop. Mitral valve opening (MO) follows immediately after minimal LV-dimension.

apexcardiogram and LV dimension can also be presented as a loop. Normally, 5–30% of total diastolic increase in dimension occurs during the down-stroke of the apexcardiogram. In patients with coronary artery disease, however, values well outside this range may be seen, with either a larger increase or a reduction in dimension (Fig. 4).

Recent investigations by Gibson and co-workers suggest, that the dimension decrease during LV relaxation is due to a regional increase in wall thickness caused by LV tension persisting, when the rest of the LV is already relaxing, whereas the abnormal increase of LV dimension during relaxation is due to regional reduction in wall thickness before the mitral valve opens (8).

ABNORMAL LEFT VENTRICULAR FILLING

The assessment of abnormal left ventricular filling is possible by analysis of the following: 1) peak LV lengthening rate; 2) left ventricular dimension change during the different phases of LV filling; 3) the time interval of the different periods of LV filling (3, 5). Each parameter alone, or in combination, has proven of clinical value in the detection of an abnormal LV filling pattern in patients with valvular heart disease, as well as in patients with LV dysfunction without valve motion abnormalities.

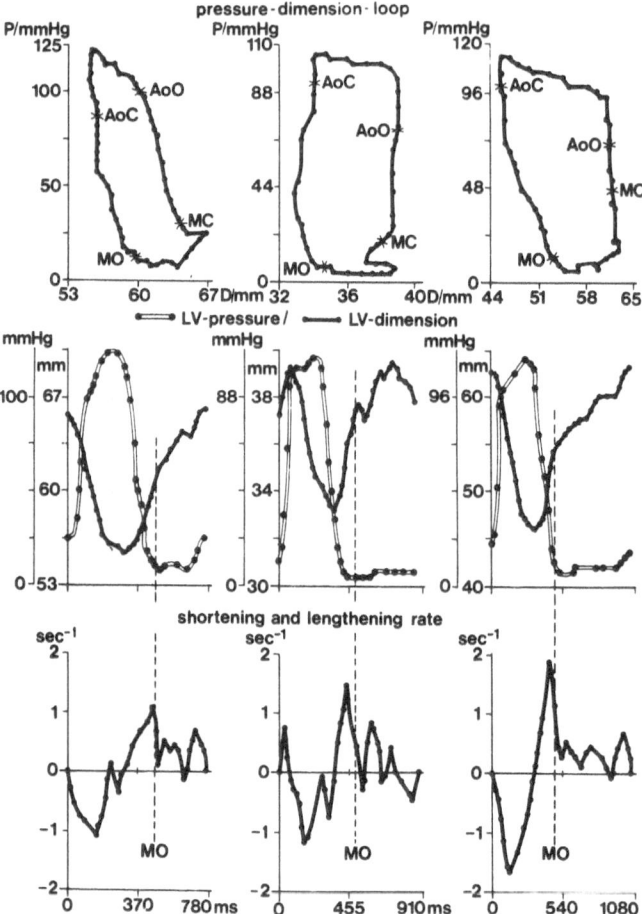

Fig. 4. Abnormal pressure dimension loops in 3 patients with ischemic heart disease. In all cases; peak LV lengthening rate precedes mitral valve opening (MO), MC = mitral valve closure, AoO = aortic valve opening, AoC = aortic valve closure.

In mitral stenosis the abnormal filling pattern is characterized by a reduction of the peak lengthening rate and a prolongation of the period of rapid diastolic filling. After successful mitral valve surgery (commissurotomy, prosthetic valve replacement) these abnormalities return to normal. The different types of valve protheses inserted in mitral position, display different filling patterns after cardiac surgery (15).

In contrast to patients with left ventricular inflow obstruction, the LV peak lengthening rate in patients with a significant left ventricular volume over-load (mitral insufficiency or aortic insufficiency) is preoperatively excessively increased and decreases markedly in the very early post-operative period (19) after successful cardiac surgery.

In the presence of left ventricular disease without primary valve dysfunction, left ventricular filling patterns can be also abnormal. In patients with hypertrophic obstructive cardiomyopathy, left ventricular systolic function is normal in the presence of an abnormal left ventricular diastolic function. Despite normal LV peak lengthening rates, the left ventricular filling pattern can be markedly disturbed, as has been shown by several investigations (11, 12, 14). In most patients with HOCM, LV rapid filling time as well as dimension increase during rapid filling are reduced, suggesting left ventricular inflow obstruction (Fig. 5).

This abnormal diastolic function is not however, specific for HOCM, as has been proved recently in our laboratory. The left ventricular filling pattern in patients with secondary LV hypertrophy due to chronic pressure overload (aortic stenosis, severe arterial hypertension) does not differ from that of patients with HOCM, and is thus not related to the specific morphological architecture only seen in patients with HOCM, as was previously suggested (10). In most patients with LV hypertrophy due to chronic pressure overload,

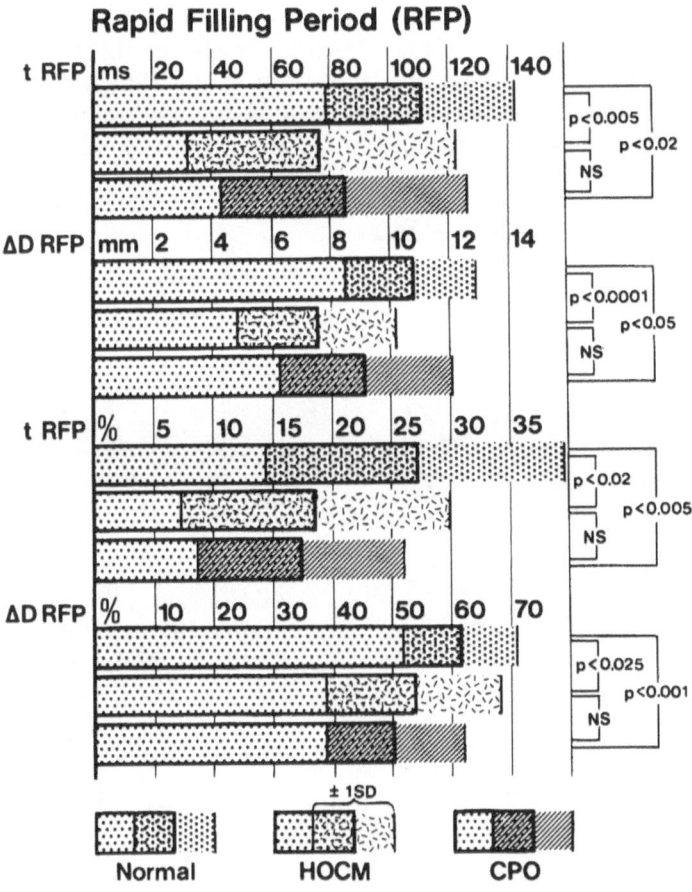

Fig. 5. Absolute and percentage dimension or time change during the rapid filling phase in normal subjects, patients with hypertrophic obstructive cardiomyopathy (HOCM) or chronic LV pressure overload (CPO).

the reduced dimension increase during the rapid filling phase can be compensated by a forceful atrial contraction with a significant greater dimension increase during atrial filling than in normal subjects (12).

Similar results – suggesting abnormal left ventricular diastolic properties despite normal left ventricular contraction – have been reported by Decoodt in patients with ischemic heart disease (2). In this study, the proportional change in diameter occurring during the rapid filling phase was reduced to a mean of 53% from one of 73% in normals, while that during atrial systole was increased to a mean of 32% as compared with 15% in normals.

Echocardiographic studies in patients treated with Adriamycin (mean dosage 360 mg/m^2) revealed that left ventricular systolic, as well as diastolic, function is disturbed when compared with normal subjects. Abnormal diastolic function is assessed by a reduced peak left ventricular lengthening rate together with relatively lower dimension increase during the rapid filling phase (Fig. 6) (13). It is suggested, that this abnormal diastolic filling pattern results from LV restriction due to an increase in LV stiffness, which might be caused by Adriamycin-associated degenerative changes in the LV.

These results reveal that the assessment of LV function by computer analysis of the M-mode echogram is a useful and reproduceable, non-invasive method of determining systolic and, especially, diastolic LV function in a quantitative manner.

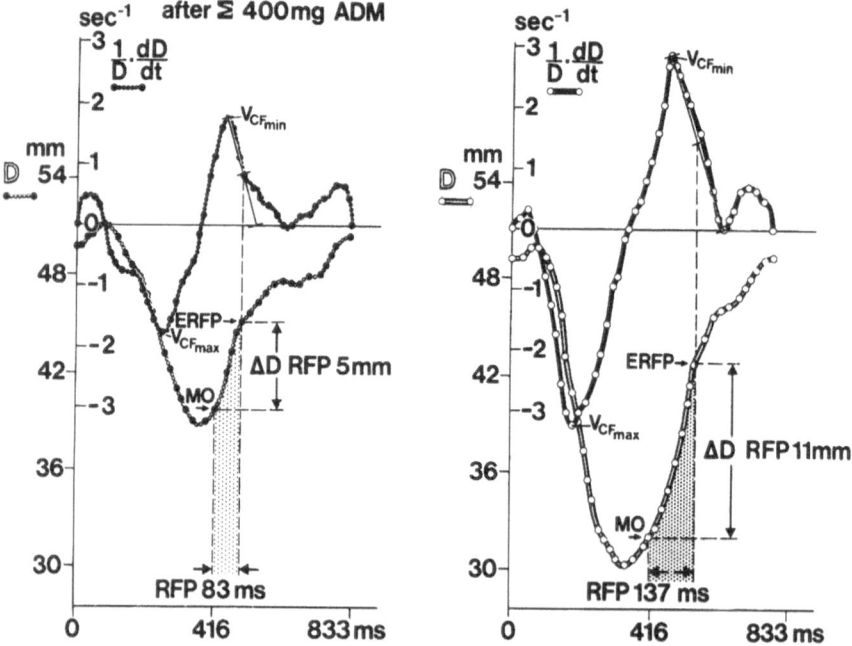

Fig. 6. Dimension-time curve of a normal subject and of a patient treated with Adriamycin (ADM). In the patient with ADM peak LV- shortening and lengthening rate are diminished. The rapid filling phase (RFP) is shorter with regard to the time interval and the dimension increase (ΔD) compared with a normal subject.

REFERENCES

1. Ahmad M, JE Sanderson, V Dubowitz, KA Hallidie-Smith: Echocardiographic assessment of left ventricular function in Duchenne's muscular dystrophy. Brit Heart J 4:734, 1978.
2. Decoodt PR, DG Mathey, HJC Swan: Abnormal left ventricular filling in coronary artery disease by automated analysis of echocardiograms. Circulation 52 II:133, 1975.
3. Decoodt PR, DG Mathey, HJC Swan: Automated analysis of the left-ventricular diameter time curve from echocardiographic recordings. Computers and Biomed Res 9:549, 1976.
4. Doran JH, TA Traill, DJ Brown, DG Gibson: Detection of abnormal left ventricular wall movement during isovolumic contraction and early relaxation. Comparison of echo- and angiocardiography Brit Heart J. 40:367, 1978.
5. Gibson DG, D Brown: Measurement of instantaneous left ventricular dimension and filling rate using echocardiography. Brit Heart J 35:1141, 1973.
6. Gibson DG, DJ Brown: Assessment of left ventricular systolic function in man from simultaneous echocardiographic and pressure measurements. Brit Heart J 38:8, 1976.
7. Gibson DG, TA Prewitt, DJ Brown: Analysis of left ventricular wall movement during isovolumic relaxation and its relation to coronary artery disease. Brit Heart J 38:1010, 1976.
8. Gibson DG, IH Dorau, TA Traill, DJ Brown: Regional abnormalities of left ventricular wall movement during isovolumic relaxation in patients with ischemic heart disease. Europ J Cardiol Suppl 7:251, 1978.
9. Prewitt TA, D Gibson, D Brown: The "rapid filling wave" of the apex cardiogram. Its relation to echocardiographic and cineangiographic measurements of ventricular filling. Brit Heart J 37:1256, 1975.
10. Sanderson JE, D Gibson, DJ Brown, JF Goodwin: Left ventricular filling in hypertrophic cardiomyopathy. An angiographic study. Brit Heart J 39:661, 1977.
11. Sanderson JE, TA Traill, MG St. J. Sutton, DJ Brown, DG Gibson, JF Goodwin: Left ventricular relaxation and filling in hypertrophic cardiomyopathy. An echocardiographic study. Brit Heart J 40:596, 1978.
12. Siegert R, P Hanrath, W Bleifeld, W Kupper, D Mathey: Abnormal relaxation and diastolic filling pattern in different forms of LV hypertrophy. Circulation 58, II:195, 1978.
13. Stein E, P Hanrath, W Bleifeld, M Garbrecht, M Müllerleile: Abnormes Kontraktions- und Füllverhalten des linken Ventrikels bei Tumorpatienten unter Adriamycin-Therapie. DMW 103:1408, 1978.
14. St. J. Sutton MG, AJ Tajik, DG Gibson, DJ Brown, JB Seward, ER Giuliani: Echocardiographic assessment of left ventricular filling and septal and posterior wall dynamics in idiopathic hypertrophic subaortic stenosis. Circulation 57:512, 1978.
15. St. J. Sutton MG, J Traill, AS Ghafour: Echocardiographic assessment of left ventricular filling after mitral valve surgery. Brit Heart J 39:1283, 1977.
16. Upton MT, DG Gibson, DJ Brown: Echocardiographic assessment of abnormal left ventricular relaxation in man. Brit Heart J 38:1001, 1976.
17. Upton MT DG Gibson: The study of left ventricular function from digitized echocardiograms. Progress in Cardiovasc Diseases XX, 5, 3/4, 1978.
18. Venco A, DG Gibson, DJ Brown: Relation between apex cardiogram and changes in left ventricular pressure and dimension. Brit Heart J 39:117, 1977.
19. Venco A, M St. J. Sutton, D Gibson: Non-invasive assessment of left ventricular function after correction of severe aortic regurgitation. Brit Heart J 38:1324, 1977.

CORRELATIONS BETWEEN AORTIC ROOT MOTION AND LEFT ATRIAL VOLUME CHANGES

G. BIAMINO, H.J. WESSEL, W. SCHLAG, and R. SCHRÖDER

The typical motion of the anterior and posterior wall of the aortic root in the direction of the anterior chest wall was recently correlated to the left ventricular stroke volume (6, 7). In contrast to this hypothesis, when analysing the pattern of motion of the Björk-Shiley aortic valve prosthesis it was noted that the closure movement of the tilting disc always precedes the end of the forward motion of the aortic root. We have, therefore, attempted to correlate the motion of this structure with other echocardiographic parameters.

Our conclusions are similar to those reported by Strunk et al. (9) and indicate that the pattern of the aortic root during the heart cycle reflects changes in volume of the left atrium.

METHOD

The studies were carried out on 82 patients (10 to 68 years, average age 54 years). In 50 cases there was no sign of aortic or mitral valve disease. In 32 patients the echocardiograms were recorded after implantation of aortic and/or mitral valve prosthesis (Björk-Shiley tilting disc valve). The M-mode echocardiograph unit was manufactured by Organon Teknika. The ultrasound frequency was 2.25 MHz. The parameters were recorded by a strip chart system (Honeywell) with chart speeds of 25, 50 and 100 mm/sec.

RESULTS

In patients in sinus rhythm who have a Björk-Shiley prosthesis in the aortic position, it is normally possible to identify six points in the echo pattern of the aortic root. The tracings of Figure 1 show that the motion of the aortic root in the direction of the anterior chest wall continues beyond closure of the tilting disc (point 3). The posteriorly directed aortic root motion (point 4) starts after the second heart sound. The steepness of the echoes of the aortic root is maximal between point 4 and 5. Between point 5 and 6 a plateau occurs, then the posterior motion accelerates again until point 1 is reached. The course of the curve between point 1 and 2 (opening of the valve) is horizontal, whereby a small wave at the first part of the first heart sound can occasionally be noted.

Charles T. Lancée (ed.), Echocardiology, 147–152. All rights reserved
Copyright © 1979 by Martinus Nijhoff Publishers bv, The Hague/Boston/London

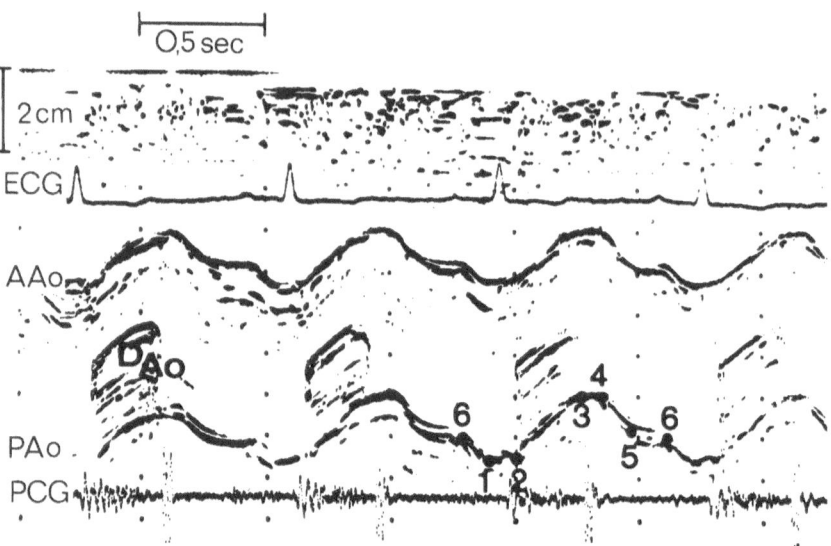

Fig. 1. Echograms of tilting Björk-Shiley valve prosthesis in aortic position. 1–6 characteristic points in the cyclical aortic root configuration. ECG: electrocardiogram, PCG: Phonocardiogram, AAo and PAo: anterior and posterior wall of the aortic root, D_{Ao}: tilting disc in the opened position.

As Figure 2 demonstrates, in some cases it was possible to record the echoes of the prosthetic tilting disc and the echoes of the normal mitral valve (DE) simultaneously. The end of the rapid filling phase is represented by point 5. The posteriorly directed motion of the aortic root from point 6 to point 1 is concomitant with the reopening movement of the anterior leaflet of the mitral valve, reflecting the left atrial contraction. This dorsally directed motion of the aortic root (from point 6 to 1) is absent in the presence of atrial fibrillation (Fig. 4), a fact also observed by other authors (3, 7, 8).

These findings indicate that the motion of the posterior wall of the aortic root is consistent with its anatomical juxtaposition and due to the dorsally directed contraction of the anterior left atrial wall. Consequently, the parallel movement of the anterior wall of the aortic root should be regarded as purely passive and only influenced by volume changes of the left atrium, independent of the course of ventricular contraction. Therefore, patients with AV-block III° were studied (Fig. 3).

Figure 3b shows that the atrial contraction influences the pattern of the anterior mitral leaflet only during the ventricular diastole. During the ventricular systole (P wave no. 4 and 6) the atrial contraction does not change the echo pattern of the mitral valve. In contrast, regardless of the phase of the ventricular cycle the left atrial contractions induce a posterior displacement of the aortic root (Fig. 3a).

Furthermore, in patients with ventricular extrasystoles (Fig. 4) the anterior displacement of the aortic root occurs independently from the opening of the

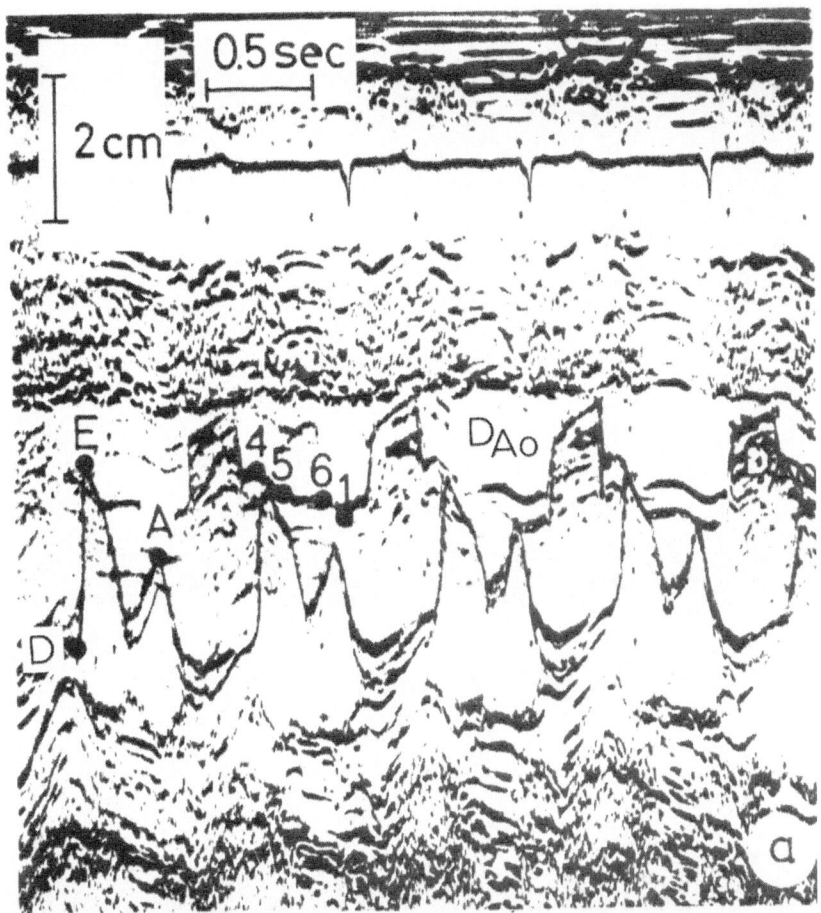

Fig. 2. Echogram of the tilting disc of the aortic valve prosthesis simultaneously with the anterior leaflet (D–E–A) of the mitral valve.

tilting disc, so that the ventral motion of the aortic root probably reflects only the antegrade, pressure passive flow from the pulmonary system into the left atrium.

DISCUSSION

The continuance of the anterior motion of the aortic root beyond aortic valve closure has been documented in several papers without particular comments (1, 2, 3, 4, 5). The echo pattern of the aortic root was subdivided simply into a systolic movement towards the anterior thorax wall and a diastolic dorsally-directed movement. With the exception of the pre-systolic posteriorly-directed displacement of the aortic root, every movement of this structure was related to the contraction course of the left ventricle.

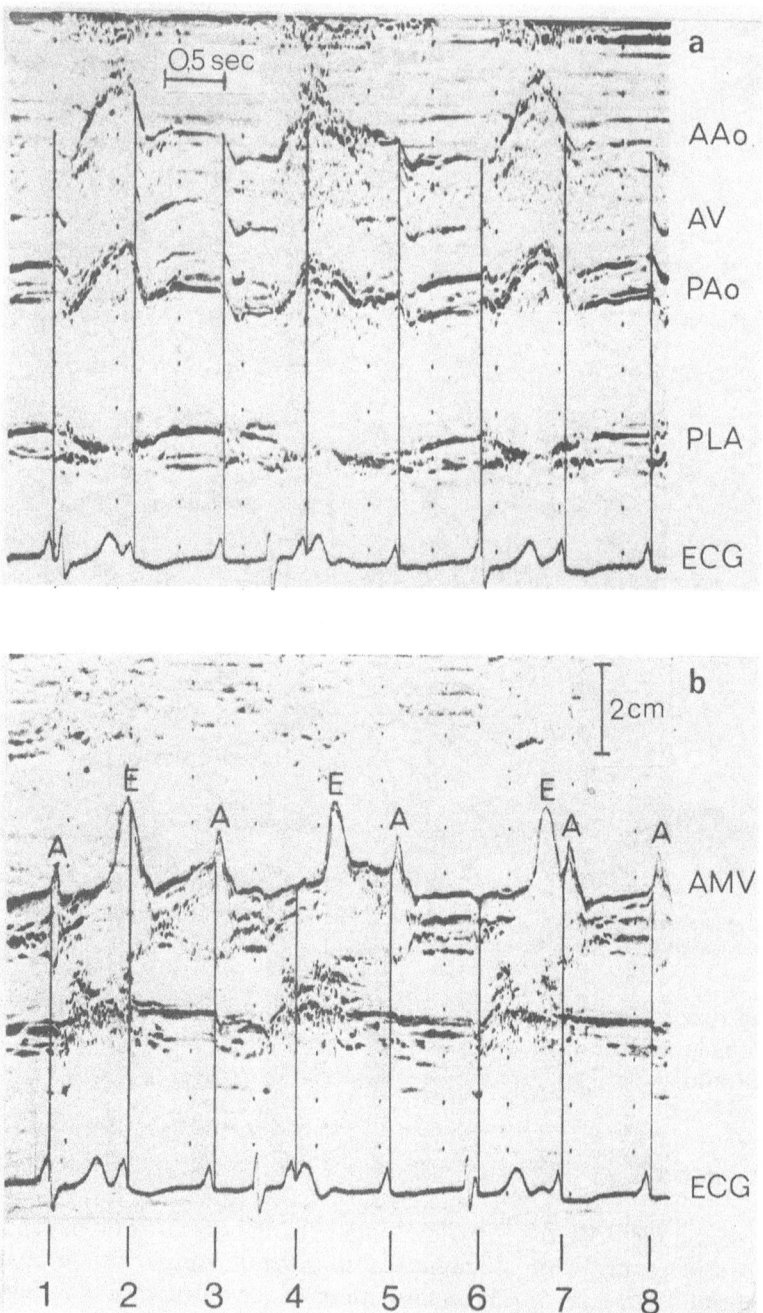

Fig. 3. Continuous echogram of the aortic root and the mitral valve superimposed in order to demonstrate the influence of atrial contraction on these two structures in the case of AV-block III°.

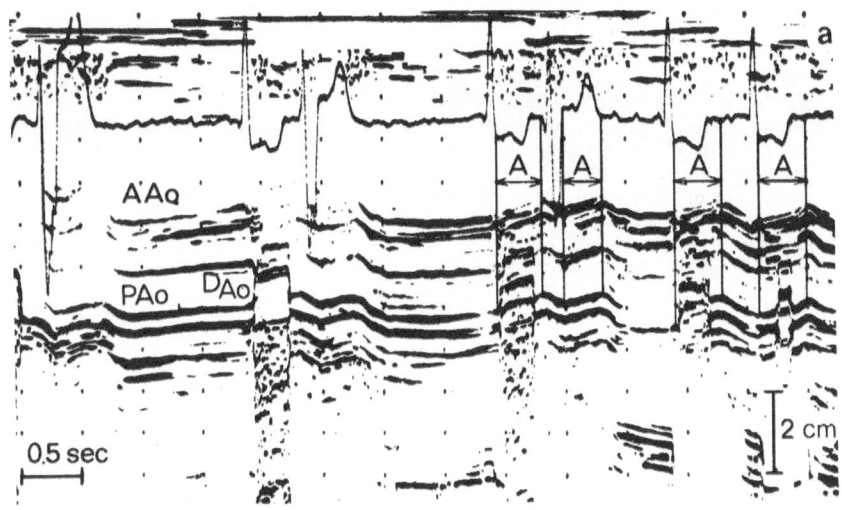

Fig. 4. Echogram of a Björk-Shiley prosthesis in the aortic position in the case of atrial fibrillation and ventricular extrasystoles.

Note that the systolic motion of the aortic valve is ventrally directed, even after an extrasystole without opening of the tilting disc. The duration of this movement (A) is influenced only little by the left ventricular ejection period.

The results presented indicate that the diastolic pattern of the aortic root is induced by the left atrium emptying into the left ventricle. Confirming the results of Strunk et al. (9), in concomitance with the opening movement of the mitral valve, the aortic root moves posteriorly (point 4) until the end of the rapid filling phase of the left ventricle (point 5). The subsequent period reflects the slow filling period. At point 6 the posterior directed movement of the aortic root accelerates again until point 1 following the left atrial contraction.

The following findings do not support the hypothesis that amplitude and duration of the anterior movement of the aortic root may be directly correlated to the ejection volume of the left ventricle: 1. The posterior wall of the left atrium moves dorsally simultaneously with the anterior displacement of the aortic root; 2. The slope of the aortic root is completely independent of the time course of the left ventricular ejection, and of the maximal aortic flow; 3. On the other hand, the aortic root demonstrates a posterior motion during atrial systole, independent from the left ventricular contraction state (Fig. 2). 4. Finally, the ventrally-directed motion of the aortic root also takes place to nearly the same degree in the case of ventricular extrasystoles without opening of the aortic valve (Fig. 4).

These findings indicate that the anterior root movement may be an expression of the left atrial filling during ventricular systole.

In conclusion, our echograms show that the aortic root motion during the heart cycle is indirectly related to the ejection capacity of the left ventricle since the pattern is influenced by changes in volume of the left atrium.

REFERENCES

1. Gramiak R et al.: Investigate Radiology 3:358, 1968.
2. Gramiak R et al.: Radiology 96:1, 1970.
3. Feigenbaum H: Echocardiography, 2nd edition, Philadelphia, Pa., Lea & Febiger, 1976.
4. Feizi Ô et al.: Brit Heart J 36:341, 1974.
5. Francis GS et al.: Brit Heart J 37:376, 1975.
6. Gehrke J et al.: Z Kardiol Suppl 2:47, 1975.
7. Pratt RC et al.: Circulation 53:947, 1976.
8. Weyman AE et al.: Circulation 50:905, 1974.
9. Strunk BL et al.: Circulation 54:744, 1976.

ABNORMAL MITRAL VALVE MOTION, SEPTAL HYPERTROPHY AND LEFT VENTRICULAR OUTFLOW TRACT OBSTRUCTION: ECHOCARDIOGRAPHIC AND HAEMODYNAMIC STUDY IN HYPERTROPHIC OBSTRUCTIVE CARDIOMYOPATHY

G. DROBINSKI, M. EUGÈNE, J.I. EVANS, and Y. GROSGOGEAT

Abnormal movement of the mitral valve observed in patients with hypertrophic obstructive cardiomyopathy (HOCM) consists of variable degrees of systolic anterior motion (SAM) towards the interventricular septum and has been recognized by angiography and echocardiography. Several explanations of its mechanism have been suggested: abnormal insertion of the anterior mitral leaflet (1), malposition of the papillary muscles (2), posterior displacement of the mitral annulus by septal hypertrophy (3) and venturi effect due to the high speed of ejection in the left ventricular outflow tract (4). A close correlation between SAM and the intraventricular pressure gradient has been demonstrated and SAM is also thought to play a part in the mechanism of mitral incompetence, the incidence of which increases with the severity of the disease (5).

The aim of this study was to define the relationship between SAM and left ventricular outflow tract obstruction and to assess the practical consequences. To this end, the results of haemodynamic investigation in 24 patients with characteristic echocardiograms of HOCM were reviewed.

MATERIAL AND METHODS

The series comprised 16 men and 8 women whose ages ranged from 27 to 72 years. The echocardiographic diagnosis of HOCM was based on the criteria established by Henry (6).
- Septal hypertrophy with end diastolic thickness: ≥ 15 mm.
- Septal/posterior wall thickness ratio: ≥ 1.3.
- The presence of SAM under basal conditions or after pharmacodynamic stress testing.

In our series SAM was observed in 13 patients under basal conditions, to a moderate degree in 5 patients but with complete apposition of septal and mitral echos in 8 patients. In the other 11 patients SAM was absent at rest but could be induced by intravenous infusion of Isoprenaline at a rate of 4 γ/mn. Betablocker therapy was stopped 48 hours before echocardiography and cardiac catheterization was carried out within 24 hours of echocardiography. In 15 patients the haemodynamic study was completed by an external carotid pulse recording from which the left ventricular ejection period, corrected for heart rate was calculated.

RESULTS

Four groups of patients were defined according to the intraventricular pressure gradient recorded during cardiac catheterization under basal conditions and after pharmacodynamic stimulation.

The deformation of the left ventricular cavity, indices of free wall function and results of external carotid pulse recording varied from group to group but septal hypokinesis was observed in all patients with a reduced systolic thickening. (average $14 \pm 8\%$).

Table 1. Results of cardiac catheterization.

Group	N	Rest	P stimulation	SAM rest	SI (ml/syst/m2)	LVEDP (mm Hg)	Age (yrs)
1	4	0	0	1/4	43 ± 12	27 ± 13	52 ± 10
2	10	0	95 ± 26	5/10	45 ± 8	10 ± 7	47 ± 13
3	6	48 ± 8	75 ± 4	4/6	47.5 ± 5.5	18 ± 5	44 ± 12
4	4	147 ± 5	–	4/4	41.5 ± 4	21 ± 8	63 ± 8

P: Left intraventricular pressure gradient.
SI: Systolic index
LVEDP: Left ventricular end-diastolic pressure.

Group I

Echocardiography showed the left ventricular cavities of patients in this group to be small (end diastolic diameter (DD) = 37 ± 3 mm). Moderate septal hypertrophy was associated with hypertrophy and hypo-kinesis of the posterior wall (end-diastolic posterior wall thickness: PWT = 15 ± 2 mm; posterior wall systolic thickening: PWST = $37 \pm 16\%$). Corrected left ventricular ejection periods calculated in 3 of these 4 patients were subnormal at rest ($92 \pm 9\%$), increased after Amyl-nitrite in 1 patient (108%) and decreased in the other two (85%).

Group II and III

The morphology of the left ventricle in patients in these two groups was similar, with a moderate reduction in the size of the left ventricular cavity (DD = 45 ± 8 mm). Moderate septal hypertrophy (SWT = 22 ± 5 mm) was associated with a normal posterior wall (PWT = 10 ± 4 mm; PWST =

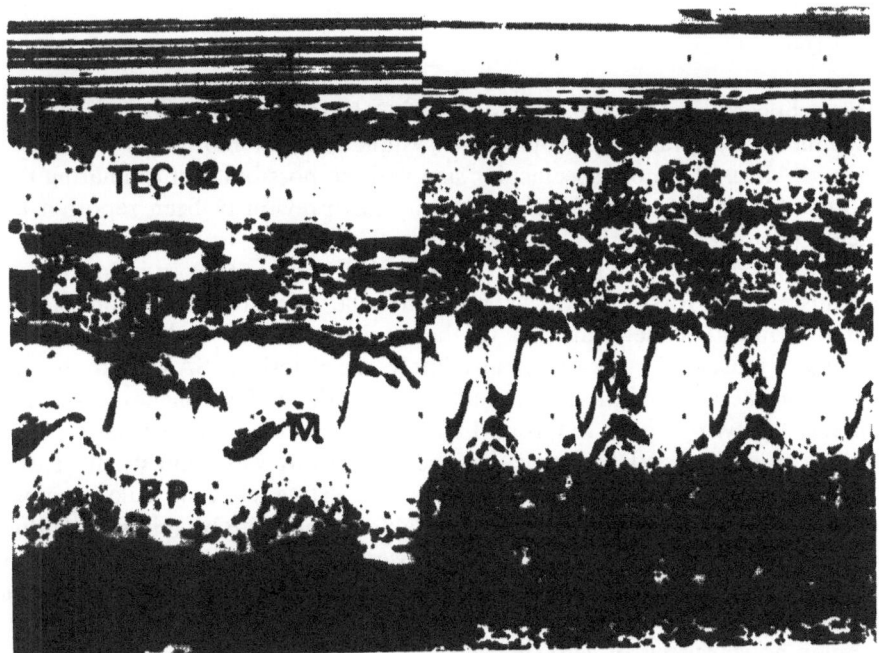

Fig. 1. SAM induced by intravenous infusion of Isoprenaline in a patient with no recordable intraventricular pressure gradient. The left ventricular ejection period decreased after inhalation of Amylnitrite.

$88 \pm 22\%$). Left ventricular ejection periods were normal or slightly increased at rest ($100 \pm 6\%$) and increased significantly in 10 out of 11 cases after Amylnitrite ($110 \pm 6\%$). An interesting finding was the inability to reproduce SAM after beta-blockade in 3 out of 4 patients in whom SAM, absent under basal conditions, had previously been induced by pharmacodynamic stimulation.

Group IV

The patients in this group had small left ventricular cavities ($DD = 35 \pm 4$ mm) and septal hypertrophy was severe ($SWT = 29 \pm 2.5$ mm). The posterior wall was also hypertrophied ($PWT = 16 \pm 4$ mm) but PWST was normal ($74 \pm 5\%$). Betablockade had no effect on the systolic motion of the mitral valve.

Two of these patients underwent myomectomy. Post-operatively the SAM and intraventricular pressure gradient completely regressed in one patient; in the other SAM was reduced and the gradient disappeared. Echocardiography also showed persistant mid-systolic closure of the aortic valves and unchanged parietal hypertrophy. The left ventricular ejection period decreased from 105 to 95%. The ventricular volumes, ejection fractions and indices of left ventricular performance remained unchanged but LVEDP was reduced from 25 to 8 mm Hg.

DISCUSSION

The echocardiographic diagnosis of HOCM depends on the presence of asymmetrical septal hypertrophy and systolic anterior motion of the mitral valve. SAM is the most spectacular sign and the possibility of estimating the intraventricular gradient from its severity has previously been reported by Henry (6).

However, an approach which takes this sign into account in isolation can be misleading. Firstly, SAM is not only due to anterior motion of the anterior mitral leaflet but also to the cordae tendinae and the posterior papillary muscle (7). Secondly, absolutely characteristic SAMs can be recorded in the absence of an intraventricular gradient. This phenomenon was observed in two patients in Group I after pharmacodynamic stimulation. The finding of decreased left ventricular ejection periods was against left ventricular outflow tract obstruction. Analysis of selective left ventricular angiography showed ventricular ejection to be almost complete by mid-systole due to the inotropic stimulation, and there were no angiographic signs of left ventricular outflow tract obstruction. The final diagnosis in these cases was not that of HOCM but of hypertrophic cardiomyopathy without obstruction. Similar appearances of left ventricular ejection with SAM and no intraventricular gradient have been reproduced experimentally with inotropic stimulation in the dog (8). The persistance of SAM and mid-systolic closure of the aortic valves on post-operative echocardiography in the absence of an intraventricular gradient may be explained by this type of left ventricular

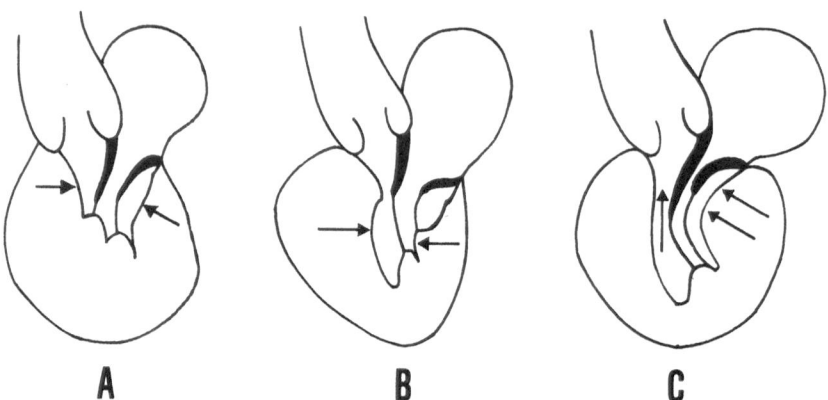

A   **B**   **C**

Fig. 2. Mechanisms of SAM.
(a):   SAM due to malposition of the papillary muscle: Obstruction due to the anterior mitral leaflet.
(b):   SAM due to apposition of the papillary muscle and interventricular septum in the mid zone
        of the ventricle.
(c):   SAM due to the energetic contraction of the posterior wall with rapid ventricular ejection.

ejection inducing SAM by the Venturi effect. This phenomenon is closely related to the quality of myocardial contraction, especially that of the posterior wall. When PWST is reduced SAM does not occur at rest and may only be induced by pharmacodynamic stimulation (Fig. 2).

From a practical point of view it is important to compare the results of echocardiography, external carotid pulse recording and cardiac catheterization in each case, in order to avoid false positive diagnosis of HOCM based on typical echocardiographic appearances after pharmacodynamic stimulation.

However, it must be emphasized that when SAM is present under basal conditions or with beta-blockade it is usually a sign of a severe form of HOCM. It is most obvious in the cases with high intraventricular gradients and severe septal hypertrophy (Group IV). Those forms with the highest gradients also have hypertrophy of the posterior wall, which nevertheless contracts normally. When posterior wall hypertrophy reaches a certain degree the percentage systolic thickening decreases. This may reflect extension of the morphological abnormalities of the interventricular septum to the posterior wall of the left ventricle (9, 10): reduced interventricular gradients and left ventricular ejection periods may then be observed (11). Finally, the fact that ventricular deformation is a major factor in the production of SAM and outflow tract obstruction is illustrated by regression of SAM after myomectomy.

The presence of SAM under basal conditions is an important sign and may be an additional argument in favour of surgical management in patients with moderate pressure gradients but who, in fact, have severe outflow tract obstruction. It signals the progression of the disease to a state of decreased ventricular compliance which is, in itself, a more significant sign of the severity of the disease than the intraventricular pressure gradient, which may vary with the haemodynamic conditions during catheterization.

REFERENCES

1. Bjork VO, G. Hultquist, H Lodin: Subaortic stenosis produced by an abnormally placed anterior mitral leaflet. J Thorac Cardiovasc Surg 41:659, 1961.
2. King JF, RL Reis, MR Bolton: Superior to inferior septal hypertrophy in IHSS. The fundamental determinant of obstruction. Circulation 47 (sup-IV): 6, 1973.
3. Calazel P, J Tricoire, JP Douzeau, P Bernadet: Etude angiographique des myocardiopathies obstructives. Essai d'evaluation du rôle du septum interventriculaire et de la grande valve mitrale dans le phenomene obstructif. Arch Mal Coeur 69:229, 1976.
4. Henry WL, CE Clark, SE Epstein: Mechanism of outflow obstruction in IHSS. Circulation 47 (sup-IV): 177, 1973.
5. Wigle ED, AG Adelman, P Auger, Y Marquis: Mitral regurgitation in muscular subaortic stenosis. Amer J Cardiol 24:698, 1969.
6. Henry WL, CE Clark, SE Epstein: Asymmetric septal hypertrophy. Circulation 47:225, 1973.
7. Rodgers JC: Motion of mitral apparatus in hypertrophic cardiomyopathy with obstruction. Brit Heart J 38:792, 1976.

8. Burford TH, AF Hartmann, TB Ferguson, RW Ferrier: The production of muscular subaortic stenosis in dogs. J Thorac Cardiovasc Surg 54:639, 1967.
9. Grossman W, LP McLaurin, JP Moss, HA Stefadouros, DT Young: Wall thickness and diastolic properties of the left ventricle. Circulation 49:129, 1974.
10. Maron BJ: Distribution of myocardial cellular defects in ASH. Differences between patients with and patients without outflow obstruction. Ann Int Med 81:669, 1974.
11. Witchitz S, JP Binet, B Philippe, A Senekies, P Chiche: Traitement d'une CMO par myotomie chez un sujet de 67 ans. Arch Mal Coeur 69:783, 1976.

ECHO-PRESSURES RELATIONSHIP BEFORE
AND AFTER HEMODYNAMIC CHANGES

ALLESANDRO GIAMBARTOLOMEI, TASSILO BONZEL,
PAOLO ESENTE, and GOFFREDO G. GENSINI

In the last few years, echocardiography has been applied to the evaluation of patients with ischemic heart disease.

Special attention has been directed to the study of left ventricular function. Ventricular dimensions and their changes are established parameters of left ventricular performance (1–4). E-F mitral valve slope and A-C interval are thought to provide information about left ventricular diastolic pressures and compliance (5–7). In this study, attention is focused on mitral valve motion parameters and left atrial dimensions since these data are easily obtainable and readily reproducible.

All tracings were recorded simultaneously with left ventricular pressures at rest and after acute hemodynamic intervention to verify the specificity and sensitivity of established echocardiographic indices and to assess new ones.

MATERIALS AND METHODS

Our patient population consisted of 25 males (age 21–70 years, mean 50.8 years) undergoing diagnostic cardiac catheterization. Twenty two patients had ischemic heart disease with significant narrowing ($>75\%$ diameter reduction) of at least one major coronary vessel and 3 had a normal cardiovascular system. In all patients, a good echographic tracing of the mitral valve, aortic root and left atrium could be easily recorded. Patients with valvular abnormalities, hypertension or ventricular aneurysm were excluded.

Echocardiograms were obtained in $30°$ left decubitus utilizing an Irex echocardiograph with a 10 mm, 2.25 mHz unfocused transducer. Tracings were recorded on an Irex Continutrace 101 multichannel recorder. High fidelity left ventricular pressures (Millar tip-transducer catheter) were recorded simultaneously at 100 mm/sec before and after left ventriculography (ANGIO) (35/50 ml Renografin 76) and sublingual nitroglycerin (TNG) (0.6 mg).

The following parameters were considered: left ventricular initial diastolic pressure (LVIDP), left ventricular end-diastolic pressure (LVEDP), atrial component of the end-diastolic pressure or atrial kick (AK), mitral valve A-C interval, AC "notch", PR minus AC interval (PR-AC) and maximal left atrial dimension (LADmax).

RESULTS

At baseline, mean LVIDP, LVEDP and AK were 7.5 ± 2.8, 15.4 ± 5.3 and 5.2 ± 3.2 mm Hg, respectively. AC interval ranged from 70 to 140 msec (mean 95 msec) and PR interval from 140 to 200 msec (mean 158 msec). Mean PR-AC was 65 ± 15 msec. A PR-AC interval ≤ 60 msec was found in 5 of 8 patients (62%) with LVEDP > 18 mm Hg and in 6 out of 17 patients (35%) with LVEDP < 18 mm Hg. An AC "notch" was observed in 7 patients: in 5 of them LVEDP was > 18 mm Hg.

Mean LADmax was 36 ± 4.7 mm, with a fair positive correlation with LVEDP ($r = 0.71$). Whenever LADmax exceeded 40 mm Hg (7 cases), LVEDP was > 18 mm Hg. When LADmax was below 40 mm (18 cases), LVEDP was < 18 mm Hg in 17 cases (1 false negative). (Fig. 1).

No good correlation was found between LVIDP, AK, and the echocardiographic parameters considered.

All left ventricular diastolic pressures rose significantly after ANGIO ($p < 0.001$) and decreased after TNG ($p < 0.001$).

LADmax exhibited a similar behavior after both interventions (p < 0.01, baseline – ANGIO; p < 0.001, ANGIO – TNG).

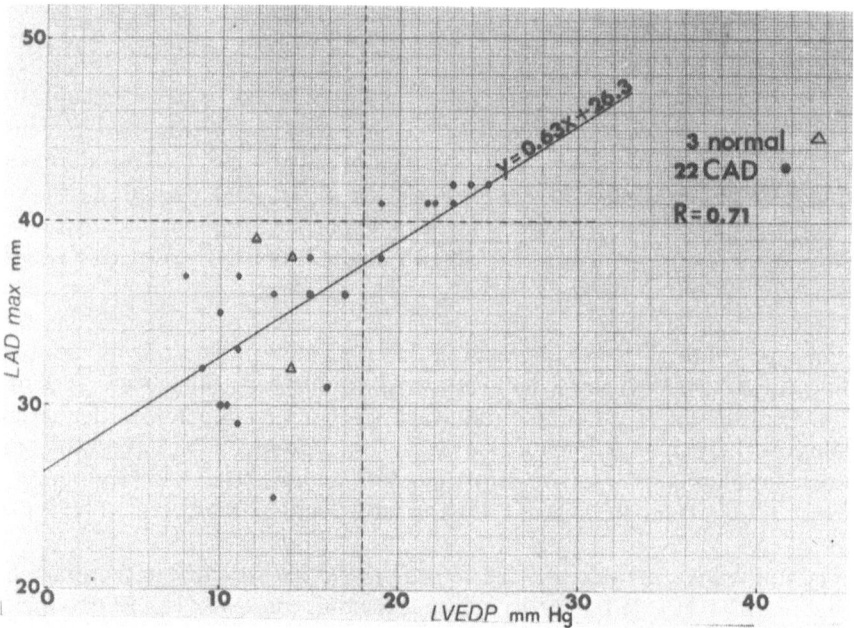

Fig. 1. Relationship between maximal left atrial dimensions (LADmax) on the ordinate and the left ventricular end-diastolic pressure (LVEDP) on the abscissa in our group of patients. The correlation coefficient and regression equation are shown. The dashed lines drawn from an LVEDP of 18 mm Hg and LADmax of 40 mm separate patients with large left atrium and high LVEDP. No false positive (upper left quadrant) and only 1 negative (lower right quadrant) were found.

The 8 patients with LVEDP > 18 mm Hg showed no or minimal change in LADmax following ANGIO.

AC and PR intervals widened significantly after ANGIO and decreased after TNG (p <0.001 and <0.005, respectively). Consequently, PR-AC interval showed changes of questionable significance after ANGIO (p <0.1) and TNG (p <0.05).

After ANGIO, the presence of AC "notch" was observed in 16 patients (LVEDP range 19–42 mm Hg). AC "notch" was never seen after TNG.

DISCUSSION

Feigenbaum and co-workers (7) found that delayed mitral valve closure (increased PR-AC interval) was a good indicator of elevated LVEDP. This early work was performed on patients with valvular heart disease receiving digitalis. Later studies failed to find a correlation between PR-AC and LVEDP in patients with ischemic heart disease (8–10). There is general agreement, however, that an AC "notch" is a fairly reliable indicator of increased LVEDP (11).

In this group, utilizing an arbitrary PR-AC value ≤ 60 msec as indicator of LVEDP ≥ 18 mm Hg, we found a high incidence of both false negatives and positives, even when the atrial component of LVEDP was considered. Similarly, the correlation between AC "notch" and LVEDP was not satisfactory, but, because of the small size of the group, statistical evaluation was not possible. After ANGIO, however, the incidence of AC "notch" exhibited a more than twofold increase as compared to baseline and in no instance was an AC "notch" observed after TNG. Therefore, after acute pressure changes in both directions, AC "notch" becomes a reliable indicator of LVEDP.

The hemodynamic modifications produced by contrast material and TNG shifted both PR and AC intervals in the same direction. Since the atrioventricular conduction and the echographic representation of mitral valve closure may be influenced separately in the course of acute hemodynamic intervention, the significance of PR-AC interval under these circumstances is altered.

Contrast material injection increases pre-load and most likely decreases left ventricular compliance. This results in impaired late ventricular filling and AC "notch" appears to be its echocardiographic manifestation (12). Furthermore, since TNG exerts opposite action upon left ventricular filling pressure, the absence of AC "notch" after TNG seems to offer further support to this interpretation.

In this group of patients, a fair correlation between LADmax and LVEDP was found. Most authors consider an LADmax of 40 mm or less to be normal (1, 13). All our patients with an enlarged left atrium had an elevated LVEDP (over 18 mm Hg). Only 1 patient had a high LVEDP and a normal left atrium. However, in this particular case, both values were borderline, 19 mm Hg and 38 mm, respectively.

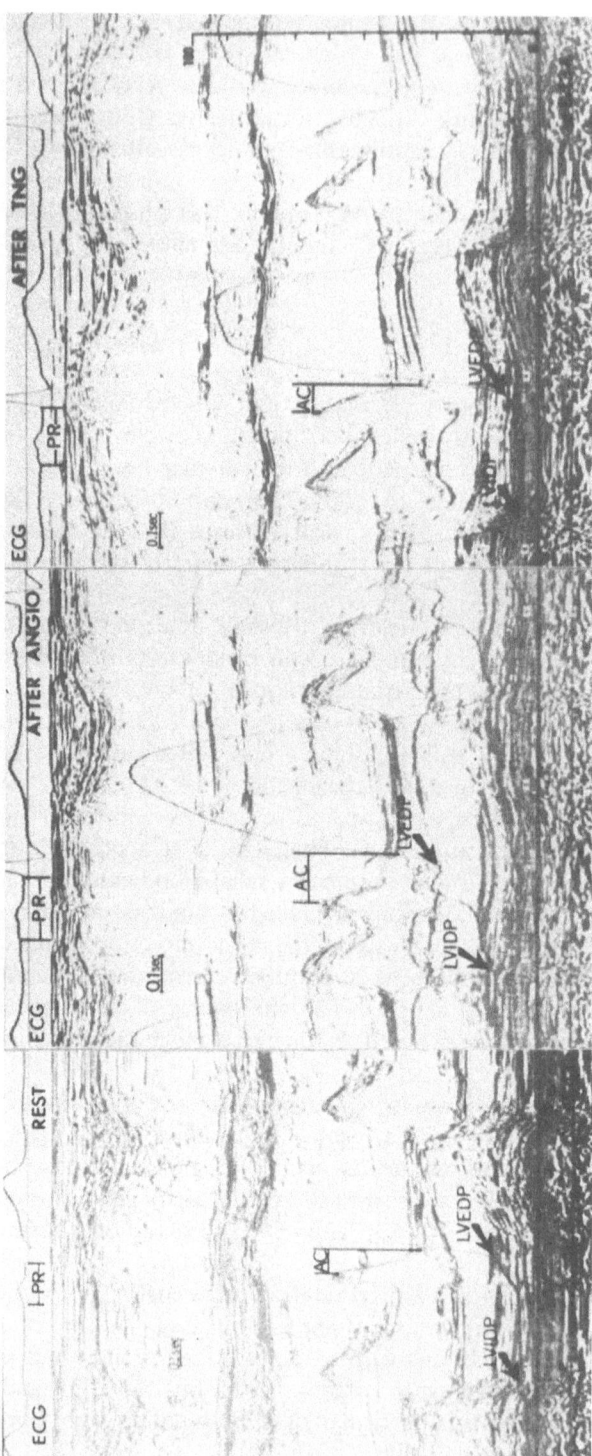

Fig. 2. Echogram of the mitral valve recorded simultaneously with left ventricular pressure in a patient with severe ischemic heart disease, at rest, after ventriculography and after nitroglycerin. LVEDP and PR-AC intervals were normal at rest, changed significantly after ventriculography and returned to normal after TNG. An evident AC "notch" was present only after angiography.

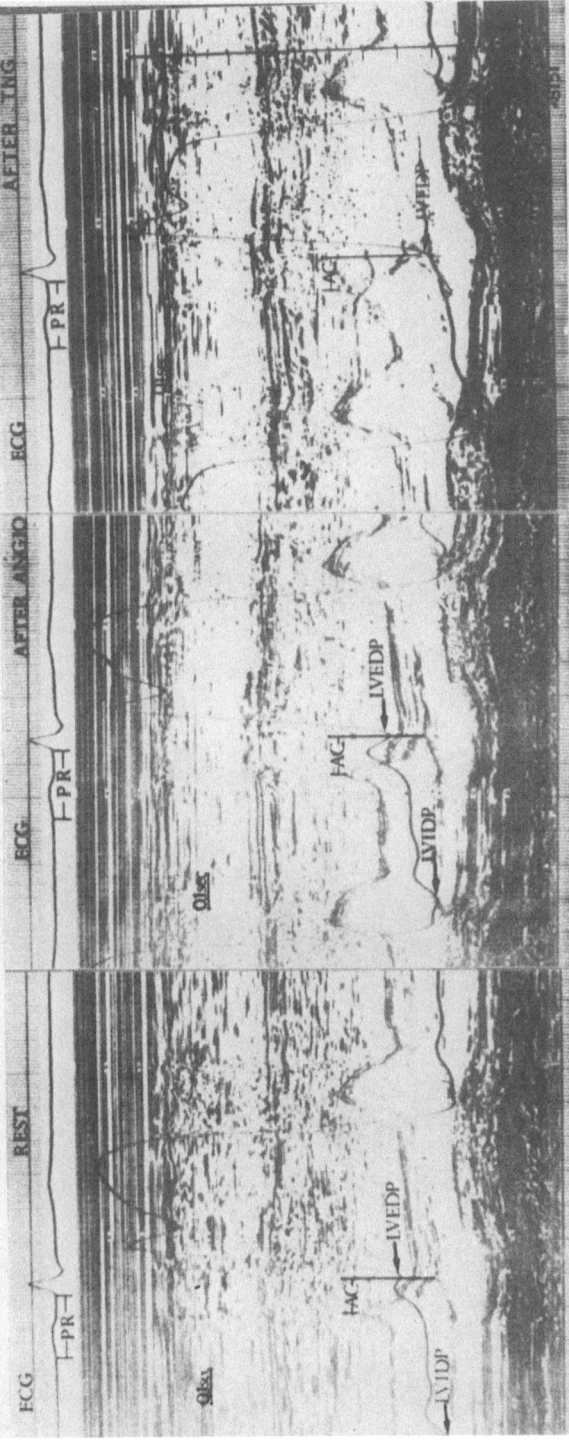

Fig. 3. Echogram of the mitral valve recorded simultaneously with left ventricular pressures in a patient with severe ischemic heart disease, at rest, after ventriculography and after nitroglycerin. The LVEDP was above 18 mm Hg at rest and after ventriculography and was normal after nitroglycerin. PR-AC interval was > 70 msec in all instances. An evident AC "notch" was present at rest and after ventriculography.

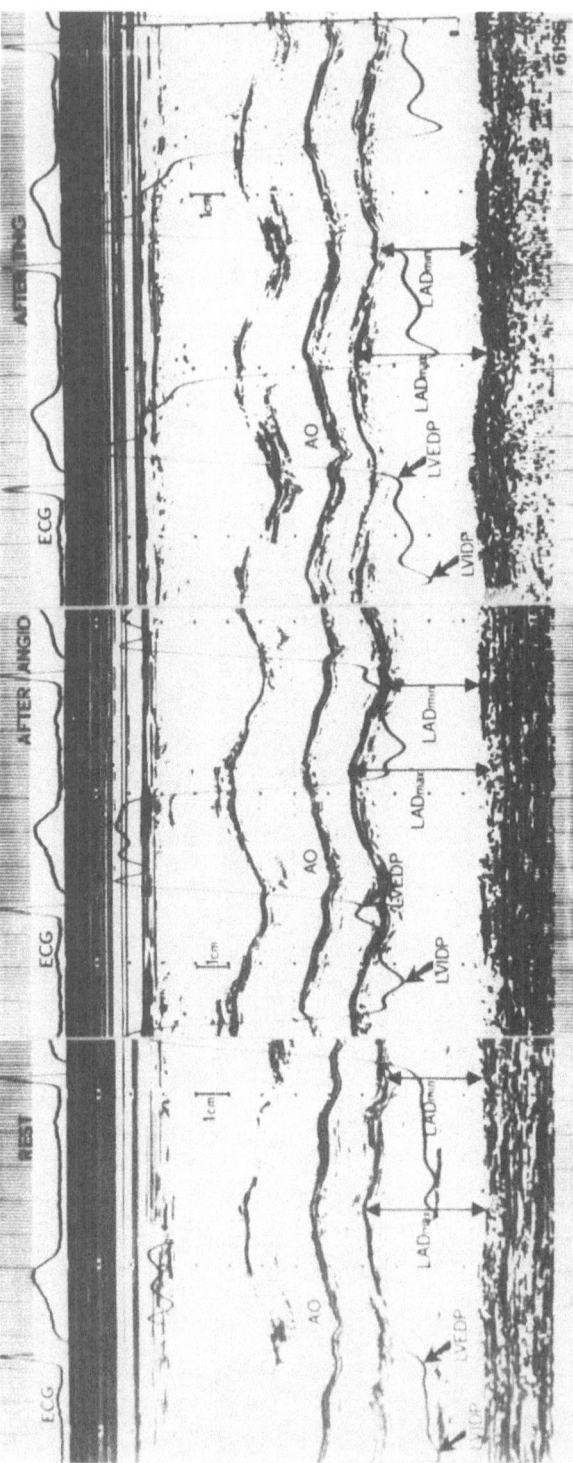

Fig. 4. Echogram of the aortic root and left atrium recorded simultaneously, with left ventricular pressures in a patient with severe ischemic heart disease, at rest, after ventriculography and after nitroglycerin. The LVEDP was below 18 mm Hg at rest, rose significantly after ventriculography and returned to baseline value after nitroglycerin. LADmax was below 40 mm at rest, increased after ANGIO and returned to normal after nitroglycerin.

This would indicate that elevated left ventricular filling pressure tends to cause left atrial enlargement and, consequently, increased LADmax is a reliable predictor of elevated LVEDP.

In this series, we observed a significant increase in LADmax in response to acute volume overload (ANGIO), promptly reversed by TNG. However, the patients with elevated LVEDP at baseline showed no change or minimal LADmax increase after volume overload. LADmax response to TNG in this group was indistinguishable from the one observed in the general population. This behavior would suggest that the normal left atrium is easily distensible, whereas the atrium exposed to chronically elevated left ventricular pre-load has a reduced compliance.

CONCLUSIONS

We conclude that 1) PR-AC does not correlate well with left ventricular diastolic pressure in patients with ischemic heart disease; 2) LADmax appears to be a useful indicator of significantly elevated LVEDP; 3) LVEDP and LADmax change in the same direction after acute interventions, but when the LVEDP is elevated, the distended left atrium does not respond to acute overload with further increase in maximal dimension.

REFERENCES

1. Feigenbaum H: Echocardiography. (2nd Edition), Philadelphia, Pa, Lea and Febiger, 1976.
2. Corya BC, S Rasmussen, SB Knoebel, H Feigenbaum: Echocardiography in acute myocardial infarction. Am J Cardiol 36:1, 1975.
3. Corya BC: Echocardiography in ischemic heart disease. Am J Med 63:10, 1977.
4. Gibson DG: Detection of incoordinate left ventricular contraction by echocardiography. In Echocardiology with Doppler applications and real time imaging. Bom N (ed), The Hague, Martinus Nijhoff, p 105–112.
5. DeMaria A, RR Miller, EA Amsterdam, W Markson, DT Mason: Mitral valve early diastolic closing velocity in the echocardiogram: relation to sequential diastolic flow and ventricular compliance. Am J Cardiol 37:693, 1976.
6. Laniado S, E Yellin, M Kotler, L Levy, J Stadler, R Terdiman: A study of the dynamic relations between the mitral valve echogram and phasic mitral flow. Circulation 51:104, 1975.
7. Konecke LL, H Feigenbaum, S Chang, BC Corya, JC Fischer: Abnormal mitral valve motion in patients with elevated left ventricular diastolic pressures. Circulation 47:989, 1973.
8. Yow MV, N Reichek: Left ventricular end-diastolic pressure and echocardiographic mitral valve closure. Circulation 51:11–51, 1975 (abstract).
9. Giambartolomei A, P Esente, T Bonzel, LF Deere, GG Gensini: Behavior of echocardiographic parameters following acute hemodynamic interventions. Circulation 58:11–52, 1978 (abstract).
10. Lewis JR, JO Parker, GW Burggraf: Mitral valve motion and changes in left ventricular end-diastolic pressure: A correlative study of the PR-AC interval. Am J Cardiol 42:383, 1978.
11. Feigenbaum H: How does a mitral valve echogram reflect left ventricular diastolic pressure? The American College of Cardiology, Advanced Echocardiography. Sept 27, 28, 29, 1978. Indianapolis, Ind.
12. Ambrose JA, J Meller, MV Herman, L Teicholz: The ventricular A-wave: a new echocardiographic index of late diastolic filling of the left ventricle. Am Heart J 96:615, 1978.
13. Haft JI, MS Horowitz: Clinical echocardiography. Futura Publishing Company Inc., Mount Kisco, New York, 1978.

EFFECT OF WOLFF-PARKINSON-WHITE SYNDROME PRE-EXCITATION ON LEFT VENTRICULAR FUNCTION, ASSESSED BY M-MODE AND CROSS-SECTIONAL ECHOCARDIOGRAPHY WITH INTRACARDIAC ELECTROPHYSIOLOGICAL RECORDING

R.P. HAYWARD and R.A. FOALE

INTRODUCTION

Reports concerning echocardiographic assessment of patterns of Left Ventricular (LV) wall motion in the Wolff-Parkinson-White (WPW) syndrome (Refs. 1–4) have provided differing accounts of the abnormalities present, thus suggesting that such abnormalities may be variable. It has not been shown how variation may be caused. These studies have, however, shown abnormalities, particularly of the interventricular septum (IVS) in Type B WPW syndromes (right-sided accessory pathway), and of the LV posterior wall (LVPW) in Type A WPW syndromes (left-sided accessory pathway).

By use of intracardiac electrophysiological recording with programmed premature stimulation (the atrial extrastimulus technique, Ref. 5), the mechanism of abnormal ventricular activation has been elucidated in WPW syndromes. The QRS complex in WPW is usually a fusion, comprising pre-excitation (the delta wave) and relatively late activation of remaining ventricular myocardium via the normal atrioventricular pathway. Theoretically, it appears probable that variations in patterns of LV wall motion previously noted may reflect variations in physiological characteristics exhibited by patients with WPW syndrome – specifically in respect of the volume and site of pre-excited myocardium. A further contributing variable may be the portion of IVS being transected by the M-mode echo beam, since it has been suggested that the IVS, during systolic motion, shows a "hingepoint". We have therefore used the cross-sectional echocardiogram to observe motion of a wide zone of the IVS, and have employed the atrial extrastimulus technique to achieve control of the degree of ventricular pre-excitation.

PATIENTS AND METHODS

Patients with Types A and B WPW syndromes and no other heart disease have been investigated by 30 and 90 degree cross-sectional echocardiography during the course of intracardiac electro-physiological investigation. Regular fixed-rate right atrial (RA) pacing has been employed, interrupted by progressively premature atrial stimulation. As prematurity of the atrial extrastimulus (A2) increases, approximating it to the previous normal paced beat (Al), increasing delay develops in the AV node but not in the bypass pathway, resulting in increasingly gross pre-excitation, until the effective refractory period (ERP) of the bypass is reached and pre-excitation is abolished. M-mode recordings were available from the sector scan record

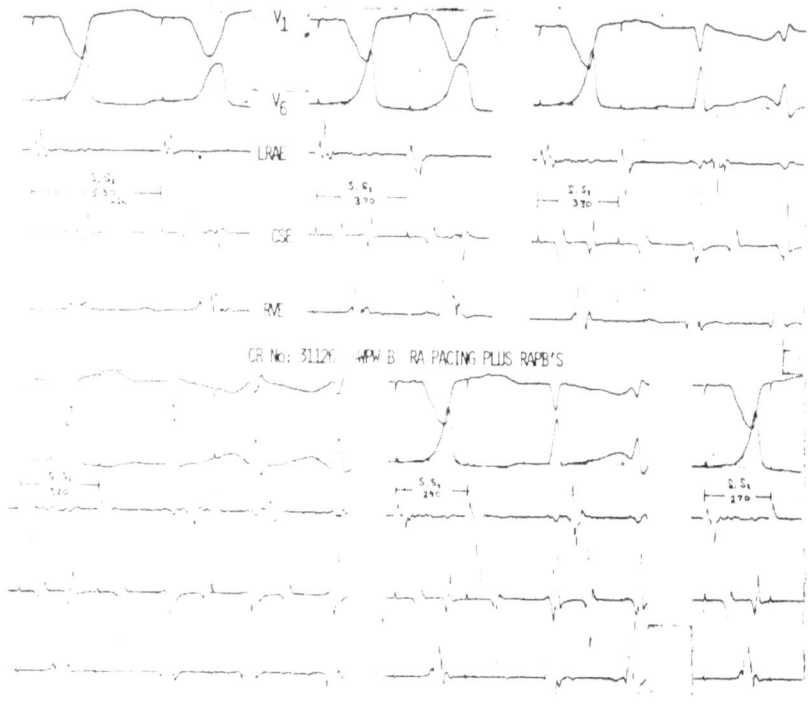

Fig. 1. Effect of increasing prematurity: pre-excitation initially enhanced, then abolished as KB ERP (350 msec) exceeded; RT induced.

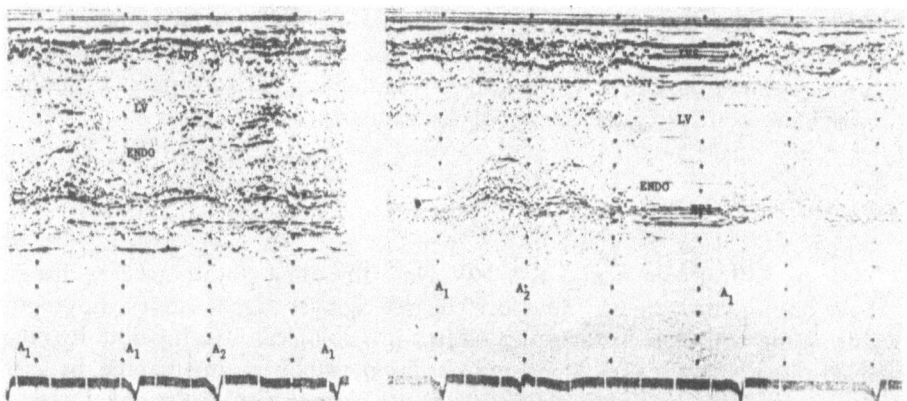

Fig. 2. M-mode print-out from sector recording in B WPW. Left sequence showing markedly premature A2, conducted with gross pre-excitation; right sequence showing similarly early A2 but without pre-excitation.

RESULTS

During study, reentry tachycardias were regularly induced by atrial stimulation and, where indicated, atrial fibrillation was also induced, so that both
arrhythmias were available for echocardiographic analysis. Figure 1 shows
typical enhancement of pre-excitation leading to Kent bypass (KB) block and
reentry tachycardia (RT) initiation in a case of Type B WPW syndrome. In
such B WPW patients, LVPW motion was normal, while the IVS showed
characteristic abnormality. With mild pre-excitation, initial posterior IVS
motion was followed by later anterior motion and final posterior end-systolic
motion. Greater pre-excitation caused more marked and prolonged early
systolic posterior motion, while sector scanning showed progressive shifting
of the septal hingeing point. Abolition of pre-excitation caused return to
more normal septal motion (Fig. 2). In Type A WPW syndromes IVS motion
was normal, while LVPW motion showed premature anterior systolic movement whose extent was also pre-excitation dependent. The net effect of
increasing pre-excitation on LV dimension change in a case of B WPW is
shown in Figures 3 and 4, the latter also showing a strong similarity between
wall motion in reentry (RT) and in the absence of pre-excitation.

DISCUSSION

This study supports the precept that abnormalities of LV wall motion in
WPW are dependent not only on the site but also on the degree of pre-
excitation. It appears that pre-excited beats are less effective than non-pre-

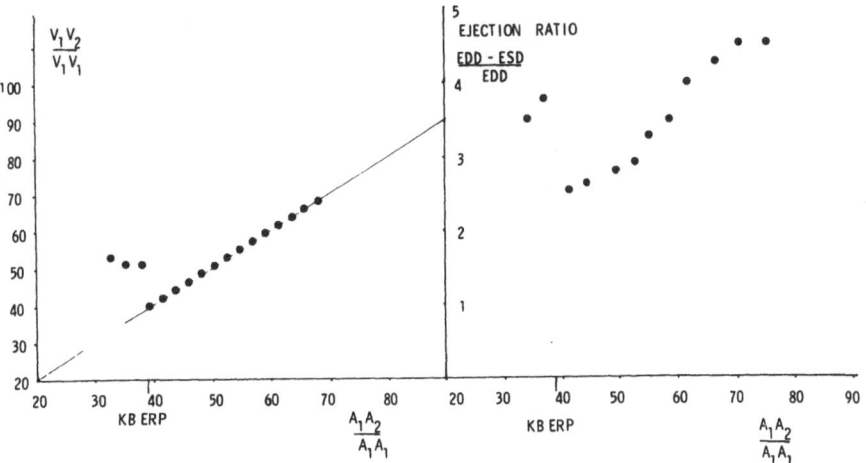

Fig. 3. Effect of progressively early A2's upon resulting ventricular complex coupling intervals
(left sequence), and on LV ejection, expressed as change in LV internal dimension. EDD = end-
diastolic dimension, ESD = end-systolic dimension, KB = Kent Bypass (Rt sequence).

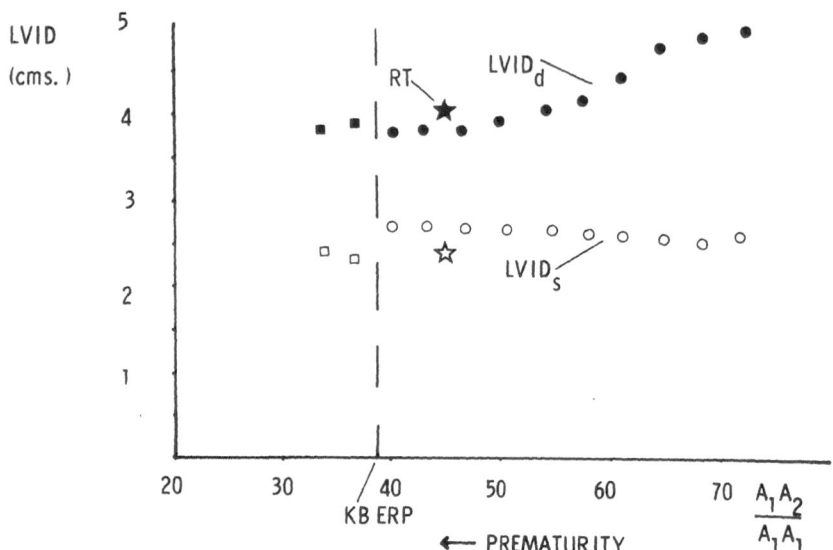

Fig. 4. Effect of prematurity on systolic and diastolic LV internal dimension (LVIDs and LVIDd), with ○ and without □ pre-excitation, and during non pre-excited reentry tachycardia (RT).

excited beats. This is not explicable solely on the basis of reduced diastolic filling with prematurity, since abolition of pre-excitation by yet more premature stimulation causes improved ejection. The role of atrial coordinated transport is being further investigated. This phenomenon may be involved in the haemodynamic deterioration seen with WPW tachycardias that cause gross pre-excitation, such classically as atrial fibrillation.

REFERENCES

1. De Maria et al.: Circulation 53:249, 1976.
2. Chandra et al.: Circulation 53:943, 1976.
3. Francis et al.: Circulation 54:176, 1976.
4. Hishida et al.: Circulation 54:567, 1976.
5. Castellanos et al.: Circulation 41:399, 1970.

ASSESSMENT OF LEFT VENTRICULAR DIASTOLIC VISCOUS FORCES BY COMBINED ECHO-PRESSURE MEASUREMENTS IN MEN

O.M. HESS, J. GRIMM, and H.P. KRAYENBUEHL

According to the traditional concept heart muscle behaves as a non-Hookean elastic material with an exponential diastolic pressure-volume relationship (1–3). However, recent studies demonstrated marked deviations from this exponential relationship, especially during the particularly filling-rate-dependent early diastole (4–7). Therefore, the purpose of the present study was to evaluate the diastolic stress-strain relationship by a simple elastic and a visco-elastic model in 6 control subjects (CO) and 14 patients with moderate to severe aortic insufficiency (AI).

1. MATERIAL AND METHODS

Twenty patients with an average age of 37 years who underwent diagnostic heart catheterization and simultaneous single-beam echocardiography were included in the present study. The patients were divided into the following 2 groups: Group 1 consisted of 6 control patients with normal left ventricular function and Group 2 of 14 patients with chronic volume overload due to moderate to severe aortic insufficiency. Aortic regurgitation fraction as assessed by thermodilution techniques averaged 61% in Group 2.

Left ventricular high-fidelity pressure measurements and single-beam echocardiography (Ekoline 20A, Smith-Kline-Instruments) were carried out simultaneously in all 20 patients. In Figure 1 an example of a pressure tracing and of an echocardiogram, recorded on an oscillograph "Electronics for Medicine" at a paper speed of 100 mm/sec, is shown.

Quantitative evaluation of the pressure tracings, and the echocardiograms was made by a computer-assisted system (PDP-11/10). In each patient the pressure and echo curves were drawn manually using an electronic digitizer and the following parameters were calculated by the computer: midwall shortening velocity, meridional and lateral wall stress, segmental power, cycle efficiency and the diastolic stress-dimension relationship.

The basic data for the assessment of diastolic function are the diastolic stress-strain relations, which were fitted to two different models, a simple elastic and a visco-elastic model:

$$\text{simple elastic model:} \quad S = b \cdot e^{k \cdot E} \qquad (M_1)$$
$$\text{viscoelastic model:} \quad S = B \cdot e^{K \cdot E} + y \cdot \dot{E} \qquad (M_2)$$

S: meridional wall stress; b and B: simple elastic and viscoelastic constant of

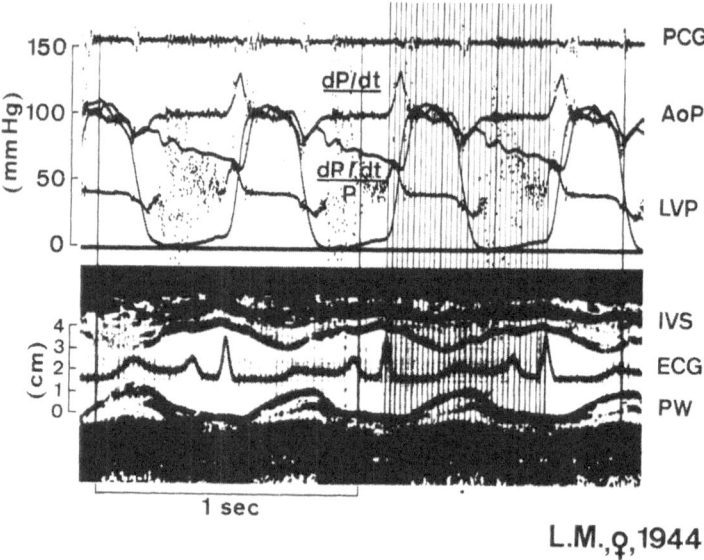

L.M.,♀,1944

Fig. 1. Left ventricular pressure-dimension relationship in a control patient with normal left ventricular function. PCG: Phonocardiogram; AoP Aortic pressure; LVP: Left ventricular pressure; dP/dt: First derivative of the left ventricular pressure; dP/dt/P: First derivative of the left ventricular pressure divided by total pressure; IVS: Interventricular septum; ECG: Electrocardiogram; PW: Posterior wall; D: Left ventricular minor axis diameter.

myocardial stiffness (intercept); k and K: simple elastic and viscoelastic constant of myocardial stiffness (slope); E: Lagrangian strain; y: constant of myocardial viscosity; Ė: midwall strain rate.

Mathematical evaluation of model 1 was done by using a semilogarithmic regression function, however, for model 2 an iteration procedure had to be used, since model 2 was characterized by 3 variables and 3 constants. The iteration was performed by replacing one of the 3 constants, usually y, by a value between 15 and 0.01, which was varied until the best curve fit, or in other words the highest possible correlation coefficient (r), was obtained. A sample calculation is given in Table 1.

Table 1. Iteration procedure for the evaluation of the viscoelastic stress-strain relationship. k and b: simple elastic constants of myocardial stiffness; r: correlation coefficient; K and B: viscoelastic constants of myocardial stiffness; y: viscoelastic constant of myocardial viscosity.

	k	b		r
simple elastic	9.1	9.75	–	0.90
	K	B	y	r
viscoelastic	8.7	7.6	15.0	0.53
	8.0	10.9	10.0	0.66
	7.4	11.5	5.0	0.84
	7.3	12.1	3.0	0.88
	7.3	12.3	2.0	0.89
	7.2	12.6	1.0	0.90
	7.2	12.8	0.5	0.91
	7.2	12.9	0.1	0.93
	6.1	16.1	0.01	0.86

Statistical comparison of the two models (b versus B and k versus K) was performed by using the nonparametric Wilcoxon signed rank sum test.

2. RESULTS

The comparison of the diastolic stress-strain data by a simple elastic and a viscoelastic model showed the following results:

	M_1/M_2 r r	M_1/M_2 b B	M_1/M_2 k K	M_1/M_2 y
CO	0.96/0.98	3.8/2.9	9.5/11.8	–/0.7
AI	0.94/0.97*	6.2/2.9**	10.4/16.4**	–/3.2

*: $P < 0.05$; **: $P < 0.02$.

An example of a simple elastic and a viscoelastic stress-strain relationship of a patient with AI is given in Figure 2. The simple elastic relationship shows appreciable deviation during early diastolic filling from the true exponential stress-strain relationship. However, after correction for the viscous influences the stress-strain relationship is more linear and the correlation coefficient for the regression equation increases from 0.96 to 0.99.

3. DISCUSSION

Rankin and co-workers (4) showed that dynamic influences are responsible for deviations from the true exponential stress-strain relationship during

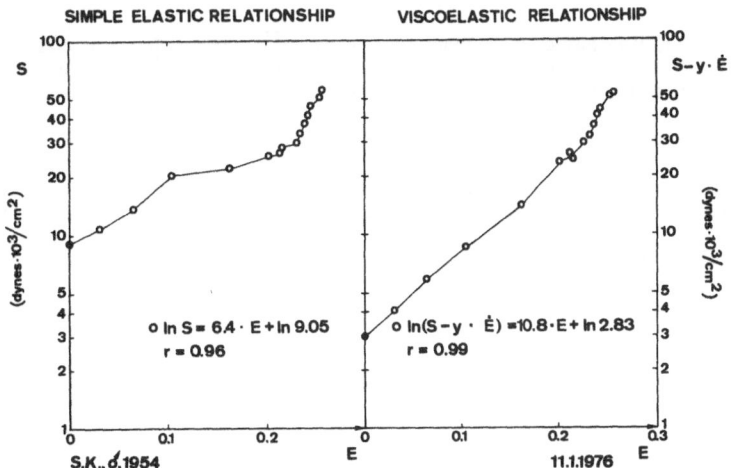

Fig. 2. Left ventricular diastolic stress-strain relationship in a patient with severe aortic insufficiency. The simple elastic relationship is shown on the right, the viscoelastic relationship on the left side. S: Left ventricular diastolic stress; E: Left ventricular diastolic strain; $S - (y \cdot \dot{E})$: Left ventricular diastolic stress minus the product of myocardial viscous constant (y) and diastolic strain rate ($\dot{E}$).

early diastole and during atrial filling in dogs monitored over long term. Therefore, the purpose of the present study was to determine, using combined echo-pressure measurements, left ventricular diastolic properties for 20 patients by applying a simple elastic and a viscoelastic stress-strain model.

Statistical comparison of the simple elastic and the viscoelastic stress-strain model showed that in the normal left ventricle viscous influences play a minor role and the difference between the simple elastic and the viscoelastic stiffness constants are small. However, in the enlarged and hypertrophied left ventricle, such as in aortic insufficiency, viscous properties are important determinants of left ventricular diastolic function, and diastolic filling characteristics in myocardial hypertrophy are determined by both elastic and viscous elements.

Correlation of the diastolic stress-strain relationship in patients with aortic insufficiency occurred mainly during the particularly filling-rate-dependent early diastole, whereas the correction during atrial filling was generally small.

One major point for the use of the viscoelastic stiffness parameters is that the viscoelastic constants of myocardial stiffness are significantly different from the simple elastic constants in patients with aortic insufficiency. Therefore, it is important that for the assessment of left ventricular diastolic stiffness the viscous influences are evaluated, because the simple elastic constants reflect a composite of elastic and viscous forces and may be misleading especially in patients with myocardial hypertrophy.

REFERENCES

1. Mirsky I: Assessment of passive elastic stiffness of cardiac muscle: mathematical concepts, physiologic and clinical considerations, directions of future research. Prog Cardiovasc Dis 18:277, 1976.
2. Gaasch WH, WE Battle, AA Oboler, JS Banas, HJ Levine: Left ventricular stress and compliance in man; with special reference to normalized ventricular function curves. Circulation 45:746, 1972.
3. Diamond G, JS Forrester, J Hargis, WW Parmley, R Danzig, HJC Swan: Diastolic pressure-volume relationship in the canine left ventricle. Circ Res 29:267, 1971.
4. Rankin JS, CE Arentzen, PA McHale, D Ling, RW Anderson: Viscoelastic properties of the diastolic left ventricle in the conscious dog. Circ Res 41:37, 1977.
5. Kennish A, E Yellin, RW Frater: Dynamic stiffness profiles in the left ventricle. J Appl Physiol 39:665, 1975.
6. Gaasch WH, JS Cole, MA Quinones, JK Alexander: Dynamic determinants of left ventricular diastolic pressure volume relations in man. Circulation 51:317, 1975.
7. Gibson DG, DJ Brown: Relation between diastolic ventricular wall stress and strain in man. Brit Heart J 36:1066, 1974.

LEFT VENTRICULAR FUNCTION AND INTERVENTRICULAR SEPTAL MOTION IN MITRAL STENOSIS: ECHOCARDIOGRAPHIC ABNORMALITIES

Z. KRAJCER, L.W. PECHACEK, V.S. MATHUR, E. GARCIA, and R.J. HALL

Previous data from our laboratory in patients with mitral stenosis (MS) studied with biplane angiography has revealed abnormalities in the contraction pattern of the interventricular septum (1). Possible determinants of abnormal septal motion in patients with isolated MS are altered left ventricular (LV) shape during diastole, impaired contractility of the septum, or the influence of right ventricular (RV) pressure. The purpose of this study was to evaluate LV function in isolated MS and to determine the underlying mechanism of abnormal septal motion by correlating echocardiographic with hemodynamic and angiographic results.

MATERIALS AND METHODS

M-mode echocardiographic studies were done in 10 normal subjects and 15 patients selected randomly from a large group that had isolated MS documented at cardiac catheterization. There were 11 females and 4 males in the MS group with a mean age of 41.4 years (range 29–60). The normal subjects had a mean age of 29.1 years (range 25–32). Multiple echographic recordings were obtained on each patient and only high quality records were included for analysis. Maximal systolic endocardial velocity (SEVM) was determined by drawing a tangent to the steepest portion of the systolic endocardial excursion of the septum and LV posterior wall (PW) and measuring slope in mm/sec (2). Maximal diastolic endocardial velocity (DEVM) was measured by drawing a tangent to the steepest portion of the diastolic endocardial excursion of septum and LVPW and measuring slope in mm/sec. Other echographic measurements included RV and LV diastolic diameter, LV systolic diameter, percent of LV minor diameter shortening (%MDS), percent of septal and LVPW systolic thickening (%T), and septal and LVPW excursion (E) during systole. A minimum of five cardiac cycles were analyzed independently for each patient by two observers. In 9 patients with atrial fibrillation the measurements were standardized using cycle lengths of approximately 0.8 sec to correspond to mean heart rate of the normal group (66 beats/min). Inter-observer variation was assessed using the paired Student's t-test. Group comparisons were done with the unpaired Student's t-test using a two-tailed distribution.

Hemodynamic measurements included cardiac index, stroke volume, pulmonary arterial pressures, mitral valve area and flow rate. Angiographic

Charles T. Lancée (ed.), Echocardiology, 175–179. All rights reserved
Copyright © 1979 by Martinus Nijhoff Publishers bv, The Hague/Boston/London

determinants included ejection fraction and analysis of septal motion on LV angiogram from the left anterior oblique projection. All values were expressed as mean $\pm$ standard error of the mean.

RESULTS

Hemodynamic and angiographic data for the 15 MS patients included mean mitral valve area of 1 ± 0.1 cm^2; mean pulmonary artery systolic pressure of 46 ± 4.7 mm Hg; mean cardiac index (Fick method) of 2.8 ± 0.17 l/min/m^2; and mean ejection fraction of 0.6 ± 0.03. LV angiogram revealed that 14 of 15 patients had hypocontractile motion of the upper third of the septum while 11 of 15 had normal motion of the lower two-thirds of the septum during systole.

Results reported by two different observers in determining echographic measurements were not significantly different. Pertinent echocardiographic findings are presented in table 1. RV end-diastolic diameter was 17 ± 1.4 mm and 18 ± 1.5 mm for the normal and MS groups, respectively with no significant difference. There was no significant difference in systolic LVPW thickening ($40 \pm 3\%$ and $39 \pm 9\%$) and systolic LVPW E (10.8 ± 0.5 mm and 11.2 ± 0.4 mm) between normals and the MS group. Eleven of 15 MS patients had an exaggerated posterior excursion of the septum in early diastole. No significant correlation could be found in the MS group between mitral valve area and DEVM or mitral valve area and SEVM of septum and LVPW.

DISCUSSION

Previous data from our laboratory have revealed that MS patients have abnormal LV shape on quantitative ventriculography as manifested by the ratio of long to short axis being lower than normal and by poor septal motion (1). In our echographic study DEVM of the septum and LVPW were significantly lower in MS patients than in normal subjects. DEVM of the septum was, however, significantly more decreased ($p < 0.001$) than DEVM of LVPW ($p < 0.05$). SEVM of the septum was also significantly lower than in normals ($p < 0.01$) while SEVM of LVPW was significantly higher than in normals ($p < 0.05$). Although the mean age of the MS group was higher than that of normals it is unlikely that this influenced the difference in echographic data since others have found no significant correlation between age and SEVM or DEVM (2).

Our observations contradict the theory based on angiographic studies done in the right anterior oblique projection that patients with MS have poor function of posterobasal LV wall (3). Some of the plausible explanations for decreased DEVM of the septum and LVPW observed in MS patients are decreased mitral valve flow rate and/or impaired LV diastolic compliance. We were, however, unable to find any significant correlation between mitral

Table 1. Echocardiographic findings.

Group	DEVM-IVS mm/sec	SEVM-IVS mm/sec	T-IVS %	E-IVS mm	SEVM-PW mm/sec	DEVM-PW mm/sec	$\frac{\text{E-IVS}}{\text{E-PW}}$	MDS %
Normals	56±5	43±2	40±2	7±0.4	49±2	125±7	0.7±0.03	37±1
Mitral stenosis	27±4	30±4	27±3	5.7±0.7	66±7	89±14	0.5±0.07	33±2
P value	<0.001	<0.01	<0.001	NS	<0.05	<0.05	<0.05	<0.02

valve flow rate and DEVM of septum (R = 0.02) or LVPW (R = 0.03). Kovick et al. (2) previously described in patients with muscular dystrophy that DEVM of LVPW was significantly impaired, presumably due to the reduced rate of LVPW relaxation. DEVM has been previously found to reflect LV contractility more accurately than SEVM (2).

Our findings show that patients with MS have significantly impaired septal motion during systole as well as diastole when compared either with LVPW in the same ventricle or the septum in normal subjects. These dynamic septal abnormalities might indicate that an asymmetric myopathic process is primarily affecting the interventricular septum. Several investigators have described decreased cardiac output and LV hypocontractility in MS (4, 5). Although it is generally thought that this is due to decreased flow rates through a stenotic mitral valve, it is obviously not the entire explanation since mitral commissurotomy usually fails to produce a significant increase in cardiac output unless there is a drastic increase in mitral valve area postoperatively (5). In our study only 2 patients had a significantly reduced ejection fraction while nine of 15 patients had a cardiac index less than 2.8 $l/min/m^2$. These findings are similar to data reported by others (4, 5).

RV volume overload was excluded as a cause of abnormal septal motion in our study by hemodynamic and angiographic findings. In addition echocardiography did not reveal evidence of increased RV diastolic dimensions. It has been shown previously that RV pressure or volume overload cause a modest decrease in both peak velocity of the contractile elements and peak changes in pressure over time (dp/dt) of the LV (6). We were unable to find any significant correlation between abnormal septal motion (decreased DVEM, SEVM, E, %T) and pulmonary artery pressures, mitral valve area, or mitral valve flow rate.

Recent observations by Weyman et al. (7) by means of cross-sectional ultrasound in patients with MS suggest that abnormal septal motion is related to inequality in early diastolic filling of the ventricles. They suggested that filling of the LV in early diastole is limited by a narrowed mitral valve while the RV fills rapidly, producing relative diastolic RV volume overload. This would result in a shift of the septum toward the LV. Subsequently, LV filling would then occur with the RV already distended, causing the LV to be less distensible and compliant. The same investigators have suggested that the early diastolic dip of the septum in MS patients is related to inequality in RV and LV filling in early diastole. This initial downward septal motion is occasionally seen in normal individuals, however, in a less exaggerated form (7).

CONCLUSION

Although the cause of abnormal septal motion is still obscure, it appears that several factors might be playing a role in this abnormality. Our study revealed that in patients with isolated MS there is a disparity in regional contractility between interventricular septum and LVPW as manifested by hypodynamic septal motion during systole and diastole.

REFERENCES

1. Garcia E, M El Guindy, VS Mathur, et al.: Ventricular geometry and function in mitral stenosis studied with biplane cineangiography (abstract). Circulation (supplement II): II–66, 1976.
2. Kovick RB, AM Fogelman, JB Abbasi, et al.: Echocardiographic evaluation of posterior left ventricular wall motion in muscular dystrophy. Circulation 52:447, 1975.
3. Heller SJ, RA Carlton: Abnormal left ventricular contraction in patients with mitral stenosis. Circulation 42:1099, 1970.
4. Ball JD, H Kopeland, AC Waltham: Circulatory changes in mitral stenosis at rest and on exercise. Br Heart J 14:363, 1952.
5. Feigenbaum H, RW Campbell, CM Wunsch, et al.: Evaluation of the left ventricle in patients with mitral stenosis. Circulation 34:462, 1966.
6. Kelly DT, HM Spotnitz, GL Beiser, et al.: Effects of chronic right ventricular volume and pressure loading on left ventricular performance. Circulation 44:403, 1971.
7. Weyman AE, JJ Heger, G Kronik et al.: Mechanism of paradoxical early diastolic septal motion in patients with mitral stenosis. A cross-sectional study. Am J Cardiol 40:691, 1977.

SYSTOLIC BLOOD FLOW PATTERN ESTIMATED FROM MULTIPLE SECTOR-SCAN PULSED DOPPLER VELOCIMETRY

J.P. LAPORTE, C. ODDOU, F. LAURENT, and P. BRUN

The interest of blood flow velocity and acceleration in the ascending aorta for the study of left ventricular performance has been previously outlined (1); though, for technical reasons, the method was not confirmed as a routine procedure. For reasons related to the anatomical location of the ascending aorta behind the sternum, a different region was selected – the left ventricular outflow tract – in order to introduce an external approach: a multiple-sector-scan, pulsed Doppler ultrasonic method. The first attempt to derive blood flow velocity fields in the human left ventricle was recently presented, demonstrating the possibility of measuring blood velocity at different locations during the ventricular fast filling phase (2). The same approach was proposed here, in order to determine, non-invasively, the blood flow velocity and acceleration fields in the ejecting left ventricle, notably in the outflow tract.

MATERIALS AND METHOD

The ultrasonic velocimeter used was P. Peronneau's pulsed Doppler system, commercialized by Alvar (F 93107 Montreuil). Doppler signals were processed, after quadrature phase detection, in order to display the frequency spectrum as a zero-crossing histogram. The time-motion echogram (Organon Teknika), the sampling zone depth, and an electrocardiographic reference were simultaneously recorded. Multi-scan images were used to control the left ventricle outflow tract location. Data were gathered from young normal volunteers. The probe was located on the thorax at two points situated in a plane containing the axis of symmetry of the left ventricular outflow tract (Fig. 1). The Doppler probe was equipped with a small collimated spotlight, whose beam indicated the direction of the ultrasonic beam. A sector was manually covered round each of the two thoracic points selected and a number of preselected zones, centred by the beam intersections were explored by using a set of different angles and depths. This preselection took into account angle and depth correction for ultrasonic beam distortion (2). Each zero-crossing histogram recorded from these zones was redrawn to give a continuous, lightly smoothed line and analysed on a digitizing tablet connected to a microcomputer.

The Doppler shift moduli were measured during the interval between Q-wave and the closing time of the aortic valves, and recorded together with the ultrasonic parameters, the sampling zone coordinates, the beam orientations and the cycle durations. All data were stored on flexible disks. Due to respiratory arhythmia and to changes in the subject's sympathetic drive during the recording period, the different cardiac cycles recorded were of unequal duration and had to be post-synchronized according to strict rules, elaborated for the ejection phase. These were derived from a separate study on the relation between ejection and cycle duration. Velocity was computed according to the following formulas:

$$\text{tg } \vartheta_1 = \frac{1}{\sin \phi} \frac{F_2}{F_1} - \cos \phi \qquad V = \frac{c}{2} \frac{F_1}{F_e} \frac{1}{\cos \vartheta_1},$$

where V is the velocity component in the observation plane, c the ultrasonic velocity in the blood, F_e the ultrasonic emitting frequency, F_1 and F_2 the Doppler frequency shifts, ϕ the angle between beams, ϑ_1 the angle between the velocity vector and one of the beams. Instantaneous velocity fields could then be plotted for any time during the ejection period. Display of these maps on a colour monitor made an accurate follow-up of the time evolution of the velocity field in different regions of the left ventricle possible. Time-motion recordings of the ascending aorta, the interventricular septum and the anterior mitral leaflet immediately below the aortic valve, were also digitized in order to be able to subtract the overall displacement of the left ventricle from the computerized velocities, and thus work with velocities in the cardiac cavity reference system. The digitizing tablet accuracy was compatible with a 400-Hz sampling rate, so that the velocity time derivative could be computed. Nevertheless, in order to obtain the dynamic blood particle acceleration taking into account convective effects, the spatial derivative of the velocity

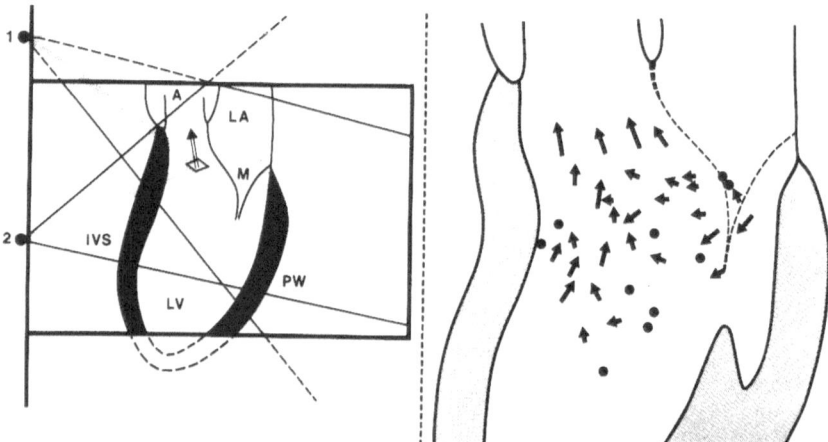

Fig. 1. The multi-sector-scan pulsed Doppler technique. The arrow indicates the velocity vector computed in a geometrically coordinated zone explored by ultrasonic beams issued from points 1 and 2. A: Aortic valve, M: Mitral valve, LA: Left atrium, LV: left ventricle, IVS: Interventricular septum, PW: Posterior wall.

Fig. 2. Preliminary mapping of blood velocity inside the left ventricle during the ejection period (150 msec after Q-wave). The arrow lengths are proportional to velocity moduli (closed circles: zero flow).

field had to be computed, even though spatial velocity field resolution was not very accurate. In some selected areas, blood particle local acceleration fields were derived from the instantaneous velocity field maps.

RESULTS

Previous results in relation to the left ventricular filling phase (2) had demonstrated, at least partially, the accuracy of a two-component velocity reconstruction in what was called a "geometrically and chronologically coordinated zone". Two characteristics were described: 1) Comparison of information obtained from independent beams, post-synchronized, did reveal a fair coordination of events. 2) Comparison between adjacent zones did reveal the absence of interference between zones: there was no evident cross talk between zones, though they were sometimes less than 5 mm apart. Similar findings could be quoted after reviewing the different ejection-phase Doppler shift recordings and velocity maps, though in a less striking way, due to the rather simple overall pattern of the ejection velocity maps. When compared to the complex left ventricular filling phase, with its transient jet stream structure followed by a recirculation phenomenon and a breaking of the jet mechanism, the overall pattern of the ejection velocity maps appeared less complicated and rather uniform. The flow field had the appearance of a potential flow induced by wall motion. No recirculating pattern was observed during the ejection phase in the different regions of the left ventricle outflow track. During ejection, the velocity vector moduli were significantly smaller than during the filling phase, when compared in the equatorial region of the left ventricle corresponding to the short axis (ellipsoid assumption); but in the subaortic region the moduli were higher, though maximal velocity remained inferior to the maximal filling velocity in the left-ventricular inflow tract. The fact that mean velocity did increase in the downstream direction seemed related to the tapering of the outflow tract. Velocity vectors near the walls appeared normal to them, and the distribution of the vector orientations suggested a tendency to converge toward the centre of mass of the ventricle. This was striking when the left ventricular posterior wall near the mitral annulus was considered: the blood velocity vectors, instead of being oriented toward the aortic or subaortic region, pointed to the opposite wall, i.e. the septum in its medial part (Fig. 2). A diphasic aspect of the Doppler shift curves, composed of two similar waves parted by a mid-systolic transient phenomenon, did appear during the ejection period in the subaortic area of the left ventricular outflow tract, with a corresponding translation on the velocity curves. The significance of the mid-systolic pattern remained unclear.

DISCUSSION AND PERSPECTIVE

We have reported here a preliminary analysis of the measurements of the detailed, instantaneous distribution of the blood velocity in the human left ventricular chamber during systolic ejection. Such measurements have been obtained using atraumic, pulsed Doppler, ultrasonic velocimetry, and were performed in close connection with multiscan echocardiographic imaging, allowing the determination of the dynamic instantaneous cavity geometry. From such data, combining the spatio-temporal derivative of the velocity fields, the blood particle acceleration field – due to unsteady and convective effects – can be derived, which may give information about cardiac performance and myocardial contractility. The pumping efficiency is revealed by mapping these accelerations, i.e. the pressure gradients inside the cavity which act at the onset of the systolic ejection, as the potential energy of the blood. If the aortic impedance could be evaluated, or if pressure at the root of the aorta was known, the potential energy could be derived. It is expected that such a fluid acceleration or pressure gradient field is highly dependant on the left ventricular efficiency.

REFERENCES

1. Noble MIM, D Trenchard, A Gus: Left ventricular ejection in conscious dogs. I. Measurement and significance of the maximum acceleration of blood from the left ventricle. Circulation Res 19:139, 1966.
2. Brun P, C Oddou, P Dantan, JP Laporte, F Laurent, P Perro: Blood flow dynamics during human left ventricular filling phase. Third International Conference on Cardiovascular Dynamics. Leiden (The Netherlands), August 27–31, 1978.

ATRIAL SEPTAL DEFECT AND PARADOXICAL SEPTAL MOTION: AN ECHOCARDIOGRAPHIC ARTEFACT

V.S. MATHUR, J.A. GARCIA, A. ALI, C.M. DE CASTRO, E. GARCIA, and R.J. HALL

The phenomenon of "paradoxical" septal motion is a well recognized echocardiographic feature in patients with atrial septal defect (ASD) (1–4). Its reported frequency in patients with ASD has varied between 38 and 94% (2, 5). This phenomenon is not specific for ASD and its presence has been described in a variety of other conditions (6). The present study was undertaken to explore the mechanisms responsible for this paradoxical motion in patients with ASD.

MATERIALS AND METHODS

Twenty patients, proven to have ASD (secundum) by cardiac catheterization and subsequent surgery, were studied with simultaneous biplane left ventricular (LV) angiography and echocardiography. The pulmonary artery pressure was normal in all patients except one. A large left to right shunt was present in every patient, the ratio of pulmonary to systemic flow being at least 2.5:1 in each instance. Analysis of LV angiograms was also carried out in 18 additional subjects with normal examinations, electrocardiograms, and chest X-rays who underwent cardiac catheterization due to atypical chest pain. Left ventriculogram, hemodynamic data, and coronary arteriograms were found to be normal in all 18 of these subjects. The end-diastolic and end-systolic silhouettes of LV and aorta were traced, and the position of the spine marked for reference in the left anterior oblique (LAO) projection. The excursion of the aorta was measured between the spine and a point just above the aortic valve (Fig. 1). Correction for magnification was made using grids placed at the point of the LV center in end-diastole. The echo transducer was held in place during ventriculography by a specially designed holder (7) and its position on the chest wall as well as its angulation and distance from the LV silhouette were measured.

RESULTS

Echocardiograms were normal in all 18 normal subjects. In the 20 patients with ASD, right ventricular enlargement was present in all and septal motion was paradoxical in 18 (Fig. 2) and flat in two.

Analysis of LV angiograms revealed that during systole (from end-diastole

Charles T. Lancée (ed.), Echocardiology, 185–189. All rights reserved
Copyright © 1979 by Martinus Nijhoff Publishers bv, The Hague/Boston/London

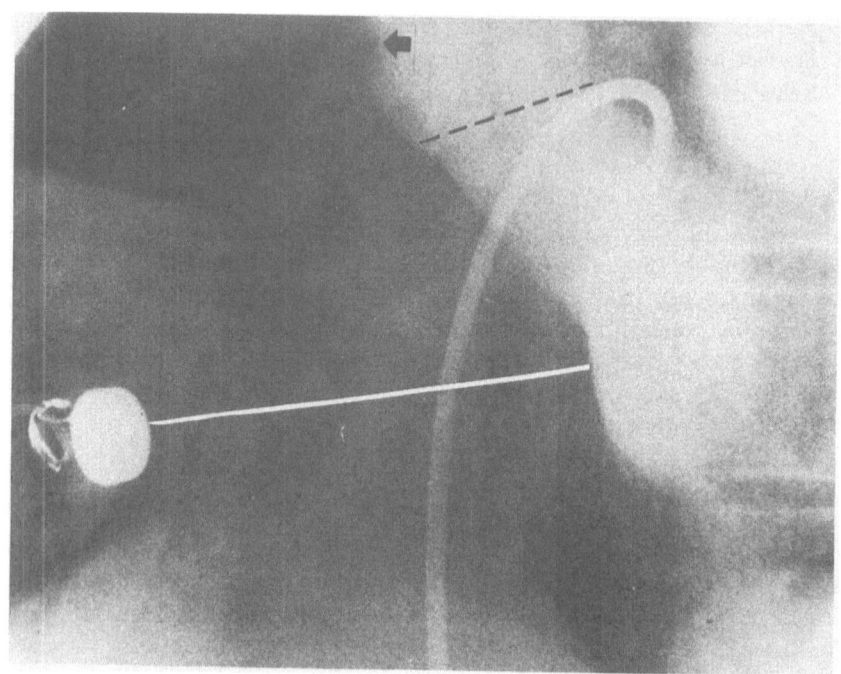

Fig. 1. LV angiogram in LAO showing aortic valve (broken line) ascending aorta (arrow) and septum. The echo transducer is on the anterior chest wall with a line depicting the direction of its beam.

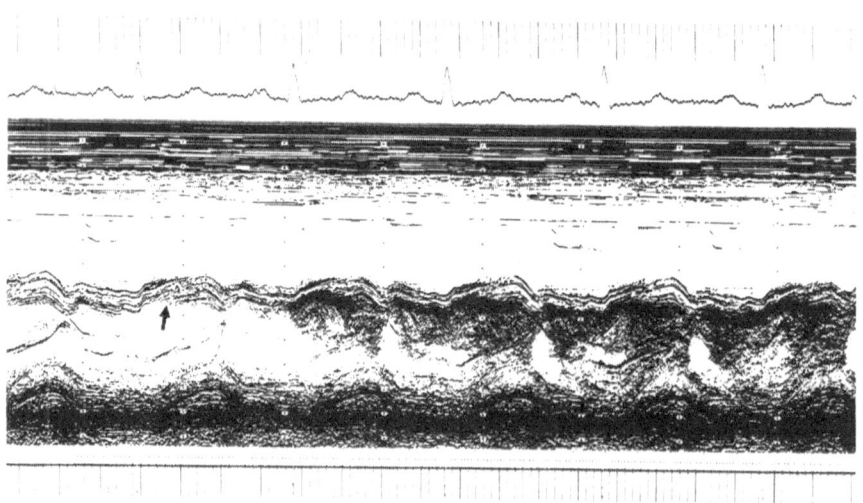

Fig. 2. Echocardiogram from the same patient recorded simultaneously reveals "paradoxical" septal motion (arrow). Contrast material injected from the LV angiogram appears as multiple echoes in the LV cavity from the third cycle onwards. Electrocardiogram is on the top and cine frame marker is near the bottom.

to end-systole) the ascending aorta and aortic valve moved anteriorly and inferiorly in both normals and patients with ASD. Anterior movement during systole was 11 ± 1 mm (mean $\pm$ SEM) in ASD patients which was 270% of anterior movement in normals $(4.1 \pm 1$ mm). The difference was highly significant $(p < 0.001)$. The inferior movement was similarly exaggerated in ASD patients $(11.4 \pm 4$ mm), being 259% of similar movement in normals $(4.4 \pm 1$ mm). The difference was also significant $(p < 0.01)$.

The location of the mid-point of the septum between aortic valve and apex was measured with reference to a fixed point (vertebral body) as well as the moving point on the ascending aorta, just above the aortic valve. In relation to the ascending aorta, mid-septum in ASD patients moved 12.3 ± 1 mm posteriorly towards the LV center during systole. This was 195% of similar movement in normals $(6.3 \pm 1$ mm, $p < 0.02)$. Net posterior movement of the mid-septum, when measured with the spine as a reference, was, however, significantly less $(p < 0.02)$ in ASD patients $(1.3 \pm 2$ mm) when compared to the normal group $(4.6 \pm 1$ mm), the net posterior excursion of mid-septum being only 28% of normals. The angle between the plane of the ascending aorta and the plane of the septum changed in a similar manner in patients with ASD and in normals. The change between end-diastole and end-systole was $10 \pm 1°$ in ASD patients and $14 \pm 3°$ in normals.

The direction of the echo beam was evaluated in relation to the septum. At end-diastole, the mid-septum was in the line of the echo beam, but during systole, due to markedly exaggerated anterior and inferior motion of the aortic valve, the relationship changed in ASD patients much more than in normals. At end-systole, a different part of the septum, near the left ventricular outflow tract, was in the line of the echo beam. Although the distance between the echo transducer and mid-septum increased with systole, the distance between the echo transducer and the part of the septum in the line of its beam decreased, producing the "paradoxical" septal motion.

DISCUSSION

M-mode echocardiographic patterns depend in part on the distance of the echo transducer from the echo interface. If the echo beam is reflected by the same point of a cardiac structure throughout the cardiac cycle, the resulting echo pattern truly reflects the systolic and diastolic excursions of that structure in relation to the echo transducer. If, however, during a cardiac cycle, there is movement of the entire heart, then the echo patterns depend on the systolic and diastolic excursions of that particular structure as well as the overall cardiac motion. In patients with ASD and large left to right shunt, the pattern of "paradoxical" septal motion is well recognized and has been attributed to right ventricular volume overload (2, 3). However, in some patients this pattern can persist even after complete surgical correction (3, 9), thereby suggesting that other mechanisms are involved. It has also been pointed out that smaller shunts and association of several other anomalies may result in the absence of this classical "paradoxical" septal motion (6).

The present study provides an explanation for this phenomenon in patients with ASD, large left to right shunt and right ventricular volume overload. Our angiographic findings show that the true motion of the interventricular septum is "normal" in these patients with ASD. The septum moves normally towards the center of the left ventricle with systole, just as it does in normals. This is evident by studying the relationship of the septum with the aortic valve and ascending aorta as seen in the LAO projection. The posterior excursion of mid-septum in relation to the ascending aorta is in fact even more than in normals. Why then does the echocardiographic pattern suggest that the septum is moving anteriorly in systole? There are two factors that produce this artefact: (1) the overall movement of the entire heart is grossly exaggerated, a logical consequence of greatly increased right ventricular stroke volume; and this results in (2) alignment of different parts of the septum in diastole and systole in the path of the echo beam coming from a stationary echo transducer fixed to the chest wall. As the normal anterior excursion of aortic valve and ascending aorta is greatly exaggerated in patients with ASD, being 200–300% of normals, it neutralizes the normally occurring posterior septal motion. Consequently, the net septal motion in space is less than in normals (1.3 ± 2 vs 4.6 ± 1). The exaggerated inferior motion of the aortic valve results in alignment of a relatively cephalad portion of the septum in the echo beam during systole. The cephalad portion of the septum is always anterior to the mid portion of the septum in patients with ASD and a large shunt due to a large right ventricle and posterior displacement of the LV. The overall result is that the distance between echo transducer and septal interface shortens in systole even though the septum does not truly move anteriorly. This produces the familiar and classical pattern of "paradoxical" septal motion.

CONCLUSION

The septum in ASD moves normally in relation to the ascending aorta and LV center during systole. The exaggerated anterior motion of the aortic valve and aorta partly neutralizes the normal posterior excursion of the septum and the exaggerated inferior systolic motion alters the relationship of echo transducer and heart resulting in alignment of a cephalad and anteriorly located part of the septum against the transducer in systole. The result is systolic reduction in distance between transducer and septal interface and the familiar pattern of "paradoxical" septal motion.

REFERENCES

1. Popp RL, SB Wolfe, T Hirata, et al.: Estimation of right and left ventricular size by ultrasound: A study of the echoes from the interventricular septum. Am J Cardiol 24:523, 1969.

2. Diamond MA, JC Dillon, CL Haine, et al.: Echocardiographic features of atrial septal defect. Circulation 43:129, 1971.
3. Kerber RE, WF Dippel, FM Abboud: Abnormal motion of the interventricular septum in right ventricular volume overload. Circulation 48:86, 1973.
4. Radtke WE, AJ Tajik, GT Gau, et al.: Atrial septal defect: Echocardiographic observations. Ann Intern Med 84:246, 1976.
5. Lieppe W, R Scallion, VS Behar, JA Kisslo: Two-dimensional echocardiographic findings in atrial septal defect. Circulation 56:447, 1977.
6. Assad-Morell JL, AJ Tajik, ER Giuliani: Echocardiographic analysis of the ventricular septum. Prog Cardiovasc Dis 27:219, 1974.
7. Pechacek LW, U Busch, E Garcia: Radiolucent holder for echocardiographic recordings during fluoroscopy and exercise. J Clin Ultrasound 6:355, 1978.
8. Pearlman AS, JS Borer, CE Clark, et al.: Abnormal right ventricular size and ventricular septal motion after atrial septal defect closure: Etiology and functional significance. Am J Cardiol 41:295, 1978.

THE EFFECTS OF TRAINING ON LEFT VENTRICULAR DIMENSIONS AND PERFORMANCE

A. RIGHETTI, R. ADAMEC, J. BORZYKOWSKI, G. BRANDON, A. SIMONIN, and J.C. DIDISHEIM

Although several studies have demonstrated the development of ventricular hypertrophy in animals following physical conditioning (1), few data exist concerning the effects of exercise training on ventricular dimensions and performance in man. The purpose of this study was then to assess, non-invasively, the changes in cardiac structures and performance in subjects undergoing regular daily training.

MATERIAL AND METHODS

Eighteen normal male subjects (13 soccer players and 5 cross-country skiers) volunteered for this study. All participants, ranging in age from 16 to 28 (mean age: 22 years), had a normal clinical history, physical examination and resting ECG. A maximal exercise test and an echocardiogram were done prior to, and after a mean of 2.4 months of 2 hours daily jogging and running as part of their regular training. Maximal exertion was performed on a cyclo-ergometer and maximal oxygen consumption (VO_2 max) was calculated by Astrand's nomogram (2). Echocardiography was performed the day following the exercise test in the supine position by the same operator using a commercially available echograph (ECHOPAN KS, Siemens). The standard technique was employed to obtain reproducible echocardiograms of the left ventricle at the level of the chordae tendinae and echo measurements were calculated as previously described (3). Echocardiograms and cyclo-ergometric data were analysed blindly by two independent observers.

RESULTS

Following the physical training VO_2 max increased in all but one subject. The mean value for the 17 subjects increased from 52.6 ± 3 (SE) to 59.5 ± 2 ml O_2/kg/min ($p < 0.001$). In one well trained participant, the VO_2 max (60 ml O_2/kg/min) was unchanged after training. The mean heart rate decreased but not significantly from 59 to 57. The following echocardiographic parameters represent the mean values of 17 subjects who improved their VO_2 max during the training period.

Left ventricular end-diastolic dimension increased significantly from

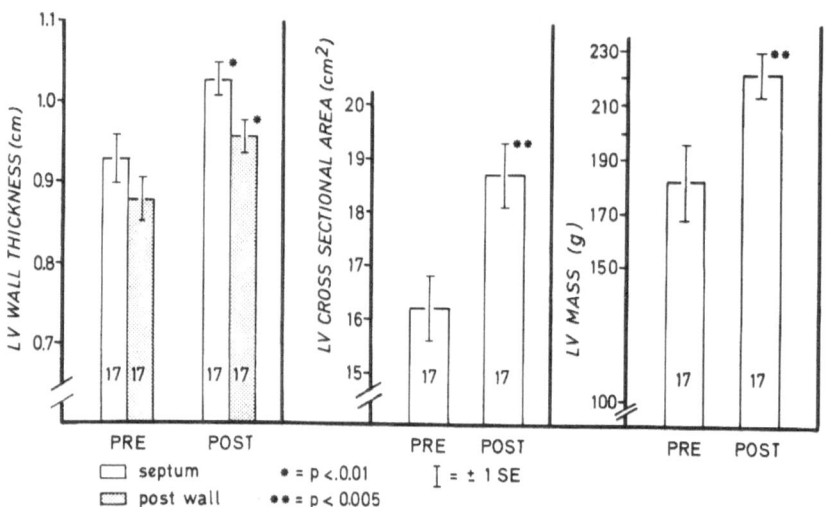

Fig. 1. Mean changes in left ventricular septal and posterior wall thickness (left panel), left ventricular cross-sectional area and left ventricular mass (right panel) during the exercise training. Bars indicate mean ± standard error.

46.7 ± 1.1 to 51.0 ± 0.7 mm ($p < 0.001$). However, left ventricular end-systolic dimension and right ventricular end-diastolic dimension remained unchanged after the training. Left septal and posterior wall excursions during systole increased from 5.0 ± 0.3 to 6.1 ± 0.3 mm ($p < 0.001$), respectively from 10.4 ± 0.3 to 11.2 ± 0.2 mm ($p < 0.01$). A greater left ventricular wall thickness was observed following the training period. The septal thickness increased from 9.3 ± 0.3 to 10.3 ± 0.2 mm and the posterior wall thickness from 8.8 ± 0.3 to 9.6 ± 0.2 mm, both ($p < 0.01$). In the 17 subjects who improved their VO_2 max after training, cross sectional area and left ventricular mass increased more dramatically from 16.2 ± 0.6 to 18.7 ± 0.6 cm^2 and from 184 ± 14 to 222 ± 8 g, both ($p < 0.005$) (Fig. 1).

Echocardiographic ejection fraction remained unchanged after the training period. However normalized septal velocity from 0.35 ± 0.02 to 0.41 ± 0.02 sec^{-1}, and mean normalized circumferential fiber shortening from 1.08 ± 0.03 to 1.21 ± 0.04 increased significantly, both ($p < 0.005$).

CONCLUSIONS

Echocardiographic measurements of left ventricular dimension, mass and performance have been shown to correlate closely with cineangiographic measurements (4). Since each subject was used as his own control some technical limitations were avoided. Maximal oxygen uptake was utilized as a method for determining the level of physical improvement after exercise training. Although no direct measurement of O_2 uptake was done, previous studies have shown the good correlation between the measured and the calculated values (2). In this study 17 of the 18 subjects increased their VO_2 max following a mean of 2.4 months of daily training; echo changes were assessed only in these 17 subjects. Although a few subjects had disparate values in the post-exercise echo measurements, the trend for the group was generally well defined; therefore we reported the results as the mean value of the group. Following the exercise training, left ventricular end-diastolic dimension, LV thickness, LV cross-sectional area and LV mass were all significantly increased. These results are in accordance with the data of others who observed similar cardiac changes in athletes and subjects after exercise conditioning (5, 6). The ejection fraction increased but not significantly, however the significant increase in post-exercise values of the mean Vcf and normalized septal velocity may well represent a definite improvement of cardiac performance in our study population.

REFERENCES

1. Wyatt HL, JH Mitchell: Influences of physical training on the heart of dogs. Circ Res 35:883, 1974.
2. Åstrand PO, K Rodahl: Textbook of work physiology. McGraw-Hill Book Company, New York, p 624, 1970.
3. Righetti A. M Crawford, R O'Rourke, H Schelbert, P Daily, J Ross, Jr.: Interventricular septal motion and left ventricular function after coronary bypass surgery. Am J Cardiol 39:372, 1977.
4. Troy BL, J Pombo, C Rackley: Measurement of left ventricular wall thickness and mass by echocardiography. Circulation 45:602, 1972.
5. Roeske WR, RA O'Rourke, A Klein, et al.: Noninvasive evaluation of ventricular hypertrophy in professional athletes. Circulation 53:286, 1976.
6. DeMaria AN, A Neumann, G Lee, W Fowler, DT Mason: Alterations in ventricular mass and performance induced by exercise training in man evaluated by echocardiography. Circulation 57:237, 1978.

D. APPLICATIONS IN CARDIAC VALVE STUDIES

SECTOR SCANNING AND M-MODE
IN AORTIC ROOT AND VALVE DISEASE

R. GRAMIAK and N.C. NANDA

Two-dimensional real-time echocardiography has been available for a number of years and has shown clinical utility in the diagnosis of various lesions involving the aortic valve and root. A comparison of the diagnostic efficacy of real-time imaging to M-mode has not been accomplished, since precise, controlled comparison would require independant examination by individuals equally skilled with each modality and using a variety of equipment to eliminate experimental bias. Qualitative comparisons, on the other hand, are being made by all who use both techniques in echocardiography. Our purpose in this presentation is to relate our impressions using both M-mode and sector scanning over a 2 year period in evaluating the common conditions which affect the aortic root and valve.

MATERIAL AND METHOD

We have examined approximately 3000 patients over this 2 year interval by both techniques including acquired and congenital lesions. Each subject was first studied by conventional M-mode, using a previously described system which features a Picker ultrasonoscope Model 103 and a 35 mm camera which operates as a strip-chart recorder. Following the M-mode examination, a two-dimensional sector scanner (Picker), which produces a sector up to 60° in width and provides frame rates up to 60 per second, was used to verify the M-mode findings, to seek additional information about the disease process, and to survey the heart in search of unsuspected lesions. In most instances, the sector scan examination was recorded on video tape and in all cases a description of the real-time examination was noted. The sector scan data was used during review of the M-mode film record and incorporated into a final diagnostic evaluation.

ULTRASONIC FINDINGS

M-mode echocardiography is a sensitive detector of calcification involving the aortic leaflets (1) and is equal in this regard to sector scanning. However, the findings are more difficult to interpret when small solitary calcific deposits are present. The record will usually contain some strong echo sources within the root but it is usually also possible to demonstrate slender

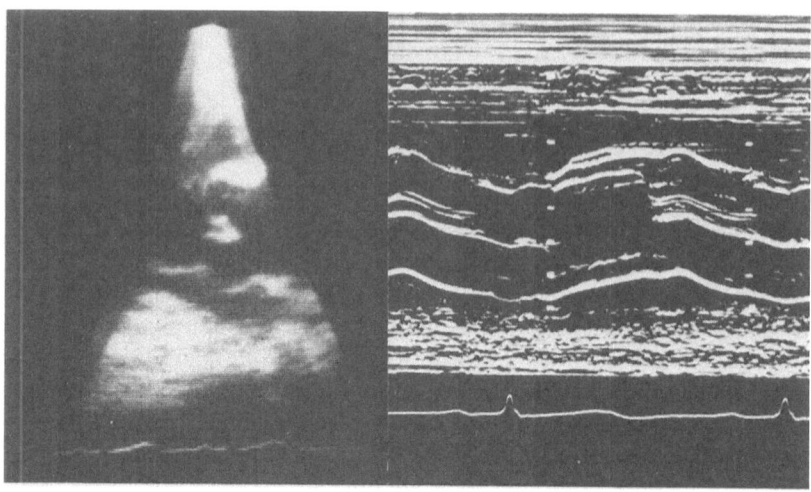

Fig. 1. The long axis view of the aortic root and valve (left) reveals thickened and highly reflective valve leaflets in diastole. In short axis, the calcification involved the right and left coronary cusps. The M-mode study (right) shows some indications of valve leaflet thickening but neither the specific location on particular cusps nor the size of the calcification can be identified.

aortic leaflets which move normally. The examiner is left to decide whether these intermittent strong echoes are real and whether they may be of significance to the patient (Fig. 1).

With heavy valvular calcification, it is often difficult to determine the extent of valve cusp mobility. When aortic regurgitation is present, M-mode can be relied upon to show the presence of diastolic fluttering of the mitral valve, whereas this information is not regularly derived during real-time scanning.

The two-dimensional method shows clear superiority over M-mode when small or solitary calcifications are present. The cusp of origin may be accurately identified and involvement of a commissure is readily seen. When calcification is more profound and cusp excursion restricted, a better appreciation of the extent of involvement and of orifice size is obtained, though quantification has not been possible in our experience.

Vegetations involving the aortic valve are probably detected as well with M-mode as with two-dimensional scanning (2). In occasional cases, M-mode has provided valuable information, especially in patients whose past medical history is confusing and in whom repeated blood cultures are negative. The demonstration of subtle diastolic fluttering of the mass or else a partially destroyed leaflet has been a valuable finding, since this never occurs in calcific aortic valve disease. The motion resolution of real-time systems is inadequate to demonstrate this phenomenon (Fig. 2).

Two-dimensional scanning provides information not obtainable in M-mode in those cases in which the motion of the mass is wild or erratic, or when the vegetation is large and extends for some distance from the cusp of origin. The multiple images obtained with variation in the examining plane

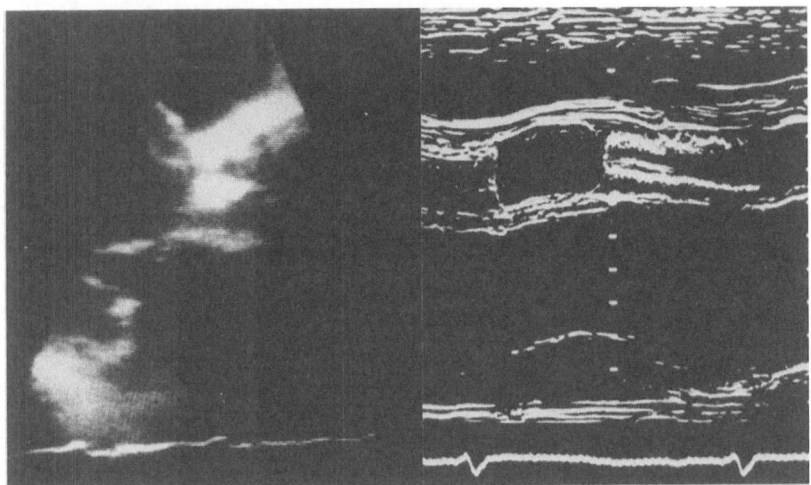

Fig. 2. The diastolic long axis frame shows a bulky mass attached to the aortic valve leaflets. A history of previous rheumatic heart disease suggested calcific aortic valve disease. The M-mode study demonstrates a subtle diastolic fluttering of the mass indicating its soft nature. Blood cultures were positive to support the ultrasonic diagnosis of a vegetation.

allow a more accurate evaluation of the size of the vegetative mass, so that better estimates of progression or regression of the lesion during therapy can be made. As with localized calcifications, the vegetation can be localized to a specific cusp to demonstrate the relationship to the orifices of the coronary arteries. Though we cannot demonstrate a higher detection rate, examiner confidence is greater, within the limitations of the method, when the findings are normal since there is more assurance that all of the valve has been inspected.

M-mode echocardiography has been disappointing for the evaluation of dysfunction of prosthetic aortic valves, probably because the poppet moves across the beam so that its motion is impossible to characterize. Two-dimensional echocardiography would appear to overcome this limitation but has also been disappointing in this application and has shown no additional information as compared with M-mode. The reason for this disappointment may be the orientation of the reflecting surface of the poppet which does not represent the portion making contact with the cage. Also, the strong reflecting characteristics of the components of the prostheses will tend to enhance the low amplitude reflection produced by the periphery of the beam, thereby emphasizing beam width and degrading lateral resolution. M-mode may be more advantageous in the detection of valvular or paravalvular leaks by demonstrating mitral valve fluttering in diastole or changes in septal motion.

In congenital aortic stenosis, two-dimensional studies readily demonstrate the domed aortic valve in systole and the restricted orifice can also be seen in long axis views (Fig. 3) (3).

Properly placed short axis planes will reveal the orifice of the stenotic valve whose area is shown with sufficient clarity in some instances to permit

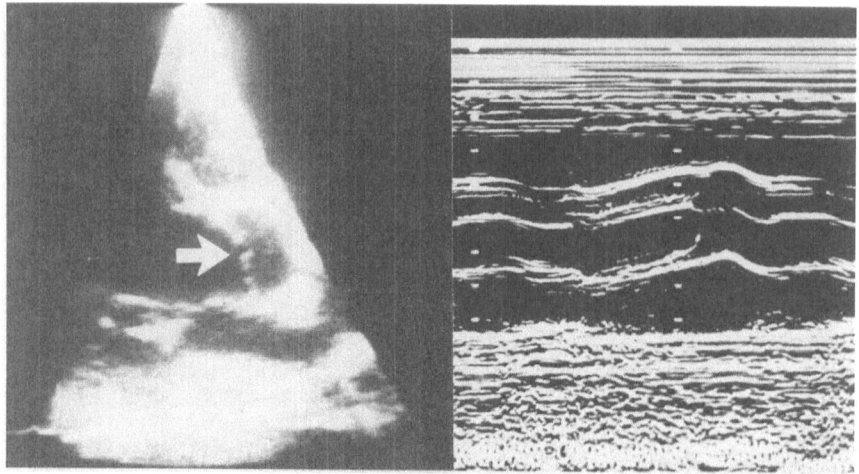

Fig. 3. A long axis view shows the aortic valve doming upward in systole with a small central orifice (arrow). In short axis, typical bicuspid leaflet anatomy was seen. The M-mode shows only asymmetry of valve leaflets and no indication of orifice size.

measurement of valve areas. M-mode has been widely recognized as deficient for these purposes since the congenitally stenotic aortic valve usually shows a motion pattern indistinguishable from normal. When the aortic valve is bicuspid, two-dimensional imaging provides superior information concerning the anatomy of the lesion. A single, usually S-shaped, line of closure identifies the biscuspid valve, anatomic asymmetry of the cusps is demonstrated, and folds at the line of closure may be seen. Thickening of leaflet edges is identified as a non-varying pattern through systole and diastole. Orifice size, again, can be appreciated. M-mode may not be as specific diagnostically since we have encountered instances of asymmetry, especially when the aortic root is dilated, but have been successful in showing the presence of 3 normal cusps, a reliable finding for ruling out the presence of a bicuspid aortic valve.

In aortic root dissection, M-mode may be somewhat superior to two-dimensional studies for demonstration of the dissected intima in the aortic root (4). In a few instances, the low amplitude echoes originating in the intima could be seen on M-mode but could not be imaged with the sector scanner. However, the real-time system allows visualization of more of the ascending aorta and suprasternal studies have demonstrated dissection spaces to reinforce the ultrasonic diagnosis. This may be of some use in recognizing false positive findings at the aortic root level, since we have seen additional linear echoes paralleling the posterior aortic wall in both M-mode and two-dimensional study in patients who were not clinically suspect of aortic root dissection. The sources of these false positives is not apparent at this time.

The two-dimensional diagnosis of aneurysm of the aortic root appears easier and more rapid, especially when the aneurysm is large. M-mode findings may be very confusing when the aorta reaches a diameter of 7 cm or more, particularly to an examiner not highly skilled in M-mode. The two-dimensional image appears to be more reproducible, so that greater confidence is achieved in following lesions to assess changes in size. The extent of involvement is more apparent since anatomically correct images of a greater portion of the ascending aorta, aortic arch, and even of the descending aorta, may be obtained with real-time imaging.

M-mode echocardiography is clearly superior is the detection of subaortic stenosis by demonstration of early systolic preclosure of the aortic valve (5). We have not been able to recognize this finding in two-dimensional echocardiography. However, the subaortic membrane or diaphragm is seen more often in sector scanning than in M-mode, though our success rate is probably less than 25% of proved cases. Similarly, abnormal aortic valve motion in the presence of IHSS, low output, or in mitral regurgitation is usually unnoticed in the two-dimensional study.

DISCUSSION

Real-time, two-dimensional scanning of the aortic root and valve is an important addition to the armamentarium of the echocardiographer and has already shown several conditions in which it is superior to M-mode in the evaluation of abnormalities. A comparison of the salient features of each technique will provide a basis for the understanding of their individual advantages and disadvantages.

M-mode is a non-anatomic presentation and, therefore, contains no useful information about adjacent structures, those which are oriented along the line of sight of the beam, or which may move across the beam. However, M-mode offers superior temporal resolution so that rapid structure motion is readily recorded. Signal processing in M-mode emphasizes weaker echo sources and generally gives a crisper appearance, making measurements easier. Dropouts and reverberating clutter present a greater problem than in two-dimensional imaging. The transducer is smaller, easier to manipulate, and somewhat more flexible in orientation.

Two-dimensional systems, on the other hand, present images which are anatomically familiar and which present structures lying parallel to the beam in their true anatomic configuration and motion. This fact alone is responsible for the superiority of two-dimensional imaging over M-mode in study of the aortic valve and root. The value of this anatomic display advantage can be judged by the fact that we are increasingly using two-dimensional studies at the bedside and not performing M-mode, except in a restricted number of instances. Were we compelled to choose between the two modalities for all of echocardiography, our unanimous choice would be real-time sector scanning. It would be imprudent, at this time, to dismiss M-mode echocardiography as a clinical tool. Certainly, the concept of high temporal resolution will continue to play an important role in the evaluation of heart disease. Whether it is retained in its present display format or incorporated into the two-dimensional image remains to be determined as new systems appear. For the present, the ideal technique appears to be a combination of both methods, preferably with the M-mode obtained from a reference two-dimensional display.

REFERENCES

1. Gramiak R, PM Shah: Echocardiography of the normal and diseased aortic valve. Radiology 96:1, 1970.
2. Busch UW, E Garcia, LW Pechacek, CM de Castro, Jr, RJ Hall: Cross-sectional echocardiographic findings in vegetative aortic valve endocarditis. Cardiovascular Diseases, Bulletin of the Texas Heart Institute 5:328, 1978.
3. Weyman AE, H Feigenbaum, JC Dillon, S Chang: Cross-sectional echocardiography in assessing the severity of valvular aortic stenosis. Circulation 52:828, 1975.
4. Matsumoto M, H Matsuo, T Ohara, Y Yoshioka, H Abe: A two-dimensional echoaortocardiographic approach to dissecting aneurysms of the aorta to prevent false-positive diagnoses. Radiology 127:491, 1978.
5. Davis RH, H Feigenbaum, S Chang, LL Konecke, JC Dillon: Echocardiographic manifestations of discrete subaortic stenosis. Am J Cardiol 33:277, 1974.

RELIABILITY OF M-MODE AND CROSS-SECTIONAL ECHOCARDIOGRAPHIC CRITERIA FOR THE DIAGNOSIS OF MITRAL VALVE DISORDERS

R.L. POPP

INTRODUCTION

At this point, approximately five years after the introduction of two-dimensional ultrasonic imaging devices, we are just beginning to become critical of the method. Initially, we were obliged to perform ultrasonic studies on patients with known valvular heart disease in order to teach ourselves what to expect in such patients. The first reports simply documented the ability of dynamic ultrasonic imaging systems to record the cardiac structures in health and disease (1). Then attempts at quantitation of the abnormalities were made and, subsequently, this information was applied prospectively to patients in the clinical setting. Obviously, the confirmation of a strong clinical suspicion in one's own patient, through observation of M-mode or cross-sectional echocardiography, is one matter, while it is quite another situation to prospectively interpret M-mode or cross-sectional echocardio-grams in the absence of appropriate clinical information. Thus it becomes increasingly important to question and document the reliability of M-mode and cross-sectional echocardiography in the diagnosis of mitral valve disorders. There are many specific clinical situations in which the ultrasonic studies can sort out which, of several possibilities, is the etiology of the patient's condition. This discussion is organized to focus on specific conditions of the mitral valve apparatus and mention the relative strengths of M-mode and two-dimensional echocardiography in recognizing conditions.

NORMAL MITRAL VALVE FUNCTION

The pattern of normal mitral valve motion on M-mode echocardiography is extremely well documented and well understood. Two-dimensional echo-cardiography (2D) has added several pieces of information, which have clarified and augmented M-mode records of the normal mitral valve. First, these 2D studies have shown the anterior and posterior leaflets normally separate during early diastolic opening, which accounts for the normal posterior leaflet motion seen on M-mode studies. In addition, the systolic position of the anterior and posterior leaflets is better understood with two-dimensional echo and the multiple reflections from each leaflet seem to cause less possible diagnostic confusion than they produce on M-mode studies. That is, one can see multiple reflections from the anterior mitral leaflet as well as the posterior leaflet in the normal patient, and in the normal patient the position of the anterior and posterior leaflet is rather clear, because of the anatomic continuity of each structure when visualized with 2D methods. Another important feature of 2D echo is the identification of the mitral and the tricuspid valves in the normal (and in the patient with inverted ventricles). The mitral valve is consistently displaced further from the cardiac apex toward the base of the heart, as compared with the tricuspid valve. By giving attention to the central fibrous body recorded in the apical four-chamber view, one can easily differentiate the anatomic mitral from tricuspid valve. (See Fig. 1.)

It is fair to say that 2D echocardiography is superior to M-mode echo-cardiography in judging a given mitral valve completely normal. This is because one may observe a much larger area of the mitral valve apparatus for abnormalities and then consider the valve to be normal in the absence of any abnormalities.

RHEUMATIC MITRAL VALVE DISEASE

After nearly 25 years experience documenting the abnormal pattern of the rheumatic mitral valve by M-mode echocardiography, 2D echo has little to add for the simple diagnosis of most patients with classical clinical presenta-

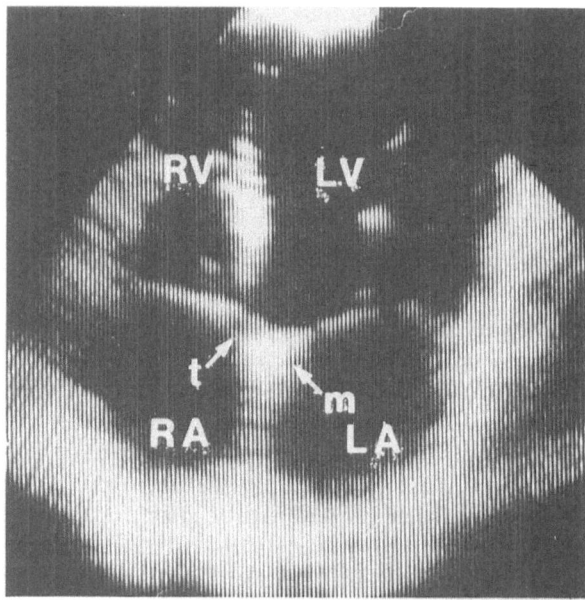

Fig. 1. Apical, four-chamber cardiac image, including both atrio-ventricular valves. The tri-cuspid valve (t) is closer to the cardiac apex, at the top of the figure, than is the mitral valve (m). The central fibrous body is between the two arrows. Echoes from the interventricular septum are shown between the right ventricular (RV) and left ventricular (LV) chambers. RA = right atrium, LA = left atrium.

tions of rheumatic mitral disease. Nevertheless, 2D echo has augmented the M-mode echo in quantitation of mitral orifice area in such patients, and has separated valves with a "square wave" anterior mitral leaflet motion due to non-rheumatic causes from the true rheumatic valves. M-mode echocardiography has been used as a very rough gauge of severity in the past, but recent studies have shown that it is not a good tool for precise quantitation of mitral orifice area; it may be quite misleading in some cases (2). Initial reports of 2D echo quantitation of mitral valve area gave extreme accuracy compared with cardiac catheterization data or areas measured at surgery (3, 4, 5). Subsequent experience has confirmed that 2D echo is superior to M-mode for quantitation of valve area, but that the degree of accuracy varies from laboratory to laboratory. At least three factors contribute to this variability. The first is the care with which these initial studies were performed. There are a great many technical factors to be appreciated when attempting quantitation of these very small orifice areas. The position of the transducer on the chest wall must be directly over the mitral valve orifice. The short axis image must pass directly through the orifice with perfect alignment, not at some angle through the valve. The level of the imaging plane must be just cephalad to the level of the papillary muscles and chordae tendineae to be at the apex of the "funnel-like" mitral valve structure. With the transducer properly located, and properly directed, the instrument must be adjusted to an optimal level of gain, reject, etc., so that there is sufficient signal to provide continuity of echoes around the circumference of the valve orifice, while not over-amplifying the signals to the point of their blending together and blooming on the oscilloscope to produce an artificially small orifice. While other factors are involved, these are the most critical ones, coupled with the exact mode of measurement of the image. Beyond these technical factors, we can appreciate how the patient load of a given laboratory will affect the amount of time taken to measure each patient study. There will be some point at which the increased experience of a high volume laboratory will be offset by the pressure of time, reducing the care with which any given patient's study is measured. Finally, other important variables will affect individual data: the specific instrument in use in a given laboratory and the amount of "feed-back" given by the standard invasive methods. Obviously, one must get to know the optimal use of one's instrument. Equally important, is the knowledge of the accuracy of the cardiac catheterization data and angiographic methods at a given institution, as well as the reliability of the numbers and information supplied by one's surgical colleagues. It is necessary to continue checking on the accuracy of these methods locally, before true reliability can be stated. (See Fig. 2.)

In our own use of these methods at Stanford, we find we are quite able to differentiate patients with what we consider critical mitral stenosis from those without critical stenosis, using a value of 1 cm^2 valve orifice area as the critical value. In measuring extremely small areas, we believe we cannot be more accurate than saying that valve orifice area is in the range of 0.4–0.7 cm^2 for example, or the valve area is 1.2–1.5 cm^2. So far, we have not had a

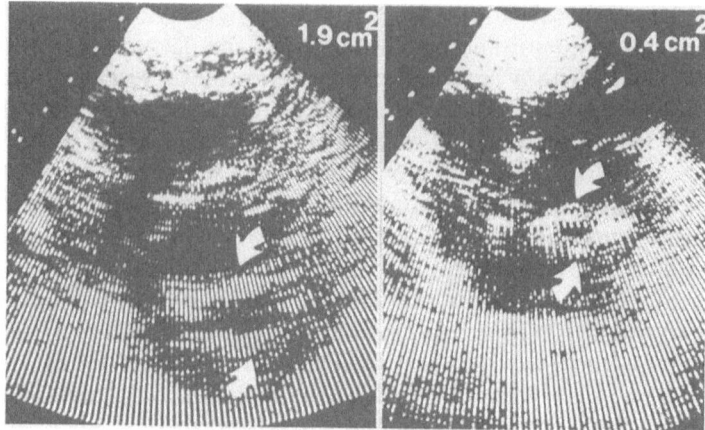

Fig. 2. Parasternal short axis cardiac images through the minimal mitral valve orifice chosen for measuring mitral valve area, in patients with rheumatic mitral valve disease.

Left panel, orifice measured 1.9 cm²; right panel, orifice measured 0.4 cm². Arrows indicate anterior and posterior leaflets. Orifice area is considered to be the central black area within the leaflet echoes.

situation in which a patient was judged to be in the critical range and accurate catheterization denied this. Much more commonly, there is associated mitral regurgitation, which invalidates the angiographic and catheterization data while the echocardiographic data is correct. In fact, we find 2D echo best serves the patient when making outpatient assessment of symptoms. We believe that two-dimensional echo can reliably and accurately differentiate the critical valve orifice, which goes together with symptoms, from the non-critical orifice present in the patient having symptoms from other causes.

MITRAL VALVE PROLAPSE

In many patients we prefer to look at the M-mode echocardiogram rather than the 2D image in order to judge whether the patient has mitral valve prolapse. This seems to be due to difficulty in assessing the dynamics of motion, the position of the mitral valve relative to the annulus, and the lack of easy quantitative methods for application to two-dimensional images (6). The M-mode criteria for mitral valve prolapse have proven quite reliable and useful in our hands. The two-dimensional method has permitted us greater flexibility in deciding which parts of the valve can best be recorded in order to find the pattern of prolapse on M-mode records. Those instruments which allow simultaneous visualization of the two-dimensional image and M-mode print out through a section of the valve are extremely nice for this purpose. Additionally, two-dimensional echocardiography has led us to suggest that there may be two factors, at least, in the generation of the M-mode pattern of prolapse. The first of these is actual elongation, redundancy and thickening of the valve leaflet structure. This is seen as multiple echoes with extremely large excursion of the leaflets throughout the imaging field. Secondly, there may be some patients, whose leaflets are not particularly elongated or thickened, in whom the posterobasal myocardium has an exaggerated "curling" motion toward the apex; this hypermobility of the annulus area causes the leaflet to bow towards the atrium at end-systole. Such valves look quite different from the redundant ones on 2D images and yet may give clear criteria of prolapse on M-mode studies. The significance of this segregation of possible etiologies is not clear at the moment. (See Fig. 3.)

Obviously, because the anatomy is well seen with 2D echo, false positive patterns of prolapse are better differentiated from true positive patterns (for example in the presence of pericardial effusion).

RUPTURED CHORDAE TENDINEAE

M-mode patterns associated with flail mitral valve leaflets have been reported. These may be quite distinctive, with chaotic motion of the mitral valve leaflets and extra echoes moving about within the field. Nevertheless, the majority of the patients we see present the problem of deciding whether there is a flail leaflet or simply a leaflet with extreme redundancy and prolapse, without detachment of the chordae. For this purpose, the M-mode echocardiogram usually has very poor reliability. Unfortunately, the 2D echocardiogram does not clear this up as well as might be expected. In a few cases, the 2D image shows a leaflet everting toward the atrium with systole and/or shows extra echoes flying about within the field, indicating portions of the valve and chordae tendineae. In the short axis images of some patients there is such an extreme motion of one section of the valve, compared with other sections, that we can assume detachment of this portion. In most patients, we are still unable to differentiate an extremely redundant leaflet from one which is partially detached.

VEGETATIONS AND MASSES

The excessive and bizarre echoes present on M-mode echocardiograms in patients with vegetations and masses often provide very striking and accurate diagnoses. The patient benefit resulting from such records has been quite gratifying for all those doing echocardiography. We now recognize that the size and location of the vegetation are important factors for registration with M-mode methods. Two-dimensional echocardiography provides a larger area for sampling of the valve and cardiac chambers than that available by M-mode. Thus one can decide where an echo mass is located, the shape of the mass, and whether this is a localized set of echoes or simply a uniform, diffuse increase in valve echoes. (See Fig. 4.)

Here again, the actual instrument used will partially determine the reliability and accuracy of this application. Instruments that provide true brightness-modulated images are best for this purpose. The subjectivity involved in

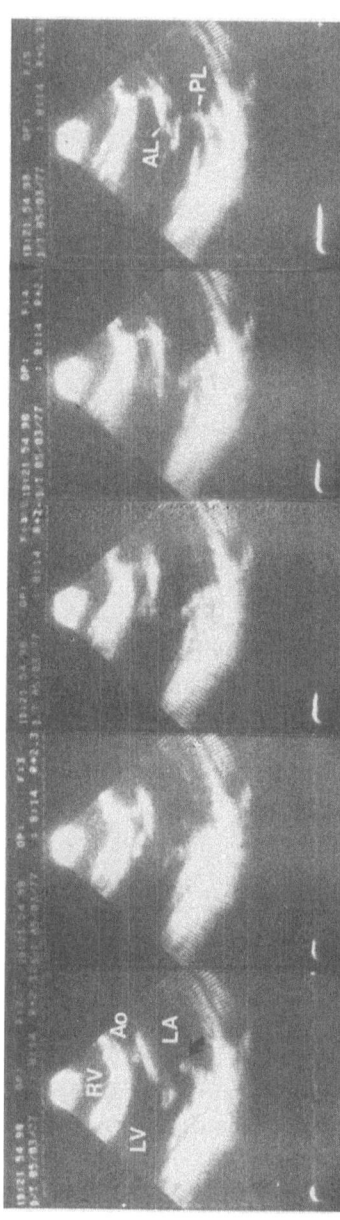

Fig. 3. Sequential parasternal long axis cardiac images, from endsystole to the subsequent early systole (left to right), in a patient with thick echoes from the mitral anterior leaflet (AL) and elongated posterior leaflet (PL). This suggests the first type of mitral valve prolapse mentioned in the text. LV = left ventricle; RV = right ventricle; Ao = aorta; LA = left atrium.

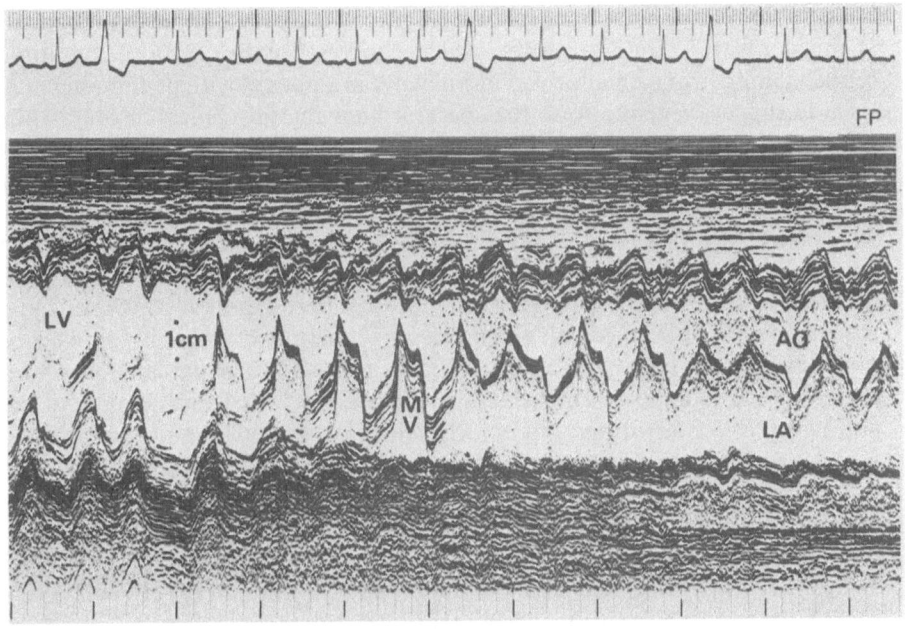

Fig. 4A. M-mode sweep from the level of the left ventricle (LV) to the level of the aorta (Ao) and left atrium (LA). Multiple bright echoes are shown in the area of the mitral valve (MV). It is not possible from such a record to accurately distinguish a diffusely reflective valve from a valve containing a discrete mass.

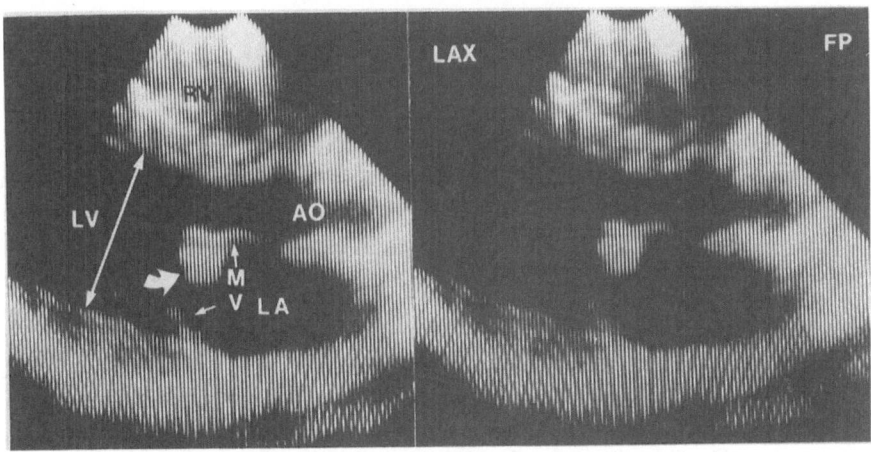

Fig. 4B. Parasternal long axis image from the same patient as in Figure 4A. Note the localized mass (fungal vegetation), indicated by the large arrow, attached to the anterior mitral valve leaflet. RV = right ventricle. For other abbreviations see Figure 4A.

interpreting two-dimensional echocardiography is a real and notable problem in this context, in both a positive and negative sense. For example, multiple echoes coming from a malformed mitral valve in a patient with pneumonia may seem to suggest vegetations to the operator knowing the clinical history, while the same image, observed by someone not being aware of the presence of fever etc., may be seen as a rheumatic valve. Thus, false positive and false negative readings are more likely in this area than in many others and caution is warranted. Nevertheless, this is one of the most important applications of 2D echocardiography because of the extreme illness of the patients under study and the relative contra-indication of invasive studies for further diagnosis. In some patients we have observed valvular masses in the setting of sepsis, in the absence of murmurs of valvular regurgitation or stenosis. In other patients, in whom there was hemodynamic embarrassment because of valvular dysfunction, the ability of 2D echocardiography to accurately assess both the masses and the ventricular dynamics has let us recommend surgery without angiography or catheterization. When one can image "valvular vegetations" in a patient with acute bacterial endocarditis, surgery will be indicated in the majority of such cases. Recent experience has shown that some of these patients can be treated medically with partial, and occasionally complete, resolution of both congestive heart failure and the abnormal echoes after treatment.

For non-bacterial masses, such as intracardiac tumors, the location of the mass is easily assessed by two-dimensional echocardiography. This location and judgment of the origin of the mass may affect thinking on the nature of the tumor and the approach and timing of surgical intervention. We have experience in avoiding invasive tests prior to surgery, with excellent outcomes in over ten cases.

OTHER CONDITIONS

Several specific abnormalities of the mitral apparatus can be appreciated by M-mode and 2D echocardiography. These include calcification of the mitral annulus, hypertrophic cardiomyopathy, dilated cardiomyopathy, and mitral valve motion affected by aortic regurgitation. Calcification of the mitral annulus is well documented by M-mode echocardiography and is quite obvious on 2D studies. This finding provides less diagnostic problems using two-dimensional methods versus M-mode records. We less commonly worry about pericardial effusion, or improperly identify these annulus echoes with two-dimensional studies than we do with M-mode. Mitral regurgitation resulting from hypertrophic cardiomyopathy gives very little difficulty be-cause of the distinctive character of the 2D images and the well known classic features of hypertrophic cardiomyopathy on M-mode echocardiograms. Nevertheless, in those patients in whom the diagnosis is not expected clinically, 2D echo more clearly illustrates this condition than does M-mode, in our experience. Mitral regurgitation in the setting of cardiomyopathy may

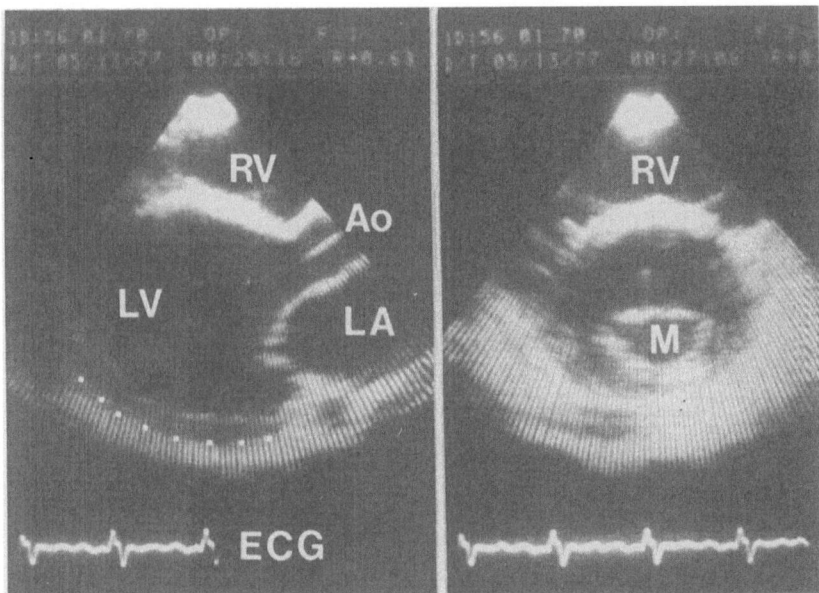

Fig. 5. Parasternal long axis (left panel) and short axis cardiac images in a patient with a dilated or congestive cardiomyopathy, and a murmur of mitral regurgitation. Note the enlarged globular Left Ventricle (LV) and Left Atrium (LA) relative to the Aorta (Ao), which is 3.5 cm in diameter. This is a pattern of primary myopathy if the ventricular contraction is poor. The circular echo-free area between the LV posterior wall and LA posterior wall is a dilated great cardiac vein or coronary sinus.

The white squares indicate the posterior wall epicardium. RV = right ventricle; M = mitral orifice; ECG = electrocardiogram.

present a therapeutic problem when deciding about surgery in such patients. Both M-mode and 2D studies can very reliably differentiate those patients with primary cardiomyopathy (extremely low degree of ventricular contraction) having secondary mitral regurgitation, from those patients with primary mitral regurgitation (well preserved left ventricular contraction) presenting a secondary clinical picture of cardiomyopathy. The two-dimensional methods have the advantage of assessing the entire ventricle so one can better appreciate segmental wall motion abnormalities associated with "papillary muscle" dysfunction mitral regurgitation, while the M-mode echo serves as a convenient means for quantitating the fractional shortening, ejection fraction, or other parameter of ventricular function. (See Fig. 5.)

Finally, with aortic regurgitation, the high frequency vibrations of the mitral valve are best seen on M-mode echocardiograms. Similarly, timing early closure of the mitral valve, due to acute and severe aortic regurgitation, is best done with M-mode echo. High frequency vibrations can be appreciated with 2D echo and localized areas of such "buzzing" may be appreciated with this method. In general, however, the M-mode is superior for this purpose.

REFERENCES

1. Bom N, PG Hugenholtz, FE Kloster, J Roelandt, RL Popp, RB Pridie, DJ Sahn: Evaluation of structure recognition with the multiscan echocardiograph. Ultrasound in Med and Biol 1:243, 1974.
2. Cope GD, JA Kisslo, ML Johnson, VS Behar: A reassessment of the echocardiogram in mitral .stenosis. Circulation 52:664, 1975.
3. Henry WL, JM Griffith, LL Michaelis, CL McIntosh, AG Morrow, SE Epstein: Measurement of mitral oriface area in patients with mitral valve disease by real-time, two-dimensional echocardiography. Circulation 51:827, 1975.
4. Nichol PM, BW Gilbert, and JA Kisslo: Two-dimensional echocardiographic assessment of mitral stenosis. Circulation 55:120, 1977.
5. Wann LS, AE Weyman, H Feigenbaum, JC Dillon, KW Johnston, RC Eggelton: Determination of mitral valve area by cross-sectional echocardiography. Ann Int Med 88:337, 1978.
6. Gilbert BW, RA Schatz, OT Von Ramm, VS Behar, JA Kisslo: Mitral valve prolapse two-dimensional echocardiographic and angiographic correlation. Circulation 54:716, 1976.

M-MODE AND TWO-DIMENSIONAL ECHOCARDIOGRAPHIC FEATURES OF PORCINE VALVE DYSFUNCTION

MOHSIN ALAM, SIDNEY GOLDSTEIN, ARMANDO MADRAZO, DONALD MAGILLIGAN, and JEFFREY B. LAKIER

In this paper we describe the M-mode echocardiographic features in eight patients and the two-dimensional (mechanical sector scanner) echocardiographic features in five patients with aortic or mitral porcine xenograft valve dysfunction.

MATERIAL AND METHODS

The clinical features of eight patients with nine glutaraldehyde-fixed porcine valves are summarized in Table 1. In addition, twenty-four patients judged clinically to have normally functioning porcine valves were also studied echocardiographically.

Of the nine dysfunctioning valves, three became stenotic and seven manifested regurgitation (Table 1). Three of seven patients with valve insufficiency (Cases 3, 7 and 8) had a past history of bacterial endocarditis, treated with antibiotics alone, with subsequent negative blood cultures. The valves from all patients were examined after surgical replacement (seven patients) or autopsy (one patient). Echocardiographic features of porcine valve dysfunction were related to the gross anatomic abnormality in all of the valves (Table 2).

Table *I*. Clinical and hemodynamic details of patients with porcine valve dysfunction.

Case No.	Age (yrs) & Sex	Valve position	Duration of implant (mo)	Murmur	Hemodynamics
1	57 M	A	11	AI	NP
2	37 F	A	42	AI	4 + AI
3	69 F	A & M	34	AS; MS	AVA 0.4 MVA 0.5
4	27 M	M	68	MI	4 + MI
5	16 M	M	60	MI	NP
6	30 F	M	65	MI, AI	4 + MI
7	50 F	M	52	MI	4 + MI
8	24 M	M	54	MI, MS, AI	2 + MI, MVA 0.7 1 + AI

A = aortic, AI = aortic insufficiency, M = mitral valve, MI = mitral insufficiency, NP = not performed, AVA = aortic valve area (cm²), MVA = mitral valve area (cm²).

Charles T. Lancée (ed.), Echocardiology, 213–217. All rights reserved
Copyright © 1979 by Martinus Nijhoff Publishers bv, The Hague/Boston/London

Table 2. Correlation of echo and gross findings in porcine valve dysfunction.

Case No.	M mode and 2 D echo features of porcine valve			Gross valve tissue findings
	thickening	Fluttering	Systolic prolapse	
1+		−	−	Thickened and vegetations.
2+		−	−	Thickened and vegetation
3+		−	−	Thickened, stenotic with calcific nodules.
4+		+	+	Torn, flail and thickened
5+		+	+	Torn, Flail, thickened and calcific nodules.
6+		+	+	Torn, flail, thickened and calcific nodules.
7−		+	+	Torn and flail
8+		+	−	Torn, thickened, stenotic calcific nodules.

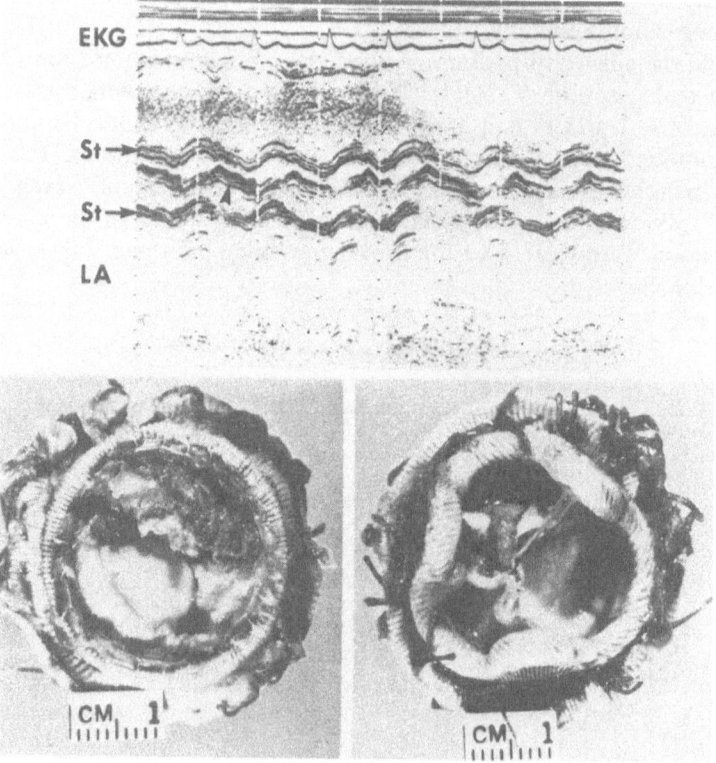

Fig. 1. Patient 1. *Upper panel,* M-mode echocardiogram of aortic xenograft valve. There is a marked increase in systolic and diastolic cusp echoes (arrowhead) with loss of cusp detail. *Lower panel,* gross appearance of the porcine aortic valve. Multiple vegetations and thickened valve cusps are seen. EKG = Electrocardiogram; LA = left atrium; St = stents.

RESULTS AND DISCUSSIONS

M-mode echocardiographic features

Generalized thickening with loss of normal cusp detail was observed in two patients with vegetative endocarditis on their aortic valves (Cases 1 and 2). The thickening was seen in systole and diastole, and these findings were confirmed at operation (Fig. 1). Generalized thickening of the cusps was also noted in patients 3 and 8, who had stenosis of the valve in the mitral position that was confirmed at operation (Fig. 2).

Localized fuzzy, fluttering echoes on the valve cusps occurred in all five patients with porcine mitral insufficiency. In the two patients with associated aortic regurgitation of the native aortic valve (Cases 6 and 8) these localized

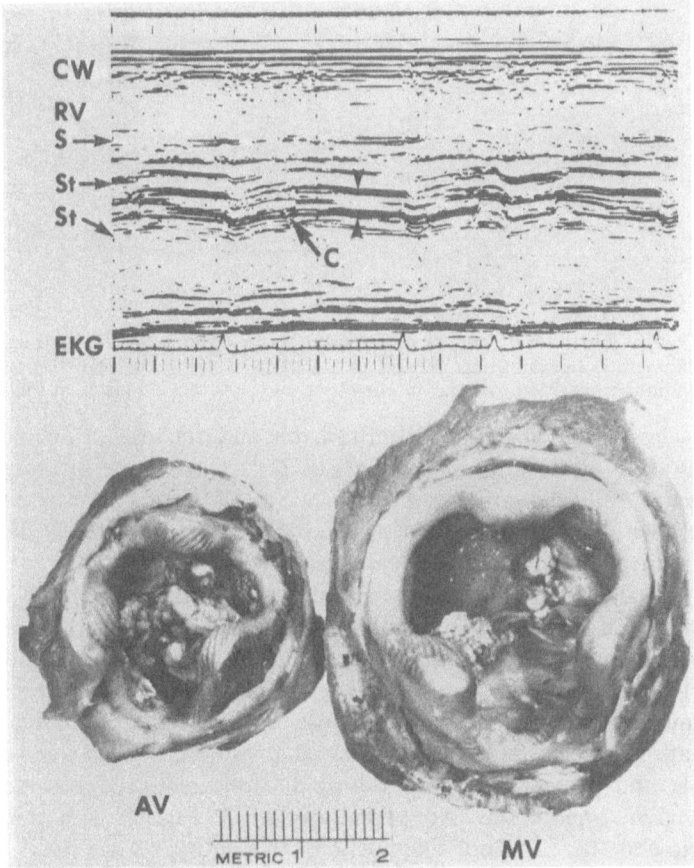

Fig. 2. Patient 3 with stenosis of porcine mitral valve. Upper panel; M-mode echocardiogram. A thin diastolic echo (arrow) of the opening of the valve cusp (C) is visualized. This echo is in fibrous continuity with thickened diastolic cusp echoes (arrowhead). The diastolic slope of the stents (St) is also reduced. Lower panel, gross appearance of porcine aortic valve (AV) and the porcine mitral valve (MV). Note the thickening and calcific nodules on both valve cusps. CW = chest wall; RV = right ventricle; S = septum; other abbreviations as in Figure 1.

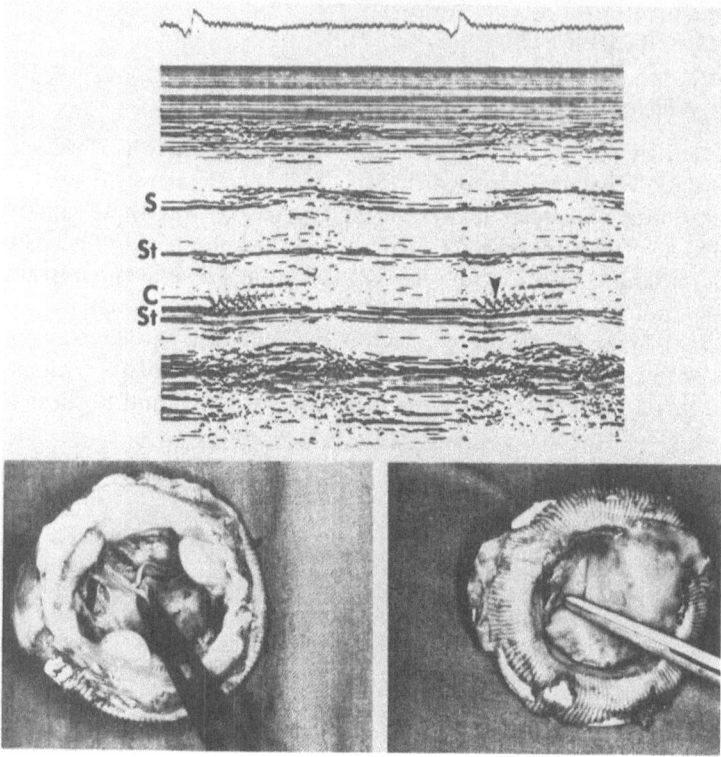

Fig. 3. Patient 7 with severe porcine mitral insufficiency. *Upper panel*, M-mode echocardiogram. Note the systolic fluttering (arrowhead) of the cusps. *Lower panel*, gross appearance of the porcine mitral valve. Note the tear in one of the cusps. Abbreviations as in Figure 1 and 2.

fuzzy echoes were observed in both systole and diastole; in one patient (Case 7), they were noted only in systole (Fig. 3). A tear in one or more cusps was observed in all five valves at operation. Systolic fluttering was never seen in patients with clinically normal porcine valves and adequately demonstrated porcine cusps on M-mode echocardiography.

Systolic fluttering was diagnostic of a torn and flail porcine cusp and is probably due to a high velocity regurgitant jet across the torn and unsupported cusp margins. With native aortic valve regurgitation diastolic fluttering may occur in a normal mitral valve. However, in both patients with flail mitral porcine leaflets and those with associated native aortic regurgitation, the fluttering on the mitral prosthetic leaflet was seen in both diastole and systole. Reduced mitral diastolic slope of porcine stent was observed in one of the two patients (Case 3, Fig. 2) with porcine mitral stenosis and therefore not diagnostic of this entity.

Two-dimensional echocardiographic features

Multiple dense echoes on the valve cusp were observed in four and of five patients with mitral valve insufficiency (Fig. 4). These echoes were shown at

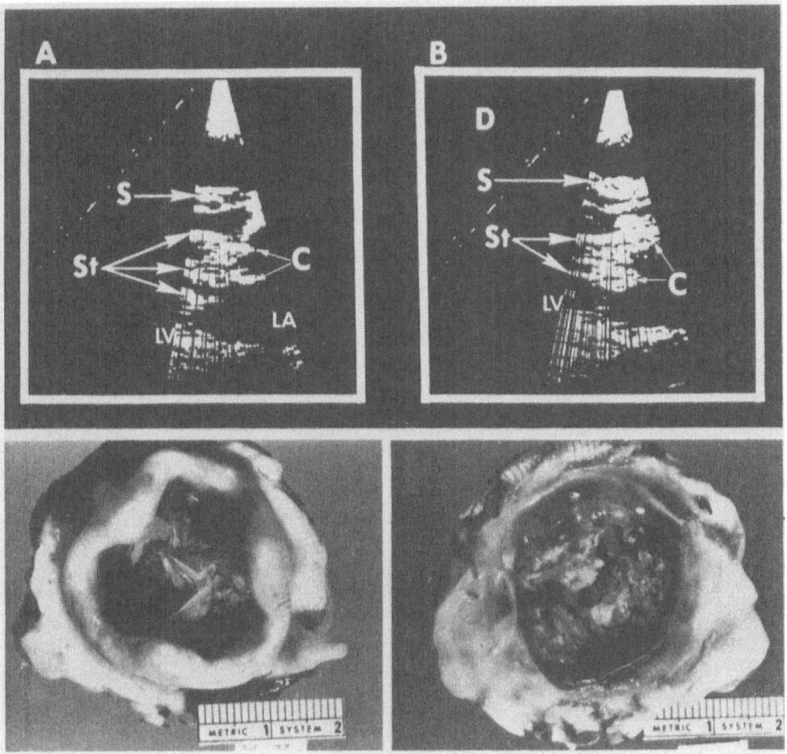

Fig. 4. Patient 5 with severe porcine mitral insufficiency. *Upper panel*, two-dimensional echocardiogram in systole (A) and diastole (B). Note the thickened dense cusp echoes (C) and the presence of these echoes in the left atrium (LA) during systole. *Lower panel*, gross appearance of the porcine mitral valve. Note marked thickening and calcific nodules, which correspond to the dense cusp echoes in upper panel. The cusps are also torn. Abbreviations as in Figures 1 and 2.

operation to be due to thickening of, or calcific nodules on, the cusps. Systolic echoes of the cusps were noted in the left atrium in four out of five patients with mitral insufficiency suggestive of torn and flail porcine cusps (Fig. 4). Tears in the cusps were demonstrated at operation in all five patients.

In conclusion, both modes of echocardiography were of value in identifying degeneration and dysfunction of the porcine xenograft valve.

ECHOCARDIOGRAPHIC ASSESSMENT OF INFECTIVE ENDOCARDITIS ON HANCOCK XENOGRAFT

G. CONVERT, J. GILETTI, and J. DELAYE

The valvular prosthesis represents a considerable improvement in the treatment of valvular heart disease. However, beneficial results of the intervention may be precluded by various complications, such as infective endocarditis. This paper reports a case of vegetative endocarditis with a Hancock xenograft bio-prosthesis in the mitral position, for which echocardiography permitted a precise diagnosis to be made.

CASE REPORT

In February 1976, a 21 year-old woman was admitted to our hospital with a rheumatic, mitral disease, categorized as being class III (NYHA). Catheterization showed a severe mitral insufficiency with atrial fibrillation and circulatory consequences (cardiac index 1.53 1/min/m², pulmonary hypertension 30 mm Hg, and tricuspid insufficiency). In addition, a moderate aortic regurgitation existed. A Hancock xenograft was implanted in the mitral position and tricuspid annuloplasty was performed (April 1976). The immediate status was excellent and 3 months later sinus rhythm was restored by DC cardioversion. Anti-coagulation was interrupted 5 months after surgery. In October 1977, a routine examination noted the beneficial results of the intervention: the patient was now in class I (NYHA), without therapy. Aortic insufficiency was minimal and frontal cardiac surface (expressed as the ratio of the expected value) had decreased from 2.75 to 2.48.

In March 1978, the patient had an embolism in the left femoral artery and embolectomy was performed, after which she was admitted to our hospital. The auscultation noted an unchanged aortic insufficiency, and an occasionally weak diastolic rumble. In addition, a systolo-diastolic pericardial rubbing was noted. Temperature was 39 °C. An enlarged spleen was palpable. The clinical diagnosis of infective endocarditis was confirmed by blood cultures, positive for streptococcus viridans (6 times out of 6 cultures).

During the hospitalization, she complained of severe headache and of photophobia. The neurologic examination was otherwise normal. Carotid arteriography disclosed a complete obstruction of the left internal carotid. The diagnosis was thus infective endocarditis, due to streptococcus viridans, complicated by femoral and cerebral embolisms. Echocardiography was performed during the septic phase, but after the embolisms. It showed (Fig. 1) a normal appearance of the Hancock valve: diastolic opening was typical and

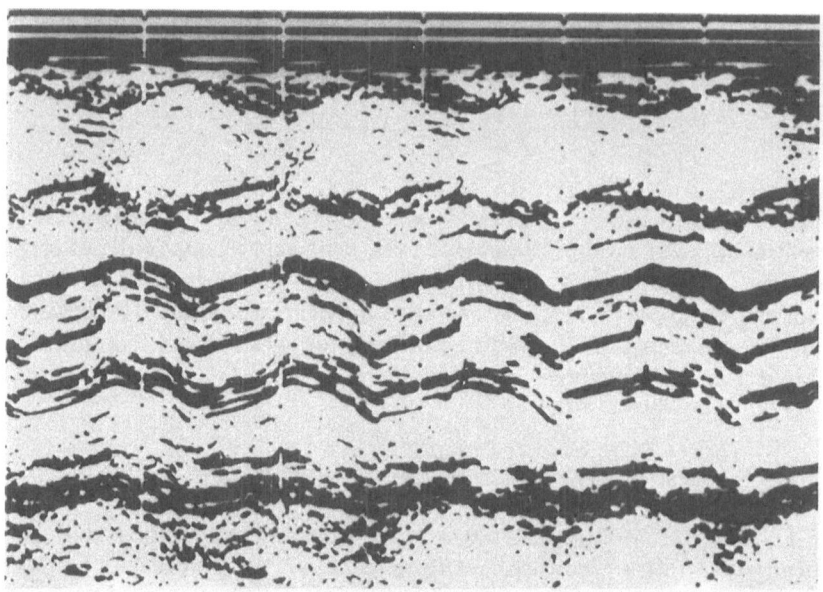

Fig. 1. Normal appearance of the Hancock valve in mitral position.

diastolic motion of the valve cusps was similar to the systolic motion of a native aortic valve. Paradoxical motion of the septum was observed. The aortic valve cusps were thickened and were apparently free of vegetation.

Antibiotic therapy (Gentamycin 120 mg per day, penicillin 32 million units per day) was continued for six weeks. The patient left hospital on oral antibiotics. She returned for routine examination one month later: the cardiac status was stable, and blood cultures were negative. In June 1978, she developed a new episode of fever (38.5 °C). A diastolic murmur of aortic insufficiency was noted and mitral regurgitation was also found, with a third heart sound. The cardiac surface had increased from 2.07 in May to 2.48. Atrial fibrillation had recurred. All the blood cultures were negative, but the sedimentation rate was high (100 mm) together with a raised white blood cell count (10,500). The echocardiogram (Fig. 2) showed important alterations. A left ventricular volume overload was noted. The internal dimension of the left ventricle was still normal. Pericardial effusion was present. The aortic valve cusps were unchanged, but the motion of the Hancock valve cusps was considerably altered: the opening of the anterior leaflet seemed normal, but the posterior leaflet displayed thick echoes, with multiple vibrations, and these echoes decreased the diastolic opening diameter. The conclusion of this examination was therefore that the bio-prosthesis was obstructed and that there was a left ventricular volume overload due to either the aortic or the mitral regurgitation.

Cardiac catherization was performed. Mean pulmonary wedge pressure

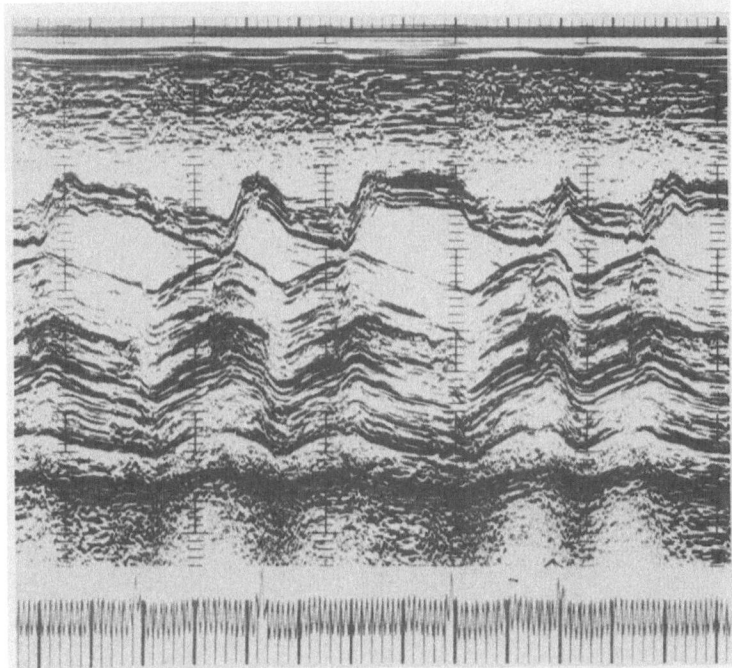

Fig. 2. Vegetations occluding the Hancock valve during diastole.

was raised (23 mm Hg), with a prominent V-wave, suggesting mitral regurgitation. Pulmonary pressure was considerably higher (87/39, mean 60
mm Hg). Cardiac index was moderately decreased (2.23 l/min/m^2). Aortic
angiography showed a moderate degree of aortic insufficiency. Cineangiography in the pulmonary artery showed moderate dilation of the left
atrium, with a prolonged presence of the contrast medium in the left atrium.
The left ventricle was not catheterized due to suspected aortic vegetation. A
decision was made to perform surgery to replace the Hancock valve and to
examine the aortic valve. The intervention was performed on June 26, 1978.
The Hancock valve showed severe damage, the cusps were thickened and
multiply perforated. The posterior leaflet had the typical appearance of
vegetation on the free edge. Vegetations also involved the annulus and
protruded into the left ventricular cavity (Fig. 3).

Histological study of the prosthesis showed severe alteration of two cusps:
one of them was covered by fibrinous exudation. The valvular tissue was
eosinophyl, and its appearance comparable with fibrinoid necrosis. Between
this valvular skeleton and the exudation, there was a polymorphic infiltration:
polynuclear cells, histiocysts, and numerous giant cells. The general aspect
was compatible with the diagnosis of chronic infective endocarditis. The
bacteriological tests were negative.

The Hancock valve was replaced by a Starr prosthesis. The aortic valve

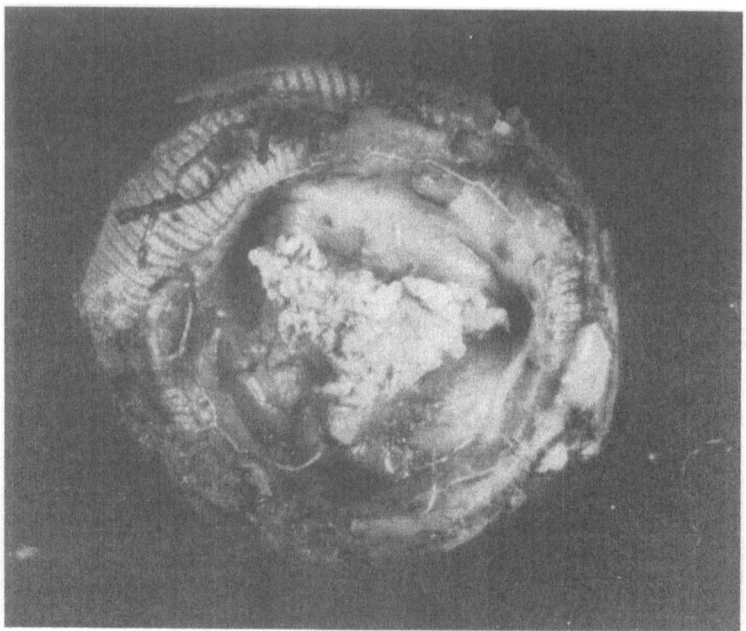

Fig. 3. Macroscopic aspect of the prosthesis, viewed from the left atrium.

leaflets showed a thickening in the non-coronary cusp with some degree of prolapse, and a correction of this valve was performed. The status was good, both immediately post-surgical and 6 months after.

DISCUSSION

Echocardiography is a very good method for the diagnosis of valvular vegetations (1, 2, 3). Being a non-invasive method it can even be performed in patients with active infective endocarditis. Diagnosis of vegetation is based on previously described criteria (1), and this technique permits the diagnosis of vegetations 2 mm thick or less. Hence echocardiography should be performed systematically, whenever one suspects infective endocarditis. Roy et al. (2) found the usual pattern of valvular vegetation in 69% of their patients presenting with an infective endocarditis.

The echocardiographic appearance of the Hancock valve in the mitral position was described by Bloch et al. (4). The authors noted a diastolic motion comparable with the systolic one observed in native aortic valves. This motion is inscribed between the two strong echoes of the annulus. So, on a good quality echo, it is possible to pick up such valvular abnormalities as thickening or vegetation. It is well known (Ferrans et al., 5), that porcine valves do not have endothelialization and that, after two years, the collagen fibers begin to dissociate. If we follow these authors, it seems reasonable to raise some question as to the durability of this type of valve. This cannot be answered from any clinical study as none, as far as we know, have yet involved a follow-up duration of as much as 5 years (6, 7).

Arshaff and Bloor recently reported sequellae of bacterial infection in Hancock valves, but the macroscopic apect was quite different from the usual vegetation observed on natural valves (8).

Hence, this case provides three valuable pieces of information:
- the inert material of Hancock valves can be damaged by infection with vegetation in the same way as the natural valves. In our case, the extensive vegetations led to a stenosis with hemodynamic consequences. Antibiotic therapy proved to have an efficacy rarely seen in cases of infective endocarditis on other artificial protheses (9, 10);
- echocardiography enables the diagnosis of vegetation to be made. The patterns are comparable with those observed in native valves. In the case reported, vegetations appeared after the acute infective episodes, and the first echo showed a normal appearance of the bioprosthesis;
- embolisms are not uncommon with this type of valve and are more frequent during the first post-operative year (11). This case emphasizes the utility of looking systematically for an infective endocardial disease whenever a patient with a valvular prosthesis presents with an embolism.

REFERENCES

1. Dillon JC, H Feigenbaum, LL Konocke, RH Davis, S Chang: Echocardiographic manifestations of valvular vegetation. Amer Heart J 86:698, 1973.
2. Roy et al: Spectrum of echocardiographic findings in bacterial endocarditis Circulation 53:474, 1976.
3. Thomson KR et al.: The reliability of echocardiography in the diagnosis of infective endocarditis. Radiology 125:473, 1977.
4. Bloch WN, JM Felner, C Wickliffe, PN Sambas, RC Schlant: Echocardiogram of the porcine aortic bioprosthesis in the mitral position. Amer J Cardiol 38, 3:293, 1978.
5. Ferran VJ, TL Spray, ME Billingham, WC Roberts: Structural changes in gluteraldehyde porcine heterografts used as substitute cardiac valves. Am J Cardiol 41:1159, 1978.
6. Mc Intosh CL, LL Michaelis, AG Morrow, SB Itscoitz, DR Redwood, SE Epstein: Atrio ventricular valve replacement with the Hancock porcine xenograft: a five year clinical experience. Surgery 78:768, 1975.
7. Horowitz MS, DJ Goodman, TS Fogarty, DC Harrison: Mitral valve replacement with the gluteraldehyde preserved porcine heterograft clinical hemodynamic and pathological correlations. J Thorac Cardiovasc Surg 67:885, 1974.
8. Arshaff M, CM Bloor: Structural alterations of the porcine heterograft after various duration of implantation. Amer J Cardiol 41:1185, 1978.
9. Arnetti EN, WC Roberts: Prosthetic valve endocarditis: clinicopathologic analysis of 22 necropsy patients with active infective endocarditis involving natural left-sided cardiac valves. Amer J Cardiol 38:281, 1976.
10. Quenzer RW, LD Edwards, S Levin: A comparative study of 48 host valve and prosthetic valve endocarditis cases. Amer Heart J 92:15, 1976.
11. Rabago G, J Fraile, NG Vega, T Moreno, V Campos: Mortality and complications in the use of Hancock's valves. Transactions of the European Society of Cardiology, Vol. I, No. 1, 018.

DIRECT ASSESSMENT OF AORTIC VALVULAR STENOSIS BY CROSS-SECTIONAL ECHOCARDIOGRAPHY

A.B. DAVIES, R.A. FOALE, and A.F. RICKARDS

INTRODUCTION

Measurement of aortic valve stenosis using M-mode echocardiography has been attempted by indirect methods, such as the measurement of left ventricular wall thickness to left ventricular cavity dimension ratio (1) or by defining the relationship between aortic cusp separation and the posterior movement of the aortic root (2). The severity of stenosis has been assessed more directly by measuring systolic cusp separation (3). This however, may be misleading as a stenosed valve is often domed and distorted and the single echo beam may pass through the base rather than the apex of the domed cusps. All methods have limitations in quantities of severity although it is accepted that an abnormal M-mode appearance does indicate an abnormal aortic valve. Cross-sectional echocardiography supplies additional spatial orientation and in children has been used to measure aortic cusp separation (4). In adults the orifice of the stenosed valve is often irregular in shape. This study attempted to measure directly aortic valve orifice area using cross-sectional echocardiography in a group of patients with aortic valve stenosis.

PATIENTS AND METHODS

Sixty four patients (age range 4.5 to 65 years) with aortic stenosis were studied; 24 of these patients had undergone cardiac catheterization within the preceding months.

Cross-sectional echocardiagrams were recorded using a 30° mechanical sector scanner*, M-mode tracings being taken simultaneously. The aortic valve was observed in both the long and short axes and with the latter transducer position multiple recordings were taken to visualise aortic valve orifice. Where possible direct measurement of the systolic valve area was determined using a calibrated grid.

RESULTS

It was possible to measure the systolic valve orifice area in 36 of the 64 patients studied. Of this group 24 patients had recent catheter data available (Fig. 1).

*Smith Kline Instrument Company Limited.

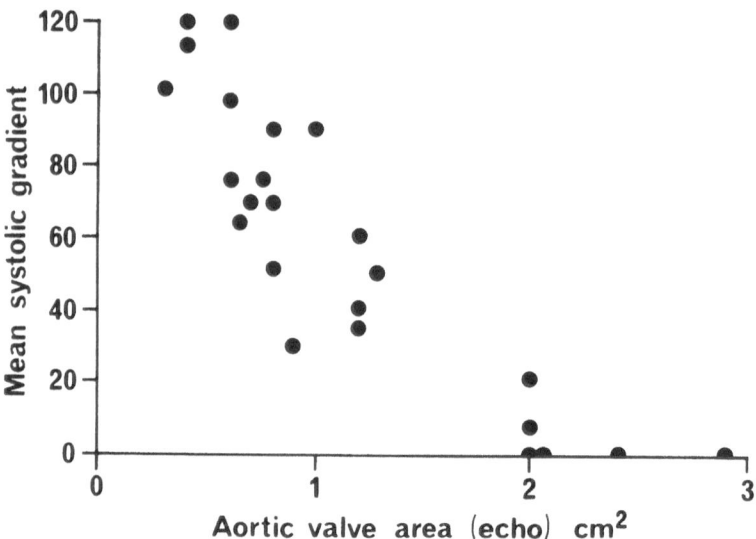

Fig. 1. Graph demonstrating the relationship between the aortic valve orifice in 24 patients measured echocardiographically and mean systolic gradient obtained at catheterization ($r = 0.89$ $p \ll 0.001$).

There was good correlation ($r = 0.89$) between systolic aortic gradient at catheterization and the estimated aortic valve orifice area. The graph demonstrates a simple exponential relationship described by the equation

$$\text{Mean Systolic Gradient} = 180.9 \; e^{-1.37 * \text{area}}$$

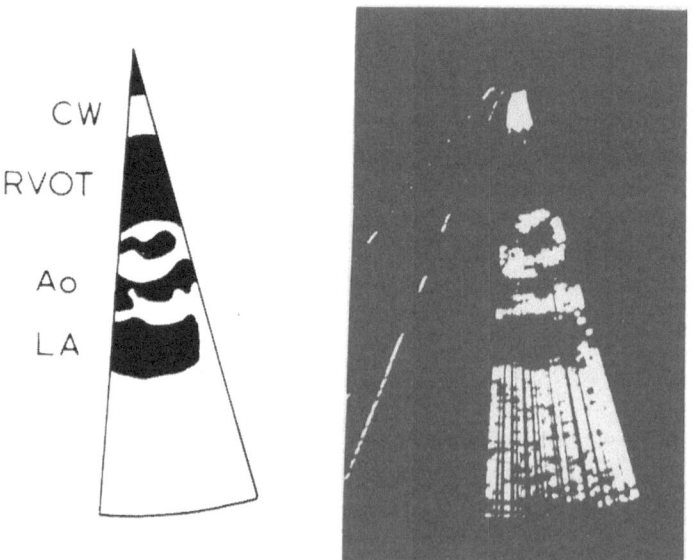

Fig. 2. Stop-frame image of a bicuspid aortic valve in diastole, short axis view with a diagramatic representation (left) showing a single thickened asymmetric closure line. CW = chest wall. RVOT = right ventricular outflow tract, AO = aorta, LA = left atrium.

In this group 7 patients had the appearances consistent with a bicuspid aortic valve with a single and eccentric diastolic closure line (Fig. 2) when the aortic root was viewed in the short axis. This was consistent with the clinical and angiographic diagnosis. In 3 patients, 3 symmetrical cusps were seen clearly and this was confirmed at surgery. In the remaining 14 patients of this group, distortion and thickening of the valve cusps excluded determination of the morphology of the valves although the valve area was measurable.

Twelve patients with clinically mild aortic stenosis, in whom the orifice area was measured, had not been catheterized and in this group 7 had the appearance of a bicuspid aortic valve consistent with the clinical diagnosis. Visualization of 3 valve cusps was possible in the remaining 5 patients (Fig. 3).

It was not possible to measure the aortic orifice area in 28 patients, 10 of whom had heavy multiple echoes within the aortic root consistent with calcification and these were confirmed as having severe aortic stenosis at cardiac catheterization. The remaining 18 subjects were considered poor echo subjects.

DISCUSSION

In patients with measurable aortic valve orifice areas good correlation existed when compared with data obtained at cardiac catheterization. The apparent exponential nature of the curve (Fig. 1) relating aortic valve orifice

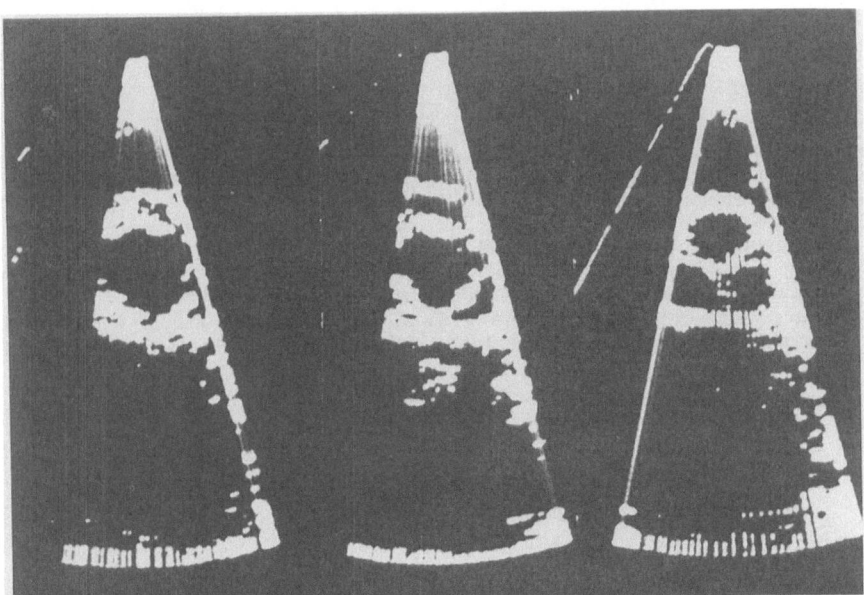

Fig. 3. Image of a tricuspid aortic valve in short axis view demonstrating symmetrical closure in diastole: the cusp opposing the aortic wall in systole.

area to mean systolic gradient is consistent with results obtained using other methods for estimating aortic valve area. The patients in whom it was not possible to measure the aortic orifice size consisted of 3 groups. Firstly, 18 of the initial group of 64 patients were considered poor echocardiographic subjects in that clear definition of the anterior mitral leaflet-posterior aortic wall continuity was not possible. Secondly, cusp distortion and thickening with calcification occurred generally in those patients with severe aortic stenosis; at surgery the valves were observed to have extremely distorted orifices often with shelving projections. Thirdly, a younger group of patients with mild aortic valve disease had highly mobile and non-thickened cusps. It was not possible to define the limits of the orifice in these patients. In our experience with a control group of normal subjects, 3 symmetrical cusps may be seen in less than 50% of cases.

In 21 of the initial group of 64 the morphology of the aortic valve could be defined and estimations as to the nature of the valve were consistent with the clinical or operative findings. This group tended to be those patients with clinically mild or moderate aortic stenosis.

CONCLUSION

In more than half of the patients studied it was possible to determine directly the aortic valve orifice area using short axis visualization of the aortic root. It was also possible to provide information about the morphology of the aortic valve in selected cases.

REFERENCES

1. Aziz KU, A Van Grondell, MH Paul, AJ Muster: Echocardiographic assessment of the relationship between left ventricular wall and cavity dimensions and peak systolic pressure in children with aortic stenosis. Am J Cardiol 40:775, 1977.
2. Reeves WC, NC Nanda, R Gramiak: The relationship between aortic valve closure and aortic root motion. Radiology 127:751, 1978.
3. Chang S, S Clement, J Chang: Aortic stenosis: Echocardiographic cusp separation and surgical description of aortic valve in 22 patients. Am J Cardiol 39:499, 1977.
4. Weyman AE, H Feigenbaum, RA Hurwitz, DA Girod, JC Dilton: Cross-sectional echocardiographic assessment of the severity of aortic stenosis in children. Circulation 55:773, 1977.

PRE- AND POSTOPERATIVE ECHOCARDIOGRAMS IN PATIENTS WITH DISCRETE TYPE SUBAORTIC STENOSIS

M. ERIJMAN, J. GLASER, and B. VIDNE

During the last 10 years, 14 patients (7 males and 7 females) with discrete type subaortic stenosis (Type I), were operated upon at our hospital. Their ages ranged between 9–38 years. The preoperative clinical findings, echocardiograms and catheterization results were compared to those found postoperatively. The time lapse between the surgery and the echocardiographic examination ranged between 5 to 120 months, with a mean time of 49 ± 6 months. The ECG in most of the patients did not change significantly; only one patient developed postoperative LBBB.

On physical examination, a harsh systolic murmur, maximal at the apex, was found in all the patients, both pre- and postoperatively; a diastolic murmur suggesting aortic insufficiency developed in 4 of the patients and increased in two others; in 4 of the patients the initial diagnosis was a possible small VSD.

Preoperative echocardiographic examination was performed in 6 of the patients whereas postoperative echocardiography was carried out in all of

Table 1. Pre- and postoperative cardiac catheterization results.

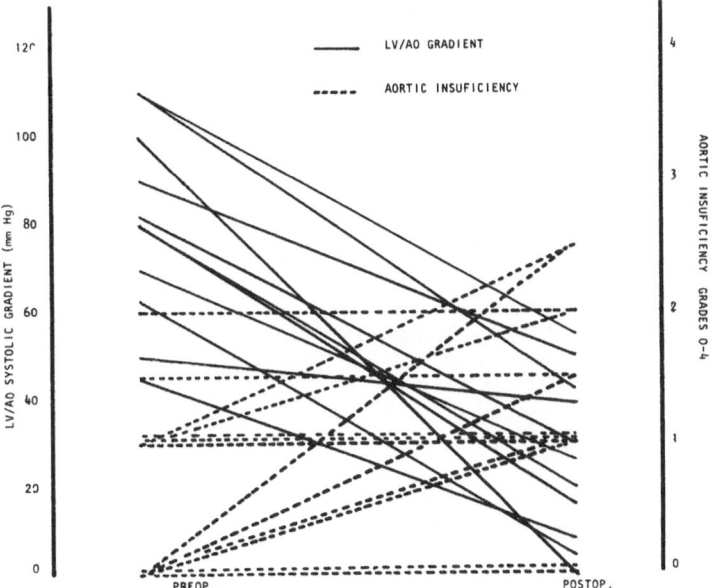

230 M. ERIJMAN ET AL.

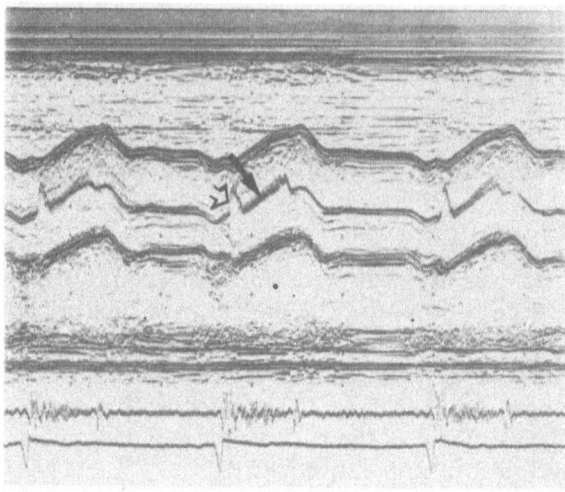

Fig. 1. Postoperative aortic valve echogram in a patient who had a sub-aortic membrane resected. The valve shows early closure (open arrow) and systolic flutter (black arrow), suggesting residual membrane and continuing valve damage. The simultaneous phono shows a harsh systolic murmur and an early diastolic murmur of AI.

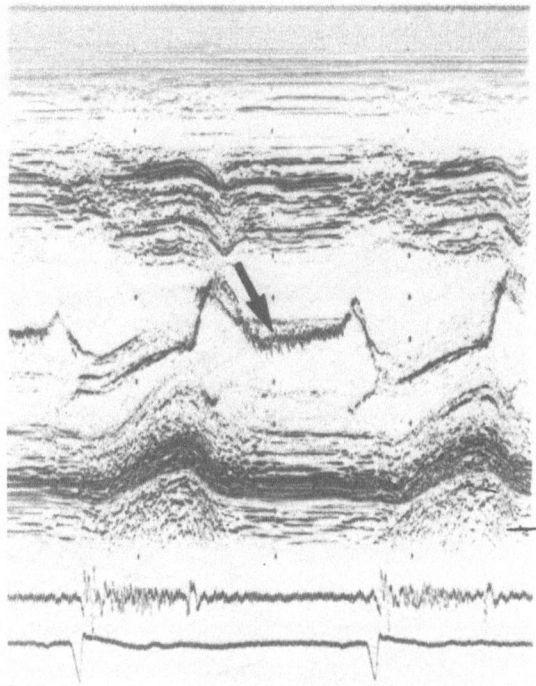

Fig. 2. Postoperative mitral valve echogram in the same patient as in Figure 1 showing diastolic flutter of the anterior mitral leaflet (black arrow), suggesting a significant degree of aortic insufficiency.

them. Findings suggesting postoperative residual membrane (early closure and/or vibrations of the aortic valve) were found in all of the patients, and signs of aortic insufficiency (mitral valve diastolic flutter) in 12 of the 14 patients on postoperative examination. Pre- and postoperative cardiac catheterizations were performed in 12 of 14 patients. The systolic gradient across the LV outflow tract decreased significantly in all the patients, ranging from 45 to 110 mm Hg before surgery with a mean of 75 ± 3 to 0–55 mm Hg with a mean of 29 ± 1, postoperatively.

Aortic insufficiency (AI) at a grade of 0–2/4 was found at the preoperative catheterization in 8 of the 14 patients (57%). Postoperatively, 12 patients presented insufficiency of the aortic valve 1–3/4 (85%). In 6 of the patients the AI increased as compared to the preoperative period and in the remaining patients, it did not change. No patient showed any signs of decreased AI.

In all patients, the LV/Ao gradient decreased whereas the AI increased in 6 and did not decrease in the rest. In 4 patients there was no AI preoperatively, and at the postoperative period there was AI of $1-2\frac{1}{2}/4$.

These results demonstrated that, although surgery was successful in releasing the LV outflow tract obstruction, it did not prevent the development of valvular aortic insufficiency of increasing severity.

We suggest that the continuous long-standing aortic valve flutter as shown in repeated echocardiograms, is a possible cause of the deterioration of the valve. This flutter is most probably due to residual membrane left by the surgeon. Although not enough to cause a significant obstruction it is enough to create a jet of blood which strikes the aortic valve continuously. Echocardiography was found to be an extremely sensitive tool in the diagnosis and follow-up of patients with the discrete type of subaortic stenosis, with varying amounts of stenosis and insufficiency.

REFERENCES

1. Chandraranta Pan, LS Cohen: Pre- and postoperative echocardiographic features of discrete subaortic stenosis. Cardiology 61:181, 1976.
2. Kelly DT, E Wulfsberg, RD Rowe: Discrete subaortic stenosis. Circulation 46:309, 1972.
3. Laurenceau JL, JM Guay, S Gagne: Echocardiography in the diagnosis of subaortic membranous stenosis (Abstr.) Circulation 48: Suppl. IV.
4. Newfeld EA, AJ Muster, MH Paul et al.: Discrete subvalvular aortic stenosis in childhood: Study of 51 patients. Am J Cardiol 38:53, 1976.
5. Zvonimir K, O Fulvio, WP Leonard et al.: Early systolic closure of the aortic valve in patients with hypertrophic subaortic stenosis and discrete subaortic stenosis. Am J Cardiol 41:823, 1978.

DETECTION OF TRICUSPID REGURGITATION WITH PULSED DOPPLER ECHOCARDIOGRAPHY

F. FANTINI and A. MAGHERINI

The diagnosis of tricuspid regurgitation (TR) is often difficult to make with certainty, whether on the basis of clinical findings, of right cineangiography or of both. M-mode and two-dimensional echocardiography give only indirect, non-specific indications relating volume load of the right ventricle. Some promising results, obtained by means of a combined contrast/two-dimensional echocardiographic examination, have been reported recently (1). Pulsed-Doppler echocardiography (PDE) has proved to be a valuable technique for evaluating blood flow characteristics at specific locations within the heart and great vessels (2). Information given by this technique is primarily qualitative. It is possible to recognize the direction of flow relative to the ultrasonic beam and the type of flow – laminar versus turbulent – within the sample volume. The purpose of this work is to illustrate the application of PDE to identify TR.

MATERIAL AND METHODS

A group of 37 patients was selected according to clinical and hemodynamic findings. It was composed of 11 patients with acquired TR, 3 with tricuspid stenosis, 1 with Ebstein's anomaly, 4 with partial A-V canal, 1 with left ventricular to right atrial communication, 8 with atrial septal defect (ASD) and 9 with ventricular septal defect (VSD). Most of the patients with congenital malformations were controlled after surgery.

Echocardiographic examination was carried out using an M-mode device, a two-dimensional phased-array ultrasonograph and a pulsed-Doppler apparatus (ATL 500A). In each patient, the central venous velocity tracing (CVVT) was recorded. The transducer was positioned on the suprasternal notch and the ultrasonic beam was directed downward, to the right and posteriorly, until a typical venous flow sound was heard. The velocity profile recorded in this area normally presents a negative wave (a) corresponding to atrial contraction and two positive waves, one occurring during ventricular ejection (s) and the other during the rapid-filling phase of ventricular diastole (d). This tracing is the reverse of that described by Kalmanson et al. (3), who direct the beam upstream, against the direction of blood flow in the jugular vein. The transducer was located on the precordium, after having identified the tricuspid valve echoes, and the tricuspid flow velocity tracing (TFT) recorded in each patient by selecting a proper depth for the sample volume, it was easy to record the TFT behind valve echoes, into the right atrium, and within the inflow tract of the right ventricle. The TFT reflects the velocity flow pattern through the tricuspid valve. In normal cases it shows a characteristic M-shaped diastolic profile. Turbulent flow is characterized by a wide band of acoustic frequencies, producing a murmur-like sound at the audio amplifier and a dispersion of dots on the graphical display, the "time interval histogram" (4).

RESULTS

All patients with TR showed turbulent flow behind the tricuspid valve echoes. In some cases, a signal indicating a systolic flow from the right ventricle to the right atrium was detected. The two types of tracings were often recorded in the same patient at slightly different locations or with different gain setting. The direction of flow is more difficult to detect when the blood flow is more disturbed (Fig. 1, left).

CVVT usually showed the absence of an s-wave or else a positive systolic wave, indicating a backward flow within the great veins during systole. The shape and the timing of CVVT were similar to the jugular venous tracing (Fig. 1, right). When tricuspid stenosis was present, turbulent flow was detected within the inflow tract of right ventricle during diastole (Fig. 2, left).

Turbulent flow behind the tricuspid leaflets was also detected in patients with partial A-V canal and cleft mitral valve, in the case with left ventricular-right atrial communication and in 2 cases with VSD and patent tricuspid commissurae. CVVT did not show a backward flow in these cases. The evaluation of the direction of flow within the inflow tract of the right

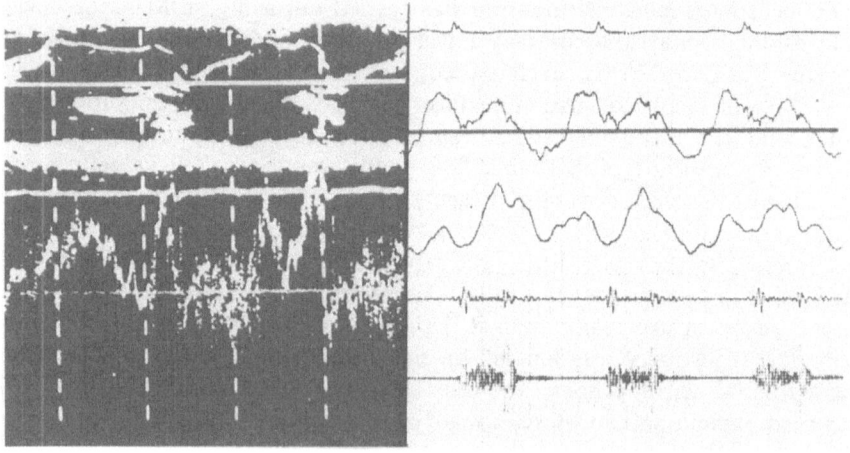

Fig. 1. Left: TFT in a case of TR; right: CVVT (top) and jugular phlebogram in a patient with TR (the horizontal line indicates zero flow).

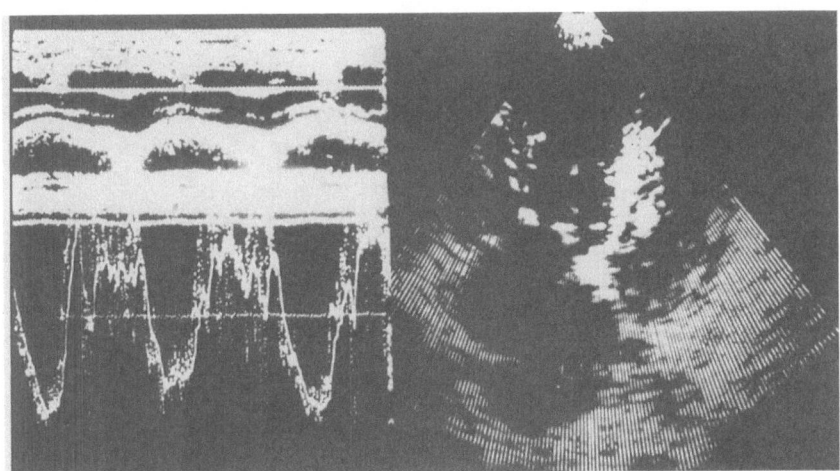

Fig. 2. TFT (left) and two-dimensional echocardiogram (right) in a patient with TR and stenosis (carcinoid syndrome).

ventricle, or through the tricuspid valve, might be helpful in identifying the presence of TR in these cases.

Patients with ASD showed rapid flow behind the tricuspid leaflets during end-systole and proto-diastole. CVVT had a characteristic pattern in these patients.

As a conclusion, we wish to emphasize that PDE complements M-mode and two-dimensional echocardiography and constitutes a useful technique for the diagnosis of TR.

REFERENCES

1. Lieppe W, VS Behar, R Scallion, JA Kisslo: Detection of tricuspid regurgitation with two-dimensional echocardiography and peripheral vein injection. Circulation 57:128, 1978.
2. Baker DW, SA Rubenstein, GS Lorch: Pulsed Doppler echocardiography: principles and applications. Am J Med. 63:69, 1977.
3. Kalmanson D, C Veyrat, C Derai, CH Savier, M Berkman, P Chica: Noninvasive technique for diagnosing atrial septal defect and assessing shunt volume using directional Doppler ultrasound. Brit Heart J 34:981, 1972.
4. Lorch G, SA Rubenstein, DW Baker, T Dooley, H Dodge: Doppler echocardiography: use of a graphical display system. Circulation 56:576, 1977.

MITRAL VALVE PROLAPSE WITH AORTIC ROOT DILATION: AN ECHOCARDIOGRAPHIC STUDY

L. HUMBLET, V. BAUDINET, and P. COLLIGNON

1. INTRODUCTION

The few reported anatomical observations of mitral valve prolapse (MVP) have demonstrated the presence of degenerative changes and mucopolysaccharide accumulation (mucoid or myxomatous degeneration) 4, 5, 6, 12). Similar lesions may also be seen at the level of the aortic valve (10) and aortic root (8, 9); they increase in frequency with advancing age (11, 13) and seem to be devoid of specificity (13). A comparison with the forme fruste of Marfan's syndrome has been made (14) on the basis of similar sites and nature of anatomical abnormalities.

Reviewing the abundant literature on MVP, the absence of aortic root dilation in patients without Marfan's syndrome is most intriguing. It is thought that the mean age of the explored populations studied was probably too low to allow for the aortic lesions to become manifest.

Eighty one patients of different ages presenting with a MVP were therefore investigated with the intention to depict aortic root dilatation, unrelated to the Marfan's syndrome.

2. MATERIAL AND METHODS

2.1. MVP group

Eighty one patients with MVP were selected on the basis of the simultaneous presence of a non ejection click (with or without systolic murmur) and of typical echocardiographic signs (2.7). A chest X-ray, resting and exercise electrocardiograms were obtained in all cases.

2.2. Control group

Ninety one patients without evidence of cardiovascular disease were examined to obtain control data for the aortic root dimensions in relation to age.

2.3. Echocardiograms

All investigations were performed by the same investigator using the M-mode and an Echocardiovisor 01-Organon Technika with probes 2, 25 MHZ having a diameter of 13 mm and focalized at 50 and 75 mm.

Recordings were made on a Honeywell L.S.6 at speeds of 25 and 50 mm/sec. The patients were lying on their back or slightly on their left side (30°). The probe was placed at the left sternal edge so as to obtain a complete mitral valve echo in a plane strictly perpendicular to the thoracic surface. In order to avoid false positives, the prove was never displaced superiorly. All measurements were taken according to the recommendations made by Feigenbaum (3). The aortic dimensions were thus expressed in terms of aortic index (AI), taking into account the body surface area.

3. RESULTS

3.1. *Control group*

With a view to assess the changes of the AI in relation to age, our control subjects were subdivided into 3 subgroups (Table 1). Amongst these 91 patients, the extreme values of the AI were between 14 and 21.7 mm/m². The normal distribution of AI in relation to age is illustrated by Figure 1.

Table 1.

	N	$\overline{\text{Age}}$	Range	$\overline{\text{AI}}$	Range	σ	Conf. Int. 5%
Control 1	31	20.8	16–25	16.8	14–20.1	±1.72	±0.6
Control 2	30	30.8	25–39	17.57	14–21.7	±1.81	±0.65
Control 3	30	45.8	40–61	18.48	16.1–21.7	±1.7	±0.61

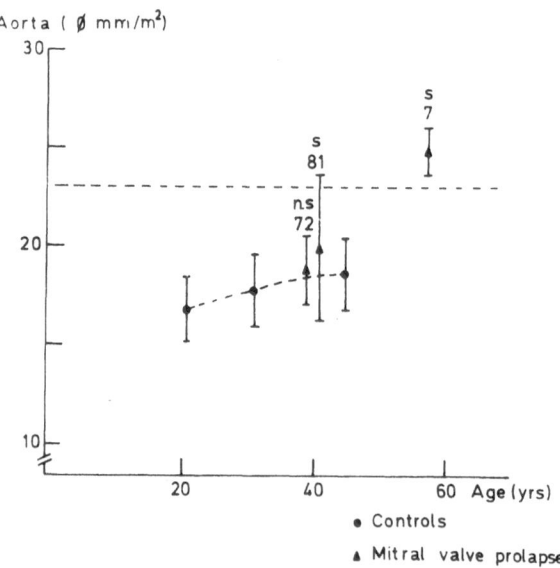

Fig. 1.

3.2. *MVP group*

This 81 patients group is made up of 30 men and 51 women. The average age is 40.6 years (extremes from 5 to 68 years). The mean AI is 20.6 mm/m$^2 \pm 3.69$ and significantly differs from the control group of similar ages ($p = 0.001$). In view of this, we tried to determine a discriminating value of the AI which could separate a group with MVP and normal AI and a group with MVP and abnormal AI. Seventy two patients with an AI < 23 mm/m^2 were found. The mean AI in this group was 19 mm/m$^2 \pm 1.76$ and was not different from control values. Nine patients with an AI $\geq$ 23 mm/m^2 were disclosed. Two of them had a Marfan's syndrome (5 years, male, AI: 25 mm/m^2 and 35 years, female, AI: 37 mm/m^2). The remaining 7 had no clinical signs or familial history of the syndrome; their mean AI was 24.84 mm/m$^2 \pm 1.16$. (Fig. 1).

These 7 patients (8.6%) are further defined by a comparison with the 72 control subjects (88.9%) (Table 2).

Mitral insufficiency manifested itself in each case by a holo- or telesystolic murmur, present chronically and devoid of the characteristics of ruptured chordae. The rhythm disturbances were depicted on resting or effort electrocardiograms and consisted of VPB's (24 cases), SVPB's and VPB's (5 cases), SVPB's (3 cases), or atrial fibrillation (2 cases). The echocardiographic features of the mitral and aortic valves failed to show any significant difference between the 2 groups. No instance of bicuspid aortic valve or aortic insufficiency was observed. The only discrepancies between the two classes consist of differences in age and sex distributions. A similar observation was made for the age and sex distribution of left anterior hemiblock. This fact deserves to be underlined and justifies further investigations of the differences in ageing changes according to sex.

4. CONCLUSIONS

Echocardiographic evaluation of patients with MVP permits to identify a small group of individuals with MVP and aortic root dilatation (8.6%). These

Table 2.

MVP Marfan excluded	AI < 23 mm/m^2	AI $\geq$ 23 mm/m^2	P
N	72	7	–
Mean age (years)	39.7	57.8	< 0.001
Male	23	6	< 0.01
Female	49	1	
Mitral insufficiency	7	3	= 0.01
Left anterior hemiblock	2	2	< 0.01
Rhythm disorder	31	4	NS

patients are devoid of the Marfan's syndrome; they are recruited after 50 years of age and show a clearcut male predominance. They have a greater incidence of mitral incompetence and left-sided conduction defects.

These observations are in accordance with previous anatomical (13) and pathological (8) reports which stressed the relationship between myxomatous valvular degenerescence and ageing and the relative rarity of aortic lesions which preferentially affect male individuals. Our results are also in keeping with previous descriptions of latent myxomatous lesions of the aortic media which are associated with mitral changes and may reveal themselves by an acute aortic dissection (9). This clinical study corroborates the idea that myxomatous lesions are the aspecific manifestation of a progressive degenerative disease which may simultaneously involve several structures within the heart.

REFERENCES

1. Brown OR, H Demots, FE Kloster, A Roberts, VD Menashe, RK Beals: Aortic root dilatation and mitral valve prolapse in Marfan's syndrome. Circulation 52:651, 1975
2. De Maria A. J King. H Bogren, J Lies, D Mason: The variable spectrum of echocardiographic manifestations of the mitral valve prolapse syndrome. Circulation 50:33, 1974.
3. Feigenbaum H: Echocardiography, Lea and Febiger, 2d edition, 1976.
4. Fernex PM, C Fernex: La dégénérescence mucoïde des valvules mitrales. Ses répercussions fonctionnelles. Helvet. med. Acta. 25:694, 1958.
5. Frable WJ: Mucinous degeneration of the cardiac valves, the floppy valve syndrome. J Thorac Cardiovasc Surg 58:62, 1969.
6. Jeresaty RM: Mitral valve prolapse – click syndrome. Prog Cardiovasc Dis 15:623, 1973.
7. Markiewicz W, J Stoner, E London, S Hunt, R Popp: Mitral valve prolpase in one hundred presumably healthy young females. Circulation 53:464, 1976.
8. McKay R, MH Yacoub: Clinical and pathological findings in patients with floppy valves treated surgically: Circulation: supplement III. 47, 48, 63, 1973.
9. McKay R, MH Yacoub: Acute aortic dissection and medial degeneration in patients with floppy mitral valves. Thorax 31:49, 1976.
10. O'Brien KP, GC Hitchcock, BG Barratt-Boyes, JB Lowe: Spontaneous aortic cusp rupture associated with valvular myxomatous transformation. Circulation 37:273, 1968.
11. Pomerance A: Ageing changes in human heart valves. Brit Heart J 30:687, 1967.
12. Pomerance A: Ballooning deformity of atrioventricular valves. Brit Heart J 31:343, 1969.
13. Pomerance A, MJ Davies: The pathology of the heart, Blackwell scientific publication, 67, 1975.

QUANTITATION OF AORTIC REGURGITATION BY A PERCUTANEOUS 128-CHANNEL DIGITAL ULTRASOUND DOPPLER INSTRUMENT

R. JENNI, W. HÜBSCHER,
M. CASTY, M. ANLIKER, and H.P. KRAYENBUEHL

A newly developed 128-channel pulsed ultrasound Doppler instrument with digital signal processing permits a non-invasive analysis of the blood stream in larger vessels within a range of about 10 cm (1). It utilizes a microcomputer and provides quasi-instantaneous velocity profiles at 0.016 sec intervals

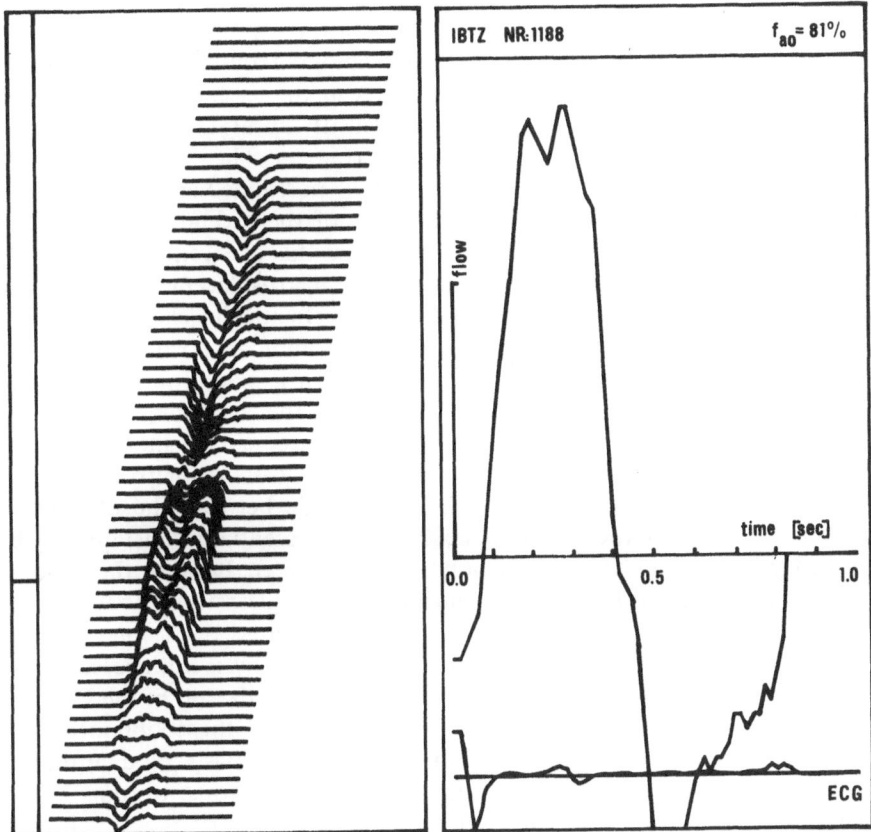

Fig. 1. Velocity profiles and volume flow pattern in the ascending aorta of a patient with severe aortic insufficiency. The profiles on the left have been averaged over 12 heart cycles and recorded at 0.016 sec intervals. The flow pattern on the right represents the result obtained by assuming that the volume flow rate is at any instant proportional to the extremal velocity in the corresponding profile. The units for velocity and flow are arbitrary as the angle between ultrasound beam and axis of the ascending aorta was not evaluated.

which may be averaged over 8–16 heart cycles. To compute the volume flow rate pattern the vessel cross-section is assumed to be circular and the velocities in each of the channels are considered as constant within the corresponding half-annulus of the lumen. One of the potential applications of this instrument in cardiology appears to be the non-invasive determination of the regurgitation fraction f_{ao} in patients with aortic insufficiency (A.I.). Theoretically f_{ao} is defined as (2):

$$f_{ao}(\%) = \frac{TSV - SV}{TSV} \cdot 100,$$

where TSV is the total stroke volume and SV the net forward stroke volume. If the coronary blood flow can be disregarded, one may approximate f_{ao} as the ratio of back flow to total forward flow in the ascending aorta during a cardiac cycle. Such volume flow quantifications require on one hand a continuous recording of the velocity profiles in the ascending aorta during several heart beats, and on the other, a sufficiently accurate evaluation of the flow on the basis of the recorded profiles (Fig. 1). The first of these two requirements implies that the transducer can be positioned and oriented such that the ultrasound beam intersects the axis of the ascending aorta at all times and that the angle between the beam and this axis remains essentially constant, even though the aorta exhibits rhythmic displacements during the heart cycle. The second presupposes that the velocities in each of the half-annuli within the lumen of the aorta are constant as postulated for the volume flow computation (1). When the transducer is placed appropriately at the suprasternal notch and aimed carefully at the ascending aorta, it is possible to assess the fullfilment of the first requirement by monitoring the temporal variations of the lumen diameter which can be inferred from the pulse echoes and velocity profiles. That the angle between the ultrasound beam and the axis of the ascending aorta remains essentially constant may be verified with the aid of an ultrasound sector scanner. Because the ratio of back flow to forward flow is independent of this angle as long as it remains unchanged, there is no need for its evaluation. Whereas the second requirement appears to be generally met in healthy subjects, this is not necessarily so in cases of A.I. because the f_{ao} values determined with the aid of the Doppler instrument can differ by much more than 15% from those obtained conventionally in the catheterization laboratory on the basis of quantitative ciné-angiography and Fick's method of measuring cardiac output. Yet, if one assumes that the volume flow rate in the ascending aorta is at any instant proportional to the maximum velocity in the corresponding velocity profile during forward and backward flow, one arrives at f_{ao} values which correlate rather well with those determined conventionally in the catheterization laboratory. This has been shown in 16 patients with mild to severe A.I. who were subjected to catheterization. The Doppler values of f_{ao} agreed within $\pm 15\%$ with the corresponding invasive f_{ao} (Fig. 2). Hence, this preliminary investigation indicates that f_{ao} may be obtained non-invasively with sufficient accuracy from the velocity profiles in the ascending aorta.

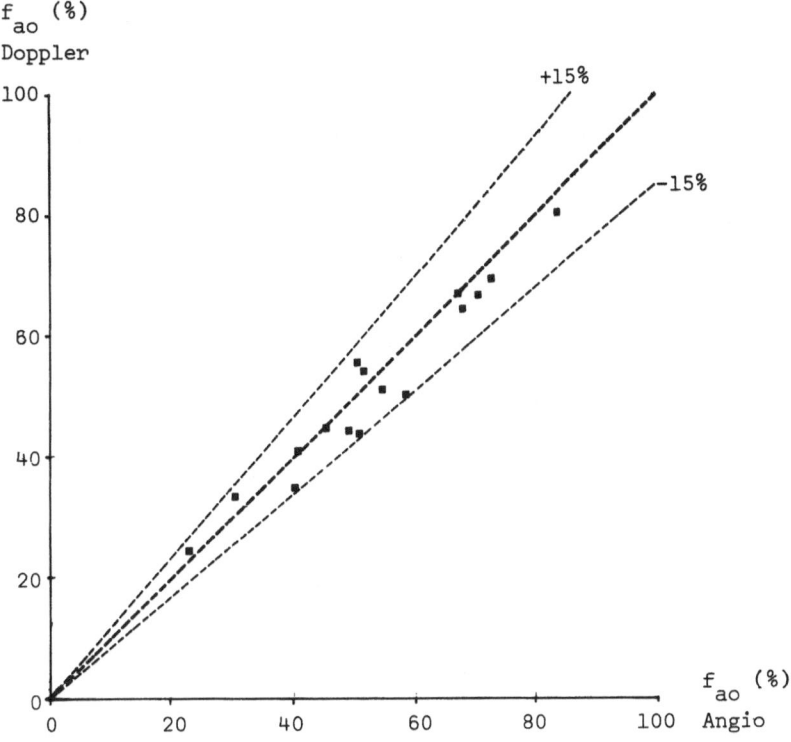

Fig. 2. Comparison of the f_{ao}-values determined non-invasively by means of the ultrasound Doppler instrument and with those obtained by quantitative cinéangiography.

REFERENCES

1. Anliker M, W Hübscher, R Jenni: Design and clinical evaluation of a 128-channel ultrasonic flow meter. Inserm 78:111, 1978.
2. Sandler H, HT Dodge, RE Hay, CE Rackley: Quantitation of valvular insufficiency in man by angiocardiography. Am Heart J 65:501, 1963.

MECHANISM OF SYSTOLIC ANTERIOR MOTION IN PATIENTS WITH HYPERTROPHIC OBSTRUCTIVE CARDIOMYOPATHY EVALUATED BY PHASED ARRAY SECTOR-SCANNING

M. KLICPERA, O. PACHINGER, P. PROBST, and F. KAINDL

The aim of our study was to analyse the anatomy and pathophysiology in patients with hypertrophic obstructive cardiomyopathy (HOCM). Special interest was given to the underlying mechanism of the echocardiographic finding of "systolic anterior motion of the mitral valve'. (SAM) to prove the concept that the development of an intraventricular gradient is due to systolic apposition of the anterior mitral valve leaflet (AMVL) toward the hypertrophied interventricular septum (IVS) thus creating left ventricular outflow tract (LVOT) obstruction.

PATIENTS AND METHODS

Fifteen patients with angiographically proven HOCM were studied non-simultaneously with a commercially available M-mode ultrasonoscope and a dynamically focused wide-angle phased array sector-scanner. Two-dimensional (2-D) studies were performed in ventricular long and short axis as well as from the apex in about 50%. Adequate images could be achieved in almost every patient, high quality pictures in 11 patients (73%).

Results

Hemodynamic data obtained in these 15 patients are listed below. Ten patients revealed a mean gradient of 77 ± 9 mm Hg at rest, 5 patients after provocation of Brockenbrough response. None of the patients without a basal gradient demonstrated mitral regurgitation (MR).

	gradient	n	LVEDP	MR
15 patients	without provocation	10	26.6 ± 5.1	5/10
	with provocation	5	18.0 ± 4.2	0/5

Echocardiographic studies revealed:
1) Asymmetric septal hypertrophy (ASH) in 14 patients with maximal thickness above the mitral coaptation point, involving up to 50% of the LV-circumference (extending to the anterolateral and inferior wall), marked concentric hypertrophy in 1 patient.
2) Large papillary muscles, positioned closer to the IVS in the long axis view of the left ventricle.

3) Forward positioning of the mitral valve (MV) during the whole cardiac cycle with no significant change in the MV-posterior wall distance during ventricular systole.
4) SAM is primarily caused by systolic forward motion of chordae tendineae against the IVS and by partially upward motion in front of the MV, aggravated by amyl nitrite.
5) SAM occurred below the narrowest part of LVOT.

DISCUSSION

The M-mode finding of SAM has been widely accepted as an abnormal systolic motion of the AMVL toward the IVS (Fig. 1). Several 2-D echocardiographic studies have supported this contention, postulating that the abnormal AMVL-motion contributes to the LVOT-obstruction and the development of an intraventricular gradient (1, 2). Our observations are not totally compatible with these reports. Like other authors (3, 4) we were never to find significant participation of the mitral leaflets in the systolic anterior motion of intraventricular structures. Our findings suggest that these reflect mainly chordae tendineae, rather than the tips of the mitral leaflets themselves (Figs. 2, 3), even though it is very hard to exactly define the insertion of the chordae tendineae on the valve leaflets. However, it seems likely that a systolic anterior motion of chordae tendineae produces abnormal traction on the mitral leaflets thus pulling them along toward the IVS. This has been shown in angiographic studies (5, 6) and certainly is responsible for the high incidence of MR.

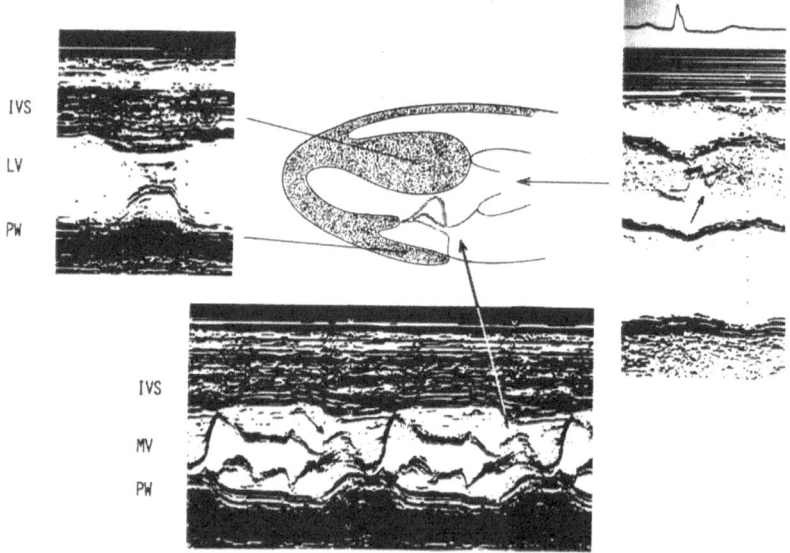

Fig. 1

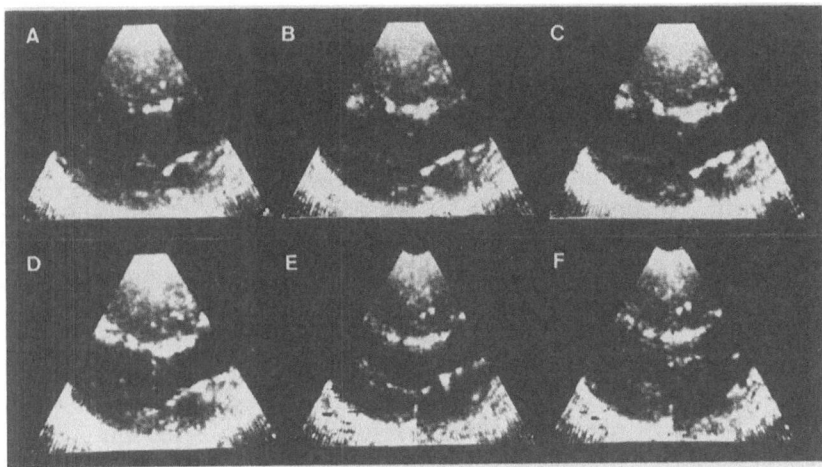

Fig. 2. Visualization of MV-movement by sequential 2-D images of the cardiac cycle (A-E systole, F diastole).

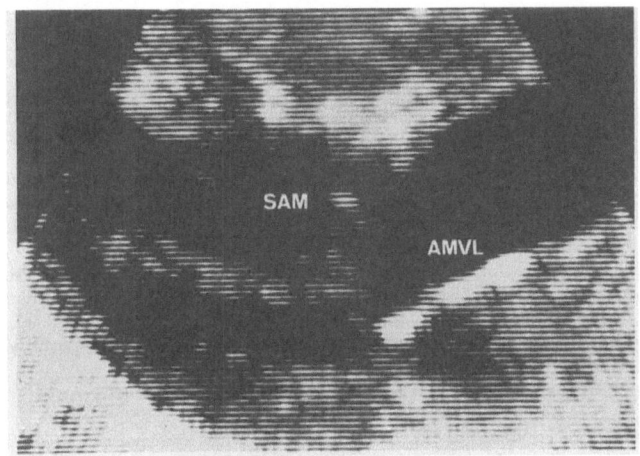

Fig. 3. 2-D image of MV-apparatus in mid-systole (enlargement of Fig. 2B).

In one of our patients with hypertrophic cardiomyopathy we found an abnormal systolic motion of the mitral apparatus on the echocardiogram suggestive of LVOT-obstruction, but could not provoke a gradient at catheterization. This observation was reported by King et al. and Rossen et al. 1974 (7, 8), who have demonstrated that even a simultaneous recording of the echocardiogram and of the left ventricular and aortic pressures has shown no gradient at the time when an obvious systolic anterior movement was present. Rodger (4) referred to the fact that the SAM on M-mode echocardiogram is represented by a complex of echos with different motion patterns in the majority of cases, rather than by a single echo. After additional 2-D studies with a multiple element echo system Rodger postulated the interposition of the posterior papillary muscle and chordae tendineae between the AMVL and IVS. In our studies we never could find the contribution of the papillary muscles but could clearly demonstrate abnormal systolic motion of chordae tendineae toward the IVS and upward in front of the MV. Our findings suggest that SAM on M-mode is produced by displacement of chordae tendineae, which traverses the sound beam at certain phases of the cardiac cycle; this could be demonstrated by selecting one beam from the 2-D sector for a simultaneous M-mode recording.

CONCLUSIONS

1) The MV does not play an active role in LVOT-obstruction
2) LVOT-obstruction is caused by ASH and forward positioning of MV.
3) SAM is due to systolic displacement of chordae tendineae, whereas a significant anterior motion of the AMVL could never be observed.
4) SAM is caused by a Venturi effect and hydrodynamic forces, generated by the exaggerated contraction of LV.

REFERENCES

1. Henry WL, Clarc ECh, Griffith JM et al.: Mechanism of left ventricular outflow obstruction in patients with obstructive asymmetric septal hypertrophy (IHSS). Am J Card 35:337, 1975.
2. Weyman AE, Feigenbaum H, Hurwitz RA et al.: Localization of left ventricular outflow obstruction by cross-sectional echocardiography. Am J Med 60:33, 1976.
3. Cohen MV, Teichholz LE, Gorlin R: B-scan ultrasonography in idiopathic hypertrophic subaortic stenosis-Study of left ventricular outflow tract and mechanism of obstruction. Brit Heart J 38:595, 1976.
4. Rodger Ch: Motion of mitral apparatus in hypertrophic cardiomyopathy with obstruction. Brit Heart J 38:732, 1976.
5. Simon AL, Ross R Jr, Gault JH: Angiographic anatomy of the left ventricle and mitral valve in idiopathic hypertrophic subaortic stenosis. Circulation 36:852, 1967.
6. Adelman AG, Mc Loughlin MJ, Marquis Y et al.: Left ventricular cineangiographic observations in muscular subaortic stenosis. Am J Card 24:689, 1969.
7. King JF, DeMaria AN, Miller RR et al.: Markedly abnormal mitral valve motion without simultaneous intraventricular pressure gradient due to uneven mitral-septal contact in idiopathic hypertrophic subaortic stenosis. Am J Card 34:360, 1974.
8. Rossen RM, Goodman DJ, Ingham RE et al.: Echocardiographic criteria in the diagnosis of idiopathic hypertrophic subaortic stenosis. Circulation 50:747, 1974.

CRITICAL EVALUATION OF THE PULMONARY VALVE ECHOCARDIOGRAM: USEFULNESS AND LIMITATIONS OF E-F SLOPE MEASUREMENTS

F. ORZAN, Z. KRAJCER, V.S. MATHUR, L.W. PECHACEK,
E. GARCIA, and R.J. HALL

Since the original report on the echocardiographic detection of the pulmonary valve was published (1), several studies have extended our knowledge of the appearance of this valve in health and disease (2, 3). Abnormality of the motion of the pulmonary valve in the early part of diastole (reduced E-F slope) has been reported to be a useful indicator of pulmonary arterial hypertension (PAH) (4, 5). A study involving 123 subjects was undertaken to determine its specificity and reliability in determining the presence and severity of PAH.

MATERIALS AND METHODS

The E-F slope of the pulmonary valve echocardiogram was analyzed in 26 normal, healthy volunteers and 97 patients with various forms of heart disease, who underwent cardiac catheterization within 24 hours, and in whom a satisfactory pulmonary valve echo could be obtained. Only patients with sinus rhythm were included. Patients were divided into four groups according to pulmonary artery (PA) pressure. Group I consisted of six patients with severe pulmonary valvular stenosis with a mean gradient of 70 mm Hg across the valve and diastolic PA pressure of < 12 mm Hg. Group II consisted of 24 patients with definite heart disease but normal PA pressure (diastolic < 12 mm Hg and mean < 20 mm Hg). The 37 patients in Group III had mild to moderate PAH; the diastolic PA pressure was between 13 and 25 mm Hg and mean PA pressure was between 21 and 40 mm Hg. Group IV was made up of 30 patients with severe PAH (diastolic PA ≥ 26 mm Hg and mean PA ≥ 40 mm Hg. The average PA mean pressures for the Groups I to IV were 11.8 ± 0.7, 16.4 ± 0.6, 28.5 ± 1.0 and 57.2 ± 2.1 mm Hg, respectively. Measurements of the E-F slope were made in a manner similar to the one described by Weyman et al. (4) and an example is shown in Figure 1.

RESULTS

The E-F slope values during quiet respiration are plotted in Figure 2 and the mean and range presented in table 1. Although there was some overlap between normals and patients, the mean values were significantly less in all patient groups, irrespective of the presence or absence of PAH. The least

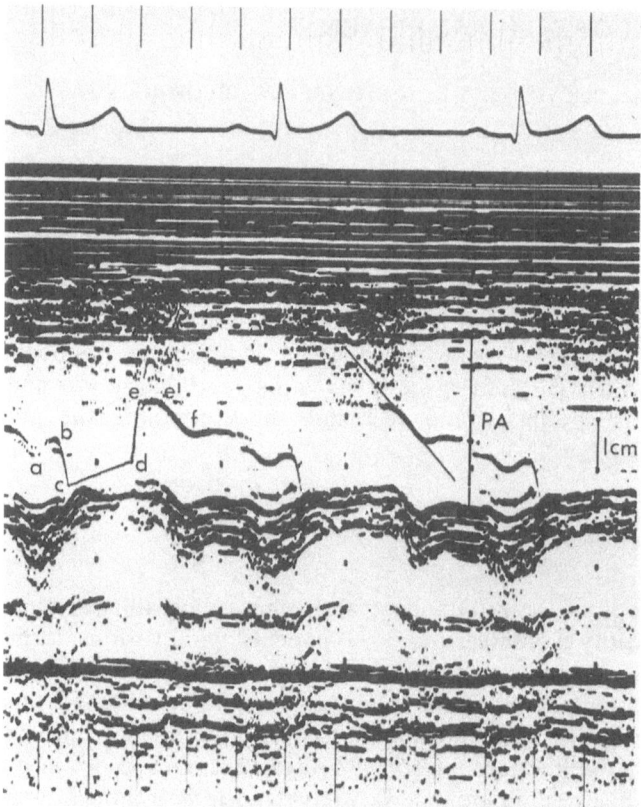

Fig. 1. Echogram of posterior cusp of pulmonary valve showing measurement of E-F slope. Systolic motion of the valve has been retouched in the first complex.

value for E-F slope was found in patients with pulmonary stenosis with the lowest PA pressure. No significant correlation was found between the magnitude of E-F slope and PA mean pressure, PA diastolic pressure, PA resistance and cardiac index, the R values being 0.2, 0.23, 0.14 and 0.14, respectively. In 17 normal subjects, in whom inspiratory and expiratory recordings could be made, the E-F slope increased with inspiration (54.6 ± 4.2 to 68.9 ± 5.4 mm/sec, $p < 0.02$). Significant inspiratory increase was not found in six patients with pulmonary stenosis (9.4 ± 3.4 to 10.7 ± 3.7 mm/sec) or 17 partients with severe PAH (7.2 ± 2.2 to 8.9 ± 2.7 mm/sec).

DISCUSSION

This study revealed that the average E-F slope of the pulmonary valve is significantly reduced not only in patients with PAH, but also in patients with various other cardiac disorders. In each of our patients with pulmonary

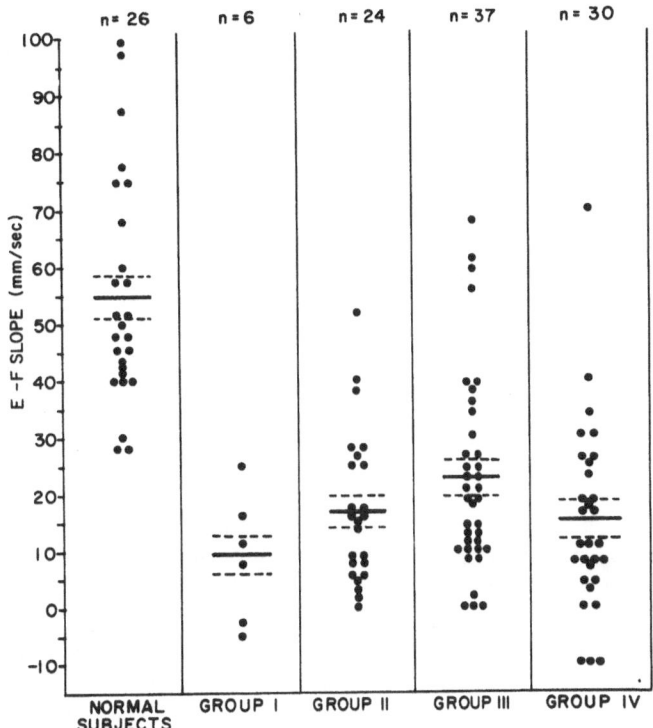

Fig. 2. The E-F slope data in normal subjects and groups I-IV are plotted with mean and standard error of the mean.

stenosis, the slope was flatter than normal, being negative in three, and all the values were below normal range, thus allowing complete separation of this group from normals (p < 0.001). We are not proposing this as a screening test for pulmonary stenosis, as better and more reliable noninvasive methods exist already; but the demonstration of a normal E-F slope should be considered strong evidence against the diagnosis of valvular pulmonary stenosis. This observation was intriguing because patients with pulmonary stenosis have no PAH and the PA pressure was lower than normal in each instance. The decreased E-F slope in these patients may be related to a relatively insignificant effect of the early and mid-diastolic filling of the right

Table I Echographic results of pulmonary valve E-F slope.

	No.	Range	Mean ± SEM	p*
Normal subjects	26	28 to 100	55 ± 4	–
Pulmonary stenosis	6	−5 to 25	9 ± 3	<0.001
Heart disease, no PAH	24	0 to 52	17 ± 3	<0.001
Mild-moderate PAH	37	0 to 68	23 ± 3	<0.001
Severe PAH	30	−5 to 70	15 ± 3	<0.001

*p = difference between normals and other groups.

ventricle on the motion of the stiff pulmonary valve. We can also speculate that the decreased E-F slope may be the result of decreased compliance of the hypertrophic right ventricle with consequent reduction in the rate of diastolic filling.

Another surprising observation was the severely decreased E-F slope in those patients with heart disease whose PA pressure was normal (Group II). Although the values overlapped with normals in some cases, the average for this group was significantly lower than normal ($p < 0.001$). In a recent publication, Hada et al. (6) pointed out that by higher positioning of the echo transducer and the resultant tilt, the diastolic slope can become flatter or even negative in patients with normal PA pressure, mimicking PAH. While this may be a partial explanation in some instances, it cannot account for all of our observations. We did not encounter a negative slope in any of our 26 healthy volunteers and did not record a slope less than 28 mm/sec in any normal subject. The slope ranged between 40 and 100 mm/sec in 23 of our 26 normals. We do not know the precise mechanisms involved in altering the E-F slope in these patients. Because PAH was not a factor in this group, other factors like diastolic compliance of the right ventricle, diastolic filling rate, stiffness of the valve, heart rate, respiration, tilt of the transducer and others may have played a role in these patients.

The reduced E-F slope in patients with PAH has been well described (4, 5) and our data confirms this observation. We were, however, unable to document a positive correlation with the degree of PAH using systolic, diastolic or mean PA pressure; neither could we find a correlation with pulmonary arteriolar resistance or pulmonary flow. Additionally, the E-F slope was in normal range in 15 of 67 (22%) patients with PAH. We, therefore, find that, although the majority of patients with PAH have reduced E-F slope, it is neither a very specific nor sensitive test, and does not reflect the severity of PAH.

The variability of the E-F slope with phases of respiration has been previously described (4, 5). Our observations of absence of a significant inspiratory increase in patients with pulmonary stenosis as well as severe PAH may provide additional clues when these diagnoses are suspected.

SUMMARY AND CONCLUSIONS

Measurements of the diastolic E-F slope of the pulmonary valve have been made in 123 subjects and correlated with hemodynamic data. Our observations reveal that (1) a reduced E-F slope should alert one to suspect some heart disease. (2) If the E-F slope is less than 28 mm/sec, a normal heart is unlikely. (3) Absence of inspiratory increase in patients with low E-F slope is suggestive of heart disease. (4) Generally, the E-F slope is reduced in patients with PAH, but a normal slope does not exclude PAH. (5) The magnitude of the slope, does not correlate with the degree of PAH, resistance or flow. (6) A reduced E-F slope is not specific for PAH and can be frequently found in patients with heart disease with normal PA pressure. (7) A reduced E-F slope should be considered an important feature in echocardiographic diagnosis of significant valvular pulmonary stenosis.

REFERENCES

1. Gramiak R, NC Nanda, PM Shah: Echocardiographic detection of the pulmonary valve. Radiology 102:153, 1972.
2. Weyman, AE: Pulmonary valve echo motion in clinical practice. Am J Med 62:843, 1977.
3. Shah PM: Echocardiography of the aortic and pulmonary valves. Prog Cardiovasc Dis 20:451, 1978.
4. Weyman AE, JC Dillon, H Feigenbaum, et al.: Echocardiographic patterns of pulmonic valve motion with pulmonary hypertension. Circulation 50:905, 1974.
5. Nanda NC, R Gramiak, TI Robinson, et al.: Echocardiographic evaluation of pulmonary hypertension. Circulation 50:575, 1974.
6. Hada Y, T Sakamoto, T Hayashi, et al.: Echocardiogram of the pulmonary valve: Variability of the pattern and the related technical problems. Jap Heart J 18:298, 1977.

ECHOCARDIOGRAPHIC DETECTION OF MITRAL REGURGITATION (MR) IN MITRAL VALVE PROLAPSE (MVP)

A.S. PEARLMAN, R. GENTILE, S.A. RUBENSTEIN, T.K. DOOLEY, and D.W. FRANKLIN

One of the major complications associated with mitral valve prolapse (MVP) is mitral regurgitation (MR) (1–3). However, confirmation of MR and accurate assessment of its severity both require left ventricular angiography, a procedure that is not performed in the majority of patients with MVP; hence, the true prevalence and distribution of severity of MR in a group of unselected patients with MVP is unclear.

Pulsed Doppler echocardiography (PDE) detects disturbances of intracardiac blood flow based on frequency shifts induced by these disturbances in pulsed, reflected ultrasound (4). As a non-invasive method that appears to be useful in detecting MR (5), PDE should be ideal for studying the prevalence of MR in patients with MVP. Furthermore, we postulated that more widespread evidence of disturbed intracardiac flow might indicate more severe MR. Accordingly, we studied patients with suspected MVP, in whom angiographic confirmation was available, to determine the ability of PDE to identify and estimate the severity of MR in these patients. The PDE criteria established in this way were then used to study the prevalence and severity of MR in a group of unselected, consecutive patients with MVP.

MATERIALS AND METHODS

Patients

Left ventricular and selective coronary cineangiographic studies were performed in 50 patients with suspected MVP. Five patients were found to have significant coronary artery disease, and were excluded from further analysis since abnormal left ventricular wall motion could influence systolic motion of the mitral apparatus. The 45 remaining patients formed Group I; 22 were men and 23 women, and age ranged from 26–76 (mean 49) years. Left ventricular cineangiograms were recorded in the 30° right anterior oblique projection, and were inspected for evidence of MVP. MR was graded as absent, mild, moderate, or severe according to a modification of standard angiographic criteria (6). Thus, angiographic grade 1^+ MR was designated as mild, grade 2^+ as moderate, and grades 3–4^+ as severe.

Group II consisted of 137 patients referred over a consecutive period of 45 months with M-mode echocardiographic evidence of MVP. Patients with cardiac conditions associated with a high prevalence of MVP (such as atrial

Charles T. Lancée (ed.), Echocardiology, 255–260. All rights reserved
Copyright © 1979 by Martinus Nijhoff Publishers bv, The Hague/Boston/London

septal defect, mitral stenosis, or hypertrophic cardiomyopathy) were excluded, since in such patients MR may be due to the associated condition and not due to MVP *per se*. Fifty-seven patients were men and 80 were women; age ranged from 18 to 76 (mean 42) years.

Clinical parameters including age, sex, presence and character of a systolic murmur, and duration over which a murmur was known to have been present, were tabulated and studied to determine if any were predictive of the presence and severity of MR.

All patients in both groups underwent echocardiographic studies. Standard M-mode echocardiograms were recorded, using a 2.25 or 3 MHz transducer and an ATL 600B ultrasonoscope and fiberoptic recorder. MVP was considered present if mid-to-late systolic mitral leaflet motion away from the echo transducer, or holo-systolic "hammocking" associated with reduplication of systolic mitral echoes, was recorded (7). Inferior transducer angulation, which can cause the appearance of holosystolic leaflet sagging in the absence of MVP (8), was avoided. MVP was tabulated as absent, mid-systolic, or holo-systolic based on the M-mode records, and was considered to be holo-systolic in patients in whom both mid- and holo-systolic prolapse was detected in different complexes. Left ventricular and atrial dimensions and mitral opening (DE) amplitude was also measured (9).

PDE studies were performed with a 3 MHz transducer and an ATL 500A range-gated pulsed Doppler unit. The transducer was placed in a left parasternal interspace and directed towards the mitral valve; the Doppler sample volume was positioned in the left atrium just behind the anterior

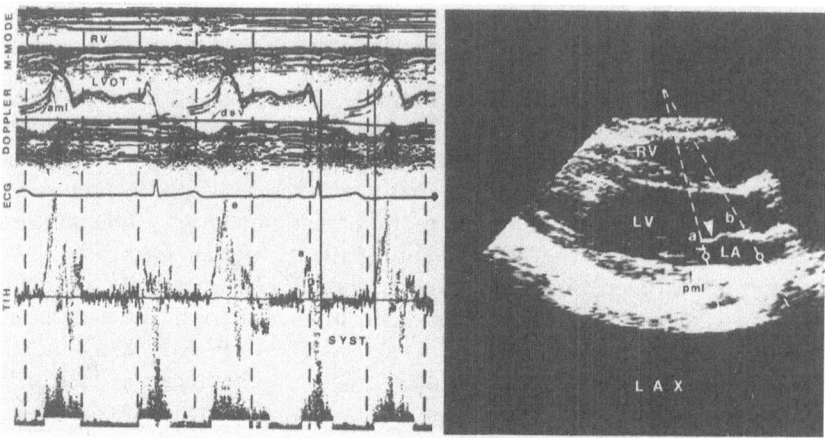

Fig. 1. Right: long axis (LAX) stop-frame showing position of Doppler sample volume (dsv). Dotted lines show two Doppler beam directions; circles on these lines show dsv position. Position "a" just cephalad to mitral valve, "b" behind aortic root. RV = right ventricle, LV = left ventricle, LA = left atrium, white arrow = anterior mitral leaflet, black arrow = posterior leaflet (pml). Left: time interval histogram (TIH) from position "a" in patient with *no* MR. LVOT = LV outflow tract, aml = anterior mitral leaflet. Positive deflections in TIH represent flow *towards* transducer, so e and a = diastolic LA outflow into LV. Note absence of systolic flow during systole (SYST).

mitral leaflet (Fig. 1, right panel, position a). Further superomedial angulation of the Doppler beam allowed investigation of blood flow patterns within the left atrium distant from the mitral valve (Fig. 1, right panel, position b). The output of the pulsed Doppler unit was converted to an audio signal and recorded, along with the Doppler A-mode signals, on video-tape. Doppler output was also printed on the strip-chart recorder in a "time-interval histogram" format (10) (Fig. 1, left panel). MR was considered to be present when evidence of systolic flow was detected posterosuperior to the mitral valve.

RESULTS

Of the 45 patients in Group I, 30 had angiographic evidence of MVP, while 15 had no MVP detected angiographically. Two additional patients without MVP by angio did have M-mode echo evidence of MVP; both underwent mitral valve replacement (for severe MR), and myxomatous degeneration of the mitral valve was noted in both instances. MR was angiographically absent in 13 (41%) of these 32 patients with MVP, mild in 6 (19%), moderate in 4 (12%), and severe in 9 (28%). Evidence of MR was found by PDE in every patient with MR demonstrated by angiography, but in none of those without angiographically detected MR (Fig. 2). Moreover, mild, moderate, and severe degrees of MR could be classified correctly, with 2 exceptions, by echo findings. Thus, all 6 patients with angiographically mild MR demonstrated a localized systolic flow disturbance present just posterosuperior to the mitral valve but not behind the aortic root (Fig. 3, top), while all 9 patients with angiographically severe MR demonstrated disturbed systolic flow at multiple sites in the left atrium (Fig. 3, bottom), *plus* enlargement of

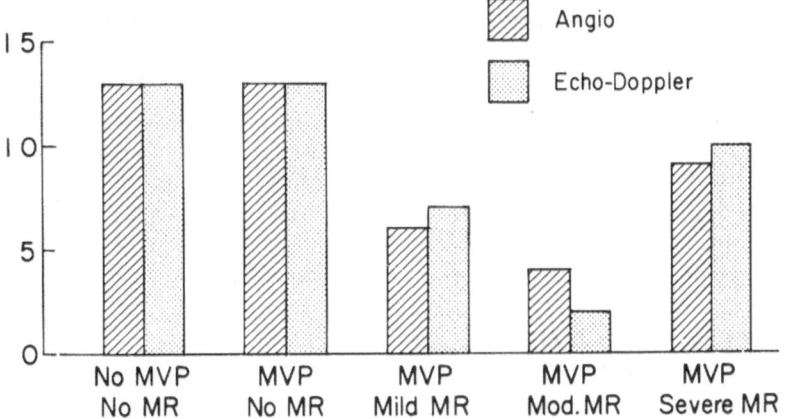

Fig. 2. Detection of MR by PDE, compared to angio findings. Number of patients in each category denoted by height of each bar. Two patients with MVP and moderate MR by angio were mis-classified by PDE; see text.

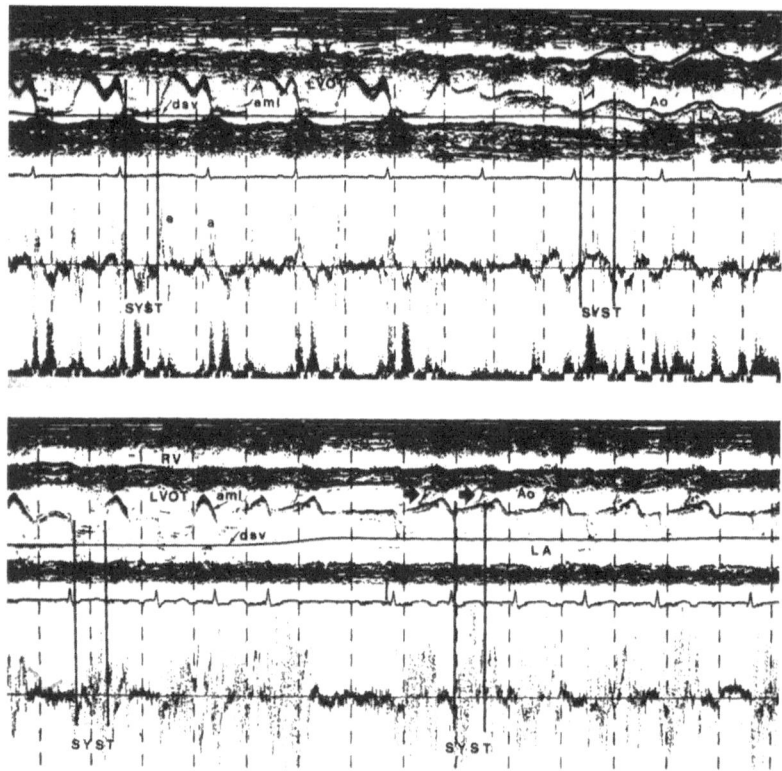

Fig. 3. Top: TIH in patient with mild MR; labels as in Figure 1. Note systolic flow *into* LA
(negative deflection) on left side of panel, but absence of such flow behind aortic root (Ao).
Bottom: TIH in patient with moderate MR. Heavy arrows = aortic leaflets. Note systolic flow
into LA at both mitral valve and aortic root levels.

both left ventricle and left atrium. Of 4 patients with moderate MR by
angiography, 2 demonstrated echo abnormalities of intermediate severity, in
that systolic flow disturbances were present at multiple sites in the left atrium,
in the *absence* of dilatation of both left heart chambers. However, 1 patient
with angiographically moderate MR had only a localized flow disturbance
(mild MR) by PDE; in this patient, the echo study preceded the catheterization by 1 year, so that the possibility of progression of disease cannot be
excluded. In 1 other patient with moderate MR by angiography, diffuse flow
disturbance *and* enlargement of both left heart chambers (severe MR) was
recorded by echo. Using the echo criteria described above, 86% of patients
throught to have mild MR by echo, all with moderate MR, and 90% of those
with severe MR were classified correctly (Fig. 2).

Clinical and M-mode echo parameters were less predictive of the presence
of MR. Audible mid-late systolic murmurs were detected in occasional
patients without MR. While the great majority of patients without MR had
mid-systolic prolapse, several of these patients did demonstrate holo-systolic
MVP. Finally, anterior mitral leaflet excursion was less than 25 mm in our

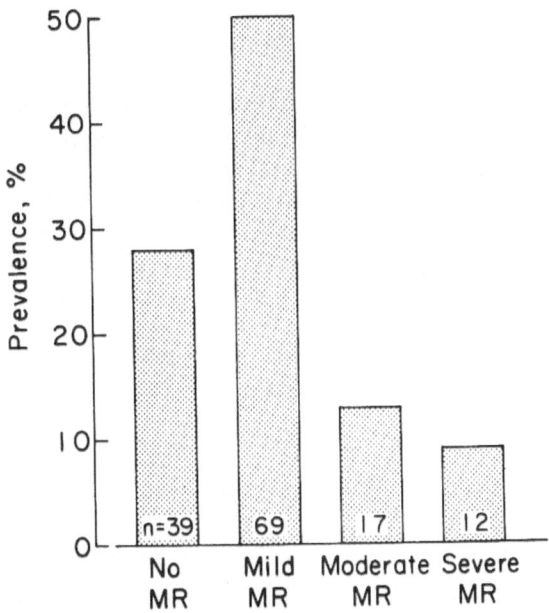

Fig. 4. Prevalence and severity of MR in consecutive patients with MVP.

patients without MVP. Increased leaflet excursion was detected in 10 (31%) of the 32 patients with MR; of these, 6 did have severe MR, but in 3 others MR was totally absent.

Of the 137 patients in Group II, MR was detected by PDE in 98 (72%) patients (Fig. 4). MR was graded as absent in 39 (28%), mild in 69 (50%), moderate in 17 (13%), and severe in only 12 (9%) patients. The severity of MR did not appear related to the pattern of prolapse, in that holo-systolic prolapse was present in 44% of patients with no MR, 59% with mild MR, 61% with moderate MR, and 46% with severe MR. Large amplitude mitral opening (D-E amplitude >25 mm), thought possibly to indicate marked mitral apparatus redundancy and thus more severe prolapse, was likewise not found to be associated with more severe MR. Thus, while 34 (25%) of the patients with MVP demonstrated large amplitude mitral opening, only 9 of these 34 patients had severe MR, while 6 had no MR.

Severe MR was detected in 12 patients, 10 (83%) of whom were over 50 years of age. While severe MR was unusual in younger patients, it was not invariable in elderly patients with MVP; thus, of 36 patients greater than 50 years of age, MR was absent in 11 (31%), mild in 8 (22%), moderate in 7 (19%), and severe in 10 (28%). Finally, although every patient with severe MR demonstrated enlargement of both left ventricle and left atrium, the absence of left-sided chamber enlargement did not always indicate trivial MR. All patients with mild or no MR had neither left ventricular nor left atrial enlargement, but normal chamber sizes were also noted in 6 (35%) of the 17 patients with moderate MR by PDE.

CONCLUSION

Our results demonstrate that PDE is extremely accurate in detecting MR in patients with MVP. This finding is of particular importance, since the presence of MR could not be predicted reliably by the presence and character of a systolic murmur, by M-mode echo parameters thought indicative of the severity of mitral apparatus redundancy, or by the presence or absence of dilatation of left heart chambers. Moreover, PDE appears to be moderately accurate in estimating the severity of MR in these patients. Thus, while the performance of serial left ventricular angiography in order to study the development and progression of MR in MVP would be impractical, PDE seems ideally suited to such long-term studies.

REFERENCES

1. Devereux RB, JK Perloff, NR Reichek, ME Josephson: Mitral valve prolapse. Circulation 54:3, 1976.
2. Ranganathan N, M Silver, TI Robinson, JK Wilson: Idiopathic prolapsed mitral leaflet syndrome: angiographic-clinical correlations. Circulation 54:707, 1976.
3. Gilbert BW, RA Schatz, OT Von Ramm, VS Behar, JA Kisslo: Mitral valve prolapse: two-dimensional echocardiographic and angiographic correlation. Circulation 54:716, 1976.
4. Johnson SL, DW Baker, AR Lute, HT Dodge: Doppler echocardiography: the localization of cardiac murmurs. Circulation 48:810, 1973.
5. Johnson SL, DW Baker, AR Lute, JA Murray: Detection of mitral regurgitation by Doppler echocardiography. Am J Cardiol 33:146, 1974.
6. Sellers RD, MJ Levy, K Amplatz, CW Lillehei: Left retrograde cardioangiography in acquired cardiac disease – technic, indications, and interpretations in 700 cases. Am J Cardiol 14:437, 1964.
7. DeMaria AN, A Neumann, G Lee, DT Mason: Echocardiographic identification of the mitral valve prolapse syndrome. Am J Med 62:819, 1977.
8. Weiss AN, JW Mims, PA Ludbrook, BE Sobel: Echocardiographic detection of mitral valve prolapse-exclusion of false positive diagnosis and determination of inheritance. Circulation 52:1091, 1975.
9. Sahn DJ, AN DeMaria, J Kisslo, A Weyman: Recommendations regarding quantitation in M-mode echocardiography: results of a survey of echocardiographic measurements. Circulation 58:1072, 1978.
10. Lorch G, S Rubenstein, D Baker, T Dooley, H Dodge: Doppler echocardiography: use of a graphical display system. Circulation 56:576, 1977.

VALIDITY OF ECHO-PULSED DOPPLER VELOCIMETRY FOR ASSESSING THE DIAGNOSIS AND SEVERITY OF AORTIC VALVE DISEASE AND PROSTHETIC VALVE FUNCTION

C. VEYRAT, N. CHOLOT, G. ABITBOL, and D. KALMANSON

Non-traumatic exploration of intracardiac and large vessel blood flow using echo-pulsed Doppler velocimetry (PDV) now makes the diagnosis and evaluation of valvular heart disease possible. First proposed by Baker and Johnson for intracardiac turbulence detection in 1973, (1) this technique was modified, the output signal being demodulated into an analog flow-velocity curve combined with a spectral display (2, 3, 4). This paper studies its application to aortic valvular disease (AVD), and prosthesis (PR) function.

MATERIAL AND METHOD

The study comprises a control group of 20 normal subjects, a group of 42 patients with AVD-12 pure stenosis (AS), 19 pure regurgitation (AR), 11 combined lesions (AS+AR) – and a group of 13 patients with aortic prosthesis (PR). The diagnosis was confirmed in all cases by left-heart catheterization (31), aortography (24), dye dilution curves (14), and/or surgery (31). The assessment of the severity of the lesions was based on a 3-grade scale. We used the ATL 500A* apparatus, including a 3 MHz PD veloci-meter, with a repetition rate of 2 to 15 KHz of very brief pulses of 1.0 to 1.5 μsec duration, associated with an A and M mode echocardiography provided with a single transducer of 1.2 cm diameter, whose principle has been described elsewhere (1).

RECORDING TECHNIQUE (Fig. 1)

Several approaches may be used complementarily; the transducer is generally best placed at the suprasternal notch. After an echo examination of the arterial (aorta and right pulmonary artery) and cardiac structures, it is possible using the PD technique, to record the flow velocity of a small blood sample (2 × 4 mm) by simply moving the velocimetric gate (G) through a depth ranging between 3 and 17 cm from the skin – usually between 5 and 10 cm for aortic arch and orifice – to obtain successive samples along the aorta. The 2nd-3rd left, and sometimes right intercostal spaces and the right

*ATL, Bellevue, Wash., U.S.A.

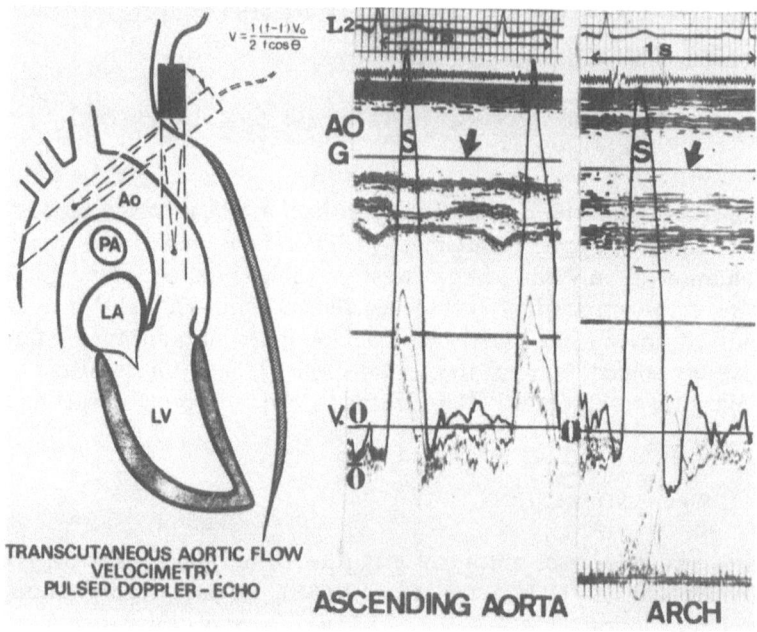

$$V = \frac{1}{2} \frac{(f-f)V_0}{f\cos\theta}$$

Fig. 1.

supraclavicular approaches may also be combined specially for aortic orifice and PR.

RECORDING OF THE TRACINGS

The tracings are recorded simultaneously with ECG (lead 2) and external frequency selected phonocardiogram (PCG), on a 8-Channel IREX* photographic recorder with patients in a reclining position with head lowered. Echo Doppler tracings include flow velocity curves (V), frequency spectrum (SP) and echo traces (ECHO), separately of simultaneously. A horizontal line (G) marks the site of the velocimetric sample.

RESULTS

The curves recorded represent flow velocity patterns without an absolute calibration. Systolic aortic forward flow velocities being considered as positive for physiological reasons, the sign of the analog curve will be artificially reversed for the aortic arch.

*IREX, Inc., Mahwah., N.Y., U.S.A.

NORMAL SUBJECTS (Fig. 1)

In the ascending aorta, the curve shows a large systolic positive wave (S) followed by a small reversal wave (R) and then keeps close to the zero line. The same pattern is displayed in the arch, with opposite sign for the spectrum frequency.

PATIENTS WITH AVD

1. *Aortic stenosis* (Fig. 2)

The main diagnostic features consist of a) pattern anomalies: the "S" summit appears flattened with a very irregular plateau, b) timing anomalies: prolonged ejection time and delayed onset of the curve at the arch. An evaluation of the severity of the lesion is possible based on the spreading of the abnormal pattern more or less farther downstream in the aorta.

2. *Aortic regurgitation* (Fig. 3)

The characteristic feature is the occurrence of a negative flow wave, during part or all diastole. The duration, depth and amplitude of this negative wave at various sites along the aorta leads to assessment of the importance of the lesions.

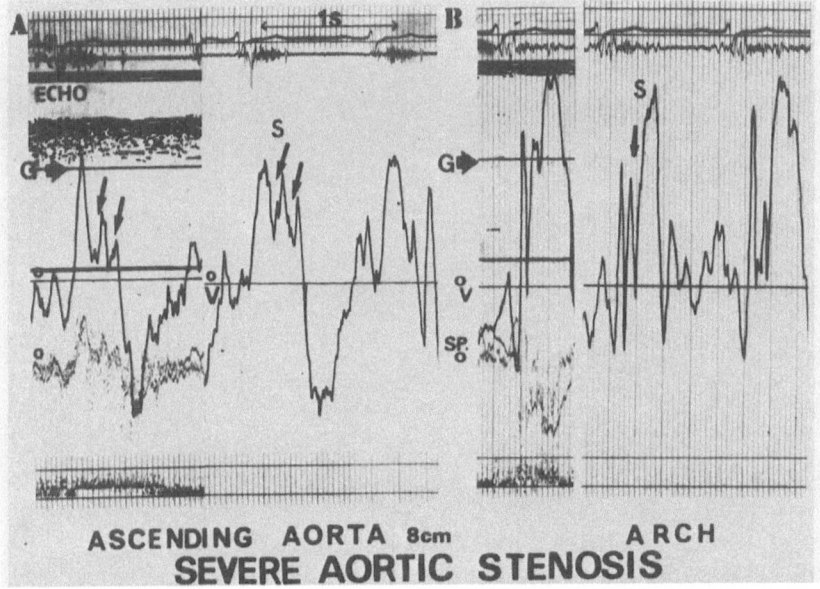

Fig. 2.

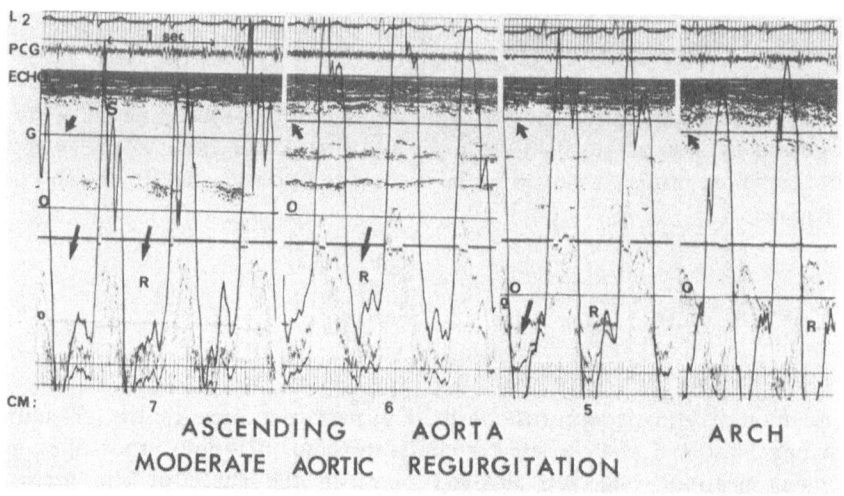

Fig. 3.

3. Mixed lesions

The curves show a combination of the above anomalies, in proportion to their respective importance.

PATIENTS WITH PR (Fig. 4, left)

With the gate set on the ball of the prosthesis, 2 thin deflections of opposite sign are recorded synchronously with the heart sounds. The aortic flow

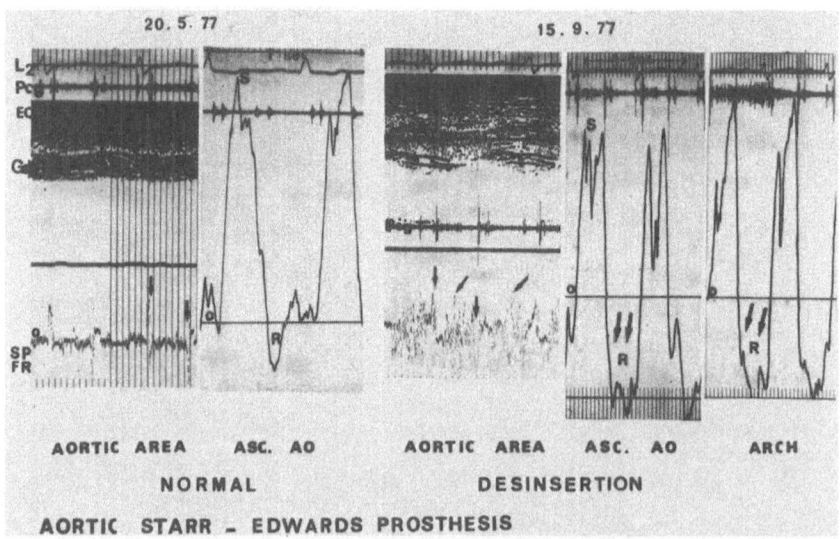

Fig. 4.

pattern may be slightly disturbed. In one case (Fig. 4, right), a sudden broadening of the spectrum and a diastolic negative wave appeared, due to paravalvular leak.

COMMENTS

Since the general problems raised by PD technique applications have already been discussed (2, 3, 4), we shall only recall that this method does not actually rely on accurate velocity measurement, but on recognition patterns and on timing data.

VALIDITY AND SIGNIFICANCE OF THE RECORDED CURVES

The remarkable similarity of the recorded curves with those of volume flow or velocity obtained using other methods in the aorta of subjects with normal or diseased valves (5, 6, 7, 8) and with PR (7), indicates their validity and their physiological and pathophysiological significance, with the proviso that the peak velocity is not adequately represented for turbulent flow. The asymmetric profile due to a stenotic valve, and the large diameter variations seen in AR, do not allow any estimation of volume flow to be made from flow velocity data. However, the velocity patterns have adequate diagnostic value for clinical requirements; in patients with AS, the indented plateau probably reflects turbulence, and the delayed curve at the arch could be related to the asymmetrically dilated supravalvular aortic segment. The diastolic negative wave in patients with AR is the graphic illustration of the regurgitant flow. As for the deflections recorded on PR, they clearly represent the velocity of closing and opening motion of the ball.

DIAGNOSIS AND PROGNOSTIC VALUE IN AVD

For diagnosis, the correlation between PDV and hemodynamical or surgical data ranges between 80% and 94% where both sensitivity and specificity for all lesions are concerned. The same applies to the assessment of the severity, with poorer assessment for AR in case of combined lesions. Discrepancies chiefly occur in cases of low cardiac output and of insufficient recording samples; a correct grading indeed requires not only knowledge of the wave form anomalies, but also of their spatial extension.

In conclusion, in spite of some limitations, the PDV provides a new, reliable, non-invasive and repeatable method for diagnosing and evaluating AVD and PR function, based on the analysis of direct blood flow disturbance data.

REFERENCES

1. Johnson SL, DW Baker, RA Lute, HT Dodge: Doppler echocardiography. The localization of cardiac murmurs. Circulation 48:810, 1973.

2. Kalmanson D, C Veyrat, A Degroote, F Bouchareine, DW Baker: Enregistrement par voie transcutanée des courbes de vélocité sanguine normales et pathologiques par la technique doppler a émission pulsée et réception démodulée, associée à l'échocardiographie. Rapport Préliminaire. CR Acad Paris 282, série D, 937, 1976.
3. Kalmanson D, C Veyrat, F Bouchareine, N Cholot: Investigation of the heart and large vessels using pulsed Doppler Flowmetry associated with echography. In: Doppler ultrasound in the study of the central and peripheral circulation, Woodcock JP, RF Sequeira (eds), University of Bristol Printing Unit, 1978, 16–29.
4. Kalmanson D, C Veyrat: Echo-Doppler velocimetry: a new non-invasive technique for diagnosing and assessing heart valve disease. In: Quantitative Cardiovascular Studies, Hwang NH, Gross and Gatel (ed), University Park Press, Bethesda Md, U.S.A., p 931–941, 1979.
5. Mennel RG, CR Joyner, PD Thomson, R Pyler, H Macvaugh: The preoperative assessment of aortic regurgitation. Cineaortography VS electromagnetic flowmeter. Amer J Cardiol 29:360, 1972.
6. Spencer MP, AP Denison: The aortic flow pulse as related to differential pressure. Circulation Res 4: 476, 1956.
7. Stein PD, HN Sabbah: Turbulent blood flow in the ascending aorta of humans with normal and diseased aortic valves. Circulation Res 39:58, 1976.
8. Tunstall Pedoe DS: Velocity distribution of blood flow in major arteries of animals and man. D.Phil., Thesis. Oxford University, 1970.

ECHOCARDIOGRAPHIC DETECTION OF AORTIC INSUFFICIENCY IN THE PRESENCE OF MITRAL STENOSIS

JOSE A. YULDE, FATIMA P. RAMOS, CAMILO I. PORCIUNCULA, HOMOBONO B. CALLEJA, and RODOLFO C. SOTO

Diastolic fluttering of the mitral valve leaflets and the left side of the interventricular septum (IVS) have been recognized as reliable indirect echocardiographic signs of aortic insufficiency (AI) (1–3). The regurgitant jet from an incompetent aortic valve can set a normal, pliable valve into vibration. However, in the presence of a rigid stenotic mitral valve, fluttering of the mitral leaflet may not be detected by echocardiography. Previous investigators have reported the rarity of mitral fluttering in mitral stenosis (MS) in association with aortic insufficiency (AI) (2–6). Fluttering of the left side of the IVS has been the only evidence of AI in these cases (4–6). No mention has been made of the effect of the severity of AI on the diastolic fluttering in the presence of mitral stenosis (MS). This study was undertaken to determine the sensitivity of echocardiography in detecting varying severity of AI in the presence of MS and how this sensitivity is affected by the severity of the associated MS.

MATERIALS AND METHODS

This study includes 74 patients with combined aortic insufficiency and mitral stenosis. Thirty patients with aortic insufficiency but without MS served as control group. There were 50 males and 54 females, with the age ranging in age from 12 to 64 years. The diagnosis in all cases was established by hemodynamic studies performed within one week of the echocardiographic examination.

All echocardiograms were obtained using a Picker Echoview 10 connected to a strip chart Honeywell Visicorder. A 2.25 MHz transducer focused at 7.5 cm with a repetition rate of 1000 impulses/sec was used in taking a complete echocardiographic sweep from the aortic root to the LV apical area in a standard manner previously described (3). The echocardiograms were reviewed for evidence of AI and MS. The echocardiographic criteria for AI used were: A. diastolic fluttering of the mitral valve leaflets, aortic valve and left side of the interventricular septum, B. left ventricular dimension and motion suggestive of LV volume overload. Site of the fluttering was noted in each case. The left ventricular end diastolic diameter (LVEDD) was measured from the left side of the IVS to the endocardium at the peak of the R wave of the accompanying ECG. The left ventricular end systolic diameter (LVESD) was taken as the shortest distance between IVS and the PW. The IVS and

Charles T. Lancée (ed.), Echocardiology, 267–273. All rights reserved

PW amplitude was measured as the vertical distance from end diastole to end systole. The echocardiographic criteria for MS were: A. diminished EF slope and B. anterior motion of the posterior valve leaflet during diastole.

All patients underwent a complete right and left heart catheterization including a left ventricular and aortic root injection performed by a standard technique. Mitral valve area (MVA) was calculated in patients with MS using the formula of Gorlin and Gorlin (10). MVA of more than 1.5 cm^2 was considered mild, 1 to 1.5 cm^2 moderate and less than 1 cm^2 severe MS.

Aortic insufficiency was graded according to Seller's criteria (11). Aortic insufficiency of 1+ was considered mild, 2 to 3+ moderate and 4+ severe. Patients were grouped according to the severity of AI: Group I, mild AI, Group II, moderate and Group III, severe, Group IV composed of AI without MS served as control. Each group of AI except Group IV is characterized further according to the severity of associated MS. The percentage of AI detection by echo was compared among the 4 groups. In addition, the echo detection on AI was compared within each sub-group of MS. The LVEDD, LVESD, IVS and PW amplitude were compared among the four groups and correlated with the severity of AI.

RESULTS

There were 32 patients in Group I, 29 in Group II, 13 in Group III and 30 in Group IV. The hemodynamic features, number of patients, sex distribution and mean age in each group are shown in Table 1.

Table 1. Features of 104 patients studied in this series.

Group	Hemodynamic features	No. of patients	Sex M	F	Mean age (years)
I	AI (Mild) +MS	32	20	12	31.58 ± 11.72
II	AI (Moderate) +MS	29	10	19	31.87 ± 8.77
III	AI (Severe) +MS	13	7	6	28 ± 12.7
IV	Pure AI	30	13	17	27.2 ± 10.7

Table 2. Number of patients in each grade of severity of MS based on computed MVA.

Group	Mild (1.5 cm^2)	Mitral stenosis Moderate (1–1.5 cm^2)	Severe (1 cm^2)	Total
I	3	5	24	32
II	3	10	16	29
III	8	0	5	13
IV	0	0	0	30

Table 3. Percentage of AI detected in each subgroup of associated MS.

Group	Mild MS	Moderate MS	Severe MS
I	3%	0%	0%
II	100%	70%	31%
III	100%	No data	100%

Of 32 patients in Group I, 3 had associated mild MS, 5 with moderate and 24 severe MS as shown in Table 1. The associated MS was mild in 3, moderate in 10 and severe in 16 in those in Group II. It was mild in 8 and severe in 5 patients in Group III.

Only one patient in Group I was positive for echocardiographic criteria for AI giving a sensitivity of 3% (Table 3). This patient has associated mild MS and fluttering was noted at the left side of the IVS during diastole as shown in Figure 1.

In Group II, 15 patients were positive for AI by M mode echocardiographic criteria giving a sensitivity of 51.7%. Three of these patients had mild MS. Fluttering was present in the left side of the IVS in all. Seven of these 15 patients had moderate associated MS whereby diastolic fluttering was observed in the left of the IVS in 3 and in the AMVL in 4. The remaining 5 patients have severe MS. Fluttering of the left side of the IVS during diastole was noted in 4 and in the AMVL in only 1 patient. Within the group 100% (3/3) of those with mild MS; 70% (7/10) of those with moderate MS; and 31% (5/16) of severe MS were positive for echo criteria for AI (Fig. 1). Representative tracing from these groups is shown in Figure 2.

All patients in Group II showed fluttering of either the AMVL or the IVS or both, giving a 100% detection of AI in this group. Diastolic fluttering of the AMVL was present in 4; of the left side of the IVS in 2; and of both

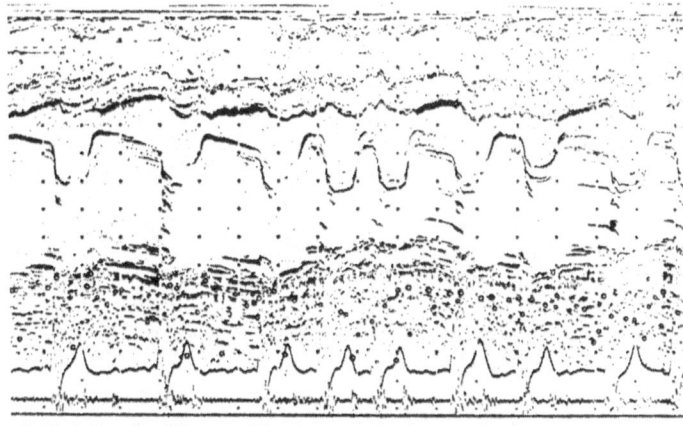

Fig. 1. An echocardiogram of a 45 year old female with mild AI and mild MS. Note the diastolic fluttering of the left side of the IVS.

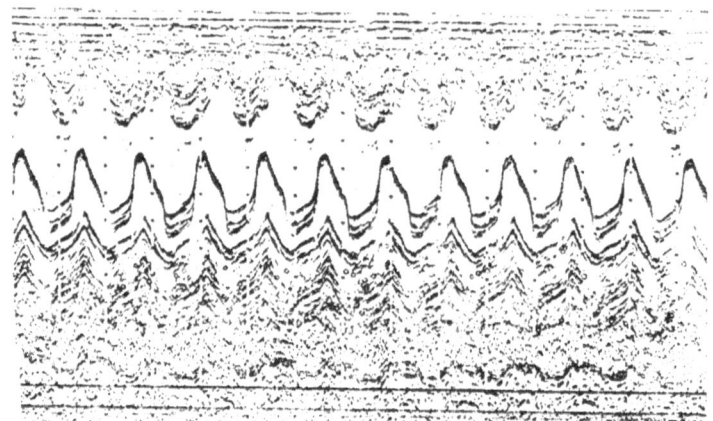

Fig. 2. Tracing from an 18 year old male patient with moderate AI associated with moderate MS showing diastolic fluttering of the AMVL.

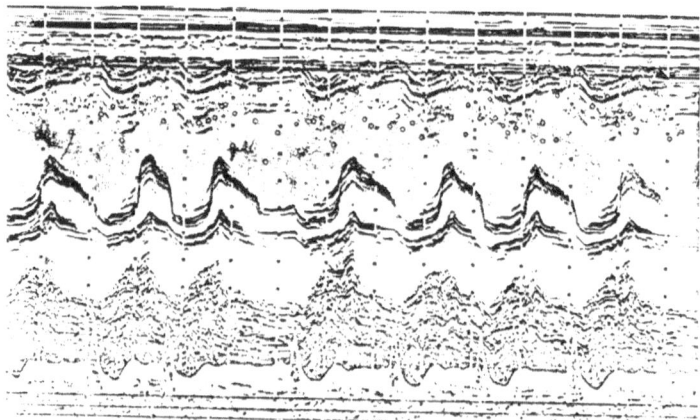

Fig. 3. Tracing from a 29 year old male patient with severe AI and mild MS showing fluttering of the AMVL during diastole.

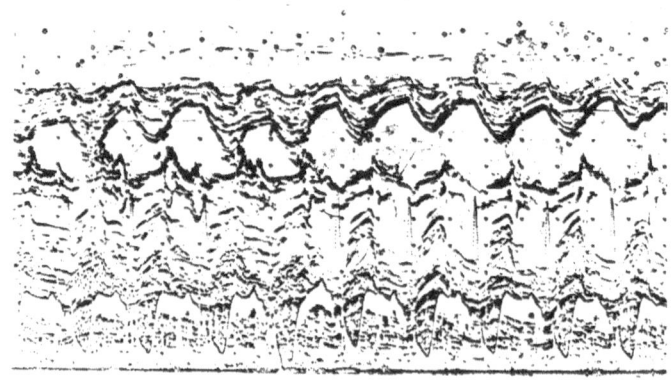

Fig. 4. Tracing from a 42 year old male patient with severe A1 showing fluttering of the AMVL and left side of the IVS.

AMVL and IVS in 2 of the 8 patients with mild MS. In 5 with severe MS, 1 has diastolic fluttering of the IVS, 2 of the AMVL and 2 of both AMVL and IVS. Figure 3 shows a representative tracing from this group of patients.

In the control group of 30 patients with pure AI, 100% detection of AI was obtained. Fluttering of the AMVL and IVS during diastole was present in 25 and of the IVS alone in 5 patients. Figure 4 shows a representative tracing.

The overall detection of AI in the presence of MS in these series is 40.6% (30/74) as compared to the 100% (30/30) in those with AI alone. The LVEDD and LVESD in Group I were still normal with a mean of 4.43 ± 0.78 cm and 3.3 ± 0.59 cm, respectively. The normal range in the laboratory is 4.61 ± 0.43 cm for LVEDD and 3.24 ± 0.51 cm for LVESD (12). The LVEDD had a mean of 4.88 ± 0.88 cm and the LVESD has a mean of 4.32 ± 0.78 cm in Group II. This is not significantly bigger than that of Group I. In group III and LVESD were significantly bigger than Group I and Group II with a mean of 10.6 ± 1.42 cm and 10.5 ± 1.85 cm, respectively. Group IV had the largest LV diameter but not significantly bigger than Group III.

DISCUSSION

The fine fluttering of the anterior mitral valve leaflets during diastole is a common echocardiographic finding in patients with aortic insufficiency (1–6). The finding that the left side of the interventricular septum can be set into vibration by an anteriorly directed regurgitant jet from an incompetent aortic valve increases the sensitivity of echocardiography in detecting this clinical condition. The mitral flutter is said to be due to a centrally and posteriorly directed regurgitant jet hitting the mitral valve leaflets. The incidence of this echocardiographic finding in aortic insufficiency varies with different series. Winsberg (2) in his series of 35 patients, noted this diastolic fluttering of the AMVL in 11 and in 5 others the fluttering was equivocal. Pridie (5) reported only 13 patients with rapid oscillations of the AMVL in 55 patients with AI. D'Cruz (4) reported 40 of 42 patients showed a fine flutter of the anterior mitral leaflet. In the series of Cope (6) of 46 patients with AI, all demonstrated mitral flutter, of whom 17 showed septal flutter during diastale. Pridie (5) in a series of 75 patients with aortic regurgitation found no correlation between the presence of mitral vibrations and the severity of the aortic reflux.

Most of these series (2, 5–6) were based on the study of aortic insufficiency in the presence of a normal mitral valve. In addition, only a few patients had complete hemodynamic studies to quantify the severity of AI. These studies have not adequately analyzed the effect of mitral stenosis on the echocardiographic detection of AI. While Pridie (5) in his series of 20 patients with this mixed valvular lesion failed to detect mitral flutter in all, no mention was made of the severity of the valvular lesions and how this affected the echocardiographic detection of AI. In Winsberg's series (2), only 1 out of the 9 patients with combined mitral stenosis and aortic insufficiency was found to have mitral flutter, but there were no hemodynamic data available to quantify the severity of the combined valvular lesions. In the series of D'Cruz (4) of 4 patients with combined lesions, only 2 manifested septal flutter. The severity of mitral stenosis or aortic insufficiency was not quantify by hemodynamic studies in all these series (2, 4–6), so that the effect of severity of aortic insufficiency in the presence of mitral stenosis in its echocardiographic detection can not be ascertained.

In our series, the severity of AI and MS was clearly defined by hemodynamic studies. Group I was composed of mild AI with 3, 5, 24 mild, moderate and severe MS, respectively. Detection of AI was made in only one patient (3%).

The stiff mitral valve leaflets in this group could probably not be set into vibrations by a small regurgitant jet from the aorta. In group II septal fluttering was observed in only 6. Ninety percent of the patients in group II had moderate to severe MS so the mitral valve may not be able to vibrate due to its stiffness. In spite of the severity of stenosis in group II being comparable with that of group I, the echocardiographic detection of AI in group II is 55%. The severity of aortic insufficiency must be responsible for its increased detection in group II. The 100% detection of severe AI in group III could be well explained by the tremendous amount of regurgitant blood setting the structures that it hits into strong vibrations. This excellent detection of AI by echo in this group of patients could be also due to the comparatively larger number of patients with mild MS (62% of the population).

Diastolic fluttering of the left side of the ventricular septum is an important echocardiographic sign in AI associated with MS (4). This sign was present in 23 of the 30 positive echocardiographic detection of AI. This is fortuitous, considering that the mitral valve fluttering could be diminished by the severity of MS. In this series mitral fluttering was present in 7 mild MS, 5 moderate and 3 severe cases. The 3 severe MS with mitral flutter were associated with severe AI. Diastolic septal fluttering may be the only clue to the presence of AI in these conditions with a markedly rigid mitral valve. In the presence of the same degree of aortic insufficiency, increasing severity of associated MS tends to diminish the echocardiographic detection of AI. This is due to the increasing stiffness of the mitral valve with increasing severity of MS diminishing its ability to vibrate when hit by the regurgitant volume of blood. Another reason is the progressive reduction in the stroke volume with increasing severity of MS, consequently also reducing the amount of regurgitant volume. The echocardiographic measurement of left ventricular dimensions has been reported to be of value in assessing the severity of aortic regurgitation (7). Several studies have shown that left ventricular diameter was significantly larger with increasing severity of A-1 (7–9). Whether these echocardiographic findings hold true in patients with combined aortic insufficiency and mitral stenosis has not been reported. Our data show that increasing severity of AI causes significantly bigger left ventricular dimension, even in one presence of MS. The group with severe AI has significantly bigger

LVEDD in spite of the associated severe MS. The LS septal and posterior wall motion are considerably hyperactive as compared with those with mild AI. These additional echocardiographic parameters can be useful in estimating the severity of AI, even in the presence of MS.

SUMMARY

The sensitivity of echo detection of AI in association with varying degrees of MS was studied in 74 patients with hemodynamic data. The sensitivity of echocardiography in detecting AI in the presence of MS is increased by the greater severity of AI. This sensitivity, however is diminished by the increasing severity of the associated MS in patients with mild and moderate AI. In severe AI, the severity of MS does not seem to affect the sensitivity of echocardiographic detection. LV dimensions and septal and posterior wall motions are helpful echocardiographic parameters in determining the severity of AI.

REFERENCES

1. Teichholz LE: Echocardiography in valvular heart disease. Prog Cardiovas Dis 17:283, 1975.
2. Winsberg F, GE Gabor, JG Hernberg , B AnWeiss: Fluttering of the mitral valve in aortic insufficiency. Circulation 41:225, 1970.
3. Feigenbaum H: Echocardiography. Philadelphia, 1976 Lea and Febiger, p 131, 1961.
4. D'Cruz I, HC Cohen: Flutter of left ventricular structures in patients with aortic regurgitation with special reference to patients with associated mitral stenosis. Am Heart J 92:684, 1976.
5. Pridie RB, R Benham, CM Oakley: Echocardiography of the mitral valve in aortic valve disease. Br Heart J 33:296, 1971.
6. Cope GD, JA Kisslo: Diastolic vibration of the intraventricular septum in aortic insufficiency. Circulation 51:589, 1975.
7. Gray HE, DW Baritt: Echocardiographic assessment of severity of aortic regurgitation. Br Heart J 37:691, 1975.
8. Stone JM, CL Haine, S Chang: Use of ultrasound to detect volume overloads of the left ventricle (abstract). Circulation 40: (suppl. 3) 196, 1969.
9. Assa Morell JL, AJ Tajik, ER Giuliani: Echocardiographic analysis of the ventricular system. Prog Cardiovas Dis 17:219, 1975.
10. Gorlin R, SG Gorlin: Hydraulic formula for calculation of the area of the stenotic mitral valves and central circulatory shunts. I Am Heart J 41:1, 1951.
11. Sellers RD, MJ Levy, K Amplatz, CW Lillehei: Retrograde cardioangiography in acquired cardiac cases: Technics, indications and interpretations of 700 cases. Am J Cardiol 14:434, 1964.
12. Yebes RB, PB Bravo, JA Yulde, CI Porciuncula, AG de la Paz, HB Calleja: Echocardiographic values in normal adult Filipinos (abstract) 9th Annual Convention, Phil Heart Asso, Legaspi City, p 65, 1978.

II

PEDIATRIC ECHOCARDIOLOGY

DEDUCTIVE ECHOCARDIOGRAPHIC DIAGNOSIS IN CONGENITAL HEART DISEASE

J. LINTERMANS

It is common practice to think about congenital heart disease in terms of predetermined entities. Echocardiography has certainly not prevented this tendency, as this technique offers the possibility of recognizing many forms of CHD directly. Indeed, much in echocardiography is pattern recognition. Overriding of the septum by an enlarged vessel brings to mind the possibility of tetralogy of Fallot; however, this ultrasonic sign can be seen in pulmonary atresia, or truncus ateriosus, or even in a Taussig-Bing anomaly. Pattern recognition is thus not sufficient. To arrive at an echocardiographic diagnosis of a complex heart abnormality, a more logical, step-by-step approach is necessary. This can be accomplished by conceptually dividing the heart into its 3 major anatomical segments: the atria, the ventricles and the great arteries. By applying this segmental approach, which has been advocated by Van Praagh, it will be possible, most of the time, to arrive at a correct ultrasonic diagnosis. A schematic outline of the diagnostic steps to be solved is given in the following table:

1. The atrial situs,
2. The location and identification of the ventricles,
3. The identification of the great arteries,
4. The ventriculo-arterial connections,
5. Presence of obstructive lesions,
6. Presence of cardiovascular shunts.

1. THE ATRIAL SITUS

As a first step, it will be necessary to establish the atrial situs. Although both atria have characteristic morphologic features, none of these features can be recognized ultrasonically. Non-invasive diagnosis of atrial situs is, therefore, routinely inferred from other features: the viscero-atrial situs, the bronchial situs and the sense of the P wave in lead D1 of the ECG. In addition, two-dimensional echocardiography allows the inferior vena cava and the right atrium to be identified, following peripheral vein injection of contrast material (1). Even if only the IVC is visualized, either to the right or to the left of the spine, the atrial situs can be inferred, knowing that the right atrium is usually concordant with, and on the same side as, the IVC. Furthermore, cross-sectional echocardiography allows a recording of the shape and location of the interatrial septum (2).

2. THE LOCATION AND IDENTIFICATION OF THE VENTRICLES

The next step in the echocardiographic diagnostic approach of a complex heart lesion is the study of the second major anatomical cardiac segment: the ventricles. Both right and left ventricle will have to be identified, their respective positions noted and their relationship with the atria determined. In addition, the existence of 2 atrioventricular valves, and of the IVS, will have to be ascertained.

The ventricular chambers themselves are not readily amenable to echocardiographic diagnosis. However, it is fairly easy to recognize the mitral valve, which is practically always an inherent part of the morphological left ventricle. At least 4 features permit differentiation of the mitral and the tricuspid valves:

(a)   the mitral to semilunar valve continuity,
(b)   the study of AV valve closure,
(c)   the "fish-mouth" appearance on cross-sectional viewing,
(d)   the level of insertion on the AV valve ring.

(a)   The mitral to semilunar valve continuity.

On the basis of their M-mode echocardiographic patterns, mitral and tricuspid valves cannot be distinguished from each other. However, AV valves can be differentiated through their relationship with the semilunar valves. As a general rule, the atrioventricular valve whose anterior leaflet is continuous with the posterior margin of a great artery, or with a semilunar valve, is the mitral. Conversely, the atrioventricular valve whose anterior leaflet is not continuous with a posterior semilunar valve is the tricuspid valve (3).

However, fibrous continuity from mitral to semilunar valve may be absent or not always evident, echocardiographically. 3 more ultrasonic features are then helpful in the recognition of the atrioventricular valves (3).

(b)   The study of AV valve closure.

Normally, the mitral valve closes before the tricuspid.

(c)   The "fish-mouth" appearance on cross-sectional viewing.

A transverse echocardiographic cross-section through the mitral valve will clearly show 2 leaflets with a characteristic opening and closing movement, giving this valve a "fish-mouth" appearance, (see Fig. 1). In contrast, a transverse section through the tricuspid valve – not always possible as this valve is positioned behind the sternum – will reveal a 3-leaflet valve.

(d)   The level of insertion on the AV valve ring.

With two-dimensional echocardiography, the level of insertion of the AV valves on the AV ring may be visualized. This may be helpful,

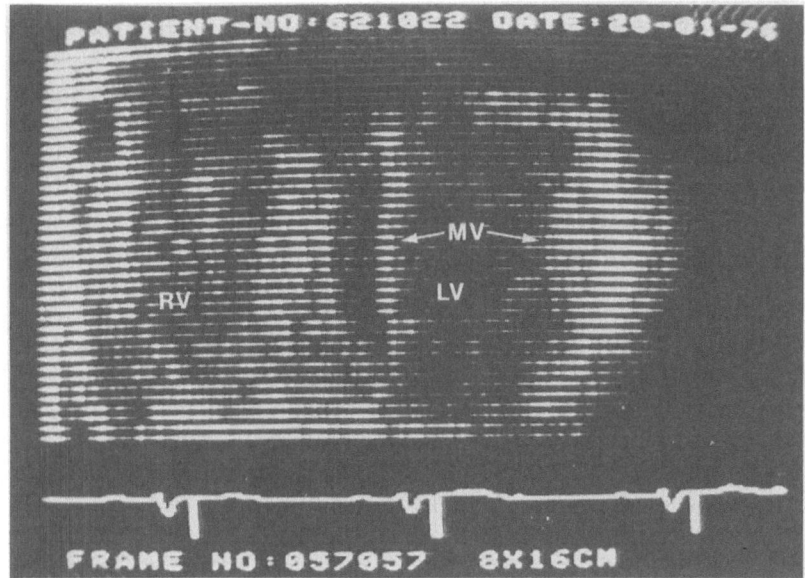

Fig. 1. Transverse cross-section through the left ventricle at the level of the mitral valve leaflets. Both leaflets are visualized (MV). The mitral valve is in an open position. In motion, this cross-section shows the characteristic "fish mouth" appearance of the mitral valve. (RV = right ventricle, LV = left ventricle).

knowing that the left (mitral) atrioventricular groove is normally slightly higher than the right (tricuspid) atrioventricular groove (4).

Once the mitral valve has been identified, respective localizations of both AV valves can be determined. Regardless of whether or not one is dealing with levo- or dextrocardia, we may assert that, if the tricuspid valve is found to the right of, and/or anterior to, the mitral valve, there has been ventricular d-looping.

Finally, atrioventricular connections can be defined.

4 possibilities exist:

– a concordant connection:
  the anatomical right atrium connects to the anatomical right ventricle;
– a discordant connection:
  the anatomical right atrium connects to the anatomical left ventricle;
– an absent atrioventricular connection;
– a double-inlet heart, through the absence of an inlet or posterior septum. This inlet, or ventriculo-bulbar septum, can be detected and distinguished by its relation to the AV valves.

3. IDENTIFICATION OF THE GREAT ARTERIES

The third question to be answered concerns the identification of the great arteries.

Short of cross-sectional echocardiography, direct ultrasonic recognition of the great arteries is difficult, as neither the aortic arch nor the pulmonary artery branches lend themselves well to conventional echocardiographic detection. M-mode echocardiographic identification of the great arteries is, however, possible and is based on indirect evidence.

To begin with, the Van Praagh loop-rule should be remembered. This is a general anatomic rule stating that, in a ventricular d-loop (or with a right-sided tricuspid valve), the aortic valve is usually to the right of the pulmonary valve. The opposite is true in a ventricular l-loop. A right-sided and posteriorly oriented semilunar valve should thus indicate a normal vascular arrangement, whereas if the right-sided valve lies anterior, d-TGA is to be suspected. Unfortunately, in ventriculo-arterial discordance, it is known that in only approximately 70% of the cases is the anteriorly-placed aorta to the right. The loop-rule should thus probably not be invoked when trying to identify the great arteries in complicated forms of transposition complexes. Other diagnostic criteria are therefore needed, such as:

(a) the cross-sectional echocardiographic recognition of the spatial re-lationship of the great arteries, at semilunar valve level or at their origin (see Fig. 2).

With cross-sectional echocardiography, using a high transverse scan, the precise spatial relation of the great arteries can be determined. If

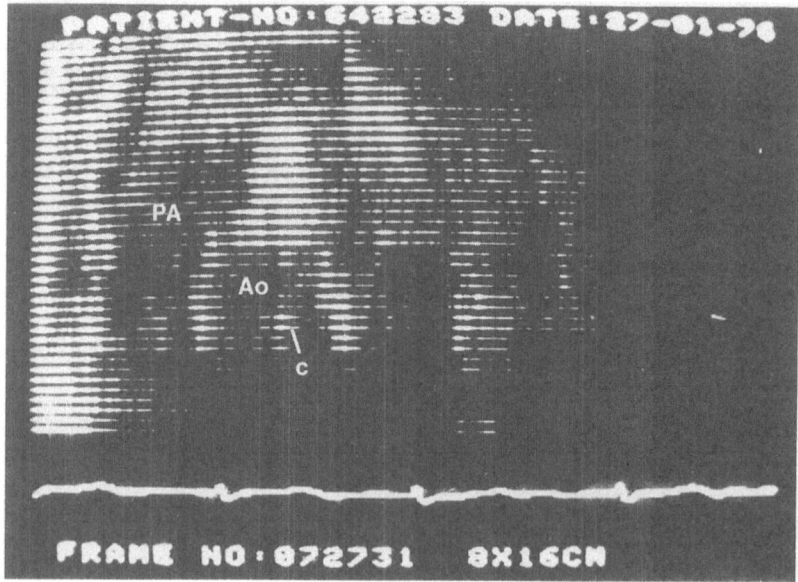

Fig. 2. Cross-section through the long axis of the right ventricular outflow tract and the origin of the pulmonary artery (PA). The aorta (Ao) is posterior to the pulmonary artery and is sectioned transversely, appearing as a circular structure. This is the normal relation between both great arteries (c = aortic cusps).

the vessels are normally related, the aortic origin will be viewed as a posterior and right-sided, circular, echo-free space, containing a central diastolic cusp echo, and the right ventricular outflow tract, which crosses anterior to it before turning posteriorly to its left as the main pulmonary artery, as a crescentic anterior and left-sided echo-free space (5). On the other hand, if the vessels are transposed so as to become parallel at their origin, they will be viewed, on a high transverse scan, as two perfectly circular spaces, opposite in orientation to the echo-free spaces observed in normal subjects (6). Indeed, the origin of the posterior vessel (the PA) is now left-sided relative to the origin of the anterior vessel. Even so, in some complex heart lesions, including L-TGA, the semilunar valves may have an apparent normal right-left and anterior-posterior inter-relationship, with a right valve in a posterior location. However, in this instance, the valve is the pulmonary, and not the aortic as in a normal heart. Even if a normal vascular relation is found, L-TGA should be suspected if, on a high transverse cross-sectional scan, 2 perfectly circular echo-free spaces are viewed.

(b) The diameters of the great arteries at the level of their ostia.

Knowing that the pulmonary ostium is always slightly larger than the aortic ostium (7) may help in arriving at a decision about vessel identification. Naturally, this criterion falls short in the presence of pulmonary obstruction.

(c) Time intervals.

The shortest ejection time generally points to the systemic ventricle, except if pulmonary vascular resistance is increased.

(d) M-mode sweep upwards from the posterior great artery.

In normal subjects, a M-mode sweep upwards from the aortic valve shows the upward continuation of both the posterior and anterior walls of the aorta. In patients with classical d-TGA, this upward sweep from the pulmonary valve will show the upward continuation of the anterior wall, whereas the posterior wall terminates abruptly at the level at which the pulmonary artery turns posteriorly (8).

The above criteria are not completely reliable for the identification of the great arteries, as they rely upon indirect evidence.

Direct identification of the great arteries is possible, though, with cross-sectional echocardiography:

(a) Detection of the aortic arch:

Aortic identification rests on the observation of the continuity between the ascending aorta and the aortic arch (2). The transducer of a real-time cardiac imaging sector scan is placed in the supra-sternal notch, and is swept from the ascending aorta to the aortic arch, or vice versa. The vessel found in continuity with the aortic arch is necessarily the ascending aorta. In addition, no arterial branches are seen to take off from this ascending vessel.

(b) Detection of the main pulmonary artery.

If the ascending aorta cannot be visualized adequately, it may be important to show branching of an artery which is, then, positively identified as the pulmonary artery (5), at least in the absence of a previous shunt procedure.

In children with d-TGA, branching of the PA can be viewed with the scanner directly transverse at valvular level and tilted to carry out a headwards sweep, as with M-mode echocardiography, in order to follow the course of the pulmonary artery.

Once the ventricles and great arteries have been identified, their connections have to be defined. This will be the next step in our diagnostic approach.

4. ASSESSMENT OF VENTRICULO-ARTERIAL CONNECTIONS

As the semilunar valves may have different relationships where any given connection is concerned, this definition may be difficult to get at echocardiographically. For instance, in transposition of the great arteries, the aortic valve is right-sided, in accordance to the loop-rule, in only approximately 70% of the cases. Nevertheless, if mitral to semilunar valve continuity is present, elucidation of the ventriculo-arterial connection should not be difficult. Barring the rare possibility of a double-outlet left ventricle, there are only 2 possibilities: a normal or concordant connection, and a transposed or discordant connection. On the other hand, if a left ventricular conus is responsible for mitral semilunar valve discontinuity, determination of the ventriculo-arterial connection may be harder to define. Cross-sectional echocardiography, because of its improved ability to display the anatomy of the ventricular outflow tracts, interventricular septum and origin of the great vessels, is then often necessary. Longitudinal scans show the relation of the mitral valve and ventricular septum to the posterior great artery; multiple transverse scans, through the outflow tracts and the semilunar valves, enable the interrelations between ventricles, IVS and the great vessels to be studied. This will permit spatial reconstruction of the three-dimensional anatomy of the heart, including a definition of the ventriculo-arterial connections. Alternatively, the transverse scanning plane can be tilted up and down, from outflow tract to great vessel origin, in order to study how the great arteries project, in relation to the IVS. This can best be illustrated by some examples: in tetralogy of Fallot, a long axis view will show the aorta overriding the septum; whereas, on short axis viewing, the septum would be seen to split the

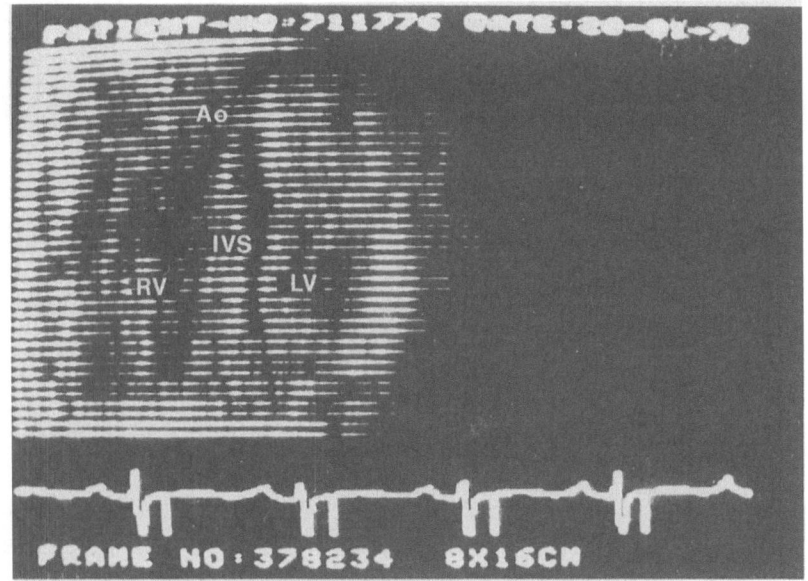

Fig. 3. Cross-section through the long axis of the left ventricle from a 5 year old boy with tetralogy of Fallot. Note the overriding of the aorta (Ao). (IVS = inter ventricular septum, LV = left ventricle, RV = right ventricle).

aorta (see Fig. 3). In double outlet RV, both great vessels will be seen to override the plane of the septum, while, on short axis viewing, both great vessels are seen to originate anterior to the septum. Contrast echocardiography may further help in defining ventriculo-arterial connections in complex positional abnormalities of the great vessels.

Four basic patterns of ventriculo-arterial connections exist:

(1) Normal or concordant connection:

The aorta arises from the anatomic left ventricle, and the pulmonary artery from the anatomic right ventricle. A normal great artery relationship will be documented most of the time, with the aortic valve posterior, inferior and to the right in relation to the pulmonary valve.

An abnormal great artery relationship is, however, possible, in the following entities:

‒ mirror-image dextrocardia:
In this situation atrial situs is inversed, there is a ventricular l-loop, and the aortic valve lies posterior, inferior and to the left of the pulmonary valve.

‒ "anatomically corrected malposition" (10).
"Malposition" here indicates an abnormal relationship between the 2 semilunar valves, classical transposition being excluded. In "anatomically corrected malposition", the aorta is connected to the

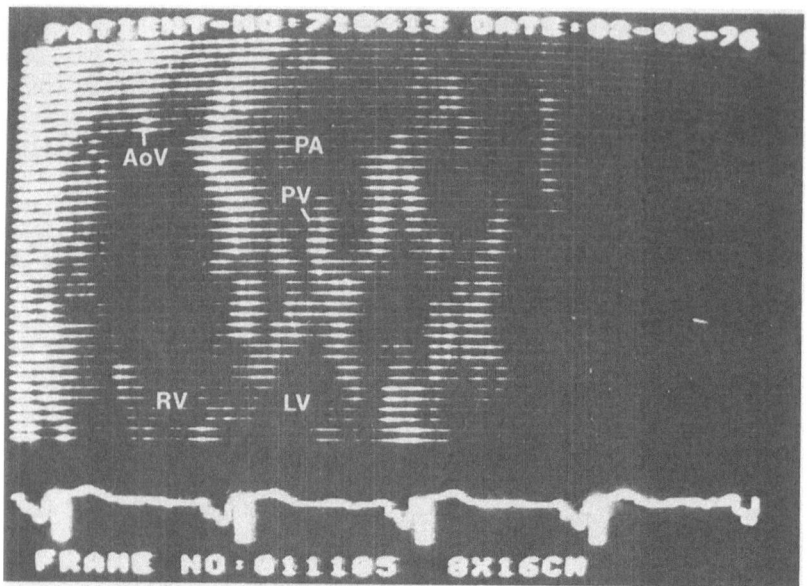

Fig. 4. Cross-sectional image of the pulmonary artery and the aorta from a 5 year old boy with transposition of the great arteries. The aortic valve (AoV) is visualized anterior and superior to the pulmonary valve (PV). The pulmonary artery (PA) is dilated (LV = left ventricle, RV = right ventricle).

anatomical left ventricle, and the PA to the anatomical right ventricle. The relationship between the 2 semilunar valves is, however, abnormal: for instance, the aorta may be to the left and anterior with respect to the pulmonary valve. Whether or not the circulation is normal will depend on the type of atrio-ventricular connection.

(2) Transposition or discordant connections:

The aorta arises from the anatomic right ventricle and the PA from the anatomic left ventricle: the great arteries are placed across the interventricular septum (see Fig. 4).

(3) Double-outlet ventricle:

Following Kirklin's definition (11), a double-outlet ventricle is defined as that condition in which more than one and a half great arteries arise from the same ventricular outlet chamber. This leaves out entities such as tetralogy of Fallot, therefore defined as a normal connection. Both great vessels may arise either from the morphologic right (DORV) or from the morphologic left ventricle (DOLV).

Entities such as single ventricle without outlet chamber could be included in this category.

The abnormal relationship between aorta and pulmonary artery is then referred to as "malposition" of the great arteries (MGA), and the position of the aorta relative to the pulmonary valve may be indicated.

(4) Single-outlet:

In this condition, a single great artery arises from the anatomic right, or anatomic left, ventricle or overrides the IVS.

Truncus arteriosus, single aortic trunk with pulmonary atresia, and single pulmonary trunk with aortic atresia are examples of single-outlet.

Atria, ventricles and great arteries have now been localized and their connections defined. Two more questions remain to be answered:
- the presence of obstructive lesions,
- the presence of cardiovascular shunts.

5. PRESENCE OF OBSTRUCTIVE LESIONS

Be it at valvular, subvalvular or supravalvular level, obstructive lesions may be diagnosed fairly easily, by both conventional and cross-sectional echocardiographic examination. Diagnosis will rely heavily upon pattern recognition, *as for instance* the documentation of ASH, SAM, premature semilunar valve closure, etc. . . .

6. PRESENCE OF CARDIOVASCULAR SHUNTS

Diagnosis of an intracardiac shunt, or a shunt at ductal level, may be arrived at in different ways:
- directly: the septal defect may be visualized directly, either by conventional echocardiography or by cross-sectional viewing
- indirectly: by noting specific secondary features such as, for instance, echocardiographic RV diastolic volume overload in hemodynamic, diastolic overloading of the right ventricle.
- by contrast echocardiography:
                       either by positive or negative contrast studies.

REFERENCES

1. Lieppe W, VS Behar, R Scallion, JA Kisslo: Detection of tricuspid regurgitation with two-dimensional echocardiography and peripheral vein injection. Circulation 57:128, 1978.
2. Dillon JC, AE Weyman, H Feigenbaum, RC Eggleton, K Johnston: Cross-sectional echocardiographic examination of the interatrial septum. Circulation 55:115, 1977.
3. Lintermans JP, WG van Dorp: Le diagnostic échocardiographique de la D-transposition des gros-vaisseaux par analyse déductive. Arch Mal Coeur 70:1337, 1977.

4. Tajik AJ, DJ Hagler, DD Mair, JT Lie: Two-dimensional real-time ultrasonic imaging of the heart and great vessels. Techniques, image orientation, structure identification, and validation. Mayo Clin Proc 53:271, 1978.
5. Houston AB, NL Gregory, EN Coleman: Two dimensional sector scanner echocardiography in cyanotic congenital heart disease. Brit Heart J 39:1076, 1978.
6. Houston AB, NL Gregory, A Shaw, DJ Wheatley, EN Coleman: Two-dimensional echocardiography with a wide angle (60°) sector scanner. Brit Heart J 39:1071, 1977.
7. Van Meurs-Van Woezik H, HW Klein, P Krediet: Normal internal calibers of ostia of great arteries and of aortic isthmus in infants and children. Brit Heart J 39:860, 1977.
8. Houston AB, NL Gregory, RN Coleman: Echocardiographic identification of aorta and main pulmonary in complete transposition. Brit Heart J 40:377, 1978.
9. Weyman EA, RL Caldwell, RA Hurwitz, DA Girod, JC Dillon, H Feigenbaum, D Green: Cross-sectional echocardiographic detection of aortic obstruction. 2. Coarctation of the aorta. Circulation 57:498, 1978.
10. Shinebourne EA, FJ Macartney, RH Anderson: Sequential chamber localization – logical approach to diagnosis in congenital heart disease. Brit Heart J 38:327, 1976.
11. Kirklin JW, AD Pacifico, LM Bargeron, B Soto: Cardiac repair in anatomically corrected malposition of the great arteries. Circulation 48:153, 1973.

NEW TECHNIQUES FOR ECHOCARDIOGRAPHIC EVALUATION OF CARDIAC ANATOMY IN CONGENITAL HEART DISEASE

DAVID J. SAHN

The outlook for infants born with serious forms of congenital heart disease has recently been significantly improved by better diagnostic, medical and surgical management techniques for congenital cardiovascular disorders. The applications of deep hypothermia, profound cold cardiac arrest, and other changes in surgical management have improved surgical mortality and outlined the necessity for accurate pre-surgical diagnosis. Nonetheless, the known risks of cardiac catheterization in infants and children which exceed those in adults, have increased the importance of non-invasive techniques, which have, therefore, had a major impact in pediatric cardiology (1, 2). The recent development of cross-sectional echocardiography and its ability to define spatial cardiac relationships, even in complex clinical conditions (3–9), has increased the applicability of ultrasound techniques in pediatric cardiology. The development and application of new views of cross-sectional echocardiography have widened the scope of the anatomy which can be evaluated non-invasively. It will be the purpose of this paper to review applicability of sequential linear array scanning systems, and sector scanners, in cross-sectional echocardiographic evaluation of cardiac anatomy, using a flow-oriented approach. This approach appears capable of defining systemic venous and abdominal relationships, pulmonary venous relationships, atrial and ventricular relationships, and the relationships of the distal outflow tracts, to completely define cardiac situs, ventricular orientation, great vessel orientation and the status of the distal outflow tracts in infants with congenital heart disease. These abilities appear to be independent of the type of instrument used, so long as it is a high resolution system, since limitations of window size are not nearly as important in pediatric patients. As such, linear arrays, especially those with electronic or dynamic focusing produce highly acceptable high resolution images, especially in small infants. The topics to be discussed as examples for the sequential approach include 1) the evaluation of abdominal situs and cardiac apex location using a water-bed-based B-scanner, 2) evaluation of inferior vena caval location, and imaging of the pulmonary veins, 3) subxiphoid visualization of the atrial cavity and interatrial septum, as well as the central fibrous body, 4) evaluation of the distal right ventricular outflow tract, that is, the position of the pulmonary artery bifurcation and the patent ductus arteriosus, and 5) suprasternal notch echocardiography for the evaluation of the distal left ventricular outflow tract. The final discussion will provide an example of how these cross-sectional anatomical views can be applied in the unborn human fetus for prenatal diagnosis and estimation of cardiac growth.

ESTIMATION OF ABDOMINAL SITUS AND CARDIAC APEX LOCATION

Infants at risk for abdominal heterotaxia with polysplenia or asplenia are often found to have severe forms of congenital heart disease. Additional, abnormalities of systemic venous drainage associated with the asplenic

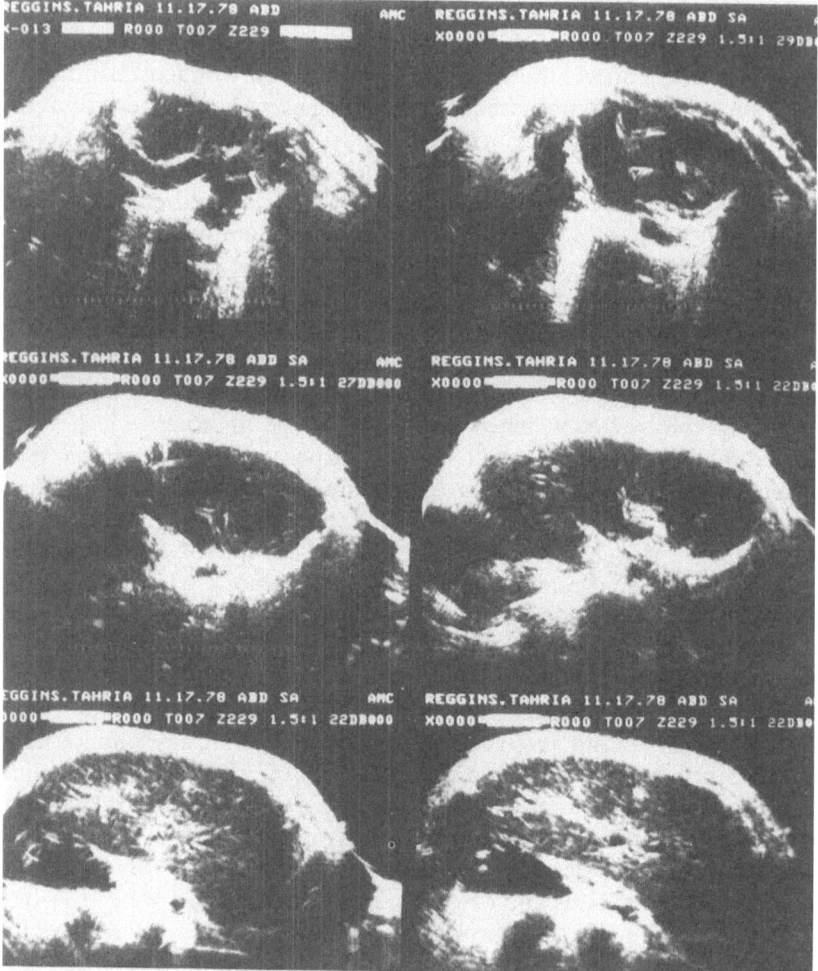

Fig. 1. Serial transverse sections, using the water-bed-based B-scanner at one centimeter increments, show a patient with a left-sided cardiac apex who has abdominal situs inversus, i.e., a left-sided major lobe of the liver and a right-sided stomach bubble. The transverse images are oriented as if we are looking up at the structures from below and therefore right-sided structures are on the left and left-sided structures are on the right. In the upper left panel a section at the level of the pulmonary artery shows the artery bifurcating to the right and left lungs. The pulmonary artery loops behind the right atrium. In the upper right panel, the right atrium is seen with the aorta occupying the central portion of the heart. The two middle views step down the level of the ventricles with the round let ventricle occupying the cardiac apex. In the lower two panels, below the diaphragm, the liver is seen as essential transverse but with its major lobe lying on the left and the stomach bubble is in behind, lying on the right.

syndromes often make it difficult to achieve adequate cardiac catheterization, especially from the lower extremities (10). Evaluation of abdominal organs and venous structures should easily be accomplished with a real-time or a B-scanning device. However, we have found that the format of the automated water-based B-scanner, initially described by Kossoff and co-workers in Australia (11), allows rapid automated, although non-real-time scanning, while infants lie quietly on the water-bed membrane. Additionally, the image format shows a complete outline of abdominal anatomy all in one exam and sequential step scans can show the relationships of liver and cardiac apex positioning, as shown in Figure 1. This can obviously be accomplished with real-time scanners, but the format shown in Figure 1 is quite pleasing and not all that dissimilar to CT scan type images.

INFERIOR VENA CAVA AND ATRIA

Having defined the anatomy within the abdomen, our next approach is to define the position of the inferior vena cava and see its continuous passage through the liver into the right atrium. This is often quite easily accomplished on a parasagittal subxiphoid view, similar to that shown in Figure 2, a drawing which documents the coronal plane anatomy in the subxiphoid view as we perform it. The transducer is placed in the subxiphoid notch and directed posteriorly, while scanning in a line between the patient's shoulders.

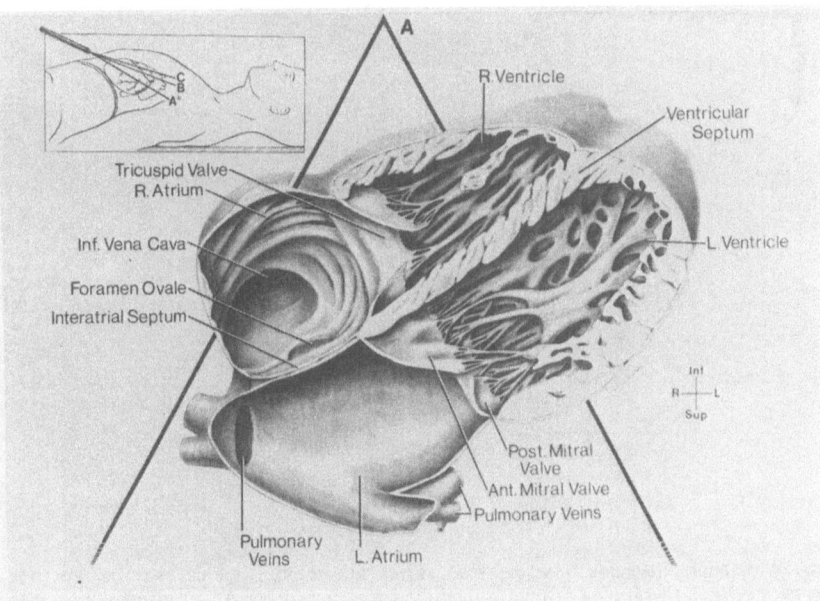

Fig. 2. Artist's rendition shows the orientation of structure images in the coronal subxiphoid four chamber view corresponding to the most posterior plane shown as "A*" in the insert. The atrial and ventricular septae are perpendicular to sound energy. The entrance of the inferior vena cava into the right atrium and of the pulmonary veins into the left atrium can be appreciated.

The heart is visualized as if inverted and viewed from behind. The inferior vena cava, and often umbilical venous remnants (in infants) and portal structures adjoining the inferior vena cava, can be easily visualized coming through the liver into the right atrium. The site of the inferior vena cava and the right lobe of the liver are usually opposite the side of the spleen, and usually define the angiographic position of the right atrium and sinus node so that they represent a very useful place to start a cross-sectional echocardiographic evaluation.

In defining atrial situs, it is likewise often useful to define the position of entry of the pulmonary veins. We have found apex positioning (12) of the transducer and subxiphoid imaging are both useful for imaging pulmonary venous structures. On apex view, the pulmonary veins can be seen obliquely

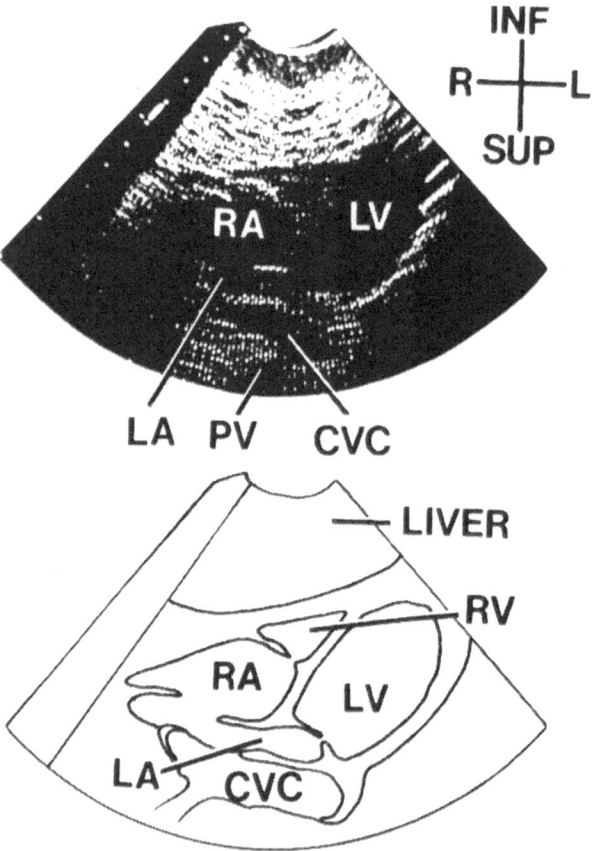

Fig. 3. Wide-angle mechanical sector scan shows a common venous chamber receiving a pulmonary vein and wrapping around behind the left atrium in the AV groove to drain into the right atrium in a patient with total anomalous pulmonary venous drainage to the coronary sinus imaged from the subxiphoid transducer location. RA = right atrium, LA = left atrium, PV = pulmonary vein, LV = left ventricle, RV = right ventricle, CVC = common venous chamber, CS = coronary sinus, TAPVD = total anomalous pulmonary venous drainage, INF = inferior, SUP = superior, R = right, L = left.

entering the left atrium posterosuperiorly. Not only can normal pulmonary venous drainage be verified and total anomalous pulmonary return ruled out by this type of view, but atrial pressure can be estimated by the curvature of the atrial septum and pulmonary venous dilation which usually accompany large left-to-right shunts and/or high left atrial pressure. In infants who are indeed found to have total anomalous pulmonary venous return, a subdividing membrane behind the left atrial cavity is usually visualized on apex and/or subxiphoid views, as shown in Figure 3 (7), and the view often allows an estimate of the position of drainage of the anomalous pulmonary veins as well, draining in this case through the coronary sinus to the right atrium, as shown in the example. Using the techniques described, the inflow regions of the heart and the atrial situs can usually be well defined. Tajik et al. (13) have defined modifications of our suprasternal notch cross-sectional echocardiographic technique, which are likewise useful for defining the anatomy of the superior vena caval system and potentially even the azygous.

EVALUATION OF THE INTERATRIAL SEPTUM

While the interatrial septum was initially described by Dillon et al. (14) in short axis, and the structure is well visualized in apex views, there is often significant echo dropout because the interatrial septum is oriented parallel to incident sound energy. Our own experience (7) has suggested that the subxiphoid position is a much more effective one for imaging the interatrial septum. The view which we use for imaging the interatrial septum is seen in Figure 2, and, visualized in this way, the septum is perpendicular to incident sound energy and imaged quite completely. Our experience would suggest that imaging of secundum, primum or even, potentially, sinus venosus ASD's can be quite successfully performed, as shown in Figure 4, when the atrial septum is imaged in this fashion. This view has been quite useful for evaluation of atrial septal defect size in patients with transposition of the great vessels, for imaging the flap torn in the interatrial septum as a result of balloon atrial septostomy, and showing the efficacy of septostomy procedures for providing interatrial mixing. In the subxiphoid view, the junction of the interatrial and ventricular septum, that is, the central fibrous body, is well imaged and ostium primum defects are easily evaluated. A natural extension for this evaluation is imaging the crest of the ventricular septum, which is likewise abnormal in patients with AV canal who have a posterior ventricular septal defect which is quite easily visualized on the subxiphoid view. As shown in Figure 5, the subxiphoid imaging usually provides definition of the complete size of the endocardial cushion defect and the distribution of mitral and tricuspid elements, as well as anchoring the tricuspid or mitral valve portions to either papillary muscles in the ipsilateral ventricle, criss-crossed into the contralateral ventricle, or attachments to the crest of the ventricular septum. As such, the cross-sectional image can provide Rastelli subtyping (15) which is often quite superior to that which can be obtained using angiography and, as shown in Figure 5, such images can be obtained quite satisfactorily with either a linear array device or with a mechanical or phased-array sector scanner.

THE DISTAL RIGHT VENTRICULAR OUTFLOW TRACT
IMAGING OF PDA'S

Recent advances in neonatology have significantly increased the survival of very small premature infants, who not infrequently have a life-threatening complication in their course, a large persistent patent ductus arteriosus (16). M-mode echocardiography, by providing an estimate of left atrial dimension, has been instrumental in the non-invasive evaluation of such infants. Nonetheless, signs of left atrial and/or left ventricular enlargement and hyperdynamic ventricular wall motion on echo are not specific findings of ductus, but often just reflect volume overload. Therefore, our endeavors with high frequency, high resolution cross-sectional imaging several years ago were turned toward direct imaging of the ductal structure itself as a distal

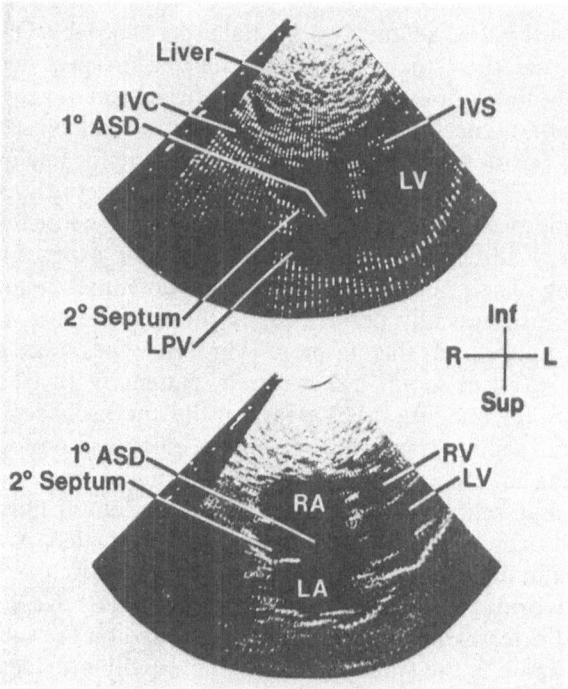

Fig. 4. Subxiphoid view shows imaging of an intact secundum atrial septum with a large ostium primum septal defect in a patient with a partial form of the AV canal. The ventricular septum is intact in the lower panel. The inferior vena cava is seen passing through the liver toward its entrance into the left atrium in the upper panel. RA = right atrium, LA = left atrium, LV = left ventricle, RV = right ventricle, 1° ASD = primum atrial septal defect, IVC = ventricular septum, other abbreviations as in Figure 3.

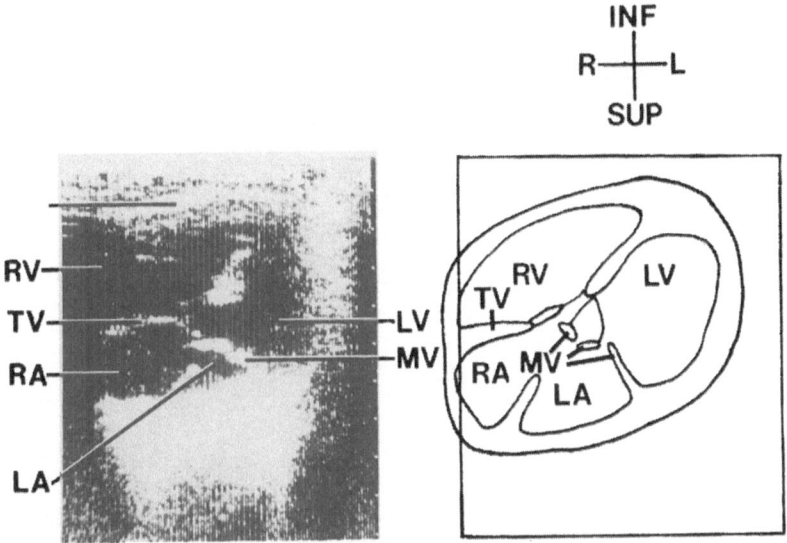

Fig. 5. A foreshortened four-chamber view from the subxiphoid location shows the distribution in the mitral and tricuspid portions of a common AV valve and the crest of the ventricular septum. The area of the ventricular septal defect as well as the crest of the ventricular septum. The area of the ventricular septal defect as well as the atrial septal defect can be imaged in this patient with a complete AV canal. Chordal attachments to the crest of the ventricular septum from the tricuspid valve are seen well. Similar attachments from the mitral valve shown in other views allowed this to be classified as a Rastelli subtype A AV canal. RA = right atrium, LA = left atrium, LV = left ventricle, RV = right ventricle, TV = tricuspid valve, other abbreviations as in Figure 3.

continuation of the right ventricular outflow tract (6). As shown in Figure 6, panel A, orienting the transducer along the line of the right ventricular outflow tract shows the spiral orientation of the aorta and pulmonary artery in normal individuals, and angling superiorly and leftward, the distal continuation of the pulmonary artery and its bifurcation can be imaged, verifying that it is, indeed, a pulmonary artery. As the scan plane is tilted superiorly and medially, the ductus arteriosus is seen as a distal continuation of the main pulmonary artery, inserting into the descending aorta. As can be seen in the drawing, the ductus itself in this view lies almost parallel to incident sound energy and the resolution of its right and left, i.e., superolateral and inferomedial walls from each other in small ductuses requires excellent lateral resolution. The image shown in panel B was obtained with a very high frequency, close-focused, 5 MHz, mechanical sector scanner which provides $1\frac{1}{2}$ mm of lateral resolution at 3–5 cm. We also often examine premature infants with an electronically-focused linear array, selected for 4 cm depth of focus position. Ductal imaging appears to be quantitative in our results compared to angiographic estimates of inner-ductal dimension, and it appears that ductal size and contour may predict, or at least allow selection of, which infants should be treated for ductal patency and which, if managed conservatively with fluid management, will have spontaneous ductal closure without intervention.

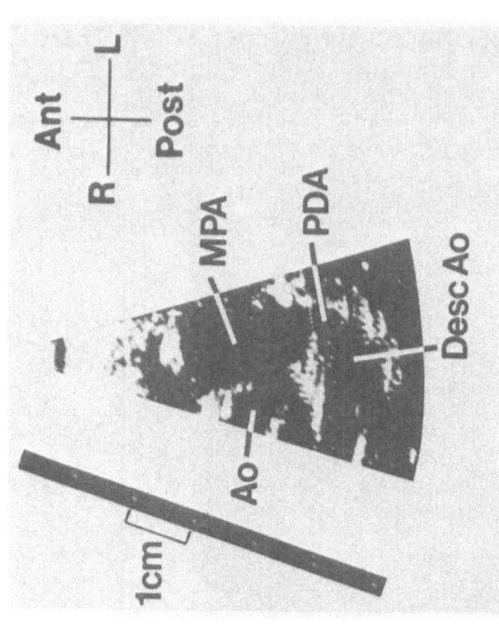

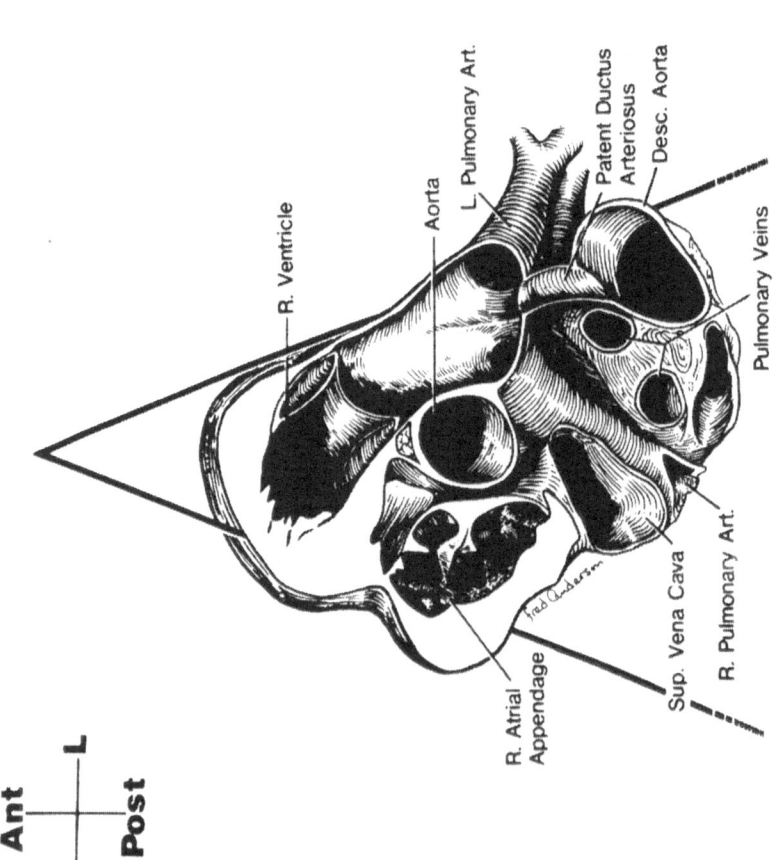

Fig. 6A. Line drawing in the plane of the right ventricular outflow tract shows the pulmonary artery bifurcation and its continuation posterosuperiorly toward the left and into the descending aorta as a patent ductus arteriosus. (Reprinted by permission of the American Heart Association from Sahn et al.: Cross-sectional Echocardiographic Imaging and Measurement of the Patent Ductus Arteriosus. Circulation 53:343, 1978.)

Fig. 6B. Stop frame image from the thirty degree, high frequency, mechanical sector scanner shows imaging of a patent ductus arteriosus running between the main pulmonary artery (MPA) and the aorta (Desc Ao). The inner dimension of the ductus measured at the dotted line is 3.5 mm.

SUPRASTERNAL NOTCH CROSS-SECTIONAL ECHOCARDIOGRAPHY FOR
IMAGING THE DISTAL AORTIC ARCH

The suprasternal notch represents an additional window for cardiac evaluation. It is probably most useful in single crystal echocardiography for
estimating the size of the transverse portion of the aorta, the right pulmonary
artery, and the superior-inferior axis of the left atrium (17), or for contrast
studies. Our previous work (5) has shown that cross-sectional echocardiography can be quite effective from the suprasternal notch, evaluating the entire
aortic arch and the anatomy of the peripheral pulmonary arteries as well.
The suprasternal notch, however, represents a relatively limited window and
appears to be most accessible with sector scan type devices, with which larger
areas of visualization can be seen from the small window. An example of a
phased-array scan showing the entire aortic arch and the vessels to the head
and neck is shown in Figure 7A, to be compared to Figure 7B, a narrow-
angle sector scan from an infant with an hourglass-shaped coarctation distal
to the left subclavian. Angiographic/echocardiographic correlations in our
laboratory (19) have suggested that this non-invasive technique can make the
diagnosis of interrupted aortic arch, predict the contour and severity of
coarctations, and suggest normally arising or anomalous vessels to the head,
neck or upper extremities. This view appears to be somewhat uncomfortable
with vibrating mechanical sector scanners and is often easier to obtain by
having a pillow placed between the patient's shoulder blades, allowing his
head to fall back, opening the suprasternal notch for access. The suprasternal
notch position will likewise be important for range-gated pulsed Doppler
application in conjunction with cross-sectional echocardiography, since it
allows imaging of ascending aorta with blood flow going directly toward the
transducer, and the descending aortic blood flow going away from the
transducer, as well as access to the central pulmonary arteries in the
mediastinum.

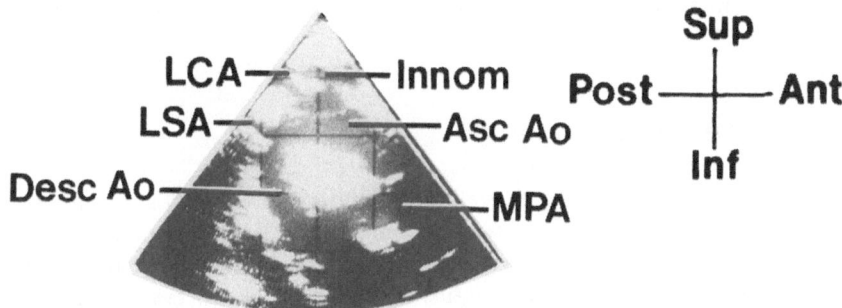

Fig. 7A. Phased-array suprasternal notch sector scan shows the anatomy of a normal descending aorta and a dilated ascending aorta, secondary to aortic valve disease. The MPA passes
underneath the aortic arch. The origin of the vessels to the head and neck, the innominate (Innom),
and its bifurcation, the left common carotid (LCA) and the left subclavian artery (LSA) are well
imaged.

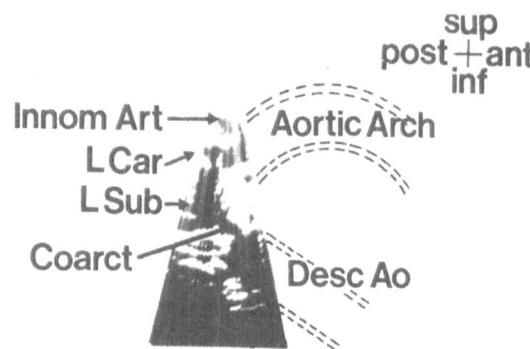

Fig. 7B. In comparison to Figure 7A, this patient has an hourglass-shaped coarctation which is imaged distal to the left subclavian artery (L Sub) with post-stenotic dilatation of the descending aorta. Innom = innominate, L Car = left common carotid.

THE COMBINATION OF VIEWS

While it was suggested that one view may be superior to another for visualizing certain structures, it is obvious that, in congenital heart disease where a great deal of anatomy has to be assessed for normality or abnormality (and indeed complicated abnormalities involve many portions of the heart), a multiplicity of views and a complete examination involving long axis, serial short axis, apical four chamber, subxiphoid four chamber, suprasternal and often right parasternal examination is necessary to outline the complete anatomy of the mediastinal portions of the cardiovascular system, most of which are accessible for evaluation by cross-sectional echocardiography. Findings suggested on single views can often be verified from completely independent angles on other views, and often allow a better understanding of echo dropout phenomena, problems of lateral resolution, as well as for verification of findings in a more definitive way, especially when they are seen on two or three views which differ widely in transducer placement location.

FETAL ECHOCARDIOGRAPHY

The understanding gained in evaluating inflow and outflow anatomy and the ultrasonic spatial relationships above and below the diaphragm and within the mediastinum have made it much easier to understand cardiac imaging studies in the unborn human fetus, where one has no control at all over transducer positioning, or over fetal positioning for that matter. Increased resolution in cross-sectional echocardiography, and increased understanding of spatial cardiac relationships among examiners, have recently increased our success rate so that we can now produce images of all four cardiac chambers, the two atrioventricular valves, the two great arteries and their semilunar valves, the great vessel relationships, the inferior vena cava, the aortic arch, and the descending aorta, as well as the ventricular and atrial septae, in approximately 95% of normal fetuses down to gestational ages of approximately 21 weeks. As shown in Figure 8, for instance, a four chamber view can be duplicated in an infant with a transducer angle which comes either down from above through the hemiaxial oblique plane, or up from below, depending upon fetal positioning within the uterus. Nonetheless, the resulting planar image is the same, although the orientation may obviously differ. Use of these concepts, along with a computerized measurement system, has allowed us to begin quantification of cardiac, vessel, chamber and wall growth patterns in normal pregnancies for comparison, for instance to hydropic fetuses or infants of diabetic mothers, and holds forth the possibility of prenatal diagnosis in the future. Our experience suggests that we may feel relatively confident in ruling out lesions such as single ventricle, pulmonary or tricuspid atresia or aortic atresia or hypoplastic left heart syndrome, as early as 20 weeks, and the images obtained suggest the possibility for future range-gated pulsed Doppler studies for studying fetal cardiac physiology.

SUMMARY

Improvements in resolution and scanning techniques have significantly enhanced the diagnostic capabilities of ultrasound, with both cross-sectional and static ultrasound techniques, for evaluation of cardiac anatomy with reference to infants and children with congenital heart disease. A greater understanding of the anatomy shown in the images has freed the cardiologist

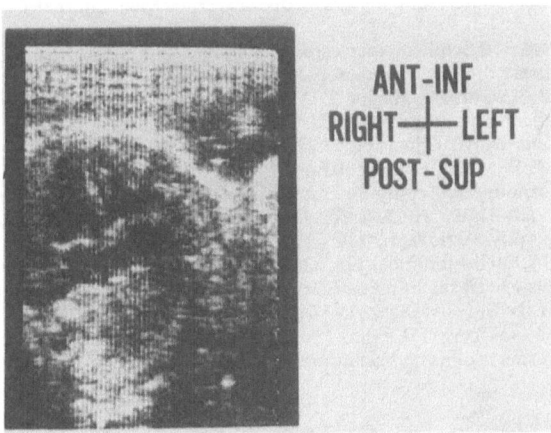

Fig. 8. A four chamber or apex equivalent view is obtained in a 33 week unborn human fetus. The right ventricle is larger than the left and is on the left. Portions of the mitral intercuspid valves are visualized in their relationship to the crest of the ventricular septum. The right and left atria are visualized well but the interatrial septum is poorly imaged. One centimeter scale markers are located to the right. The view is similar to those which can be obtained in infants after birth.

to utilize additional new views and "windows" to areas of importance away from the limited confines of the precordium for a more comprehensive evaluation of central cardiovascular anatomy.

REFERENCES

1. Sahn DJ, HD Allen, SJ Goldberg, R Solinger, RA Meyer: Pediatric echocardiography: a review of its clinical utility. Pediatrics 87:335, 1975.
2. Allen HD, LW Lange, DJ Sahn, SJ Goldberg: Ultrasound cardiac diagnosis. Ped Clin N Am 25:677, 1978.
3. Sahn DJ, HD Allen, SJ Goldberg, WF Friedman: Mitral valve prolapse in children: a problem defined by real-time cross-sectional echocardiography. Circulation 53:651, 1976.
4. Sahn DJ, WL Henry, HD Allen, J Griffith, SJ Goldberg: Comparative utilities of real-time cross-sectional imaging systems for the diagnosis of congential heart disease. Am J Medicine 63:50, 1977.
5. Sahn DJ, HD Allen, G McDonald, SJ Goldberg: Real-time cross-sectional echocardiographic diagnosis of coarctation of the aorta: a prospective study of echocardiographic-angiographic correlations. Circulation 56:762, 1977.
6. Sahn DJ, HD Allen: Real-time cross-sectional echocardiographic imaging and measurement of the patent ductus arteriosus in infants and children. Circulation 58:343, 1978.
7. Lange LW, DJ Sahn, HD Allen, SJ Goldberg: The utility of subxiphoid cross-sectional echocardiography in infants and children with congenital heart disease. Circulation 59:513, 1979.
8. Sahn DJ: Two-dimensional echocardiography. In: Echocardiography and congenital malformations of the heart, Lundstrom NR (ed) Amsterdam, Excerpta Medica, 1978, p 365–403.
9. Sahn DJ, WL Henry: Clinical applications of two-dimensional imaging in congenital heart disease. In: Advances in echocardiography, Kotler M (ed), Philadelphia, Cardiovascular Clinics of North America 9:295, 1978.
10. Ivemark BI: Implications of agenesis of the spleen on the pathogenesis of conotruncus anomalies in childhood: an analysis of the heart; malformations in the splenic agenesis syndrome, with fourteen new cases. Acta Paediatr Scand (suppl) 10:1, 1955.
11. Kossoff G, DA Carpenter, G Radovanovich et al: Octoson: a new rapid multi-transducer general purpose water-coupling echoscope. Excerpta Med Internat Cong Series No 363:90, 1975.
12. Silverman NH, NB Schiller: Apex cardiography. A two-dimensional technique for evaluating congenital heart disease. Circulation 57:503, 1978.
13. Tajik AJ, JB Seward, DJ Hagler, DD Mair, JT Lie: Two-dimensional real-time ultrasonic imaging of the heart and great vessels. Technique, image orientation, structure identification, and validation. Mayo Clin Proc 53:271, 1978.
14. Dillon JC, SE Weyman, H Feigenbaum, RC Eggleton, K Johnston: Cross-sectional echocardiographic examination of the interatrial septum. Circulation 55:115, 1977.
15. Hagler DJ, AJ Tajik, JB Seward, DD Mair, DG Ritter: Real-time wide-angle sector echocardiography: Atrioventricular canal defects. Circulation 59:140, 1979.
16. Kitterman JA, LH Edmunds, GA Gregory, MA Heymann, WH Tooley, AM Rudolph: Patent ductus arteriosus in premature infants: incidence, relation to pulmonary disease and management. N Engl J Med 287:473, 1972.
17. Allen HD, SJ Goldberg, DJ Sahn, TW Ovitt, BB Goldberg: Suprasternal notch echocardiography: assessment of its clinical utility in pediatric cardiology. Circulation 55:605, 1977.

PERCENTILES OF ECHOCARDIOGRAPHIC DIMENSIONS IN HEALTHY CHILDREN AND YOUNG ADOLESCENTS*

A population study in Dutch schools

P.J. VOOGD, H. RIJSTERBORGH, G. VAN ZWIETEN, and J. LUBSEN

INTRODUCTION

Clinically, biological measurements can be interpreted only against a back ground of knowledge about the measurement's typical value and its variability in health and disease.

It is standard practise to determine so called "normal ranges" for reference. Such ranges should be derived from measurements made in "normal" people, i.e. in people without apparent disease.

"Normal", in the sense used here, is not a homogeneous concept, for people differ in terms of age, sex, race. For many biological measurements, such attributes are unrelated to the typical value. For many others, however, there are marked relationships. Echocardiographic dimensions are an example of such relationship, since the size of the heart will depend on body size; this dependence is especially clear in childhood.

Therefore, the application of echocardiography in children requires normal ranges which depend on such attributes of the child as its age, sex, height and weight.

Previous studies either used a relatively small number of children (1, 2, 3, 4), or did not differentiate between male and female (2, 4) or dealt with a selected group of children. Also, most of the children were referred for analysis of an innocent murmur (4).

It was the purpose of the present study to investigate the relationship between echocardiographic dimensions in a group of healthy Dutch schoolchildren, and the child's age, sex, height and weight, and to determine by means of multiple regression analysis which (combination) of these attributes should be taken into account in determining reference values for each clinical application.

METHODS

Study population

The study was performed within the framework of the youth health care system in the Netherlands, which offers a medical check-up every two years. This check-up consists of a history, a physical examination and determi-

* This work was supported by the Interuniversity Institute of Cardiology (ICI), Amsterdam.

300

nation of height and weight. Haemoglobin was measured when there were complaints of tiredness or fatigue, or when pallor was noticed at the examination. Blood pressure measurements were not made. Complete records of these check-ups were available. Children with physical or mental disorders were excluded from this study. Children who were considered to have an innocent cardiac murmur were included in the study.

Echocardiographic measurements

Echocardiography was performed in 208 boys'and 224 girls. In both sex groups, the age ranged from 4–17 years and had an approximately uniform distribution (Fig. 1). The distribution of weight is shown in Figure 2.

The echoes were made in the supine position, with the subject slightly turned to the left.

An Organon Technika 03 echocardiograph equipped with a multiscan was used. After visualization of the cross-section through the long axis of the left ventricle, a single beam transducer was positioned on the chest wall in the third, fourth or fifth intercostal space; depending on the findings of the two-dimensional multiscan examination, complete M-mode scans were performed (5, 6).

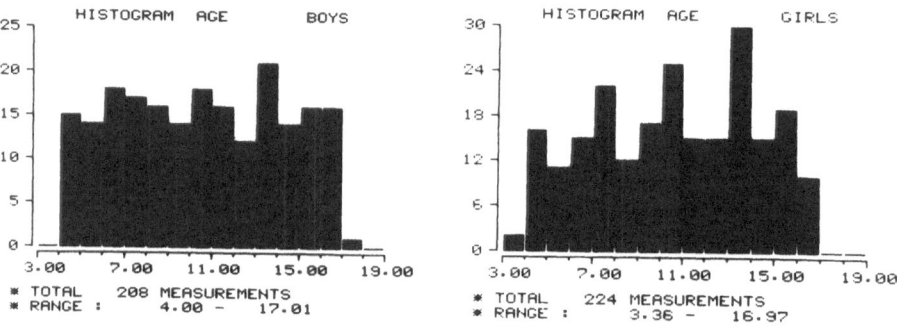

Fig. 1. Age distributions of the study population (in years).

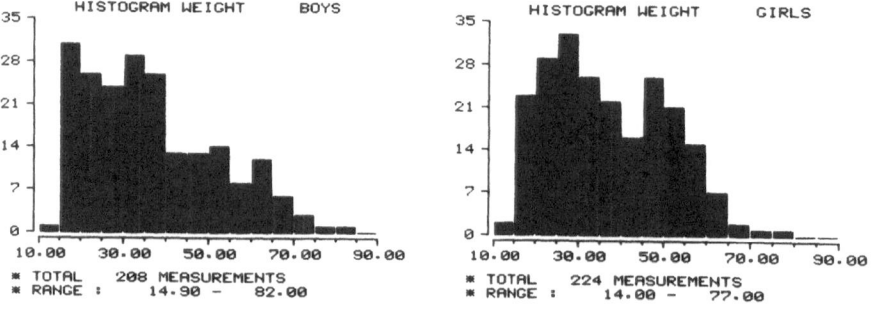

Fig. 2. Weight distributions of the study population (in kg).

The 5 MHz transducer was set in such a position that the anterior aortic wall was on the same horizontal level as the right-sided endocardium of the intraventricular septum. The following dimensions were measured: aortic (Ao) and left atrial (LA) diameter, end-diastolic (ED) inner-dimension of the left ventricle (LVID), the intraventricular septum (IVS) and the posterior wall (LVPW). Left ventricular dimensions were measured slightly caudal to mitral valve leaflet. The largest left ventricular dimension with the smallest wall thickness was taken as the true dimension.

The end-diastolic left ventricular dimensions were measured at the peak of the QRS-complex. Left ventricular end-systolic dimensions were measured at the peak upward motion of the posterior wall endocardium.

The aorta was measured in end-systole, corresponding to the most anterior position when the aortic valves were visualized. The left atrial dimension was measured at the same level.

Measurements were made at the anterior edge of the echos. Great care was taken not to incorporate the septal tricuspid leaflet into septal thickness; the LVPW endocardium was differentiated from the chordae tendinae by taking the thinnest line with the highest motion velocity. The gain was set in such a way that the epicardial-lung interface could just be visualized as separate lines.

The records were made on a Honeywell LS 6 fibre-optic recorder, at a paperspeed of 50 mm/sec, using the lowest gain setting possible. Calibration dots, derived from a stable crystal controlled oscillator, were half a second apart and 10 mm in depth.

Measurements were performed with a digitizing tablet connected to a PDP 11/10 minicomputer. The above defined measurement points on the recordings were indicated with the digitizing pen and the apropriate dimensions were computed. The computed dimensions were stored on disc, together with the other data (patient number, sex, age, height and weight) (7).

Statistical methods

To investigate the dependence of the expected values of the child's respective echo dimensions on its age, sex, weight and height, multiple regression analyses were made after logarithmic transformation of all continuous variables. Sex was entered in the regression equations as an indication variable.

The subprogram "regression" of the Statistical Package for the Social Sciences was used (8). The procedure of forward stepwise inclusion was chosen to isolate a subset of available predictor variables that would yield an optimal prediction equation with as few terms as possible. The order of inclusion was determined by the respective contribution of each independent variable to the explained variance, providing for the sequential inclusion of variables in single steps from "best" to "worst". Subsequently, as a second method, multiple regression analyses with hierarchical inclusion were performed to investigate the other relevant combinations of the independent variables.

Finally, linear regression analysis was used between log(echo-dimensions) and log(weight), for boys and girls separately.

RESULTS

Multiple regression analysis with forward stepwise inclusion of variables, showed age to be a bad independent predictor for the echo-dimensions considered in this study. This variable was never entered in the equations in the first two steps; in six cases, age was added last. In no case was the contribution of age statistically significant.

For IVS (ED), LVID (ED), LVPW (ED), LVPW (ES) and LA, "weight" proved to be the best predictor and "sex" the second best, since in forward stepwise inclusion these two variables were entered in that order. For Ao, "height" and "sex" were the two best predictors but replacement of "height" by "weight" did not materially affect the prediction. For LVID (ES) "weight" and "height" were the best predictors but the prediction was not materially affected by replacing "height" with "sex". The multiple correlation coefficients after the successive inclusion of weight, sex, height and age are given in Table 1. In all cases, the respective contributions of "weight" and "sex" were statistically significant at the 5% level.

Based on these results, it was decided to construct sex-specific nomograms on the basis of weight only. For boys and girls separately, simple linear regression equations were obtained with log(echo-dimension) as dependent and log(weight) as independent variable (Figs. 3, 4 and 5). The data-points are shown as dots. 90% of the respective echo-measurements are confined within the 5th and 95th percentile curves. The obtained simple correlation coefficients are given in Table 2. Visual inspection of the scattergrams on logarithmic scales showed apparent homoscedasticity of the residuals.

Table 1. Multiple correlation coefficients (R) after every step in the stepwise multiple regression analysis of log(echocardiographic dimension) with successive inclusion of log(weight), indicator of sex, log(height) and log(age) as independent variables.

	IVS(ED) R	LVID(ED) R	LVPW(ED) R	Ao R
log(weight)	0.681	0.826	0.714	0.784
indicator of sex	0.695	0.838	0.731	0.797
log(height)	0.696	0.840	0.734	0.801
log(age)	0.702	0.841	0.734	0.801

	IVS(ES) R	LVID(ES) R	LVPW(ES) R	LA R
log(weight)	0.586	0.753	0.696	0.583
indicator of sex	0.641	0.754	0.707	0.600
log(height)	0.644	0.756	0.708	0.604
log(age)	0.644	0.758	0.709	0.604

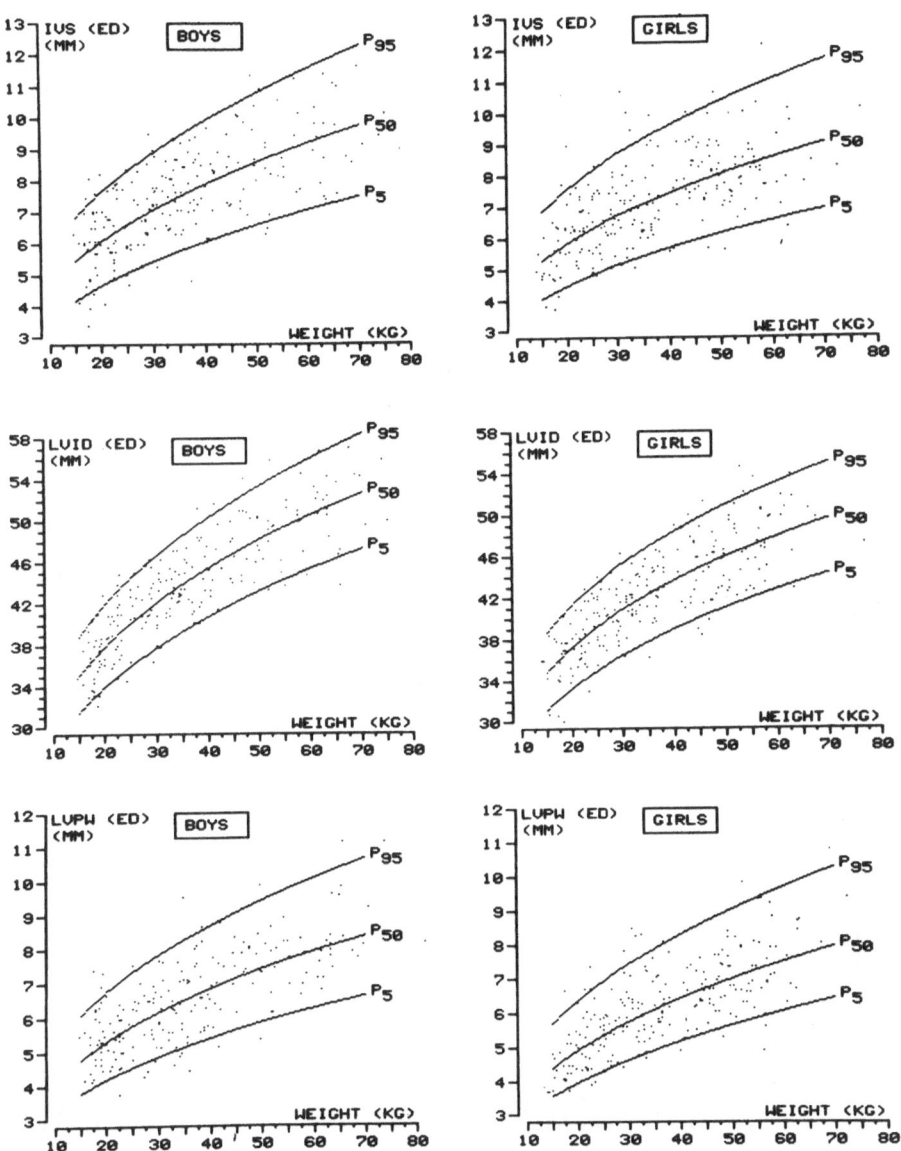

Fig. 3. Nomograms of the sex-specific percentiles of end-diastolic (ED) echocardiographic dimensions (in mm) in children, age ranging from 4 to 17 years, plotted against the child's weight (in kg). Individual measurements of 208 boys and 224 girls appear as dots.
IVS = thickness of the interventricular septum, LVID = left ventricular inner dimension and LVPW = thickness of the left ventricular posterior wall.

Therefore the log(weight) specific percentiles of the distribution of the log(echo-dimension) were determined from the distribution of the residuals.

From the result given in Table 3, the 5th, 50th and 95th percentiles may be determined for every child inside the age and weight ranges which were studied. For example: the 5th percentile of the end-diastolic left ventricular

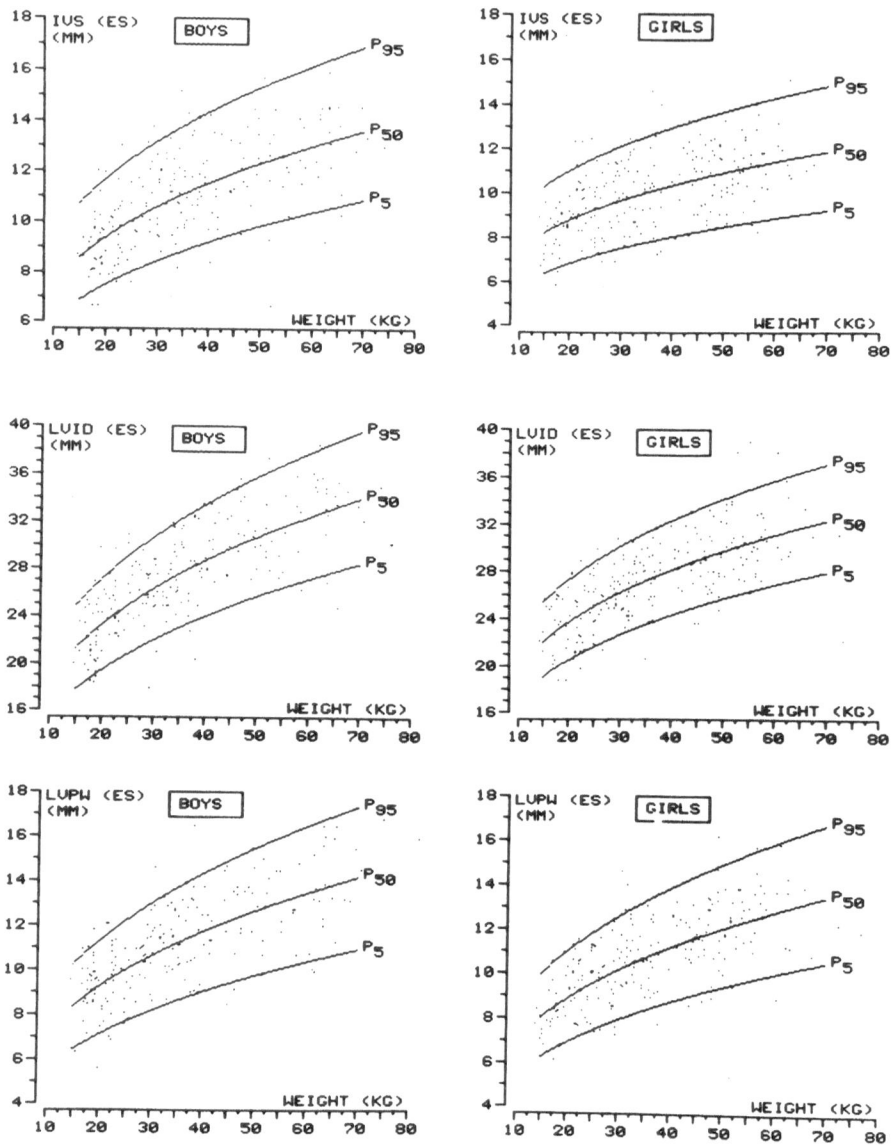

Fig. 4. Nomograms of the sex-specific percentiles of end-systolic (ES) echocardiographic dimensions (in mm) in children, age ranging from 4 to 17 years, plotted against the child's weight (in kg). Individual measurements of 208 boys and 224 girls appear as dots.

IVS = thickness of the interventricular septum, LVID = left ventricular inner dimension and LVPW = thickness of the left ventricular posterior wall.

inner dimension of a boy weighing 39.8 kg can be calculated by solving the equation $P_5 = A_5 \times (\text{weight})^B$ in which $A_5 = 15.48$, $B = 0.263$ and weight = 39.8, $P_5 = 15.48 \times (39.8)^{0.263}$ mm = 40.8 mm. The 95th percentile P_{95} of the same dimension of the boy thus = $19.13 \times (39.8)^{0.263}$ mm = 50.4 mm.

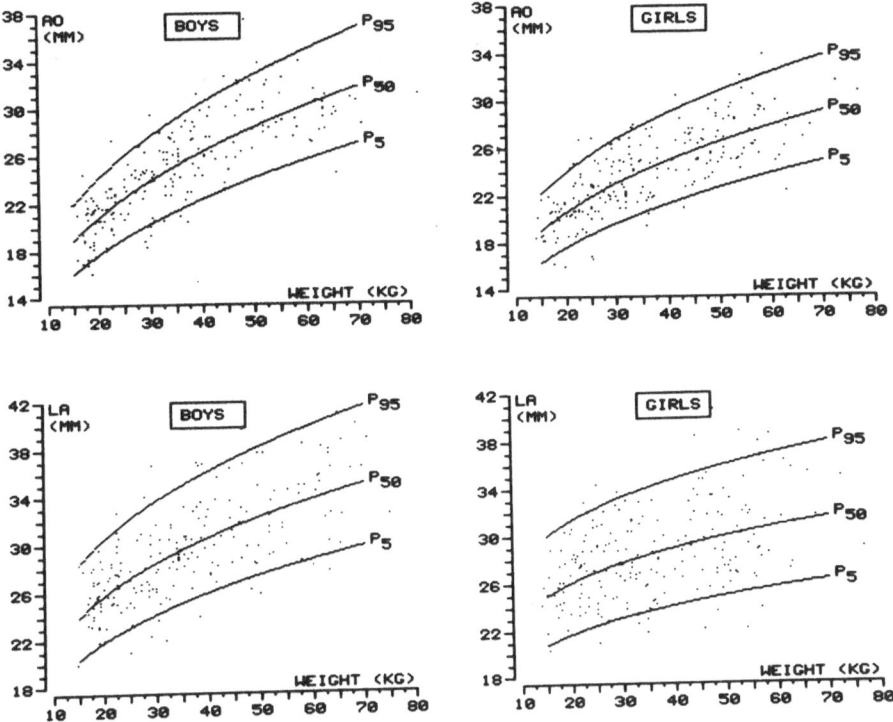

Fig. 5. Nomograms of the sex-specific percentiles of end-systolic echocardiographic dimensions (in mm) in children, age ranging from 4 to 17 years, plotted against the child's weight (in kg). Individual measurements of 208 boys and 224 girls appear as dots.
Ao = aortic root dimension and LA = dimension of left atrium.

DISCUSSION

The present study differs in a number of aspects from other studies (1, 2, 3, 4). Firstly, we have examined children without any apparent disease, a finding based on the records of the Youth Health Care system and thus they should be considered healthy.

Table 2. Correlation coefficients (R) between log(echo-dimension) and log(weight) for boys and girls respectively.

Echo parameter	Correlation coefficient	boys R	girls R
IVS(ED)		0.714	0.663
LVID(ED)		0.863	0.807
LVPW(ED)		0.715	0.734
IVS(ES)		0.673	0.545
LVID(ES)		0.776	0.732
LVPW(ES)		0.702	0.703
Ao		0.827	0.757
LA		0.716	0.456

Table 3. Derivation of the 5th, 50th and 95th percentile of echocardiographic dimensions. Tables of exponents and coefficients in the equations $P_5 = A_5 \times (\text{weight})^B$, $P_{50} = A_{50} \times (\text{weight})^B$ and $P_{95} = A_{95} \times (\text{weight})^B$ for boys (top) and girls (below) separately (weight in kg, percentiles in mm).

Echoparameter	Exponent and coefficients for boys			
	B	A_5	A_{50}	A_{95}
IVS(ED)	0.379	1.51	1.97	2.47
LVID(ED)	0.263	15.48	17.27	19.13
LVPW(ED)	0.362	1.42	1.80	2.29
IVS(ES)	0.297	3.09	3.87	4.81
LVID(ES)	0.303	7.87	9.41	10.96
LVPW(ES)	0.342	2.56	3.33	4.06
Ao	0.334	6.55	7.71	8.93
LA	0.247	10.49	12.35	14.61

Echoparameter	Exponent and coefficients for girls			
	B	A_5	A_{50}	A_{95}
IVS(ED)	0.346	1.60	2.08	2.69
LVID(ED)	0.228	16.85	18.86	20.91
LVPW(ED)	0.382	1.27	1.57	2.03
IVS(ES)	0.235	3.40	4.37	5.46
LVID(ES)	0.247	9.79	11.32	13.00
LVPW(ES)	0.339	2.51	3.21	3.98
Ao	0.272	7.86	9.18	10.67
LA	0.150	13.94	16.72	20.08

Secondly the number of children studied is significantly larger than the groups used in other studies (1, 2, 3, 4).

Finally, others also have expressed the reference values for the echo-dimensions as functions of body surface area (2, 3, 4) or weight (1, 3). The multiple regression analyses used in this study made it possible to define the exponential functions for a set of reference values with the optimal exponent and also, this method of analysis allowed us to compare the relative contributions of the different "explanatory" variables such as weight, height, sex and age.

The percentiles found in this study are roughly comparable to those published by Lundström (1), Henry (3) and Rogé (4). The percentile lines in the study of Epstein (2) do not fit with ours because, as has been stated by others (Rogé and Henry), they do not represent the percentiles of the population studied.

The main finding of this study is the observation that height and sex, or weight and sex account for most of the individual variables (sex, age, height and weight). In our study, sex has a substantial influence on reference values; contrary to Henry (3), we have therefore constructed sex-specific percentiles.

The finding that the variable "height" does not improve the correlation coefficient significantly after inclusion of weight and sex, makes it unlikely that body surface area (BSA) would give a better correlation.

This tentative conclusion is supported by the fact that the correlation coefficients between log(echo-dimension) and log(BSA) did not differ materially from the correlation coefficients of log(echo-dimension) and log(weight).

We believe that it is an obvious advantage to use a simple variable, such as weight alone, instead of a more complex one, such as BSA.

The nomograms derived in the present study are easy to use and provide reference values for the growth-related changes in echo-dimensions, however, they apply only to the well-fed children of an industrialized nation, they should not be used outside the age and weight ranges studied.

ACKNOWLEDGEMENTS

We are grateful for the enthusiastic support of M.C. Zwart-Feenstra M.D., Head of G.G. & G.D. Leiden in setting up this study. We want to express our gratitude for their very kind and efficient cooperation to I.M. Tjoa-Tam M.D., E.S. Oonk-Groen M.D., R.C. Schweizer-Lindeman M.D., A.W. Gorlee-Kroon and A. Cameraat during the study at the Gezondheidscentrum.

We very much appreciated the echocardiographic support we received from W.B. Vletter, L.K. Monsjou, C. Bernsen and W.J. Gussenhoven M.D.

REFERENCES

1. Lundström NR: Clinical applications of echocardiography in infants and children. Acta Paediatr. Scand. 63:23, 1974.
2. Epstein ML, SJ Goldberg, HD Allen, L Konecke, J Wood: Great vessel, cardiac chamber and wall growth patterns in normal children. Circulation 51:1124, 1975.
3. Henry NL, J Ware, J Gardin, SI Hepner, J McKay, M Weiner: Echocardiographic measurements that occur between infancy and early adulthood. Circulation 57:278, 1978.
4. Rogé CLL, NH Silverman, PA Hart, RM Ray: Cardiac structure growth pattern determined by echocardiography. Circulation 57:285, 1978.
5. Roelandt J: Practical echocardiography, University Press, 1975.
6. Feigenbaum H: Echocardiography, ed 2, Philadelphia, Pa., Lea and Febiger, 1976.
7. Vogel JA, G van Zwieten, N Bom, WJ Gussenhoven: Data processing of time-mode information in echocardiology. In: Echocardiology, Bom N (ed) Martinus Nijhoff Medical Division, 1977, p 335–47.
8. Nie NH, H Hull, JG Jenkins, K Steinbrenner, DH Bent: Statistical Package for the Social Sciences (2nd edition) McGraw Hill, 1975, p 320–67.
9. Gutgesell HP, M Paquet, DF Duff, DG McNemera: Left ventricular function in normal children, effects of age and heartrate. Circulation 56:457, 1977.

ACCURACY OF RANGE GATED PULSED DOPPLER ECHO FOR DETECTING THE PRESENCE AND LOCALIZATION OF LEFT VENTRICULAR OUTFLOW TRACT OBSTRUCTION IN CHILDREN

JOSE C. AREIAS, STANLEY J. GOLDBERG,
SILIJA E.C. SPITAELS, and VOLKERT H. DE VILLENEUVE

Congenital aortic stenosis is one of the more common forms of cardiac disease, accounting for an incidence of 2 to 6% (1) and acquired aortic stenosis is of considerable interest in patients beyond childhood. Accordingly, noninvasive study of the left ventricular outflow tract (LVOT) is of substantial interest. Echocardiography has become a valuable and proven method for diagnosis and management of many congenital and acquired cardiac abnormalities.

The combination of echo and Doppler allows sampling of the Doppler signal in a precise cardiac area selected by range gating the Doppler to the desired area under direct M-mode echo observation. Our purpose was to evaluate the use of the time interval histogram (TIH) of the range gated pulsed Doppler (RGPD) for separating children who had LVOT obstruction from those that had no obstruction at that level.

METHODS

Our experimental population consisted of 15 children with LVOT obstruction randomly selected from those followed at Sophia Children's Hospital of Rotterdam. The control group, aged 2 months to 15 years, consisted of 7 children with secundum atrial septal defect, 11 with ventricular septal defect and 12 with isolated pulmonary stenosis. Eight of the 15 children in the experimental group had cardiac catheterization and had cineangiographic evidence of LVOT obstruction. The 7 remaining children were not catheterized but had clinical, carotid pulse tracing and two-dimensional echocardiographic evidence of LVOT obstruction. The 30 children that served as controls were previously catheterized. In each instance a positive diagnosis was established. Each child was assigned a number and all information regarding that child was collected and analysed only according to that number. Examiners were unfamiliar with the children or their diagnosis. Children were studied without sedation. The instrumentation consisted of a second generation ATL500 and Honeywell 1856 recorder. A 3 MHz transducer was used. Doppler controls were set as follows: the highest threshold was used and Doppler gain was set to show peaks off the oscillocopic signal display. The examination performed was in many ways similar to that for a standard precordial and suprasternal echocardiogram. In each desired area, the M-mode was used exclusively to document the location of the Doppler

Charles T. Lancée (ed.), Echocardiology, 309–314. All rights reserved
Copyright © 1979 by Martinus Nijhoff Publishers bv, The Hague/Boston/London

signal and to gate the Doppler signal into intracardiac locations that were as free as possible of valve leaflets, walls or septum. Placement of the gate was also aided by the Doppler audio signal. This audio signal is in the range of 400 to 5000 Hz and corresponds to the spectrum of Doppler shifts produced by normal or disturbed flow. Because of the subjectivity of audio information, a graphic TIH of the audio was also available.

Interpretation of the numbered tracings was accomplished subsequently by evaluating randomized groups of tracings and classifying the TIH for each cardiac location and phase of the cardiac cycle as coherent or incoherent. Examples of such patterns are shown in Figures 1, 2, 3, 4. We determined in a pilot study that normal flow did not cause a TIH band width greater than 1 cm. Thus, vertical nontransient dispersion greater than 1 cm was considered true flow disturbance.

Each record was judged independently by two observers. Results of each observer were coded with the examination number. The code was broken by matching the TIH results to the previously established diagnosis.

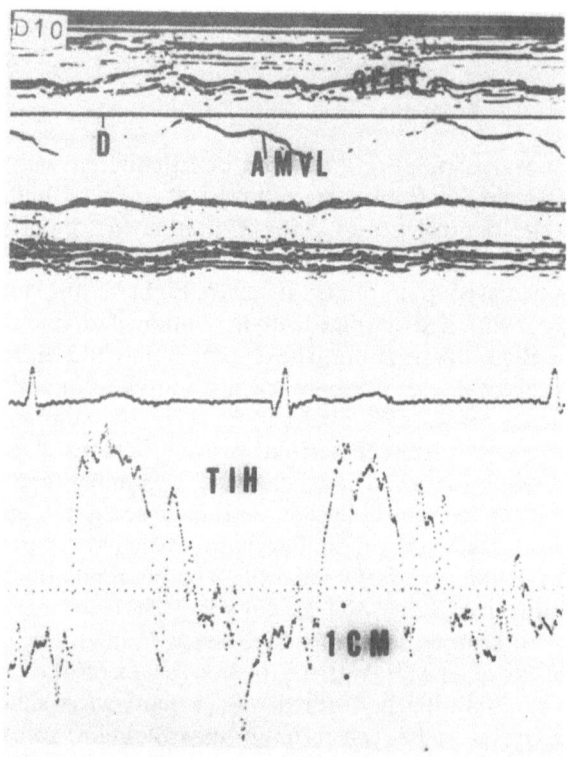

Fig. 1. The result of a normal time interval histogram (TIH) in the left ventricular outflow tract with optimal setting of the line level. (Abbreviations as in caption to Figure 4).

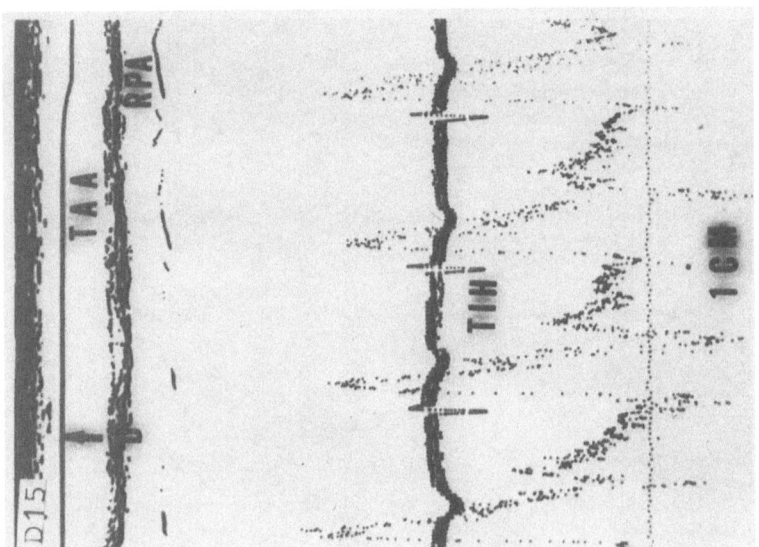

Fig. 3. The TIH of a normal transverse aortic arch with a line level again set high as demonstrated by peaks at the bottom of the picture. (Abbreviations as in caption to Figure 4).

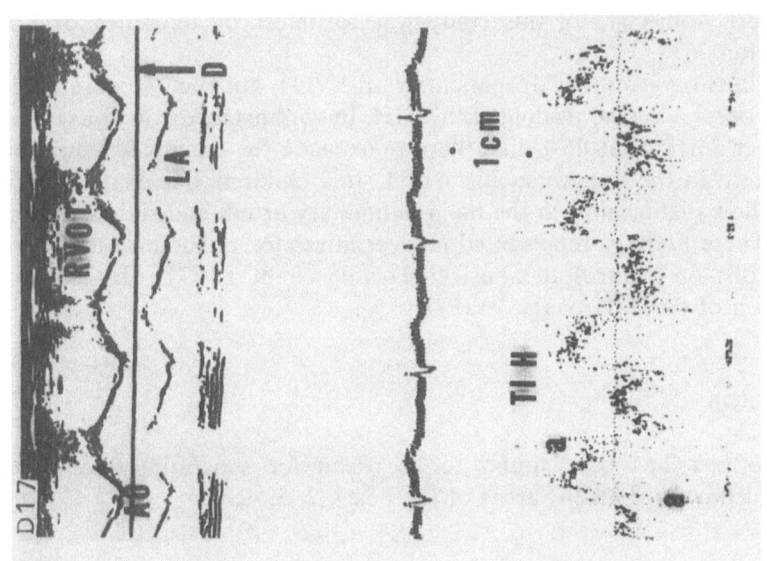

Fig. 2. The TIH of a situation in which the line level was adjusted quite high. Frequency dispersion is not so great to exceed 1 cm of displacement except at the time the aortic leaflets cross the Doppler beam. These are marked by the 'a' as a transient disturbance. (Abbreviations as in caption to Figure 4.)

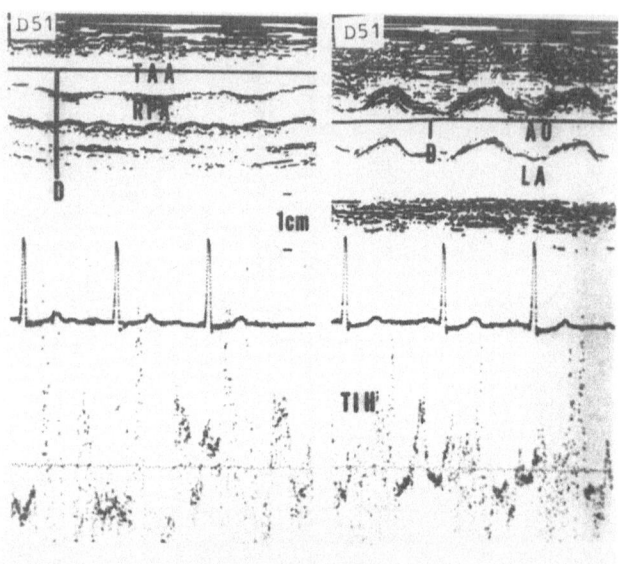

Fig. 2. Obvious dispersion of the TIH. The sample volume in the left portion is in the transverse aortic arch and in the right portion is in the main aorta.

Marked frequency dispersion occurs in systole but coherence returns in diastole. This is evidence of aortic stenosis.

Abbreviations. The position of the Doppler sample volume for each cardiac area is indicated by a "D" on the M-mode. AMVL = anterior mitral valve leaflet; SEPT = septum; RVOT = right ventricular outflow tract; AO = aorta; LA = left atrium; TAA = transverse aortic arch; RPA = right pulmonary artery.

RESULTS

The specific objective of this study was to detect the presence of LVOT obstruction.

Experimental group: all 15 patients with LVOT obstruction were detected by both observers who evaluated the TIH. In two instances, one observer did not detect aortic root flow disturbance but made the diagnosis from abnormal pattern in the transverse aortic arch. In 2 children, one examiner found systolic flow disturbance in the main pulmonary artery and right pulmonary artery. These findings represented false positives for pulmonary artery.

Controls: on control demonstrated evidence of LVOT obstruction by evaluation of the TIH of the RGPD.

DISCUSSION

Echo-Doppler has been found to be useful for separating laminar and disturbed flow in different areas of the heart (2, 3, 4, 5).

Detailed echo-Doppler theory has been previously described (6).

Briefly, a beam of ultrasound is transmitted from a vibrating crystal diagonally into the blood stream. If the ultrasound is scattered by stationary surfaces, the resulting signal will have the same frequency as the transmitted signal. In contrast, ultrasound back scattered from moving particles, such as red cells, within the blood stream will shift the transmitted frequency in proportion to red cell velocity. The magnitude of Doppler shift is determined from this difference between the transmitted and received signal, and the direction of flow with respect to the transducer can be sensed.

Two outputs are available from a RGPD. One is an audible signal that represents the frequency shift. Virtually all previous echo-Doppler studies depend solely on auditory detection of the frequency shift (2, 7). In this study we used the audio output to a limited extent during recording but the entire analysis was performed on the second output, the time interval histogram (TIH). The TIH is a simple method of approximating frequency analysis. It is formed as a series of points, one for each time period. Since most red cells in smooth flow at a given location move at approximately the same velocity and in the same direction, a narrow band of points will be inscribed on the TIH. When a disturbance exists, blood particles move in different directions and velocities creating a disorganized or incoherent pattern. The examiner's decision must be based on differentiating these two different patterns.

Diagnoses for the controls had been established previously by cardiac catheterization.

Diagnostic confirmation for the LVOT obstruction group consisted of cardiac catheterization for 8 children and two-dimensional echo-cardiographic evidence, using Weyman's method, for the remainder (8).

In each instance the LVOT obstruction was correctly identified by RGPD examination. However, for the valvular aortic stenosis the flow disturbance was not always well developed at the level just above the aortic leaflets. Better definition was usually found in the transverse aortic arch. This finding emphasises the necessity for RGPD examinations of the transverse aortic arch from the suprasternal notch.

Although the RGPD results are encouraging the technique has limitations. Quantitative information is difficult to obtain, for the interception angle is unknown. The sample volume (2×4 mm) at 3 MHz is relatively large for small children. The sample size can be decreased by increasing the echo-Doppler frequency, but this change decreases penetration. Additionally, the sample volume must be set at a selected depth, but the cardiac structures are in motion and tend to intercept the stationary sample volume. This causes artifactual dispersion of TIH. Finally, the echo signal used as a locator for the sample volume is necessarily degraded in order to obtain a useful Doppler signal.

Nevertheless the usefulness of evaluating the TIH output of a RGPD was demonstrated by this investigation under controlled circumstances.

REFERENCES

1. Lakier JB, AB Lewis, MA Heymann, P Stanger, JIE Hoffman, AM Rudolph: Isolated aortic stenosis in the neonate. Natural history and hemodynamic considerations. Circulation 50:801, 1974.
2. Johnson SL, DW Baker, RA Lute, JA Murray: Detection of mitral regurgitation by Doppler echocardiography (abstract). Cardiol 33:146, 1974.
3. Stevenson JC, I Rawabori, G Guntherof: Differentiation of ventricular septal defects from mitral regurgitation by pulsed Doppler echocardiography. Circulation 56:14, 1977.
4. Areias JC, SJ Goldberg, SEC Spitaels, VH Villeneuve: An evaluation of range gated pulsed Doppler echocardiography for detecting pulmonary outflow tract obstruction in d-transposition of the great vessels. Am Heart J 96:467, 1978.
5. Goldberg SJ, JC Areias, SEC Spitaels, VH Villeneuve: Use of the time interval histographic output from echo-Doppler to detect left-to-right atrial shunts. Circulation 58:147, 1978.
6. Baker D, G Lorch. S Rubenstein: Pulsed Doppler echocardiography. In: Echocardiography, Bom, N (ed.), The Hague, Martinus Nijhoff, 1977, p 207.
7. Johnson SL, DW Baker, RA Lute, HT Dodge: Doppler echocardiography. The localization of cardiac murmurs. Circulation 48:810, 1973.
8. Weyman AE. H Feigenbaum, RA Hurwitz, DA Gerod, JC Dillon: Cross-sectional echocardiographic assessment of the severity of aortic stenosis in children. Circulation 55:773, 1977.

VISUALIZATION OF MITRAL CLEFT IN OSTIUM PRIMUM ATRIAL SEPTAL DEFECT

A study with real-time cross-sectional echocardiography

S. BEPPU, Y. NIMURA, S. NAGATA,
Y.-D. PARK, and H. SAKAKIBARA

Mitral cleft is one of the characteristic features in endocardial cushion defect. The surgical results depend on the repair of the mitral deformities (1–4). However, up-to-now there was no way to evaluate the mitral deformities, including mitral cleft, pre-operatively or to assess the repair of the mitral valve post-operatively. Angiocardiography shows the presence of the cleft and the mitral regurgitation, but, however, gives scarcely any information about the status and motion of the leaflet and chordae tendineae (5–6). A new method is therefore needed in order to evaluate the mitral valve and its motion before and after surgery. This study was aimed at detecting mitral cleft and demonstrating motion pattern of the mitral valve, using real-time cross-sectional echocardiography.

SUBJECTS AND METHODS

Eight patients with a partial form of endocardial cushion defect were examined, 4 males and 4 females, ranging from 4 to 37 years of age. Surgery revealed that 7 patients had mitral cleft and the eighth did not. The mitral cleft was sutured in 6 patients and the valve was replaced in one. The accessory chordae was not resected.

The echocardiographs used were a Toshiba SSH-11A and a Varian V-3000, which are electronic phased-array sector scanners. Real-time images were recorded on 8 mm cine-film and by video tape recorder. The conventional M-mode echocardiograms were recorded on a Honeywell 1856 recorder using the same equipment.

The echocardiographic examinations were performed from the standard parasternal transducer position. The cross-sectional plane was set to be transverse to the anterior mitral leaflet, which plane is, for cases without this malformation, along the short axis of the heart. However, in endocardial cushion defect, the accurate transverse figure of the anterior leaflet was shown to be along the saggital section, as the right side of the mitral annulus had declined towards the apex.

RESULTS

Normally, the ultrasonic cross-section of the anterior mitral valve leaflet shows a curved pattern without interruption which is parallel to the ventricular septum during diastole and becomes straight, between the left ventricle and atrium, during systole.

Charles T. Lancée (ed.), Echocardiology, 315–318. All rights reserved
Copyright © 1979 by Martinus Nijhoff Publishers bv, The Hague/Boston/London

In endocardial cushion defect, the echo of the anterior leaflet separated into two parts in the 7 patients with mitral cleft.

Fluttering motions of the two parts were different. In patients with a large cleft, the diastolic separation was easily detected. These findings were not present in the one patient without cleft.

During systole, the echo of the two parts of the leaflet met and formed a "knot" echo at the contact point. The echo of the leaflet was not straight, but bent towards the ventricular septum with the "knot" at the point of the angle. In some patients, a thin line of echoes was detected between the knot and the ventricular septum.

Surgery revealed the presence of the accessory chordae at the site concerned. In one patient, in whom angiocardiography demonstrated severe mitral regurgitation, the echo of the anterior leaflet was almost straight and the thin line of echoes was not detected.

M-scans along the same section as the cross-sectional view showed the diastolic disappearance and the systolic multiple echoes of the anterior mitral leaflet during systole in the middle of the scan. The first finding was obtained when the ultrasound beam was directed between the two parts of the leaflet and the second corresponded to the "knot" and the thin line of echoes.

After surgery, the anterior mitral valve leaflet echo did not show diastolic separation. The "knot" echo was recorded throughout the cardiac cycle indicating the suture site. The echo pattern of the anterior leaflet was also curved as it had been pre-operatively. The thin line of echoes was also detected at the same area as before surgery. Angiocardiography demonstrated that the mild mitral regurgitation remained.

DISCUSSION

This study attempted to detect the cleft and to analyse the motion pattern of the separated parts of the arterior mitral valve leaflet in patients with an endocardial cushion defect. During cross-sectional examination, it was important to take care in selecting the proper interrogating plane.

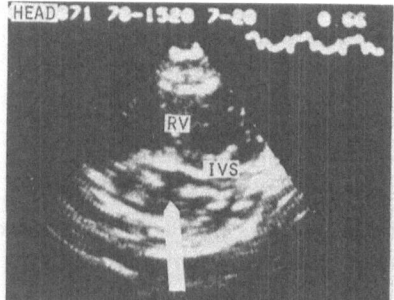 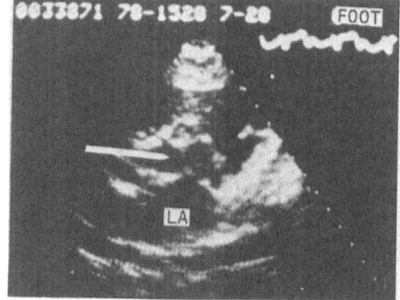

Fig. 1. The transverse figures of the anterior mitral leaflet in endocardial cushion defect. (Left) During diastole. An arrow indicates cleft. (Right) During systole. An arrow indicates the accessory chordae.

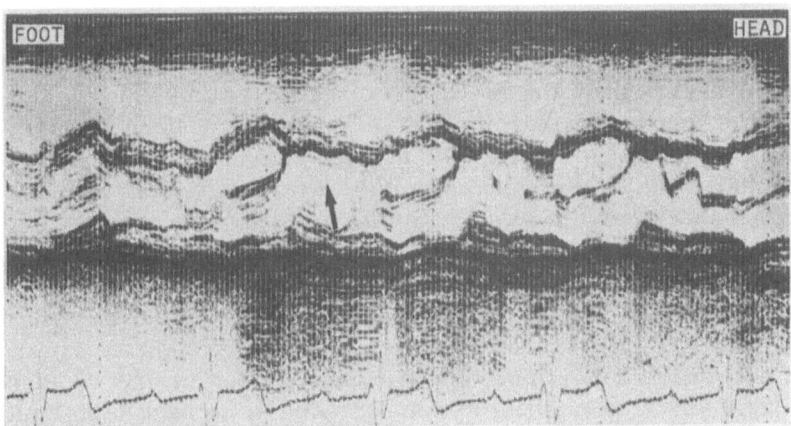

Fig. 2. M-mode scan along the transverse section of the anterior leaflet in endocardial cushion defect. An arrow indicates the diastolic disappearance of the anterior leaflet.

Cross-sectional echocardiography along the appropriate section demonstrated the diastolic separation of the leaflet in all patients with cleft. As this feature was not observed in other heart disease, it was believed to indicate the mitral cleft. It was thought that the extent of the diastolic separation corresponded to the degree of the cleft.

The "knot" echo formed at the contact site of the two parts should correspond to the non-opaque notch in the mitral area in the angiocardiogram. The thin line of echoes between the knot and the ventricular septum were thought to be the echoes of the accessory chordae.

Systolic curvature of the anterior mitral leaflet towards the septum was considered to be caused by the accessory chordae restraining the leaflet. The accessory chordae may play a role as tension chordae which prevent the edge of the cleft from prolapsing into the left atrium (7). However, these conditions may produce a gap in the coaptation between the mitral valve leaflets resulting in mitral regurgitation.

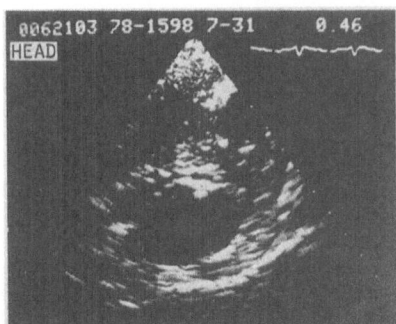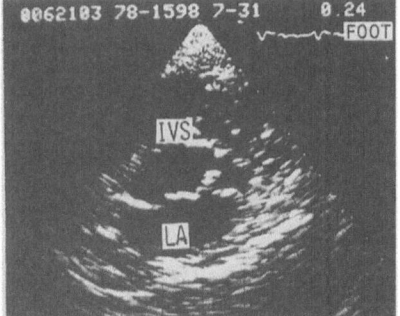

Fig. 3. The transverse figures of the anterior leaflet after surgery. (Left) Diastole. (Right) Systole.

Our patients still had slight mitral regurgitation after surgery. Echo-cardiographically, the thin line of echoes and the systolic curvature of the anterior leaflet remained as in their pre-operative condition. If the accessory chordae is functioning only as a tension apparatus, it might be redundant when the cleft is sutured (7). The anterior leaflet will be flat and coapt successfully with the posterior leaflet if the accessory chordae is resected.

As far as we know, no specific study directed itself to the observation of the deformities of the mitral valve in endocardial cushion defect. This study showed that cross-sectional echocardiography could offer useful information about mitral deformities. Although the number of patients in this study was not large, a possible procedure for mitral repair in this condition is proposed. Cross-sectional echocardiography may become an indispensable examination procedure for the assessment of mitral deformities in endocardial cushion defect.

REFERENCES

1. Braunwald NS, AG Morrow: Incomplete persistent atrioventricular canal: Operative methods and the results of pre- and post-operative hemodynamic assessment. J Thorac Cardiovasc Surg 51:71, 1966.
2. Griffiths SP, K Ellis, JO Burris, S Bumenthal, FO Jr Bowman, JR Malm: Postoperative evaluation of mitral valve function in ostium primum defect with cleft mitral valve (Partial form of atrioventricular canal). Circulation 40:21, 1969.
3. McMullan MH, DC McGoon, RB Wallace, GK Danielson, WH Weidman: Surgical treatment of partial atrioventricular canal. Arch Surg 107:705, 1973.
4. Losay J, A Rosenthal, AR Castaneda, WH Berhart, AS Nadas: Repair of atrial septal defect primum. Results, course, and prognosis. J Thorac Cardiovasc Surg 75:248, 1978.
5. Somerville J, K Lefferson: Left ventricular angiocardiography in atrioventricular defects. Brit Heart J 30:446, 1968.
6. Baron M: Abnormalities of the mitral valve in endocardial cushion defect. Circulation 45:672, 1972.
7. Edwards JE: The problem of mitral insufficiency caused by accessory chordae tendineae in persistent common atrioventricular canal. Staff Meet Mayo Clin 35:299, 1960.

CROSS-SECTIONAL ECHOCARDIOGRAPHIC FEATURES OF ANOMALOUS SYSTEMIC AND CORONARY VENOUS RETURN

R.A. FOALE, P.D.V. BOURDILLON,
J. SOMERVILLE, and A.F. RICKARDS

INTRODUCTION

Anomalous systemic venous return occurs as a co-existing abnormality in a small proportion of patients with congenital heart disease. Persistence of a left sided superior vena cava (LSVC) draining into the right atrium via an enlarged coronary sinus (CS) is the commonest anomaly (1). Recently M-mode echocardiography has demonstrated an enlarged CS when it drains abnormal systemic or pulmonary venous return (2). Cross-sectional echocardiography provides additional spatial orientation and more easily distinguishes echoes of spurious nature from those of anatomical structures. Observations using this technique were made in patients with anomalies of systemic and coronary venous return. The study also describes methods for the correct identification of these anomalies by the additional use of contrast injections into peripheral veins.

PATIENTS AND METHODS

Eleven patients (age range 6–65) with anomalous systemic venous return previously diagnosed by cardiac catheterisation were studied. A further patient with isolated congenital absence of the coronary sinus observed at coronary angiography and with therefore suspected anomalies of systemic venous return was also studied.

In 8 patients with normal cardiac connections a persistent LSVC drained to the right atrium via an enlarged CS. In one of these patients a communication also existed between the lateral part of the CS and the left atrium (LA).

In 3 patients a persistent LSVC drained to the LA direct, 2 of these patients having complex congenital heart disease and with venous return for the lower part of the body draining via an azygous system to the LSVC.

Using a mechanical sector scanner* with 30° and 81° transducer heads, cross-sectional images of the heart were recorded viewing the mitral valve in the long axis and posteriorly, the region of the atrioventricular groove. Images of the interatrial septum with right and left atria were then obtained using parasternal, apical and subxiphoid transducer positions.

*Smith-Kline Instrument Company Limited.

Charles T. Lancée (ed.), Echocardiology, 319–323. All rights reserved

Bolus injections from right and left peripheral arm veins were performed using 2–10 ml of indocyanine green. Injections were made into the femoral vein in 2 patients. The passage of resulting "contrast" echoes were then traced through the cardiac chambers, the data being recorded onto videotape and later edited directly onto 35 mm cinefilm.

RESULTS

In all patients with an enlarged CS an ovoid structure was observed in the region of the atrio-ventricular groove behind the mitral valve when viewed in the long axis (Fig. 1a). With bolus injections into the left arm this structure filled rapidly with contrast (Fig. 1b) and subsequently filling of the right

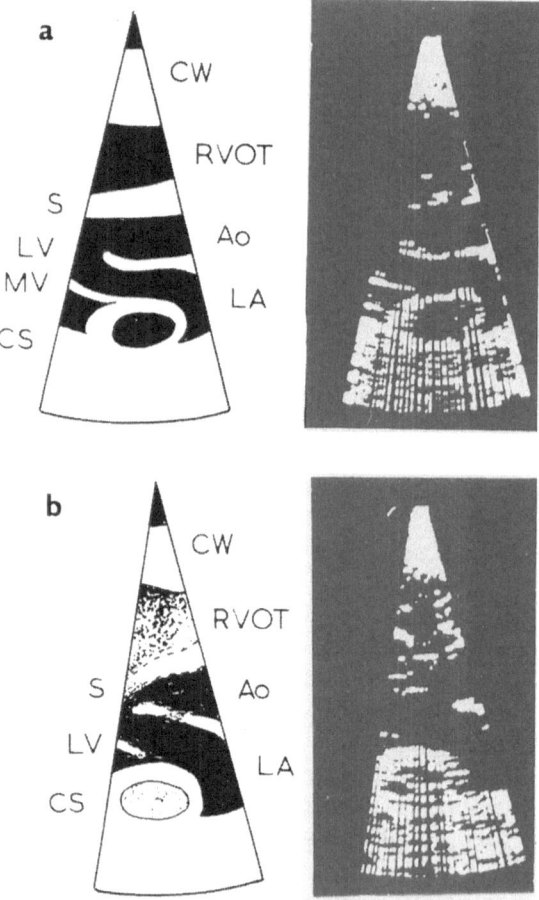

Fig. 1. Mitral valve (MV) long axis view. Coronary sinus (CS) behind mitral valve anterior leaflet. a. before contrast. b. following contrast injection from left arm. CW = chest wall, RVOT = right ventricular outflow tract, S = septum, AO = aorta, LA = left atrium.

ventricular outflow tract (RVOT) was observed. Following bolus injection from the right arm this ovoid structure failed to opacify, the RVOT only, filling rapidly. In the one patient with persistent LSVC and CS connections to the LA, rapid filling of both LA and CS was observed following injection from the left arm but not from the right (Fig. 2a, b). In the three patients with direct entry of LSVC to LA, the LA filled immediately following injection from the left but not from the right arm (Fig. 3a, b). In the patient with congenital absence of the CS and therefore suspected anomalies of systemic venous return, normal venous anatomy was demonstrated following bolus injections from right and left peripheral arm and femoral veins. This finding was later confirmed by venous angiography.

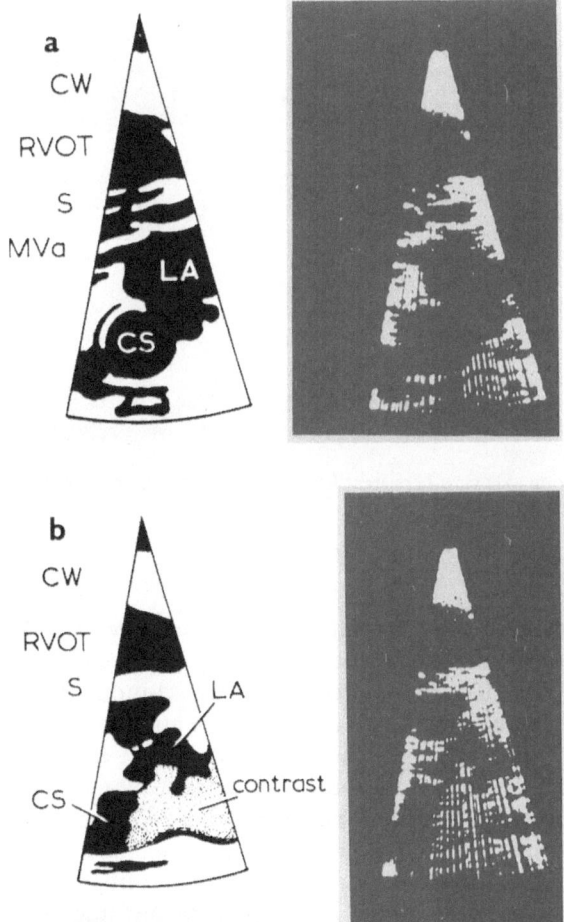

Fig. 2. MV long axis view. CS with LA connection. a. before contrast, b. following contrast injection from the left arm. Abbreviations as in Figure 1.

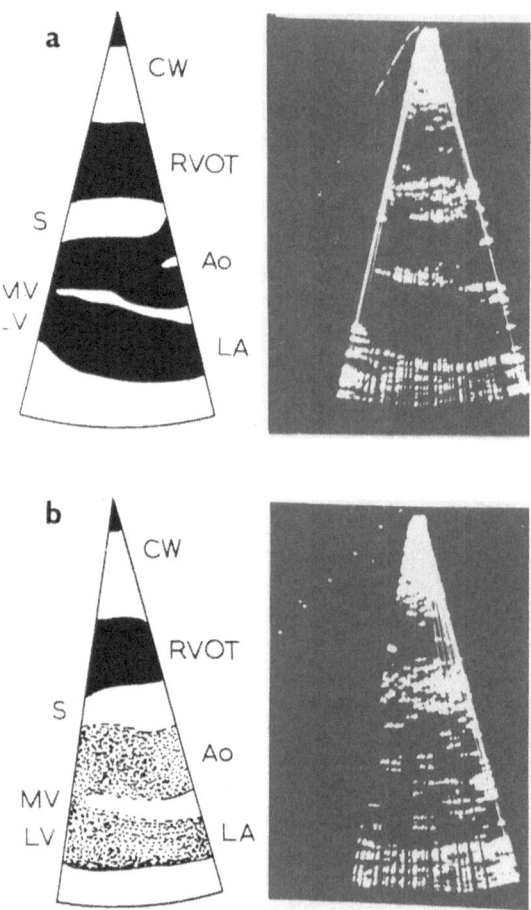

Fig. 3. MV long axis view persistent LSVC to LA direct, a. before contrast, b. following contrast injection from left arm.

DISCUSSION

A persistent LSVC in association with an enlarged CS draining to the right atrium is the commonest anomaly of systemic venous return. An enlarged coronary sinus has been identified using M-mode echocardiography as a linear echo lying posterior to the LA at the atrio-ventricular groove using the aortic valve as a reference point (1). The correct interpretation of echoes in this area may be aided by the use of cross-sectional echocardiography.

Using this technique in all patients with a persistent LSVC draining via CS to right atrium, the enlarged coronary sinus was identified as an ovoid shape in systole which rapidly assumed a circular configuration in early diastole. The ovoid flattening of the CS is presumably due to the systolic rise in intrapericardial pressure.

The additional use of bolus injections from peripheral veins whilst following the passage of the resulting echoes through each cardiac chamber allowed definition of the anatomy of systemic venous return.

SUMMARY AND CONCLUSIONS

Eleven patients with anomalous systemic venous drainage including coronary sinus abnormalities have been studied using cross-sectional echocardiography combined with contrast injections into peripheral veins.

In 8 patients with a persistent left superior vena cava draining via a coronary sinus into the right atrium, an enlarged coronary sinus was identified as lying in the posterior atrioventricular groove. In all patients a correct description of the route of systemic venous return was possible by using contrast injections. This study demonstrates the potential value of cross-sectional echocardiography, combined with peripheral vein contrast injections, in the assessment of patients with suspected anomalies of systemic and coronary venous return.

REFERENCES

1. Campbell M, DC Deuchar: The left sided superior vena cava. Brit Heart J 16:423, 1954.
2. Aziz KU, MH Paul, S Bharati, M Lev, K Shannon: Echocardiographic features of total anomalous pulmonary venous drainage into the coronary sinus. Am J Cardiol 42:108, 1978.

CONGENITAL HEART DISEASE STUDIED WITH A HIGH RESOLUTION LINEAR ARRAY SYSTEM*

W.J. GUSSENHOVEN, J. ROHMER, and C.M. LIGTVOET

Two-dimensional echocardiography has proven to be a useful non-invasive method for evaluating congenital heart disease. The strength of this technique lies in its unique ability to identify the atrioventricular and semilunar valves and the ventricular septum. Establishing the diagnosis in a wide variety of congenital cardiac malformations is often possible from this information.

A group of 300 children with congenital heart disease has been evaluated, using a dynamically focused linear array system (1). Three transducer positions, the long axis view (A), the horizontal cross-section view (B) and the sagittal right ventricular outflow tract view (C) were studied (Fig. 1), (2). Alternative transducer orientation can be carried out by tilting the transducer slightly. This is especially the case for the horizontal cross-section view, where direct information can be obtained from the ventricles and atria.

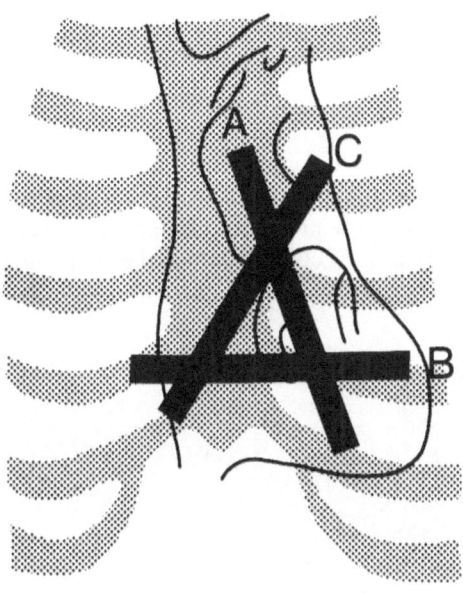

Fig. 1. This diagram shows the three positions of the transducer used for this study.

*This work was supported by the Interuniversity Institute of Cardiology (ICI), Amsterdam.

Charles T. Lancée (ed.), Echocardiology, 325–334. All rights reserved

ATRIOVENTRICULAR CANAL

Congenital defects involving the atrioventricular valves, such as partial or complete atrioventricular canal defects, were examined. The long axis view and the horizontal cross-section view offer characteristic images of these abnormalities. In partial atrioventricular canal, a narrow left ventricular outflow tract can be observed (Fig. 2). This phenomenon may be caused by the attachment of the mitral valve to the crest of the interventricular septum. In addition, a characteristic break in mitral valve echoes can be seen, representing the cleft of the valve. In the complete form of atrioventricular canal defect, there is an absence of echoes from the upper portion of the ventricular septum (3) (4). A large ventricular septal defect will give a large echo "drop-out" (Fig. 3). The single anterior atrioventricular valve leaflet is seen under the aortic root and crosses the two ventricles.

The opening of the affected valve in diastole occurs more in the direction of the right ventricle and not, as is normal, toward the left ventricular cavity itself.

Secondly, anomalies in the size of the ventricles and the atria are displayed and help to define the hemodynamic consequences of the lesions.

TRICUSPID ATRESIA

Tricuspid atresia may be described as being an absence of the right atrioventricular valve, whereby no connection between the right atrium to the corresponding ventricle is present (5) (6). The echographic view in patients with this anomaly and with normally related great vessels is characteristic (Fig. 4). The left atrium is connected to the left ventricle by the single atrioventricular valve, mitral valve. Figure 4A shows a small cavity, repre-

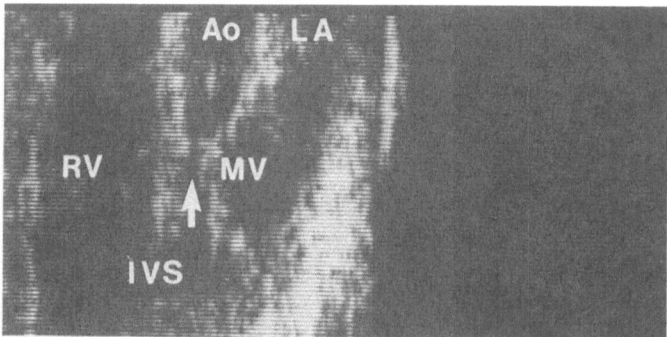

Fig. 2. Long axis view obtained from a patient with partial atrioventricular canal. The outflow tract of the left ventricle is narrow due to the apposition of the atrioventricular valve to the interventricular septum (IVS) (see arrow). (Ao = aorta; LA = left atrium; MV = mitral valve; RV = right ventricle).

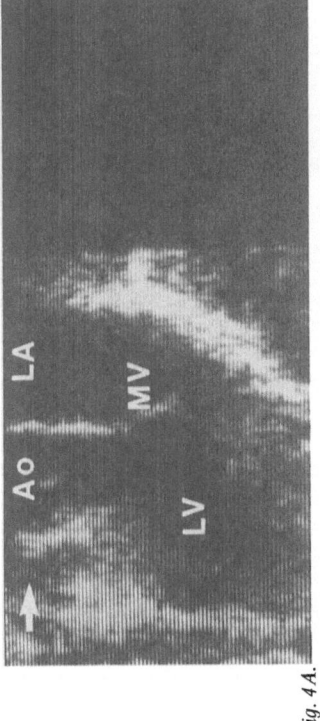

Fig. 3A.

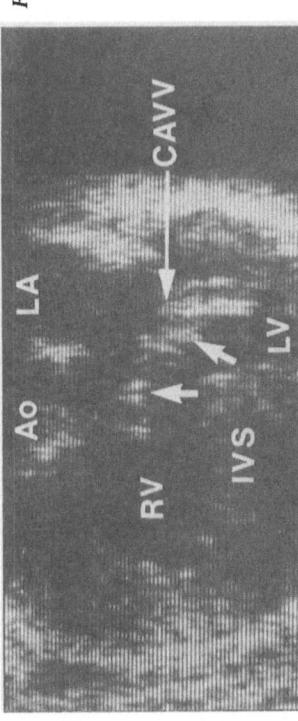

Fig. 3B.

Fig. 3A and 3B. Long axis view obtained from a patient with a complete form of an atrioventricular canal. Due to pulmonary hypertension the interventricular septum (IVS) and the anterior wall of the right ventricle became hypertrophic (A).

In Figure 3B a slightly tilted transducer was used to see the ventricular septal defect. The common atrioventricular valve (CAVV) could be seen passing this defect (see arrow).

(Ao = aorta; LA = left atrium; LV = left ventricle; RV right ventricle).

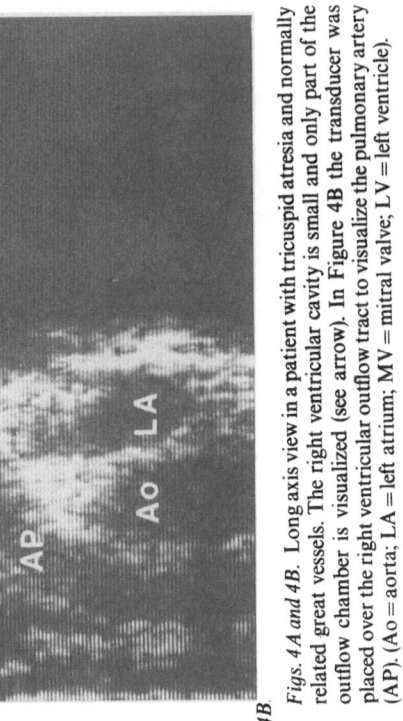

Fig. 4A.

Fig. 4B.

Figs. 4A and 4B. Long axis view in a patient with tricuspid atresia and normally related great vessels. The right ventricular cavity is small and only part of the outflow chamber is visualized (see arrow). In Figure 4B the transducer was placed over the right ventricular outflow tract to visualize the pulmonary artery (AP). (Ao = aorta; LA = left atrium; MV = mitral valve; LV = left ventricle).

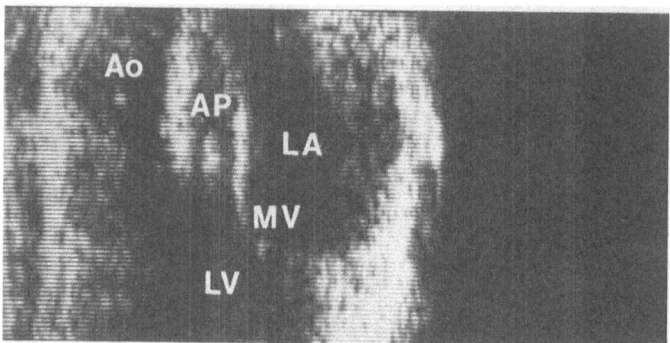

Fig. 5. Long axis view obtained from a patient with tricuspid atresia and transposition of the great vessels. No right ventricular cavity could be detected. The mitral valve (MV) was seen in the left ventricle (LV). Both great vessels arise parallel from the left ventricle. The aortic root (Ao) is located on the right side anteriorly of the pulmonary artery (AP). (LA = left atrium).

senting the outflow chamber of the right ventricle, as seen in front of the aortic root (see arrow). In order to display the normal relationship of the great vessels, the transducer was positioned over the right ventricular outflow tract (Fig. 4B). The pulmonary artery (AP) is seen, crossing the aortic root (Ao) in the direction of the left shoulder. No potential right ventricular cavity can be detected. A patient with tricuspid atresia and transposition of the great arteries is shown in Figure 5. Two great vessels, parallel to each other, arise from the main chamber – the left ventricle; a feature which is characteristic for transposition of the great vessels. No definite outflow chamber was to be detected, nor was present in this patient.

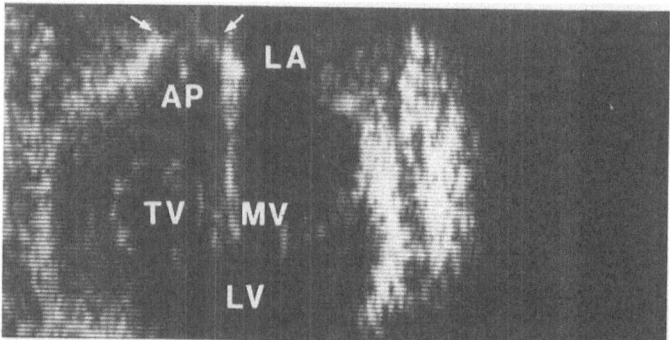

Fig. 6. Long axis view obtained from a patient with double inlet ventricle. There is no inlet septum separating the atrioventricular ostia – i.e. tricuspid (TV) and mitral valve (MV).

The great vessels were transposed. The pulmonary artery (AP) was seen posterior to the aorta and a pulmonary banding has been performed (see small arrows). The aorta was seen during real-time examination, coming from an outflow chamber.

(LA = left atrium; LV = left ventricle).

DOUBLE-INLET ATRIOVENTRICULAR CONNECTION

In a double-inlet atrioventricular connection, both atria are connected to one main chamber. A heart with this type of connection is classified by definition as univentricular (7). The echographic recognition of a double-inlet ventricle relates to the anatomic hallmark of this condition, i.e. the absence of an inlet septum separating the two atrioventricular ostia (Fig. 6). A single atrioventricular valve with large excursion is usually easily observed. Care must be taken, however, to be sure that a second, diminutive valve has not been overlooked during the examination. In some instances, a septal structure can be identified within the ventricular cavity. However, this structure usually stays remote from the atrioventricular ostia. In addition, a diminutive outlet chamber may be present. The great arteries may be normally related, dextro-transposed or levo-transposed.

EBSTEIN'S ANOMALY

Anatomically, Ebstein's anomaly of the tricuspid valve is characterized by two distinct features: distal displacement of the origin of the valve leaflets and dysplasia of the valve apparatus (8). For echocardiographic evaluation of this anomaly it is essential to understand that the spatial orientation of the valve ring has been altered. The origin of the posterior and septal part of the tricuspid valve has shifted distally into the right ventricular cavity, while the anterior tricuspid valve remains in the same anatomic position on the interface of the right atrium and right ventricle. The variability in extent of distal displacement creates a spectrum of this anomaly. The hallmark of Ebstein's anomaly is the low insertion of the septal tricuspid leaflet, which

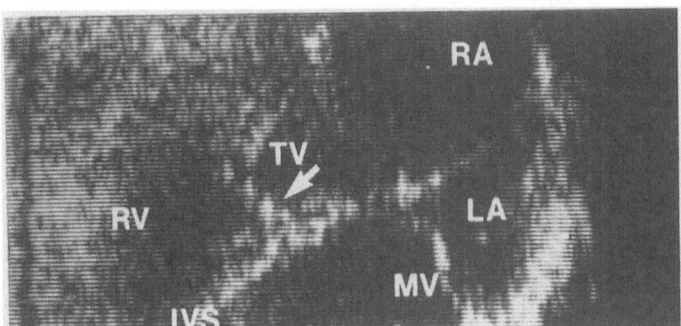

Fig. 7. Apical cross-sectional view obtained in a patient with Ebstein's anomaly. The ring of the tricuspid valve (TV) is displaced into the right ventricle (RV). The septal tricuspid leaflet is seen on the interventricular septum (IVS) (see arrow). The mitral valve (MV) can be seen in its appropriate region. The interatrial septum separates·the right atrium (RA) and the left atrium (LA).

can best be seen using two-dimensional echocardiography (Fig. 7) (9). The transducer position should be low on the apex, in a transverse cross-section slightly tilted superiorly. The additional echocardiographic features (10), such as dilated right ventricle, increased amplitude of the anterior tricuspid valve motion and, especially, the delayed closure of the tricuspid valve, when compared to that of the mitral valve, are, in themselves, non-specific. They can be seen in all cases of right ventricular volume overload.

VENTRICULO-ARTERIAL CONNECTIONS

In normal ventriculo-arterial connections, the right ventricle connects to the pulmonary artery and the left ventricle connects to the aorta. The pulmonary artery crosses the aortic root anteriorly in the direction of the left shoulder. This characteristic echo image can best be obtained with the transducer placed over the right ventricular outflow tract, and it confirms a normal relationship of the great vessels (Fig. 4B). In addition, it is possible to identify the left and right pulmonary branch.

COMPLETE TRANSPOSITION OF THE GREAT ARTERIES

In many cases of transposition of the great arteries, echocardiography relies heavily on the demonstration of altered spatial relationship of the great arteries for the diagnosis. In case of d-transposition with normal atrio-ventricular connection, the aorta is usually found to be located anteriorly and to the right of the pulmonary artery (Fig. 8) (11). The aorta can be seen over a larger area as can the pulmonary artery. The posterior wall of the

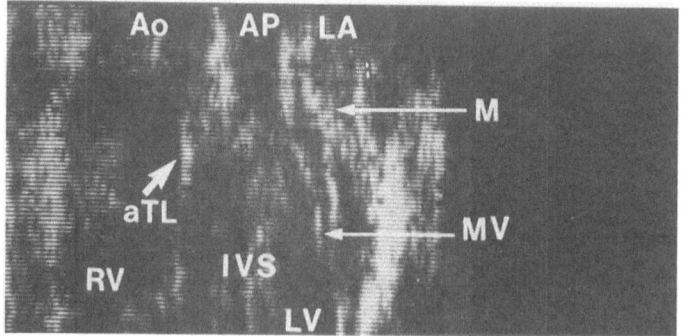

Fig. 8. Long axis view obtained in a patient with transposition of the great vessels. The great vessels both arise parallel to each other from the ventricles. The aorta (Ao) is located right and anteriorly of the pulmonary artery (AP). The Mustard baffle in the left atrium (LA) is indicated by an arrow (M).

(MV = mitral valve; LV = left ventricle; RV = right ventricle; IVS = interventricular septum; aTL = anterior tricuspid leaflet).

pulmonary artery is only seen over a small area, i.e. from the root to the separation in the left and the right pulmonary branch (Fig. 5).

After surgical correction (Mustard's procedure), the intra-atrial baffle can be observed in the left atrium (Fig. 8, see arrow). Due to the altered ventricular function, the right ventricular cavity is usually larger and globular, whereas the left ventricular cavity is small. The mitral valve may present a flutter as a result of the altered flow pattern due to the Mustard's patch.

SINGLE-OUTLET VENTRICLES

Single-outlet ventricles can be due to persistent truncus arteriosus, an aorta with pulmonary atresia, or a pulmonary artery with aortic atresia. Each anomaly can arise from a morphologically left or right ventricle, with or without an override (12).

Echo does not, however, enable us to differentiate between the types of single outlet described above.

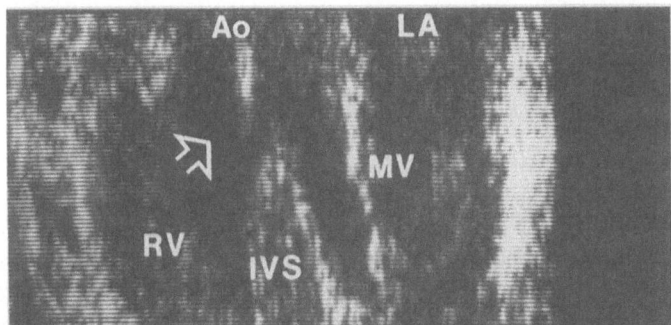

Fig. 9A.

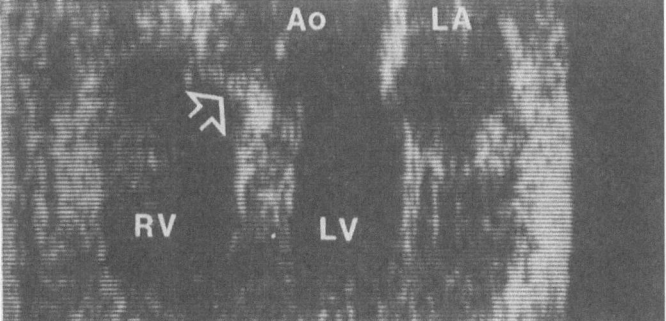

Fig. 9B.

Figs. 9A and 9B. Long axis view obtained in a patient with psuedo truncus. In Figure 9A discontinuity between the anterior aortic wall (Ao) and the interventricular septum (IVS) is clearly present (open arrow). Figure 9B is a post operative long axis view of the same patient. A patch connects the anterior aortic wall with the interventricular septum (open arrow).

(LV = left ventricle; RV = right ventricle; LA = left atrium; MV = mitral valve).

The echocardiographic demonstration of a single great artery overriding the interventricular septum is the common feature in this anomaly (Fig. 9A). The size of the ventricular septal defect can be estimated and continuity between the semilunar valve and the anterior mitral valve leaflet can always be observed. The left atrial dimension can help to differentiate patients with increased pulmonary blood flow (truncus arteriosus) from those with reduced pulmonary blood flow (pulmonary atresia with ventricular septal defect, or tetralogy of Fallot). A large left atrium suggests good pulmonary blood flow. Post-operatively, the ventricular septal patch, used to close the defect, can be identified and it is often seen as a brighter echo (Fig. 9B, see arrow).

DOUBLE-OUTLET VENTRICLE

A double-outlet connection can be defined as the situation where more than 50% of one great vessel arises from the same ventricle as does the other great vessel. Two-dimensional echocardiography accurately displays the degree of override (Fig. 10). The most reliable feature for echocardiographic diagnosis of double-outlet right ventricle is the demonstration of infundibular tissue interposed between the aortic and mitral valve (12). However, all our patients with double-outlet right ventricle had a normal mitral-aortic continuity.

ADDITIONAL FEATURES

The relative sizes of the cardiac chambers, especially those of the left atrium, left ventricle and right ventricle can easily be compared. The diagnosis of underdevelopment of the left ventricle or right ventricle can be assessed, valve prosthesis can be seen, the presence of abnormal wall thickness established.

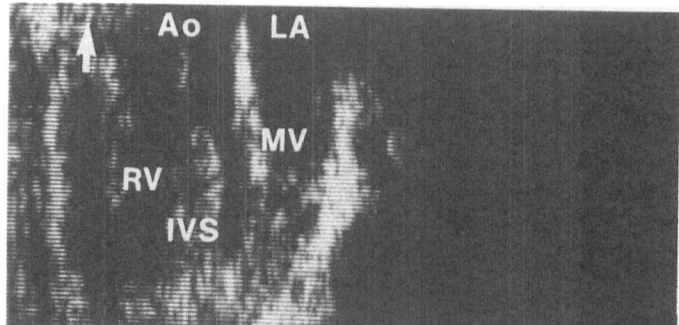

Fig. 10. Long axis view obtained from a patient with double outlet right ventricle. Both great vessels arise more than 150% from the right ventricle.
(LA = left atrium; MV = mitral valve; IVS = interventricular septum; RV = righ ventricle; Ao = aorta).
The arrow indicates the outflow tract to the pulmonary artery.

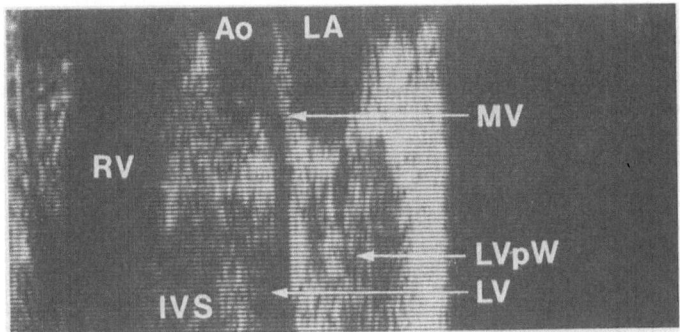

Fig. 11. Long axis view obtained from a patient with hypertrophic constructive cardio-myopathy.
(Ao = aorta; LA = left atrium; IVS = interventricular septum; MV = mitral valve; LVpW = left ventricular posterior wall; RV = right ventricle; LV = left ventricle).

An example of an extreme form of hypertrophic cardiomyopathy is shown in Figure 11. The left ventricle is extremely small.

DISCUSSION

Echocardiography has proven to be a valuable non-invasive technique in the detection of congenital malformations. The use of M-mode, especially, offered the possibility of recognizing and differentiating between many forms of congenital heart disease. The complexity and variety of congenital malformations, however, made it necessary to develop new techniques for echocardiographic examinations.

The development of cross-sectional echocardiography opened new perspectives in this field and the image quality has been considerably enhanced by recent advances in instrumentation. Applying such methods to the pediatric field, made it possible to establish the diagnosis for a variety of malformations, much more easily and more confidently than could be done using only the conventional M-mode technique.

ACKNOWLEDGEMENT

The Interuniversity Institute of Cardiology made it possible to examine the patients illustrated in this paper, in the following hospitals:
– University Hospital Leiden,
– Sophia Children's Hospital, Rotterdam.

REFERENCES

1. Ligtvoet CM, J Ridder, CT Lancée: A dynamically focussed multiscan system. In: Echo-cardiology, Bom N (ed), The Hague, Martinus Nijhoff, 1977, p 313–323.

2. Roelandt J, FE Kloster, FJ ten Cate, WG van Dorp, J Honkoop, N Bom, PG Hugenholtz: Multidimensional echocardiography: an appraisal of its clinical usefulness. Brit Heart J 36:29, 1974.
3. Rastelli GC, JW Kirklin, JL Titus: Anatomic observations on complete form of persistent common atrioventricular canal with specific reference to atrioventricular valves. Mayo Clinic Proc 41:296, 1966.
4. Sahn DJ, RW Terry, R O'Rourke: Multiple crystal echocardiographic evaluation of endocardial cushion defect. Circulation 50:25, 1974.
5. Anderson RH, JL Wilkinson, LM Gerlis: Atresia of the right atrioventricular orifices. Brit Heart J 39:414, 1977.
6. Seward JB, AJ Tajik, DJ Hagler: Echocardiographic spectrum of tricuspid atresia. Mayo Clinic Proc 53:100, 1978.
7. Anderson RH, AE Becker, JL Wilkinson: Morphogenesis of univentricular hearts. Brit Heart J 38:558, 1976.
8. Becker AE, MJ Becker, JE Edwards: Pathologic spectrum of dysplasia of the tricupid valve. Arch Path 91:167, 1971.
9. Ports ThA, NH Silverman, NB Schiller: Two-dimensional echocardiographic assessment of Ebstein's anomaly. Circulation 58:336, 1978.
10. Farooki ZO, JG Henry, WW Green: Echocardiographic spectrum of Ebstein's anomaly of the tricuspid valve. Circulation 53:63, 1976.
11. Park SC, WH Neches, JR Zuberbuhler: Echocardiographic and hemodynamic correlation in transposition of the great arteries. Circulation 57-2: 291, 1978.
12. Godman MJ: Echocardiography in the diagnosis of infundibulo truncal malformations. In: Pediatric Cardiology, Anderson R (ed), Churchill Livingstone, 1977.

ECHOCARDIOGRAPHIC STUDIES IN PATIENTS WITH TRICUSPID ATRESIA OR SINGLE VENTRICLE BEFORE AND AFTER FONTAN PROCEDURE

B. POUGET, M. TYNAN, R. ROUDAUT, A. CHOUSSAT,
M. DALLOCCHIO, and F. FONTAN

Tricuspid atresia (TA) is a rare cardiac anomaly that is not amenable to surgical reconstruction. In 1971 Fontan and Baudet (1) described a new approach for a surgical correction: the principle is to redirect the entire caval return into the lungs. A similar technique is used for patients with single ventricle (SV) with pulmonary stenosis.

TERMINOLOGY

We use the segmental approach promoted by Van Praagh and the definitions formulated by Anderson (2).
1. Atrial situs: solitus, inversus, or ambiguus.
2. Ventricular morphology: TA is a variant of primitive (or single, or common) ventricle. The chamber receiving the single AV valve is the main chamber. If there is a smaller anterior chamber, it is called the outlet chamber". The bulbo-ventricular foramen is between these two chambers:
3. Ventriculo arterial connections: Transposition is present only when the aorta arises from the outlet chamber.

METHODOLOGY

This study groups 10 patients: 6 TA without transposition of the great vessels. 2 TA with transposition and 2 SV. All of them underwent palliative shunt operations in infancy (Waterston, Blalock-Taussig, or Glenn).

The surgical technique used in the Fontan procedure depends on the anatomy. If there are normal ventriculo-arterial relations, a non valved, Dacron conduit is implanted from the right atrium to the outlet chamber. The bulbo-ventricular foramen (BVF) and one or more aterial septal defects are closed. The outlet chamber is enlarged and the pulmonary infundibular stenosis is removed. If the great arteries are transposed, an aortic homograft is used to connect the right atrial appendage to the origin of the right pulmonary artery. The ASD is closed and the main pulmonary artery is transected. The same procedure is used for SV with pulmonary stenosis.

All of our patients were studied echocardiographically (M-scan and two-dimensional) before and after surgery. A protocol was established in order to have the same examination made, as completely as possible, by several investigators. M-mode echocardiograms were obtained with a 2.25 MHz or 5 MHz focused probe. We had no problem in identifying the different cardiac structures. Nevertheless, when there was any uncertainty, we used contrast echocardiography, with systemic venous injection of indocyanine green. The characteristic flow pattern was described by Seward (3, 4) for TA; in the case of SV, it was helpful in determining the number of AV valves. 2D examinations were performed by 2 investigators using an 80° phased-array sector-scanner. The following positions were used: parasternal (long axis and transverse) apical (2 or 4 chambers) subxyphoidal and suprasternal.

RESULTS

1. *Before surgery*

We do not propose to present the characteristic features of TA or SV here. M-mode echocardiographic patterns of TA and SV were demonstrated by Chesler in 1970, and were well described by Seward and Tajik (3, 4). Absence of tricuspid valve echo, posteriorly located AV valve echo with large diastolic excursion, mitral to semilunar valve continuity and small anterior outlet chamber are the main features of TA on the M-mode. In 4 out of 6 patients we had systolic prolapse (hammock-like) of the left AV valve, within two of them a concomitant appearance of incomplete SAM. The outlet chamber was measured with great difficulty while locating the anterior endocardium was often impossible. The main chamber was measured and only relative shortening of the short axis was evaluated.

The pulmonary valve echogram demonstrated infundibular pulmonary stenosis for all our patients with TA and SV. The aortic valve was studied for systolic time intervals as a LV function index.

As Schiller pointed out (6), two-dimensional echo may provide more information in this condition. The parasternal views showed the dilatation of the left cavities and the infundibular pulmonary stenosis. Apical view of the 4 chambers clearly demonstrated the anatomic abnormalities (Fig. 1).

The right AV orifice was obliterated by a dense, thick, "linear" echo without any movement. The left AV valve had a great amplitude of motion in a large main chamber (MC). The size of the bulbo ventricular foraman could be seen, and the size of the outlet chamber was roughly estimated. The most characteristic feature, is the abnormal insertion of the IVS, far from the crux of the heart as determined by the systolic position of the AV valves and the IAS being perpendicular to them. This is compatible with the agenesis of the posterior IVS pointed out by Anderson et al. (2). Subxyphoidian views permitted the measurement of the right atrium (RA), and an estimation of its contractility. With the transducer perpendicular to the thorax, the inferior vena cava was visualized, which permitted of best visualization of the RA.

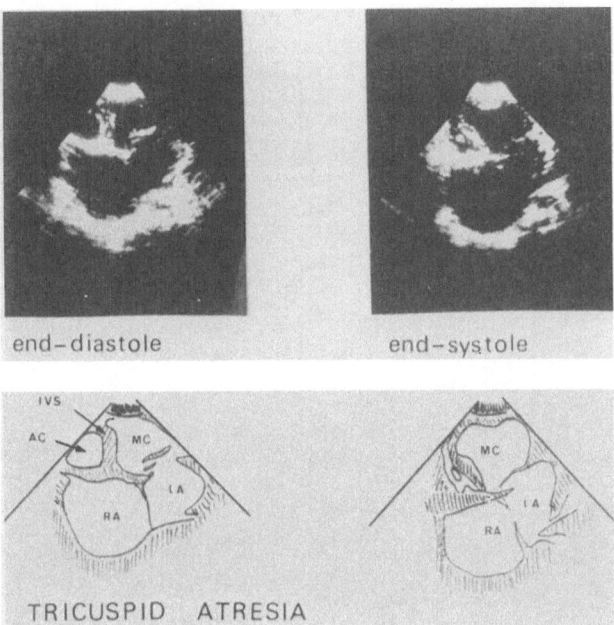

Fig. 1. This post-surgery 4 chambers view shows the abnormal insertion of the interventricular septum (IVS). The size of the four cavities can be determined: accessory chamber (AC), main chamber (MC), right atrium (RA) and left atrium (LA). The paradoxical movement of the IVS is clearly demonstrated.

2. *After surgery*

The M-mode cannot give a direct measurement of RA efficiency. Great attention was paid to the visualization of the pulmonary artery in case of an atrio-pulmonary infundibular conduit and the bio-prosthetic valves in case of an atrio-pulmonary homograft. Figure 2 is an example of a pulmonary trace. We can clearly see the valves opening twice. The first opening takes place in the ventricular diastole, soon after the end of the T wave of the ECG. This posterior movement is enhanced by the atrial systole. A short closure is coincident with the SI (prolonged) of the phonocardiogram. It then re-opens in ventricular systole. The duration of closure of the pulmonary valve is very short relative to the cardiac cycle length. Figure 3 shows the homograft pattern. Opening begins at the same time, in early diastole but is incomplete. Atrial systole allows complete opening. In contrast to the first pattern, ventricular systole is characterized by a complete closure of the valves.

2D imaging is of great value. Parasternal views allow for the appreciation of the main chamber function and the effects of right ventricular infundibulotamy. The apical 4 chamber view, as shown in Figure 1, shows the closed bulbo-ventricular foramen, paradoxical movement of the IVS, and both the enlargement and efficiency of the outlet chamber. In case of TA without

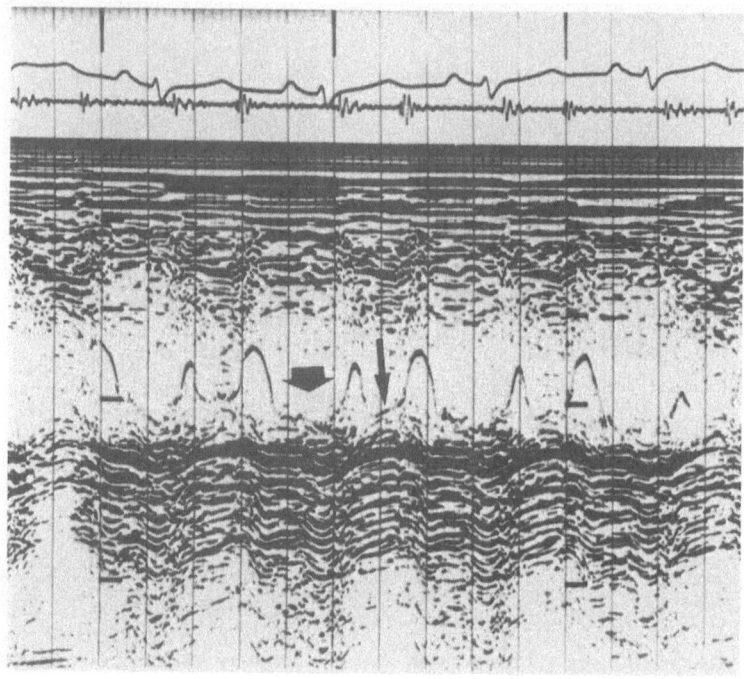

Fig. 2. Post-surgery. Pulmonary trace, in case of TA without transposition exhibits the characteristic double opening: atrial (thick arrow) enhanced by atrial systole, and ventricular (thin arrow).

transposition, a transverse view visualized (Fig. 4) the atrio infundibular conduit in front of the aortic root, with the double opening of the pulmonary valve. In the presence of an atrio-pulmonary homograft, visualization of the graft walls is difficult because they are quite parallel to the ultrasound beam. Diastolic opening of the valves is clearly seen. RA function can be assessed as described above in these two cases.

COMMENTS

Selection of these patients for surgery usually depends on criteria obtained by pre-operative cardiac catheterization and angiography.

What is the role of echocardiography? The following parameters can be assessed non-invasively: the size and contractility of the RA, which will become the right-sided pump, the relations between the ventricles and the great arteries (7), the size of the pulmonary artery and pulmonary ring (at least 75% of the aorta), the degree of subvalvular pulmonary stenosis, the size of the bulbo-ventricular foramen and an estimation of the LV function. An estimation of pulmonary/systemic resistance ratio can be made from systolic time intervals, as shown by Spooner (8). Post-surgically, echocardiography is

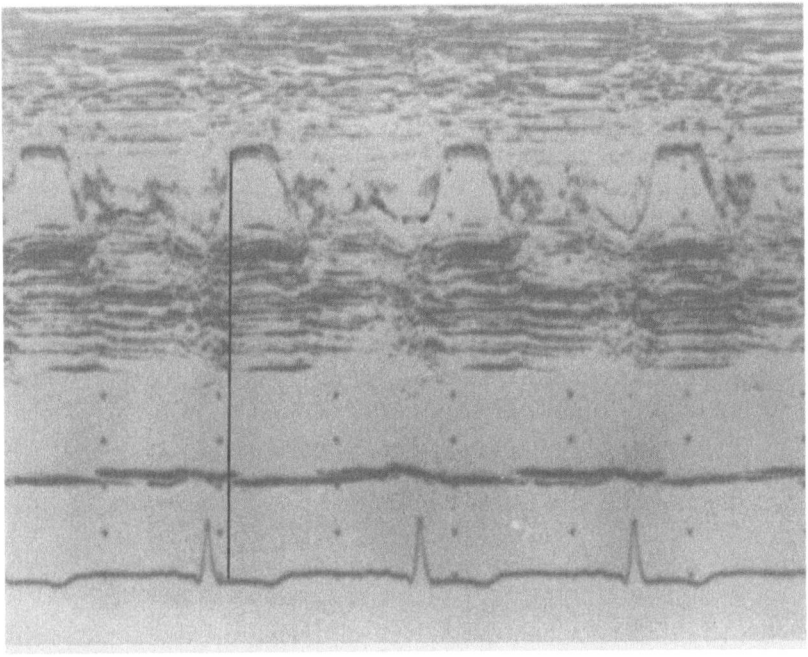

Fig. 3. The diastolic opening of the homograft valves between right atrium and right pulmonary artery is completed by atrial systole.

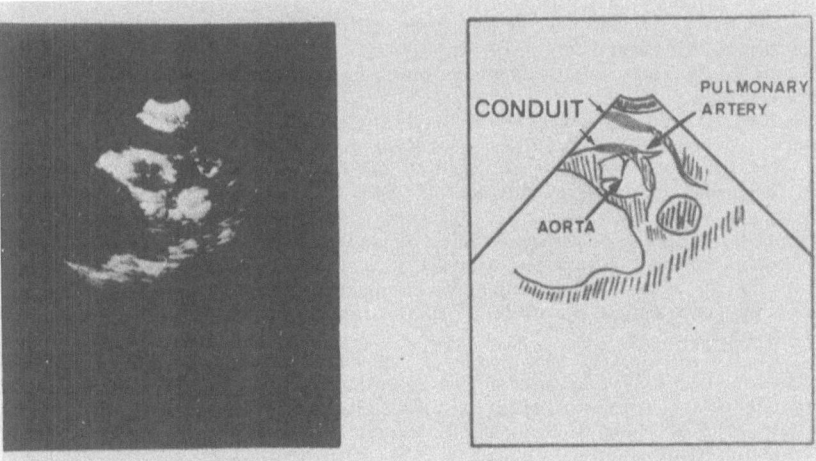

Fig. 4. A transverse cut through the heart at the level of the great vessels, permits seeing the pulmonary artery with its bifurcation. The insert of the pulmonary valves just after the dense echoes generated by the dacron atrio-infundibular conduit.

an easy way to estimate RA performance directly from cross-sectional images.

From the M-mode, indirect information is obtained by assessing the pulmonary flow from the study of the RA function. The surgical reconstruction can also be evaluated. Furthermore, in patients with TA but without transposition of the great arteries, the performance of the outlet chamber can be assessed.

In conclusion, full assessment of pre-operative status can not only be obtained by ultrasound techniques. Nevertheless, this atraumatic examination is very accurate when used to investigate anatomic abnormalities. But the surgeon needs more information: functional, pressure and resistance values. In contrast, post-operative evaluation can be made by echocardiography alone (9). Short term and long term follow-up is essential and will furnish further data on the RA physiology.

ACKNOWLEDGEMENTS

The authors wish to acknowledge the contribution of all the physicians and technicians of the non-invasive techniques laboratory (Hôpital Cardiologique du Haut-Levêque, Bordeaux) and of Maryse Frampier for typing the manuscript.

REFERENCES

1. Fontan F, E Baudet: Surgical repair of tricuspid atresia Thorax 26:240, 1971.
2. Anderson RH, JL Wilkinson, LM Gerlis, A Smith, AE Becker: Atresia of the right atrioventricular orifice. Brit Heart J 39:414, 1977.
3. Seward JB, AJ Tajik: Echocardiographic spectrum of tricuspid atresia. Mayo Clin Proc 53:100, 1978.
4. Seward JB, AJ Tajik, DJ Hagler, DG Ritter: Contrast echocardiography in single or common ventricle. Circulation 55:513, 1977.
5. Bini RM, KR Bloom, JAG Culham, RM Freedom, CM Williams, RD Rowe: The reliability and practicality of single crystal echocardiography in the evaluation of single ventricle. Circulation 57:269, 1978.
6. Silverman NH, NB Schiller: Apex echocardiography. A two dimensionnal technique for evaluating congenital heart disease. Circulation 57:503, 1978.
7. Henry NL, BJ Maron, JM Griffith: Cross-sectional echocardiography in the diagnosis of congenital heart disease. Identification of the relation of ventricles and great arteries. Circulation 56:267, 1977.
8. Spooner EW, BL Perry, AM Stern, JM Sigmann: Estimation of pulmonary/systemic resistance ratios from echocardiographic systolic time intervals in young patients with congenital or acquired heart disease. Am J Cardiol 42:810, 1978.
9. Serratto M, RA, Miller, C Tatooles, R Ardekani: Hemodynamic evaluation of Fontan operation in tricuspid atresia. Circulation 54:99, 1976.

ECHOCARDIOGRAPHIC EVALUATION OF LEFT VENTRICULAR INFLOW OBSTRUCTION IN CHILDREN USING AN 80° TWO-DIMENSIONAL SECTOR SCANNER*

CLAUDE ROGÉ, REBECCA SNIDER, and NORMAN SILVERMAN

INTRODUCTION

Left ventricular inflow obstruction (LVIO) in children can be caused by rare congenital abnormalities such as cor-triatriatum (CT), supra-valvar mitral ring (SVMR), and mitral valvar stenosis, either isolated (MS), or as part of a parachute mitral valve (PMV).

Before the introduction of echocardiography, these lesions used to be difficult to diagnose accurately before surgery or autopsy (1). M-mode echocardiography is a very sensitive technique to detect abnormalities of the mitral valve region (2 to 6), but it often does not allow differentiating between the various types of LVIO (2).

For the last 3 years, our group has been using two-dimensional (2-D) echocardiography to determine if this new technique can provide more precise anatomic diagnoses than M-mode echocardiography. This report relates our experience with 5 children who had different forms of LVIO.

MATERIAL AND METHODS

Five patients, age 8 months to 16 years, were studied. They all underwent complete M-mode and 2-D studies before cardiac catheterization. Subsequently, all of them had their diagnosis confirmed at surgery, and one, in

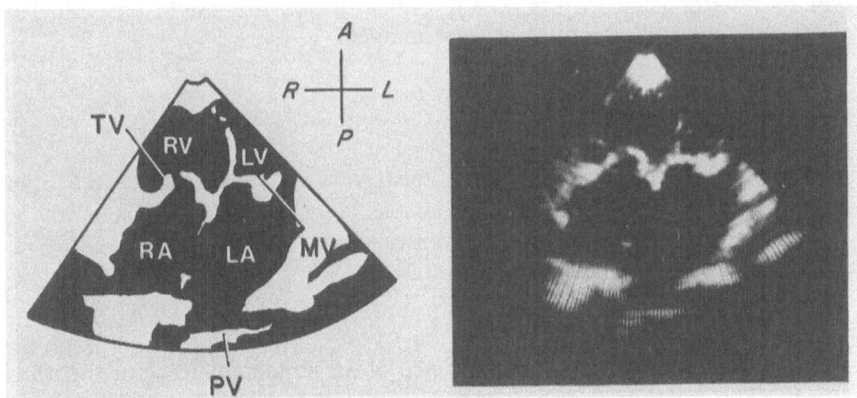

Fig. 1. Apical view on patient #1 with isolated MS.

*Supported in part by a grant from the Kaiser Foundation Research Institute.

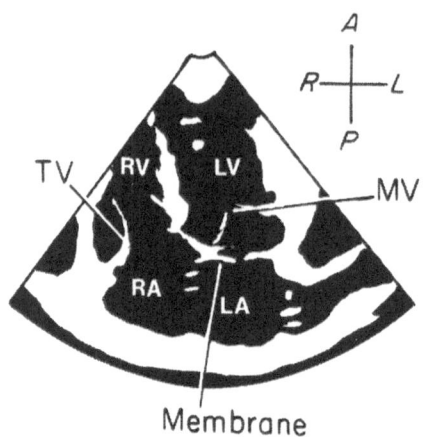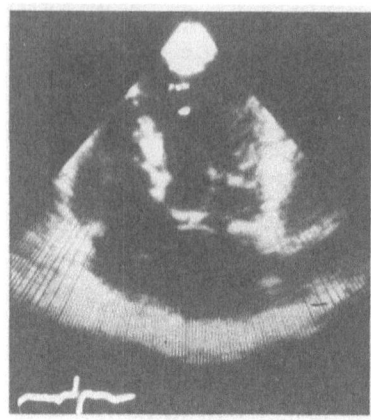

Fig. 2. Apical view on patient #5 with CT.

addition, at autopsy. Table 1 summarizes the pertinent findings for each patient.

The 2-D studies were obtained with an 80° phased array sector scanner. A 32 element transducer was used. The studies were performed in the long axis, short axis, and apical views.

RESULTS

Mitral valvar stenosis

The long axis and apical views (Fig. 1) in patient #1 showed thickened mitral valve leaflets with a decreased excursion and coarse flutter in diastole and an enlarged left atrium. No left atrial membrane could be seen. In the short axis, 2 papillary muscles were imaged.

Parachute mitral valve

In patient #2, the long axis and apical views were similar to the ones in patient #1. In the short, axis, a single, large, papillary muscle was seen arising from the center of the left ventricle.

Left atrial membranes

The 3 remaining patients had evidence of an abnormal structure in the left atrium. The position, appearance and phasic movements of this abnormal echo were identical in all 3 patients. It moved towards the mitral valve funnel in diastole and away from it in systole. In the apical view, the membrane extended behind the mitral valve leaflets and close and parallel to the valvar ring. In the long axis, the membrane was positioned obliquely between the

Table 1. Patient description.

Patient number	1	2	3	4	5
Age	13 yrs	9 mos	8 mos	14 yrs	16 yrs
Sex	F	F	F	M	M
M-mode echo:					
PMVL motion in diast.	anterior	anterior	anterior	anterior	posterior
Diast. flutter	+	+	+	+	+
'a' wave on MV	–	–	–	–	–
MVDE	decreased	decreased	decreased	decreased	normal
MVEF	decreased	decreased	decreased	decreased	normal
Lines behind MV	+	+	+	+	+
LA lines	–	–	–	–	–
Cath. diagnosis	Severe LVIO mild AS	Severe LVIO Coarct/VSD/PDA	Severe LVIO Sub AS/VSD	LVIO	LVIO
Surgical findings and procedure	Thick MV, small orifice. Replaced by porcine valve	PMV Commissurotomy PMV at autopsy	SVMR Thick MV Ring removed	SVMR Thick MV Removed	CT Removed

left atrial posterior wall and the posterior aortic root. In all 3 patients this abnormal left atrial echo disappeared after surgical excision of the membrane. The 2 patients with SVMR had an enlarged left atrium and thickened mitral valve leaflets with decreased diastolic excursion. Patient #5 (CT) had a normal appearing mitral valve and left atrial size (Fig. 2). In these 5 patients the exact nature of the LVIO could not have been inferred from the M-mode study alone, even though it was grossly abnormal in each case and pointed to an anomaly of the mitral valve region.

The 2-D study differentiated clearly patients with a left atrial membrane from patients with valvar mitral stenosis. The technique was not sensitive enough to assess fully the attachment of the membrane to the left atrial walls and CT could not be differentiated from SVMR on that basis. However, in both cases of SVMR, the 2-D study showed that the mitral valve leaflets were thickened and had decreased excursion, while in the case of CT the mitral valve apparatus was normal. The presence of a single papillary muscle on the short axis view was compatible with a diagnosis of PMV.

M-mode echocardiography is the technique par excellence for the detection of LVIO in children. We found 2-D echocardiography the best technique available to us for making the anatomic diagnosis before surgery. Improvement in the image resolution and in our skills will enhance even further the precision of this technique.

REFERENCES

1. Collins-Nakai et al.: Circulation 56:1039, 1977.
2. LaCorte et al.: Circulation 54:562, 1976.
3. Lundstrom: Circulation 46:44, 1972.
4. Lundstrom: Circulation 45:324, 1972.
5. Chung et al.: Chest 65:25, 1974.
6. Driscoll et al.: Amer J Cardiol 42: 259, 1978.

ECHOCARDIOGRAPHIC FINDINGS AND FUNCTION ANALYSIS IN INFANTS WITH ENDOCARDIAL FIBROELASTOSIS

A.A. SCHMALTZ*, Z. IBRAHIM, R.P. HEIL, and D.J. BROWN

Endocardial fibroelastosis (EFE) is characterized by an enlargement of the heart and a thickened layer of pearly whiteness covering the inner wall of the left ventricle (LV), often also of the left atrium, occasionally of the right ventricle and atrium (1). Valvular deformities or other congenital heart anomalies are present in up to 50% of cases. The incidence of EFE is one in 5000 to 6000 births, the age of manifestation is in 80% of cases during the first ten months of life. The clinical picture of these babies is that of congestive heart failure with electrocardiographic signs of left ventricular hypertrophy and repolarization abnormalities, or is determined by the associated lesions. Until now the diagnosis of this syndrome has been based on the findings of heart failure, and the angiographical features of a spherical, dilated and poorly contracting LV. This study was undertaken to offer further information for diagnosis.

SUBJECTS AND METHODS

Eight normal infants were studied, their ages ranging from 1.5 to 4.5 months (mean 3.2 months) and their body surface area from 0.25 to 0.33 m^2 (mean 0.28 m^2).

Seven infants with EFE were studied, their ages ranging from 2 to 7 months (mean 3.29 months) and their body surface area from 0.26 to 0.35 m^2 (mean 0.2 m^2) at the first investigation. The diagnosis was based on the clinical picture, heart catheterization and typical angiocardiographic findings. In one patient it was proved by autopsy. Moreover, we studied one newborn with a hypertensive crisis on the base of a renal dysplasia and a $3\frac{1}{2}$ years old boy with EFE. Their results are not included in Table 1. All subjects were studied in the supine position, using a Picker Echoview 80C with a 5 MHz transducer of 6 mm diameter. The paperspeed for the function analysis of the left ventricle was 100 mm/sec. The dimensions of the heart cavities were measured at end-diastole and end-systole, the shortening fraction was calculated as the quotient of the diameter difference of the LV divided by the end-diastolic diameter. The echocardiograms were digitized as previously described (2) at Brompton Hospital, London, using a Summagraphics digitizing tablet and a Prime 300 computer system. Instantaneous left ventricular

*Supported by a grant of German Academic Exchange Service.

Table 1. Results (mean ± standard deviation).

	LV Dimension					
	$D_{(max)}$ (mm)	$D_{(min)}$ (mm)	$Vcf_{(peak)}$ (sec^{-1})	$LR_{(max)}$ (sec^{-1})	SF (%)	LPEP/LVET
normal infants $n = 8$	20.7 ± 2.6	12.7 ± 2.5	4.66 ± 0.88	5.78 ± 1.75	35.7 ± 7.5	0.3 ± 0.04
EFE $n = 7$	35.9 ± 7.3	33.5 ± 7.0	2.28 ± 1.38	2.16 ± 0.99	11.7 ± 4.6	0.5 ± 0.05

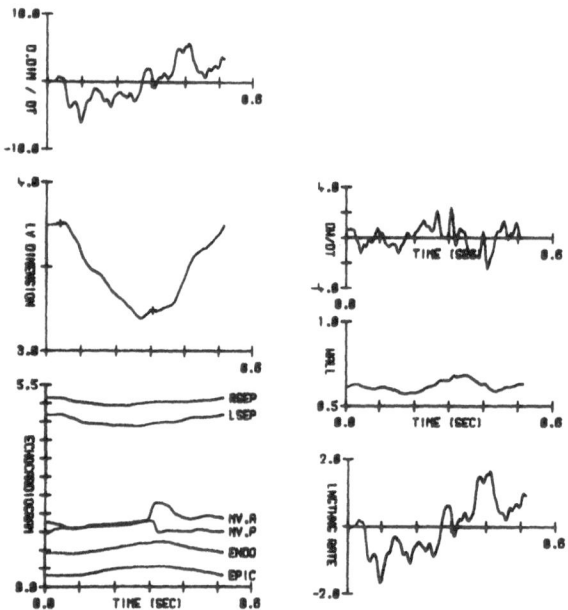

Fig. 1. Digitized left ventricular echocardiogram from a patient with EFE (for details see text).

dimension (D), its rate of change (dD/dt) and its normalized rate of change ($1/D \times dD/dt$) were derived from the echocardiogram and obtained as continuous plots over one cycle. From these plots the intervals between maximum posterior wall thickness, mitral valve opening and minimum LV cavity dimension as well as the duration of rapid increase of LV dimension and of rapid thinning of the posterior wall were measured (see Fig. 1).

RESULTS (TABLE 1)

The diameters of the LV cavity of EFE-cases were nearly twice as large as in the healthy cases. The shortening fraction was enormously reduced (see Fig.

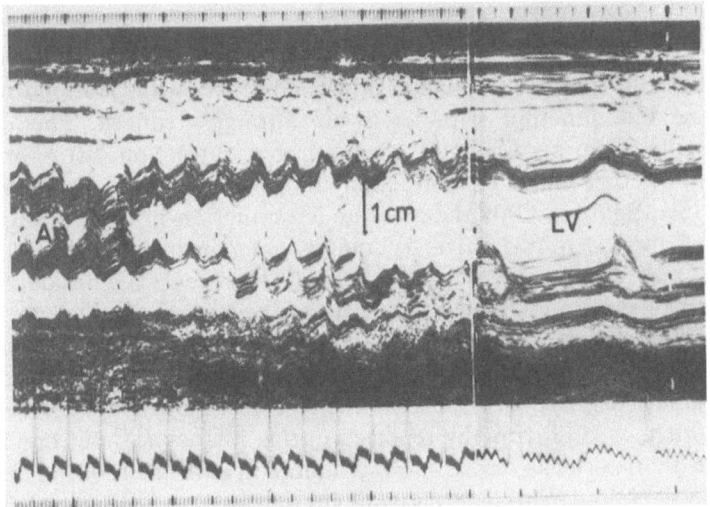

Fig. 2 Scan from the aorta (left) to the ventricle (right) in a patient with EFE.

2). Septum and posterior wall thickness were within normal limits. The mitral valve was posteriorly displaced in the LV cavity. The opening shape seemed to be very small, but the measured values of opening amplitude and early diastolic closing velocity were normal. In 4 out of 7 patients there was an abnormal septum movement during systole.

The systolic time intervals, measured from Q to the opening and from opening to closing of the aortic valve, showed a prolongation of the pre-ejection period (LPEP) and a shortening of the ejection time (LVET). The quotient LPEP/LVET of the patients was at 0.5 ± 0.11, significantly higher than in the healthy babies (0.3 ± 0.04; $p < 0.001$). Moreover, the "Q to mitral valve closing" interval was 33% shorter than the LPEP after correction for different heart rates (13% longer in normals). As with the shortening fraction, the instantaneous parameters of peak Vcf and maximum lengthening rate (LR) were significantly reduced in patients with EFE as compared with the normals: peak Vcf 2.28 ± 1.4, normal 4.66 ± 0.88 ($p < 0.05$) and LR max 2.16 ± 0.99 normal 5.78 ± 1.75 ($p < 0.01$). On the other hand, the duration of the rapid increase in dimension of the LV and of the rapid thinning of the posterior wall in EFE-patients did not differ from that in our normal group. The relation of minimum dimension of the LV, mitral valve opening and maximum thickness of posterior wall was too inhomogeneous to make any valuable statement.

The additional patients (one hypertensive case and one EFE) showed the same echocardiographic findings.

COMMENTS

The echocardiographic study of LV-function in our healthy babies showed good agreement with the results reported in the literature (3, 4).

To the best of our knowledge, the echocardiographic features of EFE have not been described in detail elsewhere. But all the reports of single cases (5, 6) agree with our findings: a dilated, poorly contracting LV with normal wall-thickness. The function parameters are strongly reduced. The computer analysis shows no predominant relaxation or contraction disturbances. The question whether the LV contraction is coordinate or incoordinate needs further investigation. Only the great underestimation of LPEP of 33% when measured by the mitral valve technique – in contrast to the 13% in our normals and the 5% reported by Sahn (7) – reveals a considerable prolongation of the isovolumetric contraction time.

The echocardiographic pattern is not diagnostic for EFE. There is neither dilatation and dysfunction, to the extent described, reported in other kinds of cardiac failure (e.g. hypoglycemia, sepsis, myocarditis and hypoxemia) nor cases of congestive cardiomyopathy reported during infancy (1). But our newborn patient with hypertensive crisis shows a limitation of the method: all the criteria for EFE were found in his first echo. But, in contrast to the patients with EFE, in whom we could not see any effect of anti-congestive therapy on the LV-function, he showed a substantial improvement within three weeks of therapy.

REFERENCES

1. Hastreiter AR, EA Fisher: Endocardial fibroelastosis. In: Moss AJ, Adams FH, Emmanouilidis GC (eds), Heart disease in infants children and adolescents, 2nd edition, Baltimore, The Williams and Williams Co., 1977, p 496f.
2. Gibson DG, D Brown: Measurement of instantaneous left ventricular dimension and filling rate in man, using echocardiography. Brit Heart J 35:1141, 1973.
3. Gutgesell HP, M Paquet, DF Duff, N McNamara: Evaluation of left ventricular size and function by echocardiography. Circulation 56:457, 1977.
4. Björkhem G: Echocardiographic assessment of left ventricular function. Europ J Cardiol 6:83, 1977.
5. Goldberg SJ, HD Allen, DJ Sahn: Pediatric and adolescent echocardiography, Chicago, Year Book Medical Publ., Inc. 1975.
6. Chung KJ, JA Manning, R Gramiak: Presentation – Association Europ Pediatr Cardiol Rhodes, 1973.
7. Sahn DJ, Y Vaucher, DE Williams, HD Allen, SJ Goldberg, WF Friedman: Echocardiographic detection of large left to right shunts and cardiomyopathies in infants and children. Amer J Cardiol 38:73, 1976.

PULSED DOPPLER ECHOCARDIOGRAPHY –
APPLICATIONS IN PEDIATRIC CARDIOLOGY

J.G. STEVENSON, I. KAWABORI, W.G. GUNTHEROTH,
S.A. RUBENSTEIN, and D.W. BAKER

Pulsed Doppler Echocardiography (PDE) complements the dimension and motion information of M-mode echocardiography by providing information concerning direction and quality of blood flow at known sites within the heart and great vessels. Since most patients seen in a pediatric cardiology setting have a blood flow abnormality, PDE has the potential of enhancing the non-invasive diagnosis in a large number of patients. Using range-gated PDE devices (1, 2), a large number of examinations have been performed on patients at the University of Washington, with some of the most useful applications being summarized here.

PATENT DUCTUS ARTERIOSUS

The PDE examination is performed from a precordial approach, Figure 1. The sample volume (SV) is placed in the right ventricular outflow tract (RVOT), and flow is followed into the pulmonary artery (MPA), with angling of the transducer towards the junction of MPA and left pulmonary artery, in search of the PDA jet. The jet may be encountered just distal to the pulmonic

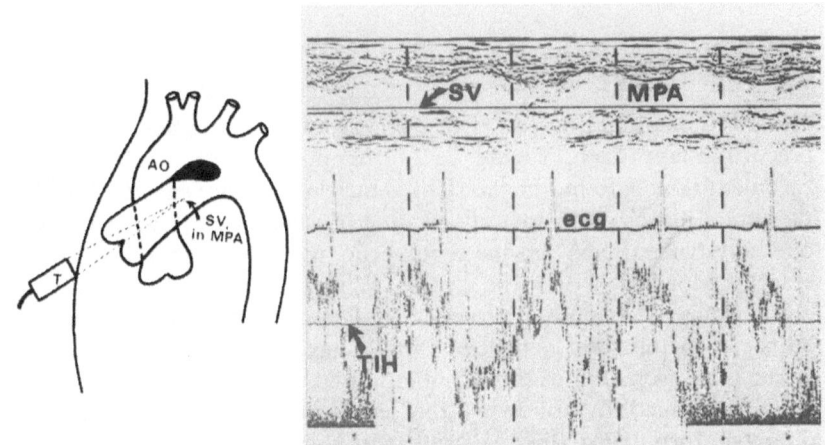

Fig. 1. Left: Approach for PDA examination Right: Flow record of PDA. Turbulent flow is indicated by dot scatter in Time Interval Histogram.

valve, or, at times, only very deep in MPA. An examination can also be done on the right pulmonary artery (RPA), from a suprasternal approach (Fig. 4), but detection of continuous turbulent flow in RPA is not specific for PDA. Most patients with PDA will be found to have continuous turbulent flow in MPA, and the flow abnormality can be shown to be ductal by finding the turbulent diastolic jet flowing into the MPA, towards the precordial transducer, Figure 1. Other systemic to pulmonic shunts do not have such directional characteristics on MPA flow. For example, Waterston and Blalock-Taussig shunts do give continuous turbulent flow in MPA, but lack the directional jet.

Our experience with PDE evaluation of PDA has been very favorable. In a series of 90 patients who had catheterization or operative determination of ductal patency, there was a 100% sensitivity of PDE detection of continuous turbulent flow in MPA, in those with PDA. In 95% of those, a specific ductal jet could be identified, and all had a proven PDA. This sensitivity and specificity has substantially aided our evaluation of patients for PDA, the largest number of whom have been premature infants. In a series of 120 such infants (3), it was found that only 21% of those with PDA had a continuous murmur, and 47% had only a systolic murmur, indistinguishable from VSD. In 32% of the infants, no murmur was heard. In all, PDE detected the ductal jet, and in 7, found evidence of VSD or mitral regurgitation, lesions which could contribute to left heart enlargement that had previously been thought to be due only to PDA. We routinely screen for such additional defects, and in surgical candidates, if PDA is the only flow abnormality do not catheterize before surgery, as long as abbreviated diastolic ductal flow does not indicate presence of pulmonary hypertension (4).

VENTRICULAR SEPTAL DEFECT

The PDE examination for ventricular septal defect (VSD) is from standard precordial approach, Figure 2. In the presence of a left-to-right shunt, turbulent flow is found in the right ventricle, and movement of the SV along the septal margin may identify an area of very rough flow, the VSD jet. Or, one may place the SV on the septal echo, move it up and down the septum, searching for flow within the septum. When the jet is found, following it into and through the septum provides a diagnosis of VSD. The presence of a harsh jet in the right ventricle is only suggestive of VSD, not specific, and could arise from for example, infundibular stenosis. Since the diagnosis of VSD is defined by following the jet through the septum, factors which diminish turbulence (large defects with little localization of VSD jet, or pulmonary hypertension limiting the shunt) have limited our ability to follow flow through the septum in some cases. Abnormal septal position, and presence of right-to-left shunts have also increased the difficulty of PDE diagnosis of VSD. In a series of 104 catheterized patients, PDE diagnosis of VSD had a sensitivity of 90%, and a specificity of 98% (5). While our current

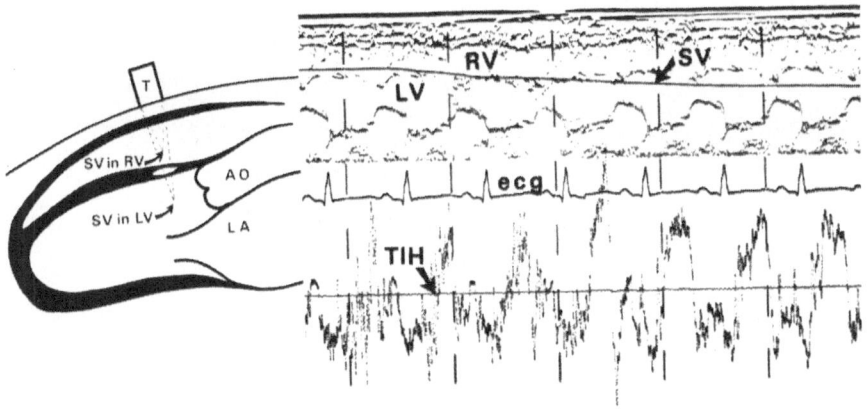

Fig. 2. Left: Approach for VSD examination. Right: flow record of VSD. Dot scatter of TIH is present in RVOT, and septum, through into LV.

experience is considerably larger, the limiting factors have prevented us from following the VSD jet through the septum in 5–10% of patients with proven VSD. In the absence of other sites of left-to-right shunt distal to the mitral valve, and absence of mitral regurgitation, we have used left atrial and ventricular dimensions, and indices of left ventricular function to provide an estimate of the magnitude of V̇SD shunt. Since PDE can detect additional defects, or exclude their presence, combined M-mode and PDE evaluation should yield a better correlation between left heart dimensions and shunt magnitude.

MITRAL REGURGITATION

The PDE examination for mitral regurgitation (MR) is from the precordial approach shown in Figure 2, but with placement of SV within the left atrium, in search of a regurgitant jet. The PDE diagnosis of MR can be made by detection of such a systolic jet posterior to the coapted leaflets, with SV clearly free of the leaflets, and then following the jet into the valve. For the recording of a flow record, the SV must be free of the leaflets, vegetations, or left atrial wall, in order to avoid artifacts within the flow record.

An estimation of severity of regurgitation may be obtained from the left atrial dimension, and to lesser degree, by assessing the depth that the MR jet can be followed into the atrium. Minor degrees of MR seem to have jets localized rather near the valve, while jets traversing the entire atrium tend to have greater regurgitant volumes. When compared to left ventricular angiocardiography in a series of 94 patients, PDE has shown a sensitivity of 95%, and a specificity of 90% in the evaluation of MR (6). Limitations include the location of the MR jet, and presence of co-existing disease. PDE appears useful also in detection of silent MR, and in evaluating the question of "catheter-induced" MR occurring at catheterization.

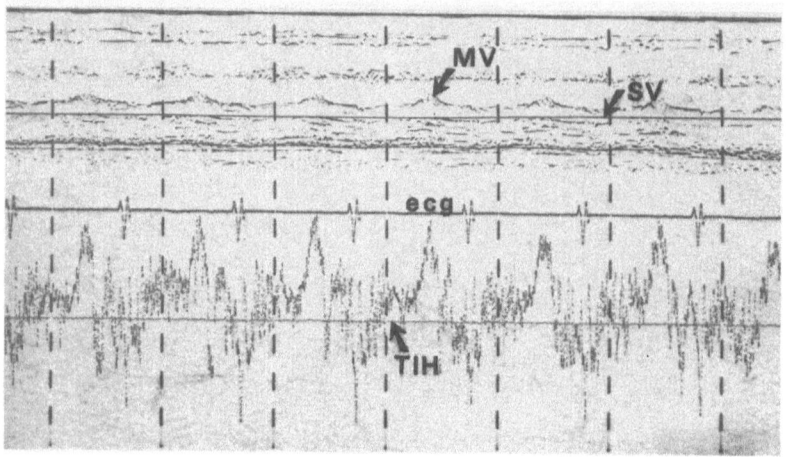

Fig. 3. Flow record of mitral regurgitation. In the TIH, the systolic dot scatter represents the turbulent MR jet.

DIFFERENTIATION OF VENTRICULAR SEPTAL DEFECT FROM MITRAL REGURGITATION

Using the approaches and diagnostic criteria above, one may easily differentiate between VSD and MR, by PDE. In a series of 40 patients in whom clinical differentiation was not possible, PDE provided a differentiation in 39, and agreed with catheterization findings in all those studied by invasive means (7). There is substantial utility in the PDE differentiation between VSD and MR, since the natural history of the two lesions differs considerably. PDE has also been useful in resolving a question of rheumatic heart disease, where the murmur of an apical VSD may have lead to a mistaken diagnosis of rheumatic MR.

DIFFERENTIATION OF MILD AORTIC FROM MILD PULMONIC STENOSIS

Differentiation of aortic from pulmonic murmurs on clinical grounds alone can be difficult, especially if the murmur stems from a mild defect. However mild, the prognosis differs. We have examined a series of children with basal ejection murmurs, in order to determine origin of the abnormal flow, and to compare the clinical criteria employed to differentiate between aortic and pulmonic murmurs. PDE examinations were done either from the precordial approach of Figure 2, examining for turbulence below, at or above the semilunar valves, or from a suprasternal notch approach as shown in Figure 4. Using PDE to determine the site of turbulent flow, it was found that the clinical criteria for differentiating between aortic and pulmonic murmurs were reasonably specific (87%), but less sensitive (70%), than PDE, (100%) (8). Since the prognosis, management and infective endocarditis considerations

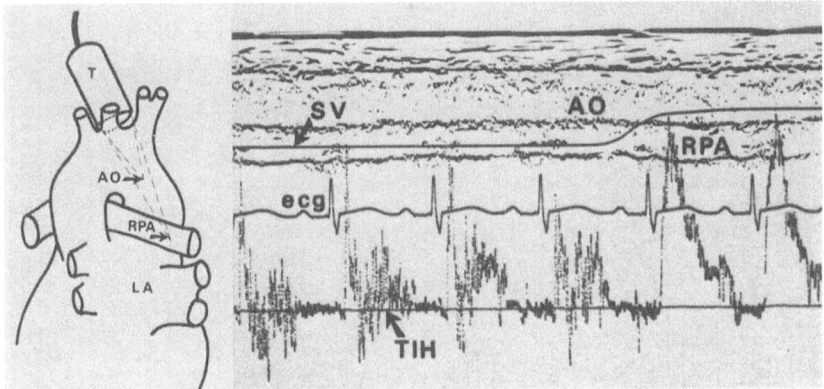

Fig. 4. Left: A posterior view of the suprasternal approach. Right: Flow record with turbulent pulmonic flow contrasted with normal aortic flow.

for these two defects are quite different, and since clinical differentiation may be difficult and imprecise, PDE appears very useful in this common clinical problem.

OTHER FREQUENT PDE APPLICATIONS

In small infants requiring palliation of cyanotic defects by creation of a systemic to pulmonic shunt, a murmur indicative of shunt function may not be heard after surgery. PDE detection of continuous turbulent flow in MPA, consistent with shunt function, may avoid needless and hazardous re-catheterization or re-operation. In patients undergoing surgery for closure of intracardiac or great vessel level shunts, we have found persistence of VSD shunting to be common for about 24 hours after surgery. Persistence of shunt beyond 48 hours suggests residual VSD. We have encountered two infants with persistent, though small volume, shunting through PDA after ligation of large PDA. A recent series has shown PDE to be useful in detection of clinically silent, but important, obstruction of systemic venous return following repair of Transposition of the Great Arteries (TGA). (9).

PDE has been useful in resolving important non-invasive diagnostic questions. The silent PDA, detected by PDE, has been mentioned. In cyanotic infants with abnormal great vessel relationships, the presumptive diagnosis may be TGA. PDE detection of ductal flow identifies the vessel receiving PDA as pulmonary artery, and can prove or disprove the presence of TGA. Figure 5 shows PDE application in the question of the "left atrial line," frequently seen during M-mode echo examinations. The line may stem from an important structure if the diagnosis is total anomalous pulmonary venous return (TAPVR), or cor triatriatum, or it may merely be an artifact. In this figure, flow characteristics posterior to the line differ from those anterior, suggesting a real structure, the proven anomalous pulmonary vein. If flow

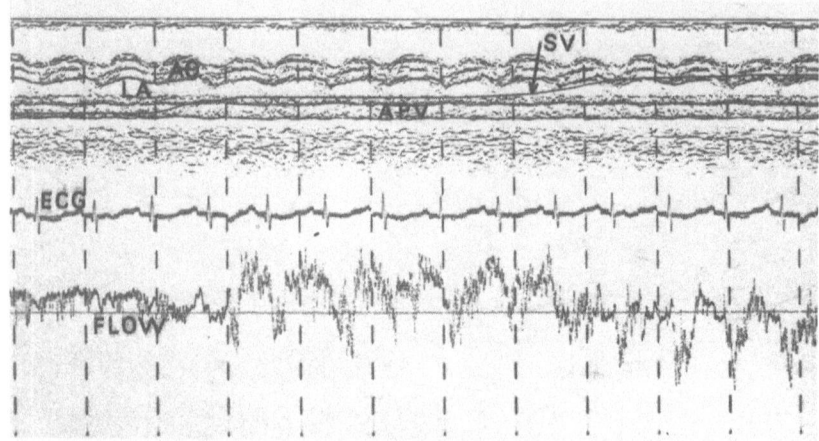

Fig. 5. Flow record of total anomalous pulmonary venous return.

characteristics are similar on either side of the line, the line is presumed to be an artifact.

CONCLUSION

Pulsed Doppler Echocardiography is a sensitive and specific non-invasive technique, well suited for the evaluation of patients with suspected blood flow abnormalities. It adds substantially to the amount, and quality, of non-invasive diagnostic information, thereby directly affecting patient management, and candidacy for invasive study or surgical intervention.

REFERENCES

1. Baker DW, SA Rubenstein, GA Lorch: Pulsed Doppler echocardiography: principles and applications. Am J Medicine 63:69, 1977.
2. Advanced Technology Laboratories Pulsed Doppler Echocardiographic Systems, Bellevue, Washington.
3. Stevenson JG, TK Dooley, I Kawabori: Patent ductus arteriosus in a neonatal intensive care unit: the utility of pulsed Doppler echocardiography. Circulation 58-2: 110, 1978.
4. Stevenson JG, I Kawabori, WG Guntheroth: Noninvasive detection of pulmonary hypertension in patent ductus arteriosus, by pulsed Doppler echocardiography. Circulation 56-3: 191, 1977 (abstract; full paper in press, Circulation 1979).
5. Stevenson JG, I Kawabori, TK Dooley, WG Guntheroth: Diagnosis of ventricular septal defect by pulsed Doppler echocardiography-sensitivity, specificity and limitations. Circulation 58-2: 322, 1978.
6. Dooley TK, SA Rubenstein, JG Stevenson: Pulsed Doppler echocardiography – the detection of mitral regurgitation. In: Ultrasound in medicine, Vol. 4, White D, Lyons EA (eds), New York, Plenum Press, 1978, p 383.
7. Stevenson JG, I Kawabori, WG Guntheroth: Differentiation of ventricular septal defects from mitral regurgitation by pulsed Doppler echocardiography. Circulation 56-2: 14, 1977.
8. Kawabori I, WG Guntheroth, TK Dooley, DE Strandness, JG Stevenson: The significance of carotid bruit in children: transmitted murmur, or vascular origin – differentiation by pulsed Doppler echocardiography. Am Heart J, 1979 (in press).
9. Stevenson JG, I Kawabori, TK Dooley, DH Dillard, WG Guntheroth: Pulsed Doppler echocardiographic detection of obstruction of systemic venous return following repair of transposition of great arteries. Circulation 58-2: 51, 1978 (abstract; full paper in press, Circulation 1979).

ASSESSMENT OF FETAL AND NEONATAL CARDIAC GEOMETRICS BY MEANS OF REAL-TIME ULTRASOUND

R. VOSTERS, J.W. WLADIMIROFF, and W.B. VLETTER

A dynamically focussed two-dimensional real-time linear array ultrasonic scanner (Organon Teknika), was used for visualization of the various fetal and neonatal cardiac structures. The frequency of the array was 3.12 MHz. Two single beam transducers were used for antenatal and neonatal M-mode recording. The frequency was 2.25 and 5.0 MHz, the diameter 13 and 6 mm respectively.

TECHNIQUES

The object is to obtain a T-M mode recording of the scanning plane, which is at right angles to the interventricular septum at the level of the mitral valve leaflets by means of a standardised technique.

The antenatal recording procedure consists of four steps:
1. the visualization of a two-dimensional cross-section of the fetal chest by means of the multi-element transducer showing spine and heart,
2. the positioning of the multi-element transducer at an angle of 45° to the antero-posterior diameter of the fetal chest in order to be at right angles to the interventricular septum,
3. the placing of the multi-element transducer in the longitudinal axis of the fetal heart at an angle of 45° to the antero-posterior diameter of the fetal chest.
    This will give the scanning plane at right angles to the interventricular septum, showing a two-dimensional image of the aortic root, the right and left ventricular wall, interventricular septum and mitral valve anterior and posterior leaflets,
4. moving the 2.25 MHz single beam transducer along this plane and produce a recording on the T-M mode.

The neonatal recording procedure is similar to antenatal procedure starting at the third step.

PATIENTS AND METHODS

In 30 normal pregnancies, varying from 34–42 weeks of gestation one antenatal examination was carried out.

In 9 patients T-M mode recordings were made:

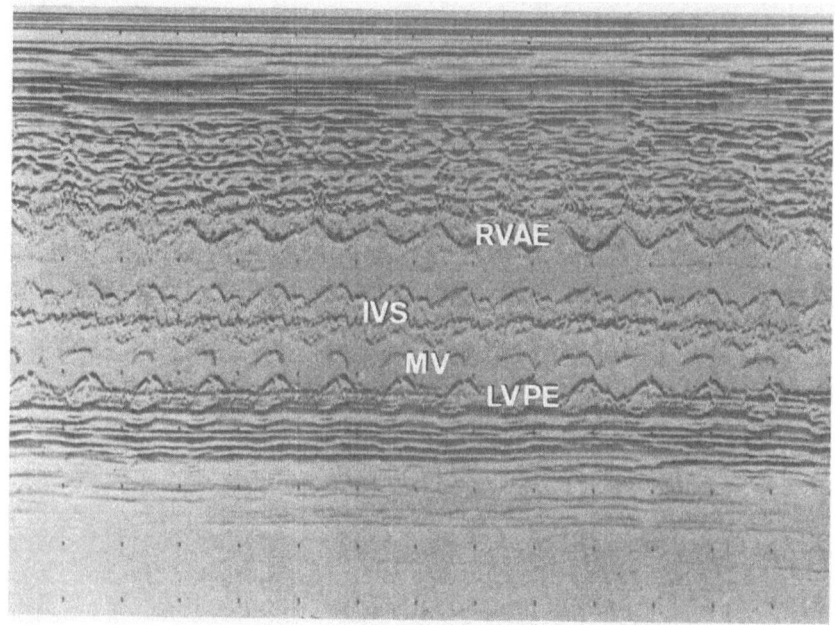

Fig. 1. Antenatal recording at 38 weeks of gestation.
RVAE: right-ventricular anterior endocard.
IVS: interventricular septum.
MV: mitral valve leaflets.
LVPE: left-ventricular posterior endocard.

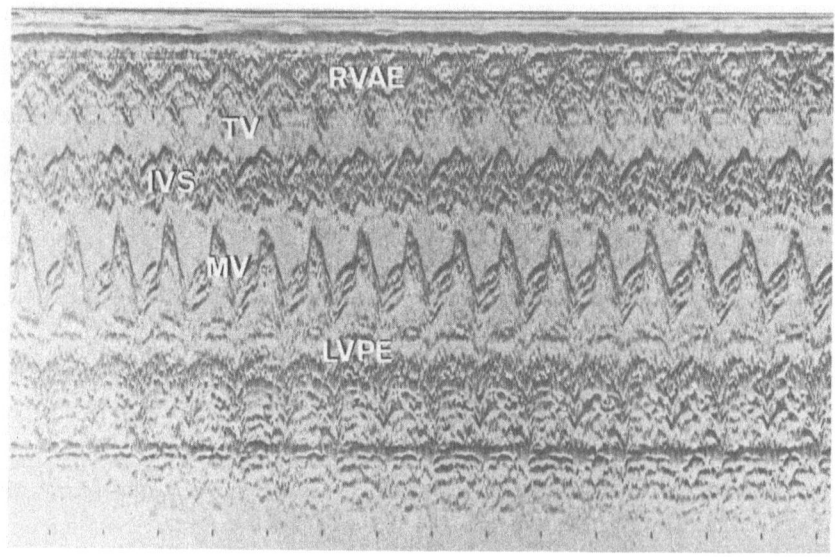

Fig. 2. Neonatal recording 2 days, postpartum.
TV: Tricuspid valve leaflets.
Note: depth-scale is changed in respect to Figure 1.

a. within 24 hours of delivery (Fig. 1),
b. within 10 min following delivery,
c. 4 hours following delivery,
d. one and two days following delivery (Fig. 2).
In each T-M mode the following measurements were performed:
- left and right ventricular dimension in the end-diastolic and end-systolic position in mm,
- interventricular septum thickness in the end-diastolic and end-systolic position in mm,
- left ventricular posterior wall thickness in the end-diastolic and end-systolic position in mm,
- left ventricular ejection-time in milliseconds determined by the time interval between end-diastole and end-systole.
- timing of the septal motion
We also calculated:
- the left-to-right ventricular ratio in the end-diastolic and end systolic position,
- two parameters expressing left ventricular wall function:
  1. fractional shortening (FS): the equation is

$$FS\% = \frac{ED - ES \text{ dimension}}{ED \text{ dimension}} \times 100\%$$

  ED = end-diastole   ES = end-systole
  2. mean velocity of fractional shortening (Vcf): the equation is

$$Vcf (sec^{-1}) = \frac{ED - ES \text{ dimension}}{ED \text{ dimension} \times ET} sec^{-1}$$

  ET = ejection time

RESULTS

In all 30 patients the antenatal left-to-right ventricular ratio is situated between 0.9 and 1.1 in 65% of the cases in end-diastole and in 60% of the cases in end-systole.
   In the 9 patients the mean values of the longitudinal data were as follows:
- the mean end-diastolic left ventricular dimension varies from 16.5 mm before delivery to 17.9 mm on the second day after delivery. The mean value for the end-systolic left ventricular dimensions ranges from 12.4 to 13.0 mm.
- the mean end-diastolic right-ventricular dimension varies from 17.0 mm before birth to 10.7 mm four hours following delivery. The mean end-systolic right ventricular dimension ranges from 15.3 mm before delivery to 9.0 mm at the end of the second post partum day,
- the mean left-to-right ventricular ratio in the end-diastolic position is 0.99 before delivery and 1.96 on the second day post partum. The mean

ratio in the end-systolic position is 0.83 before and 1.42 two days following delivery.
- the mean end-diastolic interventricular wall thickness is 3.9 mm before delivery, 2.9 mm immediately after delivery and 3.3 mm on the second post partum day. For the end-systolic interventricular wall thickness the mean figures are 4.4, 3.9 and 4.7 mm.
- a similar trend can be observed in the left-ventricular posterior wall thickness in end-diastole (3.7 – 2.4 – 2.8 mm) and end-systole (5.3 – 4.1 – 4.4 mm),
- the left-ventricular ejection time varies from 189 msec before to 213 msec one day following delivery,
- the mean fractional shortening of the left-ventricular dimension is 25.8% before and 35.8% one day after delivery,
- the mean value for the mean velocity of fractional shortening of the left ventricular dimension is 1.39 before and 1.71 one day after delivery.
- finally, septal motion appeared normal in all patients but one. In one patient there was paradoxal movement of the interventricular septum i.e. the septum was moving away from the left ventricular posterior wall during systole.

DISCUSSION

Preliminary data on fetal and neonatal cardiac geometrics have been presented. A significant increase in left-to-right ventricular index is observed. This increase occurs in the first 10 min following delivery. The values for fractional shortening and to a lesser extent for mean velocity of fractional shortening, show a tendency to increase during the 1st and 2nd post partum day, indicating a raised myocardial contraction force. More supportive data however, is needed.

III

TECHNOLOGICAL ASPECTS OF ECHOCARDIOLOGY

HISTORICAL REVIEW OF ECHO-INSTRUMENTATION

P.N.T. WELLS

The *Titanic* tragedy in 1912 was one of several incidents which led to the development of ultrasonic methods for the detection of obstacles at sea. Over the years, the early techniques have been refined so that they now have important applications in clinical diagnosis, including cardiology, as well as in sonar and non-destructive testing. Wells (1) has reviewed the progress in medical ultrasonic diagnosis which began with the work of D.H. Howry, J.J. Wild and J.M. Reid in the late 1940s and early 1950s.

1. M-MODE ECHOCARDIOGRAPHY

Their discovery of echocardiography in 1953 has recently been recalled by Edler and Hertz (2). The first echocardiograph, shown in Figure 1, was an industrial A-scope flaw detector fitted with a slit mask to allow a time-position (M-mode) recording to be made on continuously-moving 35 mm film. Some of the first recordings are shown in Figure 2.

Reid and Joyner (3) in the U.S.A. were amongst the very early echocardiographic pioneers, recording M-mode tracings on standard movie film; their 1964 equipment is shown in Figure 3.

The disadvantages of photographic recording on 35 mm film were considerable. It was a nuisance to have to wait while the trace was being

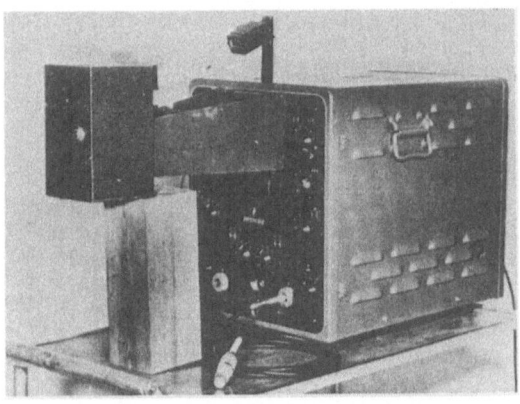

Fig. 1. The first echocardiograph, used by Edler and Hertz (2) in 1953.

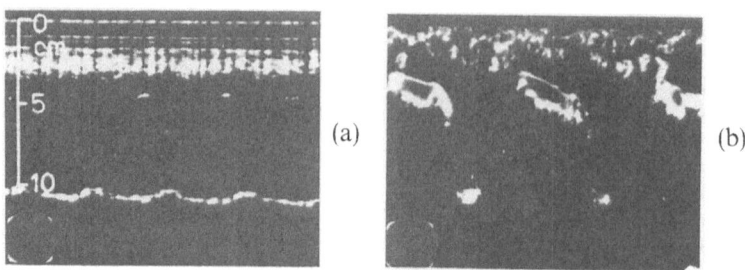

Fig. 2. Recordings of heart movements, made by Edler and Hertz (2) in 1953. (a) The first recording ever made. (b) The first recording to show mitral valve motion.

developed. This delay was avoided by the use of the time-to-voltage analogue converter, first introduced in 1961 by Edler (4), because a strip-chart recorder with instantaneous readout was employed. One of the disadvantages of this method was that only one structure could be tracked per gate, and in fact multiple-gate systems were really not developed at all. Another disadvantage of Edler's system was that the fixed time reference had to be set *beyond* the echo of interest, so that occasionally recorded structure excursions were truncated, without any indication of this being apparent on the trace. This problem was solved 5 years later by Wells and Ross (5), whose time-to-voltage analogue converter gate was set *before* the echo of interest. A solution to both problems was described in 1969 by Hertz and Simonsson (6), who 2 years earlier had developed the intensity-modulated ink-jet recorded. Their instrument was never widely used, because the advent of the fibre-optic ultraviolet recorder rendered it obsolete in echo-cardiographic applications.

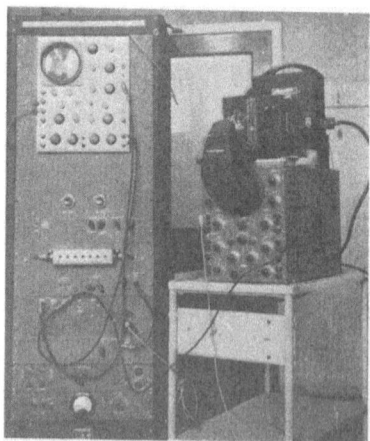

Fig. 3. Echocardiograph used by Reid and Joyner (3) in 1964.

2. TIME-OF-FLIGHT MEASUREMENT

Another very early application of ultrasound in cardiology was reported by Rushmer et al. (7) in 1956. They used two transducers, sewn on opposite sides of the myocardium, to measure the ventricular diameter in terms of the pulse transit time. Nearly 20 years later, Stegall (8) described a catheter with two transducers, designed to curl around the inside of the ventricle so that the transducers were face-to-face, thus avoiding the need for major surgery.

3. TWO-DIMENSIONAL IMAGING

3.1. *Conventional two-dimensional scanning*

Gross cardiac abnormalities, such as tumours, were shown in 1974 by Kratochwil et al. (9) to be detectable by simple scanning of the heart using an ordinary two-dimensional scanner, despite the degradation of the image by physiological movements. Moreover, carefully controlled manual scanning of the heart with a conventional two-dimensional ultrasonic scanner was shown in a review published in 1977 by Matsumoto et al. (10) to be capable of producing a kind of two-dimensional image with superimposed time-position structure movement recordings. They demonstrated the diagnostic value of this technique in abnormalities of the aortic root.

This approach of scanning the heart with a conventional B-scanner was taken further by Kossoff et al. (11), who used their 2.25 MHz multi-transducer water-bath-coupled system to make both "simple" scans (in 0.5 s or approximately 2 s) and "compound" scans (in approximately 2 s). Although the "compound" scans suffered degradation in resolution due to the movement of the heart, they afforded apparently useful "average representations". The "simple" scans showed the patterns of rapid movements of structures within the heart, rather like those of Matsumoto et al.

3.2. *"Stop-action" two-dimensional scanning*

Early in the development of cardiological diagnostic ultrasound, it was demonstrated that two-dimensional images corresponding to any desired phase in the cardiac cycle could be obtained by ecg-gating the display of a conventional scanner. King (12) was one of the pioneers of this technique, publishing his first paper on the subject in 1972. An ingenious and simple method of gating ultrasonic two-dimensional cardiac images was described in 1973 by Hussey et al. (13). They scanned the heart with a conventional diagnostic machine, but viewed the image displayed on a non-storage CRT by means of a CCTV system switched on for a short period at the appropriate phase of each cardiac cycle. Possibly the ultimate development of the "conventional" stop-action two-dimensional scanning method was that described in 1975 by Hileman et al. (14). In a single manual scanning sweep across the patient's chest, their instrument produced 9 separate images at sequential phases in the cardiac cycle, stored on the analogue scan converter of their conventional two-dimensional scanner.

As an alternative to "conventional" stop-action imaging, in 1974 Gramiak and Waag (15) described a method of rearranging M-mode recordings to construct two-dimensional images. Originally they carried out this operation by hand, but later they employed a computer.

3.3. *Intracavitary scanning*

Intracardiac probes were first used by Kimoto et al. (16); the method was described in 1964. Using ecg-gating, both two-dimensional B-scan and C-scan images were made, the latter being particularly useful for visualizing atrial septal defects. Although more recent results were reported in 1967 by Omoto et al. (17), the method has not been widely used, presumably because conventional cardiac catheterization is so much more familiar to cardiologists. The possibility of measuring the internal dimensions of the heart by multi-element transducers mounted at the tips of catheters was explored, however, by Eggleton et al. (18) in 1970 and by Bom (19) in 1972.

Returning to Japan, there has recently been a growth of interest in transoesophageal cardiac scanning. Apparatus and results were described by Hisanga and Hisanga (20) in 1978.

3.4. *Real-time two-dimensional imaging*

The possibility of producing real-time two-dimensional images of the internal structures of the living human heart *in situ* was first explored by Åsberg (21). In a paper published in 1967, he described the use of the mirror system, developed in 1963 by Olofsson (22), and which had been shown the following year by Hertz and Olofsson (23) to be capable of visualizing the *in vitro* heart, for making sequential images of the living heart. The apparatus and some of

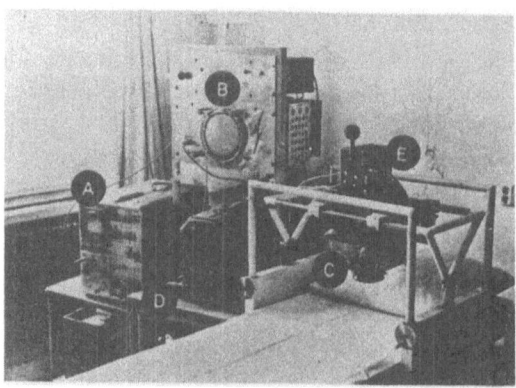

Fig. 4. The first mechanical real-time two-dimensional scanner described by Åsberg (21).

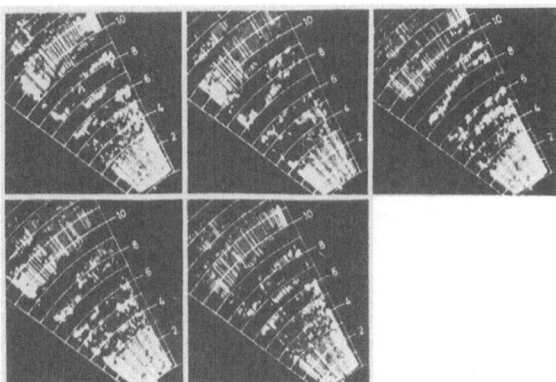

Fig. 5. Images of normal human heart, published by Åsberg (21) in 1967. The movement of the mitral valve can be followed through the cardiac cycle. Range markers in cm.

the historic scans are shown in Figures 4 and 5. Although the frame rate was only 7 s^{-1}, the principle which Åsberg demonstrated pointed the way to modern two-dimensional real-time echocardiography.

Fast mechanical scanners are now quite commonly used for real-time two-dimensional cardiac imaging. Pioneering systems were described by Flaherty et al. (24) in 1967, Patzold et al. (25) in 1970, Griffith and Henry (26) and McDicken et al. (27) in 1974, and Eggleton et al. (28) in 1975.

The first multi-element linear array scanner, described by Bom et al. (29), was tested on 18 patients in 1971. The apparatus is shown in Figure 6. Twenty transducer elements were operated sequentially to produce 20 ultrasonic lines; successive frames were interlaced to give 40 lines in the image. More recent systems have generally used a larger number of transducer elements, operated in groups to maintain good beamwidth and stepped element-by-element to give small line separation. Instruments have been described by many investigators, including Pourcelot et al. (30) and Whittingham et al. (31) in 1975.

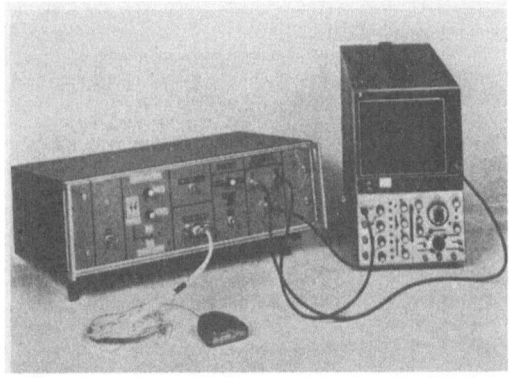

Fig. 6. The first linear array real-time two-dimensional cardiac scanner, described by Bom et al. (29), and used clinically in 1971.

Systems employing transducer arrays can, in principle, have their lateral resolution improved by synthetic focusing. A most ingenious and relatively simple method of dynamic focusing was described in 1977 by Alais and Fink (32). Instead of employing a smoothly varying amplitude grading pattern, they mimicked a Fresnel zone lens by a 3-state modulation distribution. Excellent real-time cardiac images have been obtained in this way.

The first electronically steered array system for two-dimensional ultrasonic imaging in cardiology seems to have been that of von Ramm et al. (33). Their instrument, as described in 1975, had 16 elements in an array 24 × 14 mm, operating at 1.8 MHz, as shown in Figure 7. Fixed zone focusing was used. Another system with an electronically steered array developed initially for cardiology was that of Anderson et al. (34). It used a frequency of 2.25 MHz with 32 elements in an array 13 mm long and 12 mm wide. An acoustic lens of 80 mm focal length significantly improved the lateral resolution within an 80 sector angle.

Whatever the method by which real-time two-dimensional images are produced, it is desirable to be able to record and display them in standard television format. The simplest method is to have a CCTV camera positioned in front of a conventional CRT displaying the ultrasonic scan patterns; this has been done by, for example, both von Ramm et al. and Anderson et al. Alternatively, an analogue scan converter can be used, but the system has to be used in a destructive writing mode, since the more conventional write-read-erase cycle is unsuitable for line-by-line refresh operation. So far, only one commercial scanner seems to have used this technique. Finally, the scan conversion can be achieved by writing the ultrasound data temporarily into an electronic digital memory. A description of this method was published in 1977 by Ligtvoet et al. (35).

Conventional ultrasonic pulse-echo visualization systems are limited in cardiac investigations where the penetration is up to around 150 mm, by the fact that the go-and-return pulse propagation time is around 200 μs. This sets the prf at a maximum of 5000 s^{-1}, so that the maximum frame rate is, for example, 50 s^{-1} if 100 lines are required to form a satisfactory image. By

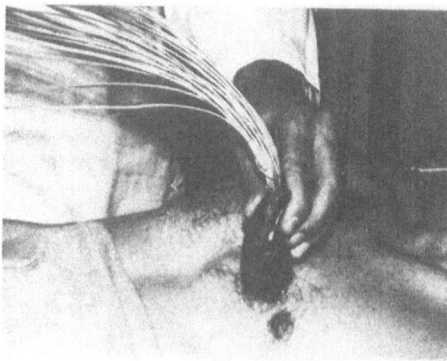

Fig. 7. Electronically steered array real-time two-dimensional cardiac scanner, described by von Ramm et al. (33) in 1975.

uniform illumination of a "slice" of tissue, it is possible, in principle, to acquire any number of lines simultaneously, thus overcoming this limitation. In practice, however, the provision of, say, 100 complete receiver chains is prohibitive both in cost and complexity. By an ingenious optical signal processing scheme, involving 2 linear arrays, one receiving echoes from within the patient and the other re-radiating the received field into a transparent medium, Torguet et al. (36) demonstrated in 1977 that high-line-density frame rates of at least 2000 s^{-1} could easily be obtained. This and similar methods deserve further investigations.

4. TWO-DIMENSIONAL ARRAYS

During the last decade, the acquisition of two-dimensional ultrasonic data has become commonplace in cardiology. In 1974, Maginness et al. (37) described their first attempts to construct a two-dimensional piezoelectric array and to use this to obtain three-dimensional ultrasonic data. Although many problems remain to be solved before fully satisfactory data can be acquired, stored, processed and displayed, this work holds great promise for the future.

5. IMAGE ENHANCEMENT

Amongst the first attempts at automatic analysis of echocardiograms was that of Griffith and Henry (38) in 1973. Successful automatic analysis requires "clean" recordings, and some evidence has been published showing that image enhancement techniques might be helpful here. In 1974, McSherry (39) reported the improvement in range resolution in echocardiography by inverse filtering implemented by digital computer. In fact, of course, the degree of improvement which can be obtained by this method is set by bandwidth and noise considerations. A marginal improvement in echocardiogram intelligibility was demonstrated as a result of moving target indicator processing, in a paper published in 1974 by Waag and Gramiak (40).

Images from a mechanical two-dimensional scanner producing 60 frames per second were digitized to 6-bit accuracy by Wixson et al. (41), who reported their work in 1975. They used a 5 MHz sampling frequency, transferring data to their computer at 100,000 samples per second. This relatively low transfer rate allowed simultaneous use of disk and tape for data storage. A two-dimensional 9-point neighbourhood averaging algorithm smoothed the B-scan images, and a pattern recognition process was proposed to identify the endocardial surface, but this has apparently not yet been shown to be completely satisfactory.

Consideration of the relatively poor lateral resolution of ultrasonic imaging systems might at first lead to the conclusion that the quality of the picture could not be increased by having lines much closer together than half-beamwidth separation. Even though such a picture contains all the available information, however, it is aesthetically unsatisfactory if the separate image lines can be distinguished. Several investigators, including Waag and Gramiak (42) in 1976, have used linear interpolation to enhance images to minimize this problem.

The results of experiments with three-dimensional echocardiography were reported in 1977 by Matsumoto et al. (43). They used a conventional water-bath-coupled scanner with ecg-gating to make stop-action scans in serial parallel planes through the heart. These scans were digitized into 128 levels and 105×80 pixels, and stored on disk. A weighted average method was used for smoothing, and each image was then reduced to two levels by using differentiation to detect boundaries. Neighbouring boundary points were then connected to construct line representations. These line representations were then displayed as stereo pairs, or used for the reconstruction of two-dimensional images in any desired plane.

6. TISSUE CHARACTERIZATION

Progress in the application of tissue characterization methods to *in vivo* cardiological problems has been disappointing, although encouraging results have been obtained in the laboratory. Three distinct approaches have been tried. The first depends on scattering measurements; for example, Gramiak et al. (44) showed that experimentally induced infarcts in dog hearts *in vitro* could be identified by relatively simple amplitude processing, and they suggested that the method might be extended to *in vivo* diagnosis by the use of a real-time scanner for guidance. Initial attempts to test this possibility, reported by Joynt et al. (45), have given encouraging results.

7. DOPPLER METHODS

In 1957, Satomura (46) published the first paper in English to describe the detection of cardiac movement by the ultrasonic Doppler effect. Ten years later, similar Russian work was reported by Lubé et al. (47). Although for a short while there was interest in simultaneous display of Doppler signals with the M-mode recording, as described by Edler and Lindstrom (48), this never became popular.

In 1974, Peronneau et al. (49) reviewed the progress which they had made since 1968 in the study of blood velocity profiles in major vessels. They had developed an 8 MHz pulsed Doppler system with 16 sequentially gated directional receiving channels, capable of generating velocity profiles with a bandwidth of 25 Hz. The system was designed for direct application of the transducer assembly to the wall of the blood vessel being investigated.

An elegant application of the continuous wave Doppler flow meter was reviewed in 1974 by Kalmanson et al. (50). Without the use of special instrumentation, abnormalities particularly of the right heart can easily be diagnosed by studying the shape of the velocity/time waveforms detected transcutaneously, for example, in the jugular vein. The continuous wave Doppler method was also shown by Light (51) to be able to give useful cardiological data by analysis of the velocity/time wave-form detected in the aortic arch by a transducer positioned in the suprasternal notch. Light used a 2 MHz system, and a bank of bandpass filters to produce a real-time display of the directional Doppler spectrum. In 1974 too, Baker et al. (52) described the visualization of the aortic arch with a pulsed Doppler system, and Benchimol and Desser (53) and Reid et al. (54) reported the measurement of coronary artery flow by means of Doppler transducers mounted at the tips of catheters. More recently, Baker et al. (55) have used a pulsed Doppler system transcutaneously to study flow within the heart, and Tanaka et al. (56) have used an M-sequence modulated ultrasonic Doppler in a similar way.

In 1977, Kay et al. (57) described a novel continuous-wave swept frequency ultrasonic echo-location system which produced dynamic auditory signals corresponding to positional changes of internal structures of the heart. The inventors claimed that this inexpensive, portable instrument allowed the 4 cardiac valves to be located with greater ease than with conventional echocardiographs. Moreover, abnormal valve motions gave characteristically different "sounds" from the normal.

8. ULTRASONIC COMPUTED TOMOGRAPHY

Preliminary experimental work on computed tomography of excised canine heart, reported in 1975 and reviewed by Greenleaf et al. (58), demonstrated that the speed of ultrasound could be mapped. Whether there are significant differences in the speeds in normal and infarcted myocardium is not yet established, and in any case it seems inconceivable that transmission ultrasonic CT imaging of the heart could be carried out adequately *in vivo*, on account of the limited access due to lung and bone.

EPILOGUE

A recent and particularly happy event was the presentation in November 1977 of the $15,000 Albert Lasker Clinical Medical Research Award to Dr. Inge Edler and Dr. Helmuth Hertz, both of Lund in Sweden, for their development of echocardiography.

ACKNOWLEDGEMENTS

All the illustrations in this paper are reproduced by kind permission of the holders of the copyrights of the original publications in which they appeared.

REFERENCES

1. Wells PNT: Biomedical ultrasonics, Academic Press, 1977.
2. Edler I, CH Hertz: J Clin Utrasound 5:352, 1977.
3. Reid JM, CR Joyner: In: Ultrasonic energy, Kelly, E (ed), University of Illinois Press, 1964, p 278–93.
4. Edler I: Acta med scand 170, suppl 370, 1961.
5. Wells PNT, FGM Ross: Ultrasonics 7:171, 1969.
6. Hertz CH, SI Simonsson: Med biol Engrg 7:337, 1969.
7. Rushmer RF, DL Franklin, RM Ellis: Circ Res 4:684, 1956.
8. Stegall HF: In: Cardiovascular applications of ultrasound, Reneman, RS (ed), North-Holland, 1974, p. 150–61.
9. Kratochwil A, C Jantsch et al: Ultrasound Med Biol 1:275, 1974.
10. Matsumoto M, T Matsuo et al.: (1977) Ultrasound Med Biol 3:153, 1977.
11. Kossoff G, WJ Garrett et al.: In: Ultrasound in medicine, vol 4, White, D and Lyons, EA (eds), Plenum Press, 1978, p 1–6.
12. King DL: Radiology 103:387, 1972.
13. Hussey M, WN McDicken, DAR Robertson: Ultrasonics 11:73, 1973.
14. Hileman RE, DE Dick, D Cooper: In: Ultrasound in medicine, vol 1, White, D (ed), Plenum Press, 1975, p 519–26.
15. Gramiak R, RC Waag: In: Ultrasonics in medicine, de Vlieger, M White, DN McCready, VR (eds), Excerpta Medica, 1974, p 244–9.
16. Kimoto S, R Omoto et al.: Ultrasonics 2:82, 1964.
17. Omoto R: Ultrasonics 6:80, 1967.
18. Eggleton RC, C Townsend et al.: IEEE Trans Sonics Ultrason 17:143, 1970.
19. Bom N: New Concepts in echocardiography, Stenfert Kroese, 1972.
20. Hisanga K, A Hisanga: In: Ultrasonics in medicine, vol 4, White D, Lyons EA (eds), Plenum Press, 1978, p 391–402.
21. Asberg A: Ultrasonics 6:113, 1967.
22. Olofsson S: Acustica 13:361, 1963.
23. Hertz CH, S Olofsson: In: Ultrasonic energy, Kelly E (ed), University of Illinois Press, 1964, p 322–6.
24. Flaherty JJ, JW Clark, HN Walgren: Dig int Conf med biol Eng 7:221, 1967.
25. Patzold J, W Krause et al.: IEEE Trans biomed Eng 17:263, 1970.
26. Griffith JM, WL Henry: Circulation 49:1147, 1974.
27. McDicken WN, K Bruff, J Paton: Ultrasonics 12:269, 1974.
28. Eggleton RC, H Feigenbaum et al.: In: Ultrasound in medicine, vol 1, White D (ed), Plenum Press, 1975, p 385–93.
29. Bom N, J Roelandt et al.: In: Ultrasonics in medicine, de Vlieger M, White DN and McCready VR (eds), Excerpta Medica, 1974, p 297–9.
30. Pourcelot L, JM Pottier et al.: In: Ultrasonics in medicine, Kazner E, de Vlieger M et al. (eds), Excerpta Medica 1975 p 54–8.
31. Whittingham TA: In: Ultrasonics in medicine, Kazner E, de Vlieger M et al. (eds), Excerpta Medica, 1975, p 59–66.
32. Alais P, M Fink: In: Acoustical holography, vol 7, Kessler LW (ed), Plenum Press, 1977, p 509–22.
33. Ramm OT von, FL Thurstone, J Kisslo: In: Acoustical holography, vol 6, Booth N (ed), Plenum Press, 1975, p 99–102.
34. Anderson WA, JT Arnold et al.: In: Ultrasound in medicine, vol 3B, White D, Brown RE, (eds), Plenum Press, 1977, p 1547–58.
35. Ligtvoet C, J Vogel et al.: Ultrasonics 15:89, 1977.
36. Torguet R, C Bruneel et al: In: Acoustical holography, vol 7, Kessler LW (ed), Plenum Press, 1977, p 69–85.
37. Maginness MG, JD Plummer, JD Meindl: In: Acoustical holography, vol 5, Green PS, (ed) Plenum Press, 1974, p. 619–31.
38. Griffith JM, WL Henry: Am J Cardiol 32:961, 1973.
39. McSherry DH: IEEE Trans Sonics Ultrason 21:91, 1974.
40. Waag RC, R Gramiak: In: Ultrasonics in medicine, de Vlieger M, White DN, McCready VR (eds), Excerpta Medica, 1974, p 239–43.

41. Wixson SE, LR Smith, JA Mantle: In: Ultrasound in medicine, vol 1, White D (ed), Plenum Press, 1975, p 363–71.
42. Waag RC, R Gramiak: Ultrasound Med Biol 2:163, 1976.
43. Matsumoto M, H Matsuo et al.: Ultrasound Med Biol. 3:163, 1977.
44. Gramiak, R, RC Waag et al.: In: Ultrasound in medicine, vol 4, White D, Lyons EA (eds), Plenum Press, 1978, p 17–22.
45. Joynt L, A Macovski, D Boyle: In: 3rd int Symp Ultrasonic Imaging and Tissue Characterization, program and abstracts, National Bureau of Standards, 1978, p 59–62.
46. Satomura S: J acoust Soc Am 29:1181, 1957.
47. Lube VM, YD Savonof, LI Yakiemenkov: Soviet Phys Acoust 13:59, 1967.
48. Edler I, K Lindström: In: Ultrasonographia medica, Bock J, Ossoinig K et al. (eds), vol III, Verlag Wiener Med Akad , 1971, p 455–61.
49. Peronneau PA, A Bugnon et al.: In: Ultrasonics in medicine, de Vlieger M, White DN, McCready VR (eds), Excerpta Medica, 1974, p 259–66.
50. Kalmanson D, C Veyrat et al.: In: Ultrasonics in medicine, de Vlieger M, White DN, McCready VR (eds), Excerpta Medica, 1974, p 278–81.
51. Light LH: In: Cardiovascular applications of ultrasound, Reneman RS (ed), North-Holland, 1974, p 325–60.
52. Baker DW, SL Johnson, DE Strandness: In: Cardiovascular applications of ultrasound, ed Reneman RS (ed), North-Holland, 1974, p 108–24.
53. Benchimol A, KB Desser: In: Cardiovascular applications of ultrasound, Reneman RS (ed), North-Holland, 1974, p 193–9.
54. Reid JM, DL Davis et al.: In: Cardiovascular applications of ultrasound, Reneman RS (ed), North-Holland, 1974, p 183–92.
55. Baker DW, DE Strandness, SL Johnson: Ultrasound Med Biol 2:251, 1976.
56. Tanaka M, M Okujima et al.: In: Ultrasound in medicine, vol 3B, White D, Brown RE (eds), Plenum Press, 1977, p 1263–77.
57. Kay L, J Boys et al.: Ultrasonics, 15:136, 1977.
58. Greenleaf JF, SA Johnson, AH Lent: Ultrasound Med Biol 3:327, 1978.

CURRENT INSTRUMENTATION

N. BOM and C.T. LANCÉE

The paper by Wells* shows the very first time-motion (M-mode) registration apparatus and the quality of some of the first cardiac recordings ever made. The M-mode technique has become widely used today, the principle still being that introduced by Edler and Hertz in 1953 (1). Real-time cross-sectional scanners were first introduced in the early seventies. Their importance is still growing and together with the M-mode facility they are the major components of the current equipment in echocardiographic laboratories. The application of Doppler, in particular pulsed Doppler, also dates back to the early seventies, and its potential to yield highly specific information of local blood flow stimulated increasing interest in this method.

This paper will review "state of the art" of M-mode systems, real-time cross-sectional imaging and Doppler techniques.

1. M-MODE RECORDING

Most recent innovations in M-mode techniques have been obtained by the introduction of new recording methods. Currently, the two best-known recording materials for M-mode registration are:

a) *direct print paper*

This is optically processed. The process method is exposure to low-level ultraviolet light to make the recording visible. This paper is typically brownish with limited image permanency. If a grey scale is defined from 0 = white to 2 = deep black, then the background is 0.2 and the maximum density is only 0.6, resulting in a limited grey scale.

b) *dry silver paper*

This type of paper has a respectably wide dynamic range. The grey scale reaches from a background of 0.15 to a maximum density of 1.4 (which is close to black). The development is based on thermal processing, either by a heat-plate or by a current through a conductive coating on the underside of the paper.

The dynamic range of dry silver paper allows an excellent recording of a "still" cross-sectional image together with a M-mode registration. An example is shown in Figure 1.

* Note: All papers, referred to by name only, are included in this book.

Charles T. Lancée (ed.), Echocardiology, 373–383. All rights reserved
Copyright © 1979 by Martinus Nijhoff Publishers bv, The Hague/Boston/London

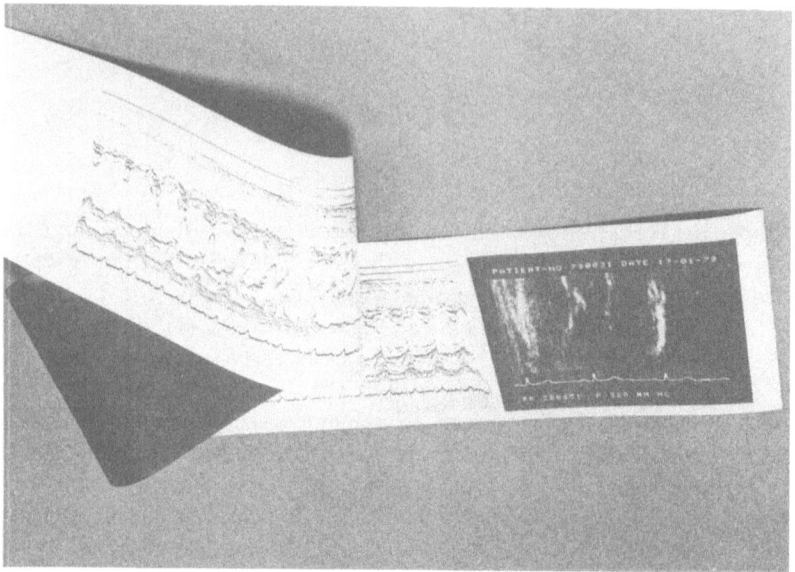

Fig. 1. Example of M-mode recording and single frame from a two-dimensional (2-D) real-time device on a strip of dry silver paper.
The 2-D image has been obtained with an additional video memory.

2. M-MODE ANALYSIS

A variety of computer-assisted analysis programs are becoming available. Most of these systems produce standardized routine outputs by processing previously recorded M-mode information. Special programs exist for the study of left ventricular echo parameters or for the accumulation of statistical information over larger series of beats. Quantized M-mode information can be obtained using a digitizing tablet and computer with the configuration shown in Figure 2.

An example of the use of computers for the analysis of M-mode data is shown in Figure 3 and 4 for a study on standardized echocardiographic dimensions of a group of school children. Once the data were entered on a routine basis, information on the population became available. An example of weight information is shown in Figure 3. The left ventricular dimensions are shown for the same group versus weight in Figure 4. A detailed description has been given in the paper by Voogd et al.

The latest developments include the possibility of reading large series of beats using a video contrast method. With this method, it is sufficient to trace the structures to be analysed with an ordinary pencil.

The subsequent input and data handling are automated. Van Zwieten et al. described this system in their paper.

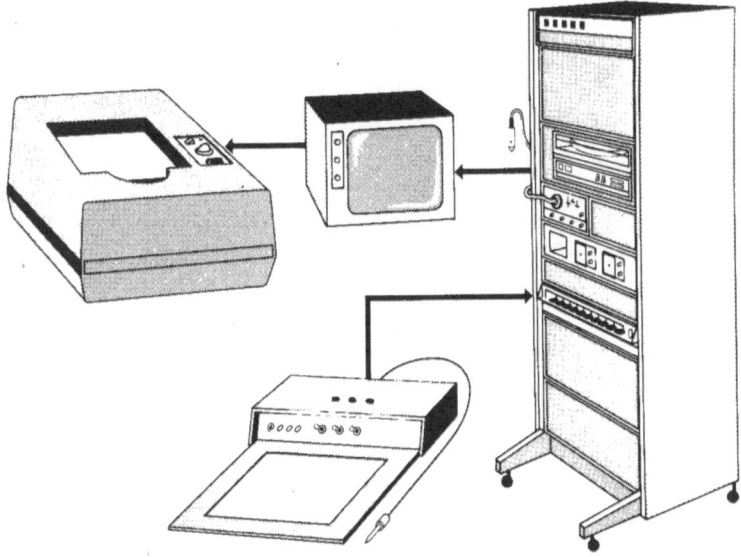

Fig. 2. Digitizing tablet with computer, monitor and hardcopy unit as used for off-line processing of M-mode data.

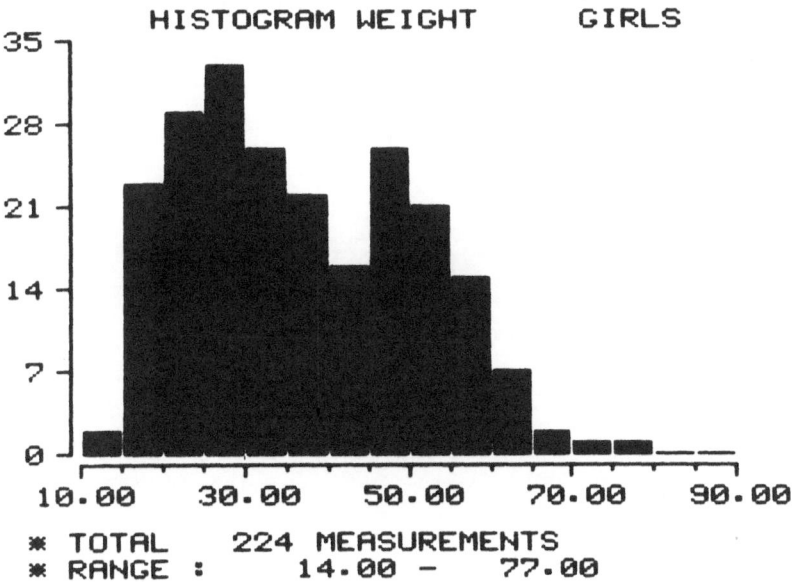

Fig. 3. Standard programs may be used to display the input data characteristics such as shown here for the weight distribution.

3. CURRENT REAL-TIME SYSTEMS

A variety of real-time imaging systems are currently in use for cardiac applications. The five most widely-used systems are indicated schematically in figure 5.

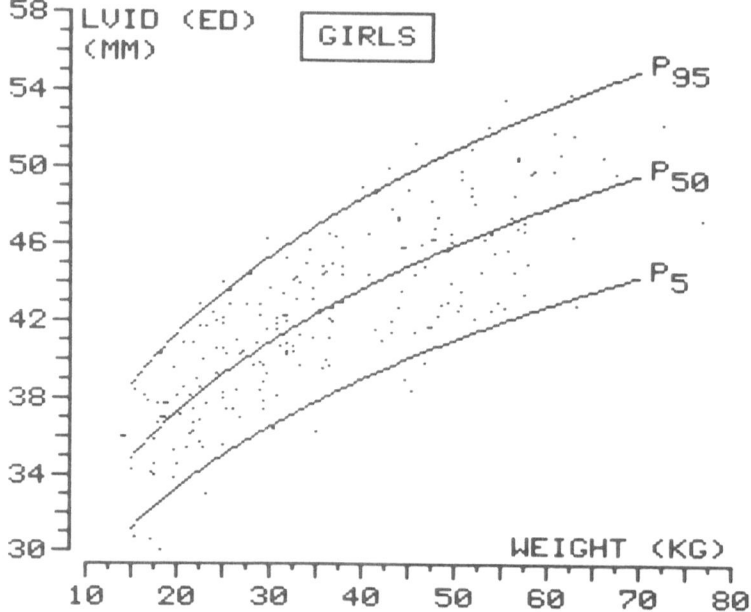

Fig. 4. Example of nomogram of percentiles of end-diastolic echo dimensions.

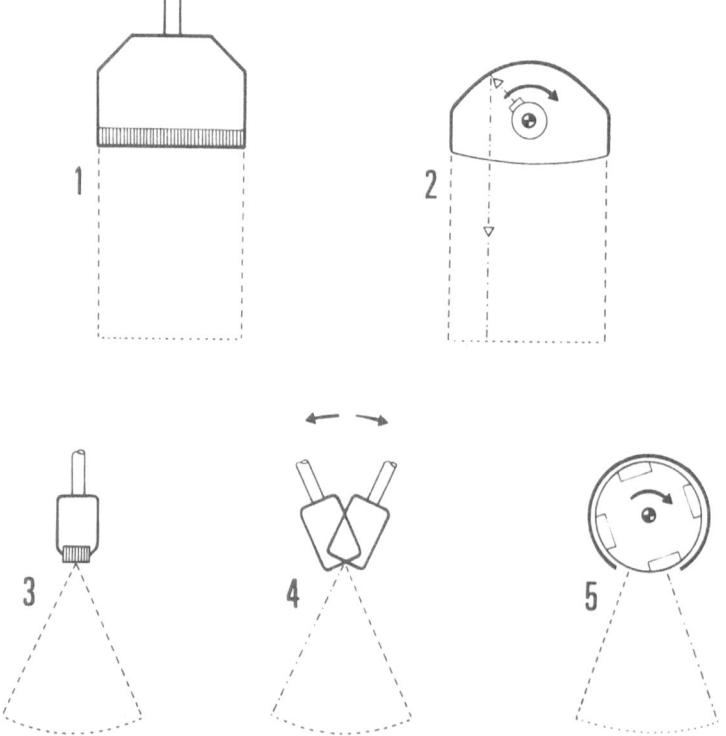

Fig. 5. Schematic drawing of present two-dimensional real time imaging principles.

1) *The linear-array system*

This frequently described principle is based on a number of elements positioned in a row. In an early application, one element was used at the time for transmission and reception. Fast switching to adjacent elements allows cardiac scanning in a rectangular format (2). One of the recent developments along these lines was the introduction of a miniaturized, battery-powered, real-time system. A photograph of this imaging device is shown in Figure 6. Details have been described elsewhere (3, 4).

If sub-groups of elements are used, instead of one element at a time, the principle remains the same but a better adaptation of the sound beam width is obtained.

2) *The mirror system*

A transducer rotates in a liquid-filled, coupling compartment, where the beam is reflected off a mirror, and a rectangular cross-section is obtained. Although this device was originally developed for obstetric use, some cardiac applications have been reported (5).

3) *The electronic sector scanner*

The principle of this system is based on an array transducer with small dimensions, where all elements are activated at the same time to form the sound beam (6). Beam deflection is introduced by appropriate differences in time delay between the individual elements. Deflection of the beam over a wide range, calls for a complex set of necessary delays. High frame rate and wedge-shaped display format are obtained with a

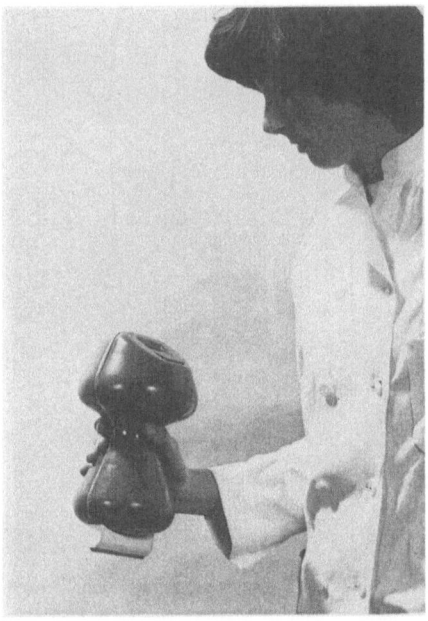

Fig. 6. Prototype of a miniaturized, battery powered real time imaging device (from: reference 4).

stationary transducer of relatively small dimensions. Continuous research is still being done, as can be seen from the papers of Burckhardt et al. and Haine et al.

4) *The mechanical sector scanner*
   A variety of such scanners exists. All systems operate with a single, circular transducer. A pivoting or rotating motion is exerted on the transducer to create a beam deflection over a sector. The beam deflection is often limited and the probe may have a tendency to vibrate. Early pivoting systems only achieved beam deflections of about 30 deg; while recent systems, like the one described by Shaw, have a range of 60 deg or more (7).

5) *The rotating wheel sector scanners*
   The rotating wheel system has a number of transducers positioned at the circumference of a revolving wheel. Each transducer is activated in front of a window. With such a system a wide angle wedge-shaped image can be obtained.

4. PRESENT DOPPLER METHODS

In cardiological applications, the most important Doppler method is the pulsed Doppler technique. The principle is explained in Figure 7. The reflected ultrasound carries a frequency shift proportional to the velocity

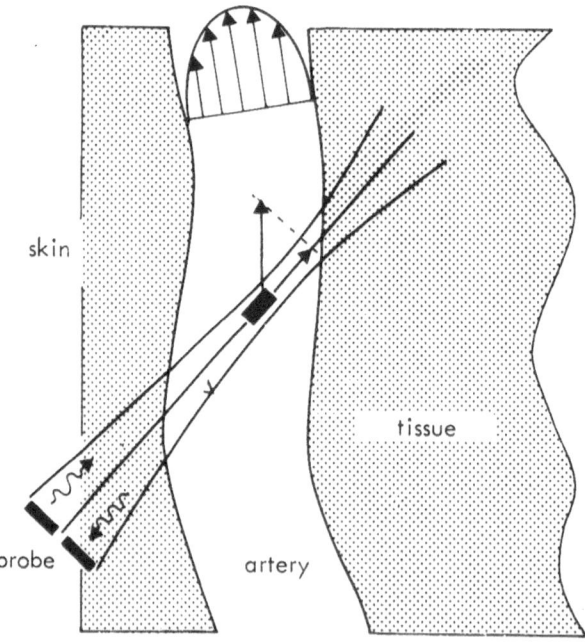

Fig. 7. Schematic drawing of the Doppler principle. Here shown to measure the velocity at a point in an artery.

vector of the reflector(s) in the beam direction and this Doppler shift thus indicates (relative) velocity.

Usually the velocity distribution is not uniform. When time-gating is used, it becomes possible to gate pulses from a particular depth and thus to calculate the Doppler shift for a number of points. By changing the gate or using multiple gating and filtering techniques, a velocity profile can be constructed. With present systems, it is difficult to obtain absolute, quantitative flow information. An example of the state of the art has been given by Brandestini et al. So far, the Doppler signal has provided information on a velocity component of blood at a particular position. The M-mode registration and two-dimensional imaging devices yield informaton on motion and on geometry of cardiac structures, respectively; and, therefore, a number of attempts have been made to combine these methods. Equipment is now available where the motion information obtained with M-mode is complemented by information on the direction and relative amplitude of blood flow at known positions within arteries or cardiac cavities. The combination of velocity information obtained using Doppler techniques with geometrical information obtained using two-dimensional ones, seems very attractive. Pourcelot describes such a combination, using a linear array, in his paper. A possible configuration has been illustrated schematically in Figure 8. However, optimal Doppler and optimal echo information require conflicting signal processing parameters, as shown in the paper of Hoeks et al.

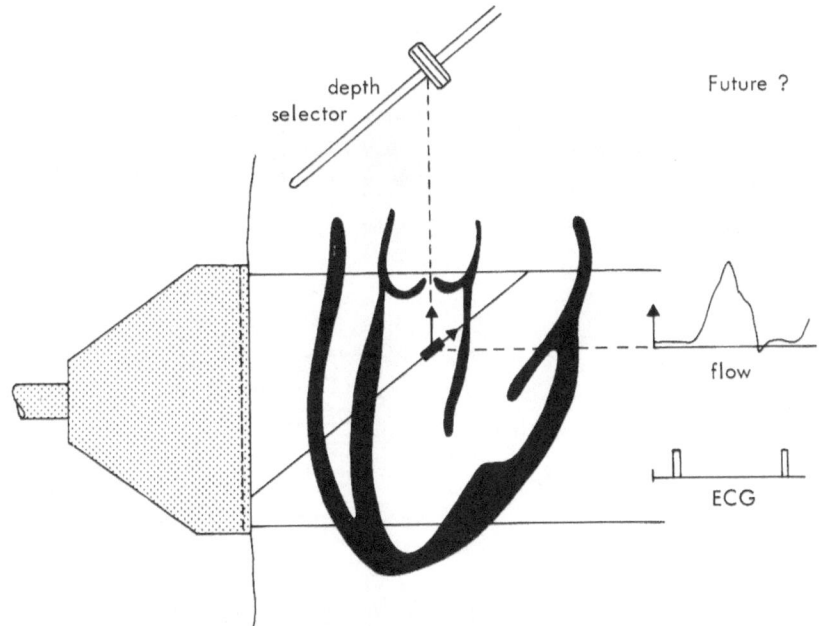

Fig. 8. Instantaneous combination of 2-D imaging and accumulation of velocity information at selected positions.

Therefore, one compromise solution might be to use a buffer memory to "freeze" a two-dimensional image of the area under investigation, then switch to optimal Doppler signal processing for a single beam within the area and, finally, incorporate the resultant Doppler information (location, beam direction and velocity) in the two-dimensional image.

5. RESOLUTION

The beam width is an important parameter, since it dictates the lateral resolution. Fixed-focus methods may improve resolution. This, however, is only valid for the focal point at a given depth. For optimal resolution, focusing should be obtained over the entire depth. Multi-element systems and

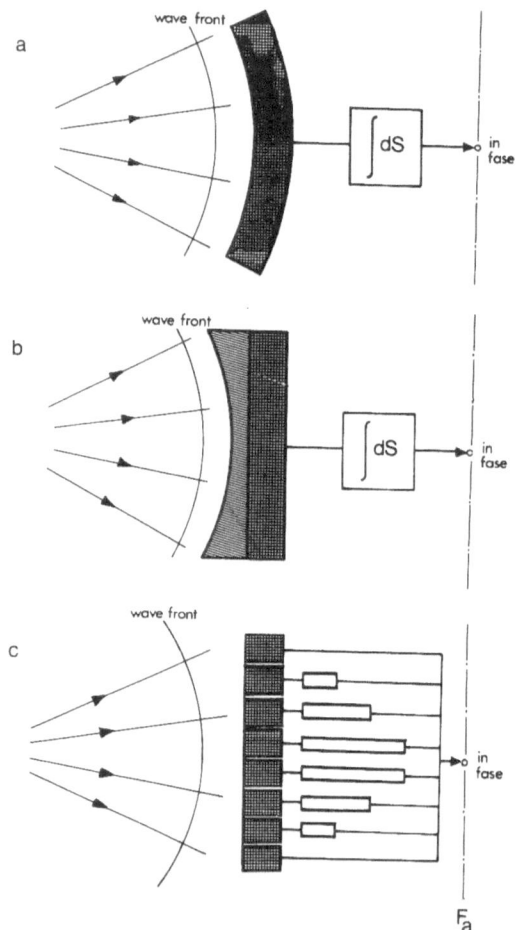

Fig. 9. A single focal point may be obtained either with a curved transducer (a), with a lens (b) or with electronic delays (c).

the use of delay lines made it possible to introduce dynamic focusing. Thurstone (8) suggested this method for electronic sector scanners. These techniques increased the need for very complex transducers, thus stimulating research in this field. Detailed analysis of array design is given in the paper by Defranould et al.

Focusing may be obtained when the transducer is subdivided into small elements and each element is given the appropriate delay so as to cause the incoming signals to be in phase as shown in Figure 9. This method can be extended to operate in the reception mode for a number of sequential focal zones. Ligtvoet et al. (9) have described a system, based on the linear array method, where six focal zones were sequentially constructed. With twelve elements for each line and accurate delay lines, high quality images are obtained.

With dynamic Fresnel zone focusing, as described by Alais (10), similar results may be obtained. This focusing is again based on a large aperture with many individual elements. In its crudest form, a three-state modulation (in phase, anti-phase or not at all) is used over the elements. This sampling approximates Fresnel zone focusing. Three zones cover the necessary echo depths adequately.

Figure 10 shows an example where the instrument on the right (B) uses a dynamic focus over the entire depth. Both instruments had a transducer frequency of (about) 2.5 MHz and were applied to the AIUM standard test object. As a first step, optimal images were obtained at very low echo intensity. Subsequently, the gain was increased by 10 dB. It can be seen that system B

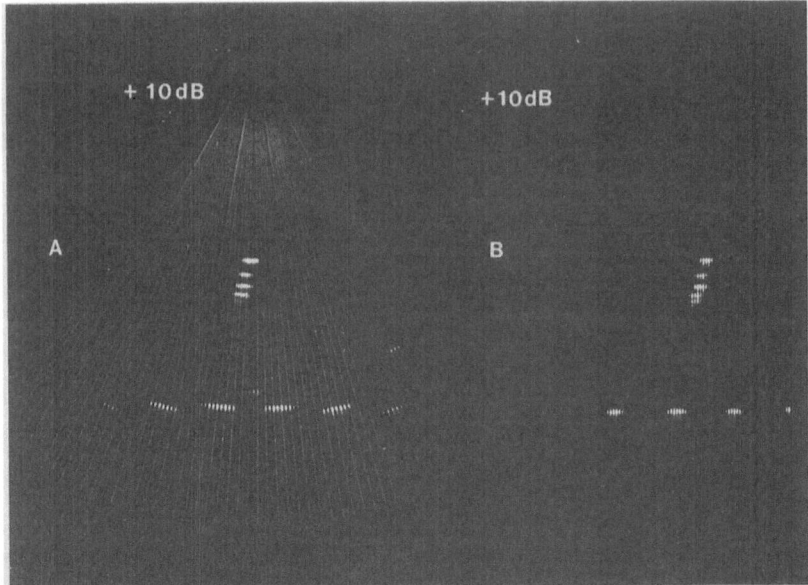

Fig. 10. Results from the AIUM test object as obtained with a system with fixed focus at 7.5 cm (A) and a system with continuous focus (B).

displays the standard relfecting rods as echoes of approximately the same width up to a great depth, while system A tends to distort echoes into a so called "banana" shape at greater depth.

It is important to understand these mechanisms, and to avoid misinterpretation due to these effects.

6. NEW DEVELOPMENTS

A linear array combining dynamic focusing and an extremely high frame rate is proposed in the paper by Delannoy et al. Computer-aided analysis of recorded time-series of cross-sectional images, as presented in the paper by Vogel et al., may provide additional diagnostic value to routine clinical investigations. The future will no doubt bring systems with dynamic lateral resolution also incorporated in the plane perpendicular to the transducer plane. So far, we have only discussed the lateral resolution within the plane of the transducer. The appearance of a real-time linear array with improved imaging of unfavourably oriented structures can be foreseen. This has been described by the author in 1971 (11) with the suggestion that it should also incorporate sets of inclined beams in the linear array method. New developments may also appear in the Doppler field. These may include a real-time, two-dimensional velocity display obtained using a multiplicity of elements and parallel processing techniques.

As Brandestini suggests, a colour display may be necessary to fuse all the data into one comprehensible image.

Although present instruments have already reached a high level of image quality, and the diagnostic importance has been widely recognized, it is to be expected that further improvements will be made.

Several technological developments may give rise to further sophistication of echo instrumentation. The impact of more, low-priced, integrated circuitry, the expected introduction of low-power flat-screen displays, these are just two examples of what the near future may bring. Even instruments with almost entirely automatic operation may soon become a practical reality.

REFERENCES

1. Edler I, CH, Hertz: The use of the ultrasonic reflectoscope for the continuous recording of movements of heart walls. Kungl. Fysiogr. Sällsk. Lund Förhandl 24:5, 1, 1954.
2. Bom N, CT Lancée, J. Honkoop et al.: Ultrasonic viewer for cross-sectional analysis of moving cardiac structures. Bio-med Engng 6:500, 1971.
3. Ligtvoet C, H Rijsterborgh, L Kappen, N Bom: Real-time ultrasonic imaging with a hand-held scanner Part I – Technical description. Ultrasound in Med & Biol, Vol. 4 p 91–92, Pergamon Press, 1978.
4. Roelandt J, JW Wladimiroff, AM Baars: Ultrasonic real-time imaging with a hand-held scanner Part II – Initial clinical experience. Ultrasound in Med & Biol, Vol. 4 p 93–97, Pergamon Press, 1978.
5. Gehrke J: Contribution of real-time B-scan echocardiography to the information about left ventricular outflow tract obstruction in hypertropic cardiomyopathy. 3rd European Congress on Ultrasonics in Medicine, Bologna, October 1–5, 1978.

6. Somer JC: Electronic sector scanning for ultrasonic diagnosis. Progress Report Medisch Physisch Instituut, August: 37–41, 1968.
7. Shaw A, JS Paton, NL Gregory, DJ Wheatley: A real-time 2-dimensional ultrasonic scanner for clinical use. Ultrasonics 14:35, 1976.
8. Thurstone FL, OT von Ramm: Electronic beam scanning for imaging. Ultrasonics in Medicine, Rotterdam, June: 43–48, 1973.
9. Ligtvoet CM, J Ridder, CT Lancée, F Hagemeijer, WB Vletter, WJ Gussenhoven: A dynamically focused multiscan system. In: Echocardiology, Bom N (ed), The Hague, Martinus Nijhoff, 1977, p 313–323.
10. Alais P, M Fink: Fresnel zone focusing of linear arrays applied to B and C echography. Acoustical Holography, Vol. 7 p 509–522, New York/London, Plenum Press, 1976.
11. Bom N: Medical Faculty Rotterdam, Dutch Patent Application nr 7104271 (31 March 1971).

A SIMPLIFIED ULTRASOUND PHASED ARRAY SECTOR SCANNER

C.B. BURCKHARDT, P.-A. GRANDCHAMP, H. HOFFMANN, and R. FEHR

1. INTRODUCTION

The phased array principle was introduced into medical ultrasound by Somer (1) and is now mainly used in two-dimensional echocardiography. In a phased array the ultrasound beam is rotated around the transducer and a sector scan is performed. The transducer typically has a width of 1–2 cm and consists of many elements, usually about 30. The rotation of the ultrasound beam is achieved by emitting the ultrasound pulses from the different elements at different instants and subjecting the received echo signals to delays, which are different for each element of the array. The principles of the ultrasound phased array are well known by now (see e.g. (1). (2)). The difference in delay τ_k between adjacent elements is given by

$$\tau_k = x_k \cdot (\sin \alpha)/c, \tag{1}$$

where x_k is the distance between elements, α is the deflection angle and c is the sound velocity.

The main problem in building an ultrasound phased array is the implementation of the delays of the received analog signals. The delay is different for each element and is also different for each beam direction. This leads to a large number of required delays. A related, although lesser problem, is the implementation of the delays of the transmission pulse. This problem is easier because in this case the signals to be delayed are digital.

This paper describes a simplified implementation of the analog signal delay system including the construction of an instrument based on this principle and the first clinical trials. The following section describes the analog signal delay. Section 3 contains a mathematical analysis of the principle used. The construction of the instrument as well as first clinical trials are described in section 4.

2. SIGNAL DELAY

In this section the simplified method of signal delay will be described. In order to make the method easy to understand we first mention a few essential facts. The maximum signal delay is several micro-seconds as can be seen by inserting typical values into equation (1). The accuracy of the delay has to be a fraction of a temporal period of the ultrasound radiation, typically 1/10 of a

Charles T. Lancée (ed.), Echocardiology, 385–393. All rights reserved
Copyright © 1979 by Martinus Nijhoff Publishers bv, The Hague/Boston/London

period if one wants low spatial sidelobes of the beam. For a typical frequency of 2 MHz the accuracy required is thus 0.05 μsec. This demonstrates that the delay has to be finely quantized. The fine quantization together with the large maximum delay account for the complexity of straightforward solutions, where tapped delay lines are used for delaying the signal.

In search of a simple method of signal delay, one finds that it is much easier to subject a signal to a phase shift than to a true delay and this is often done in phased array radars. The method has been described for a sonar system by Tucker et al. (3). This method can, however, only be used when the pulse duration is considerably greater than the maximum delay. This is not the case in medical ultrasound, where the pulse duration is 1 to 2 μsec and the maximum delay is several microseconds as mentioned before.

The essential idea for simplifying the implementation of the signal delay is to subdivide the total delay into a large, coarsely quantized delay and a small, finely quantized delay. The latter is approximated as a phase shift with an error that is now tolerable. This principle is illustrated in Figure 1. Suppose a pulse with 4 periods has to be delayed by 4.5 periods. Line ① shows the original pulse, line ② the pulse delayed by 4.5 periods. Suppose now that the coarse delay is quantized into integer periods. Therefore a delay of half a period has to be approximated by a phase shift of 180°. Line ③ of Figure 1 shows the original pulse shifted by 180° and line ④ shows the pulse which is shifted by 180° and delayed by 4 periods. Comparing line ② and line ④ we see that there is some error associated with this method which should, however, be tolerable.

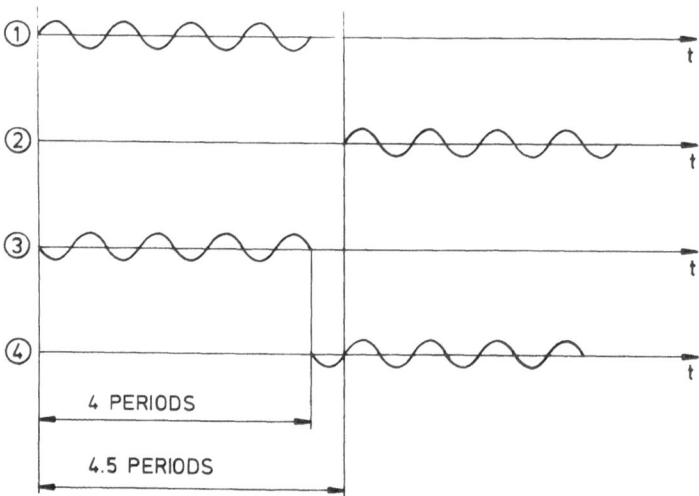

Fig. 1. Comparison of a true delay by 4.5 periods and the approximation.
  ①   Original pulse
  ②   Pulse delayed by 4.5 periods
  ③   Pulse phase shifted by 180°
  ④   Pulse phase shifted by 180° and delayed by 4 periods.

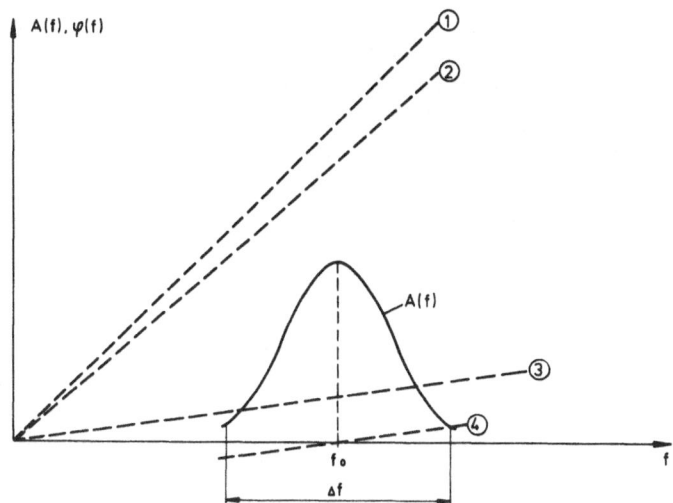

Fig. 2. Illustration for determining the error of the approximation in the frequency domain.
  ① Phase corresponding to the true delay
  ② Phase corresponding to the large, coarsely quantized delay
  ③ Phase error for the large coarsely quantized delay
  ④ Phase error for the large coarsely quantized delay combined with a phase shift.

We want to investigate the error of this approximation a little more closely. This is easily done in the frequency domain. Figure 2 shows the spectrum of a pulse centered at frequency f_0. It is well known that a delay of the pulse by the amount τ corresponds to multiplication of the spectrum with a phase factor. The phase is given by $\varphi(f) = 2\pi f\tau$. The straight line ① shows the phase corresponding to the true delay. Straight line ② shows the phase corresponding to the large coarsely quantized delay. The difference between the two gives the phase error ③. This phase error would be unacceptably large. It is, however, reduced to zero at the center frequency f_0 by means of the phase shift. The phase shift is constant over the frequency band and we are left with a residual phase error given by straight line ④. This phase error $\Delta\varphi$ is given by

$$\Delta\varphi = 2\pi\Delta\tau(f - f_0), \qquad (2)$$

where $\Delta\tau$ is the delay which is approximated by a phase shift. The error is largest at the band edges, where it is given by

$$\Delta\varphi_{\max} = 2\pi\Delta\tau(\Delta f/2) = \pi\Delta\tau\Delta f, \qquad (3)$$

where Δf is the bandwidth of the pulse. We therefore obtain for the maximum delay $\Delta\tau$ that can be approximated by a phase shift

$$\Delta\tau_{\max} = \Delta\varphi_{\max}/(\pi\Delta f). \qquad (4)$$

The possible quantization of the coarse delay is $2\,\Delta\tau_{\max}$, because the phase shift can be positive as well as negative. As an example suppose we have a bandwidth $\Delta f = 1$ MHz and accept a maximum phase error of $\pi/4$ at the band edges. We then obtain $\Delta\tau_{max} = 0.25$ μsec. This means that the large delay can be quantized into 0.5 μsec steps. At 2 MHz this corresponds to one period.

A particularly convenient means of obtaining a phase shift is by means of a mixer circuit as already pointed out in Ref. (3). The phase shift is then determined by the phase of the local oscillator signal. Figure 3 shows an implementation of the principles discussed so far for 4 transducer elements. Each transducer element is connected to a mixer. The mixer outputs are connected together in pairs. This is possible because the difference in delays is so small that they can always be connected to the same tap of the delay line. The mixer outputs are low pass filtered and connected to a bus via a demultiplexer. Each line of the bus is connected to a tap of the delay line. Note that only one delay line is used for the whole phased array.

A further attractive feature of this scheme should be pointed out. The signal which passes through the delay line has a lower frequency than the original signal. The upper frequency limit of the delay line therefore can be lower than that of a delay line which would delay the original signal. The delay of the transmission pulse is implemented in a very similar way. In this case an envelope with a coarsely quantized delay is multiplied with a continuous pulse train which has a finely quantized delay. A more detailed description of the generation of the transmission pulse will be given in section 4. A block diagram of the circuits required for each transducer element will be given in that section.

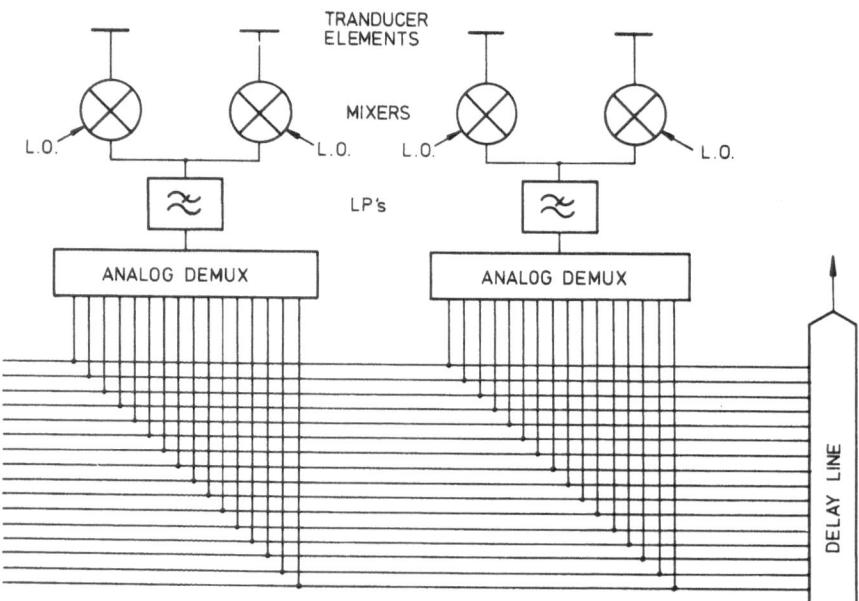

Fig. 3. Combination of phase shift and delay shown here for 4 elements of a phased array.

3. ANALYSIS OF THE SYSTEM

We will now analyse the system described in the last section. As a result of this analysis we will obtain the phase of the local oscillator signal as well as some rules for choosing the intermediate frequency and tap spacing of the delay line. Suppose we receive an echo signal $s_0(t)$

$$s_0(t) = a(t + \tau) \cos \omega_0(t + \tau). \tag{5}$$

This signal has its origin at $t = -\tau$. It must now be delayed by the amount τ such that its origin will be at $t = 0$. τ can be written as an integer number l of periods plus a fraction of a period,

$$\tau = l/f_0 + \vartheta_0, \text{ where } \vartheta_0 < 1/f_0 \tag{6}$$

and $2\pi f_0 = \omega_0$.

We can therefore write the echo signal $s_0(t)$ as

$$s_0(t) = a(t + \tau)\cos(\omega_0 t + \varphi_0) \tag{7}$$

with $\varphi_0 = \omega_0 \vartheta_0 = 2\pi f_0 \vartheta_0$. $\tag{8}$

We now mix this signal with a local oscillator signal $\cos(\omega_1 t + \varphi_1)$. After a low pass filtering we obtain the lower sideband $s_2(t)$

$$s_2(t) = a(t + \tau) \cos \left[(\omega_1 - \omega_0) t + \varphi_1 - \varphi_0\right]$$
$$= a(t + \tau) \cos (\omega_2 t + \varphi_1 - \varphi_0), \tag{9}$$

where $\omega_2 = \omega_1 - \omega_0$ $\tag{10}$

is the intermediate frequency. We now have a tapped delay line with a delay T between taps. In this delay line the signal $s_2(t)$ is delayed by $n \cdot T$ (n integer) and we obtain the delayed signal $s_{2d}(t)$

$$s_{2d}(t) = a(t + \tau - nT) \cos \left[\omega_2(t - nT) + \varphi_1 - \varphi_0\right]. \tag{11}$$

We now have

$$\omega_2 nT = m \cdot 2\pi + \varphi_2, \tag{12}$$

where m is an integer and therefore

$$s_{2d}(t) = a(t + \tau - nT) \cos (\omega_2 t - \varphi_2 + \varphi_1 - \varphi_0). \tag{13}$$

Since we want the origin of the delayed signal to be at zero we have

$$-\varphi_2 + \varphi_1 - \varphi_0 = 0. \tag{14}$$

We therefore obtain for the phase φ_1 of the local oscillator signal

$$\varphi_1 = 2\pi f_2 T \cdot n + \varphi_0 \quad \text{modulo } 2\pi \tag{15}$$

or $\qquad \varphi_1 = n\Phi + \varphi_0 \qquad \text{modulo } 2\pi, \tag{16}$

where $\Phi = 2\pi f_2 T$ (17)

is the phase shift that the signal suffers at the intermediate frequency when it is delayed one tap spacing in the delay line. n is chosen such that the delay in the delay line is as close as possible to the delay wanted,

$$|\tau - nT| \leq T/2$$ (18)

and $n = \text{int}\left(\dfrac{\tau}{T} + 1/2\right),$ (19)

where int ( ) stands for truncation to the next smaller integer.

We now want to show how the intermediate frequency f_2 and the tap spacing T are chosen to give a practical system. For practical reasons the phase φ_1 of the local oscillator signal is quantized into steps of $2\pi/m$, m integer. Therefore Φ in equation (17) should be made a multiple of such a step

$$\Phi = k \cdot 2\pi/m; \; k, \, m \text{ integers.}$$ (20)

Therefore from equation (17)

$$T = k/(mf_2).$$ (21)

Since we approximate the original delay τ by a sum of a delay and a phase shift it is practical if the delay T between taps is an integer multiple or submultiple of the original period

$$T = K/f_0, \text{ where } K = 1, 2, 3, \dots$$ (22)
$$\text{or} \quad K = 1/2, 1/3, \dots$$

Combining equations (21) and (22) we obtain

$$f_2/f_0 = k/(m \cdot K).$$ (23)

We want to illustrate this with some numerical data. Suppose the ultrasound frequency $f_0 = 2\text{MHz}$ and the bandwidth $\Delta f = 1$ MHz. As already discussed in the last section this leads to $T = 0.5$ μsec for a tolerable phase error at the band edges. Therefore $K = 1$ in equation (22). The phase of the local oscillator signal is quantized into 45° steps in order to keep the phase error small, i.e. $m = 8$. We, therefore, obtain for equation (23)

$$f_2/f_0 = k/8 \text{ or } f_2 = (k/8)f_0$$ (24)

Therefore we obtain the following possible values of f_2

$$f_2 = 0.25, \, 0.5, \, 0.75, \, 1, \dots \text{ MHz.}$$ (25)

The first value is too low because of the bandwidth of 1 MHz, the next value is possible, but has the disadvantage that the lower band edge lies at D.C. The most suitable values would be 0.75 and 1 MHz. For an intermediate frequency $f_2 = 1$ MHz we obtain for equation (16)

$$\varphi_1 = \varphi_0 + n \cdot \pi \text{ modulo } 2\pi.$$ (26)

In this case the phase φ_1 of the local oscillator is equal to the phase φ_0 of the echo signal for a delay through an even number of tap spacings and is equal to $\varphi_0 + \pi$ for delay through an odd number of tap spacings.

4. DESCRIPTION OF AN ACTUAL SYSTEM

A system was built according to the principle described so far. The following data were chosen as design goals:

Ultrasound frequency f_0:   2 MHz
Maximum deflection angle: $\pm 35°$
Number of beam directions: 128
Transducer width: 20.8 mm
Number of elements: 32
Pulse length: 2 μsec ($\Delta f = 1$ MHz)

From this we compute the following data:

Width of a transducer element: 0.65 mm
Maximum delay between two adjacent transducer elements: 0.25 μsec
Maximum delay between element 0 and element 31:   7.75 μsec

The following data were determined according to the considerations in the last section:

phase quantization of the local oscillator signal: $45°$ ... m = 8
tap spacing T: 0.5 μsec
intermediate frequency f_2:   1 MHz

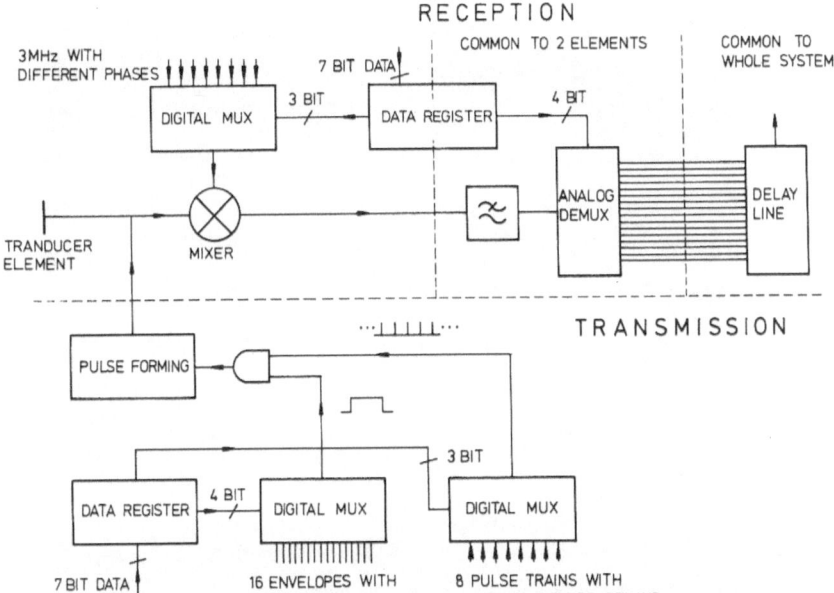

Fig. 4. Block diagram of the transmit/receive circuit of one transducer element.

The principle of delay and phase shift was already shown in Figure 3. Figure 4 shows the block diagram of the circuit necessary for each transducer element. The local oscillator signal is selected from signals with eight different phases by a digital multiplexer. The signal is low-pass filtered and applied to an analog demultiplexer which connects it to the appropriate tap of the delay

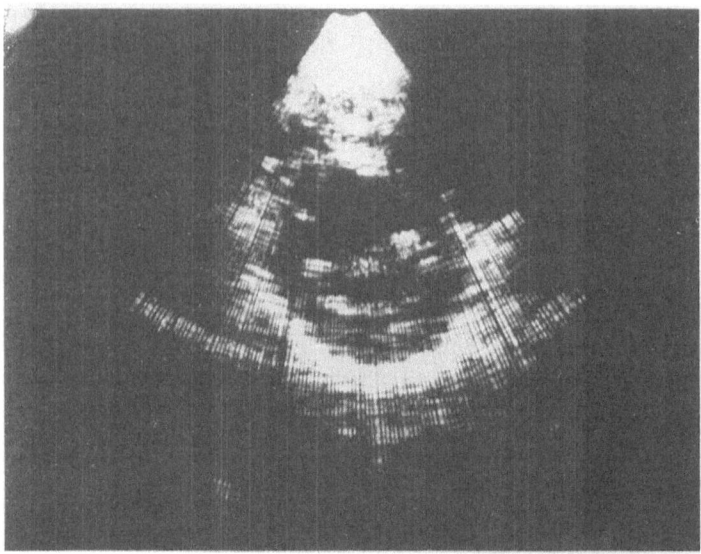

Fig. 5. Cross-section of a normal heart in the plane of the mitral valve.

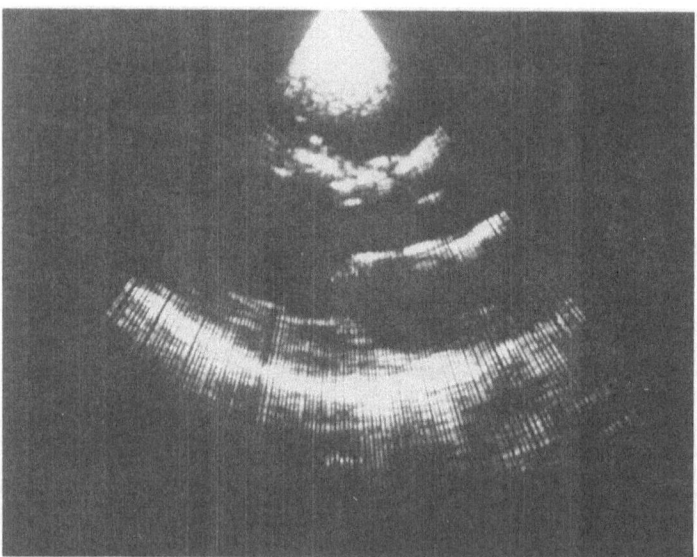

Fig. 6. Longitudinal section of a normal heart. The mitral valve as well as the aortic valve are visible.

line. The transmission pulse is generated by multiplying a continuous pulse train selected from eight different pulse trains with finely quantized delays with an envelope signal which is selected from 16 different envelope signals with coarsely quantized delays. This product is passed through an impulse forming network and applied to the transducer element. All the multiplexers are controlled by data stored in data registers. The data registers are loaded before the transmission of each pulse. The data for all the registers of the whole system are computed in a central special purpose computing unit. An additional phase shift is added to achieve weak focussing of the beam. The computation of all the data for one beam direction takes 8.5 μsec. A particular feature of the instrument is that the width of the active area is gradually increased during the reception period, i.e. for close reflectors the outer elements are inactive. The rest of the system like control unit, swept gain amplifier, display control follow design principles known from other ultrasound systems and are not described here.

The following experimental results were obtained with this system, except that the transducer only had a width of 12.8 mm and an element width of 0.4 mm. Figure 5 shows a cross-section of a normal heart at the height of the mitral valve. Figure 6 shows a longitudinal section of a normal heart. The mitral valve as well as the aortic valve are visible.

The authors would like to acknowledge the very competent experimental assistance of H.R. Wolf, P. Bauer and W. Schultz. They would like to thank Dr. D. Burckhardt and Dr. E. Grube for clinical evaluation.

REFERENCES

1. Somer JC: Electronic sector scanning for ultrasonic diagnosis. Ultrasonics 6:153, 1968.
2. Thurstone FL, OT von Ramm: Electronic beam scanning for ultrasonic imaging. In: Ultrasonics in medicine. de Vlieger M et al. (eds), Excerpta Medica, Amsterdam, 1974, p 43–48.
3. Tucker DG, VG Welsby, R Kendell: Electronic sector scanning, J Brit IRE 18:465, 1958.

ULTRASONIC ARRAY DESIGN
AND PERFORMANCE

PH. DEFRANOULD and J. SOUQUET

INTRODUCTION

Acoustical imaging obeys the fundamental laws of optics. When an object is visualized with a given system (optical or acoustical) the image obtained is the convolution of the object and the system transfer function. This is exactly what takes place when acoustical signals, reflected from a biological structure, are received by an array of transducers. The signals obtained from the transducers contain the image of the structure convolved with transfer function of both array and propagation medium. In order to reconstruct the original image, one must either perform a deconvolution (i.e. convolution with the inverse function of the system) or use a device whose transfer function does not affect convolution (e.g. a Dirac function). Deconvolution is more difficult to achieve if the number of processed points is large (high-resolution image) and if fast processing is required (real-time). An easier solution is to use a system whose transfer function is as close as possible to a Dirac function, i.e. has a broad spatial and temporal bandwidth. It is this type of approach that we have considered in this paper.

The first part of the paper describes theoretical simulations of the radiation pattern of a linear array for which focusing, beam-steering and beam-shaping can be achieved by driving each element in the array separately (1) (2). For arrays excited by short pulses, the radiation pattern can be significantly different from that obtained with narrow bandwidth radiation. We shall show two-dimensional maps of the pressure field (sagittal plane) as a function of time, based on a theory valid in the near field as well as in the far field. Special attention will be paid to the grating lobes and side-lobes and to the effects of spacing and width of elements, phase and group delay and amplitude weighting.

The simulation shows that, to get an appropriate radiation pattern, the single element transducer must have a "beam" structure with a rectangular radiating surface (small width to obtain wide angular sensitivity) acting as a perfect piston source, well coupled to water-load. We use a quarter-wave matching layer in order to obtain a broad bandwidth. The excitation of this structure by a short pulse applied to the radiating electrode (electric field parallel to thickness) gives rise to deformation in three dimensions, and no simple analytic expressions can be derived for the vibration modes. The determination of the transient response is a non-trivial problem. It can only be derived using a numerical method such as the "Finite Element" (FE) method, which requires considerable computational facilities. So, the second part of this paper is devoted to the theoretical and experimental study of the transient response of a multilayered "beam" transducer, for which we derive an analytical solution for the one-dimensional approximation.

These studies led us to build linear arrays working at 2.5 MHz. We shall describe performance and results for a 48-element array, designed for a dynamic focusing and steering system.

THEORETICAL SIMULATION OF THE RADIATION PATTERN OF A LINEAR ARRAY

The principle of the computation is shown in Figure 1. We have reduced the problem to a two-dimensional one. We assume that all the elements emit a plane wave, with uniform amplitude, limited by the lateral dimension (W) of an element (thickness expander mode). The pressure in M is the sum of all the pressures of all the emitters propagating along d_i. We have assumed the propagation medium to be isotropic and uniform. The total acoustic pressure is then given by (cylindrical case)

$$F(x, z, t) = \frac{\rho v}{\sqrt{\lambda x}} \sum_{-N}^{N} A_i W_i \frac{\sin \Omega_i}{\Omega_i} R_i(\tau_i)\, e^{j\omega \tau_i},$$

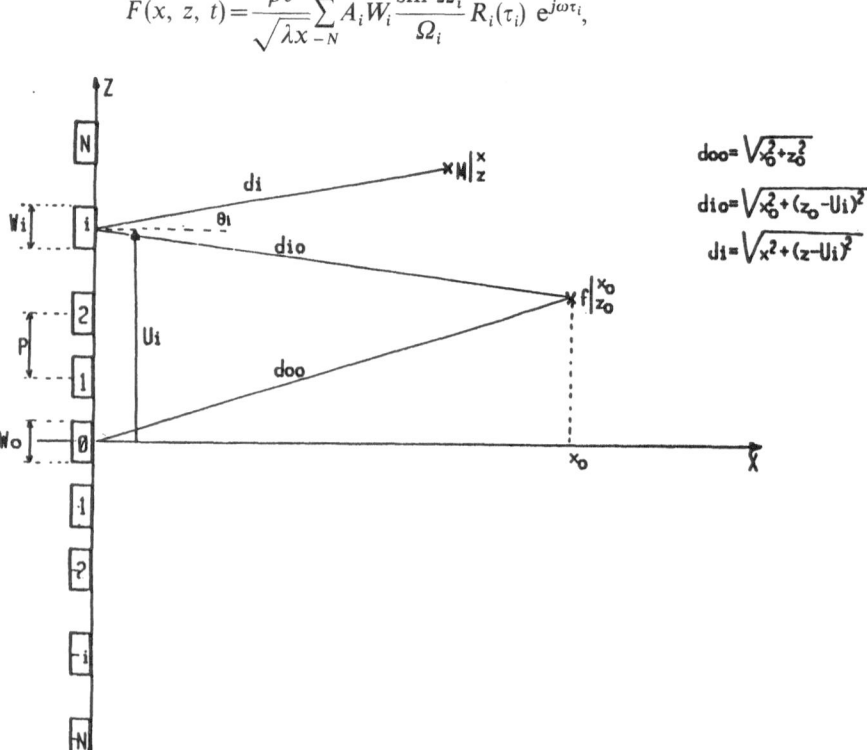

$$d_{oo} = \sqrt{x_0^2 + z_0^2}$$

$$d_{io} = \sqrt{x_0^2 + (z_0 - U_i)^2}$$

$$d_i = \sqrt{x^2 + (z - U_i)^2}$$

Fig. 1.   Schematic arrangement of the array focused at $f(X_0, Z_0)$.

where A_i and R_i (τ_i) are, respectively, the pressure amplitude and the pulse envelope at the emitter i, and

$$\Omega_i = \pi W_i \sin \theta_i / \lambda, \qquad \tau_i = t - d_i / v,$$

ω, v and $\lambda = 2\pi v / \omega$ are the frequency, the velocity and the wavelength in the propagation medium, respectively.

The following results were obtained, assuming a frequency of 2.5 MHz, water as the propagation medium and a wavelength equal to 0.6 mm ($v = 1500$ m/sec).

Figure 2 shows the modulus of the pressure field for a 24-element array

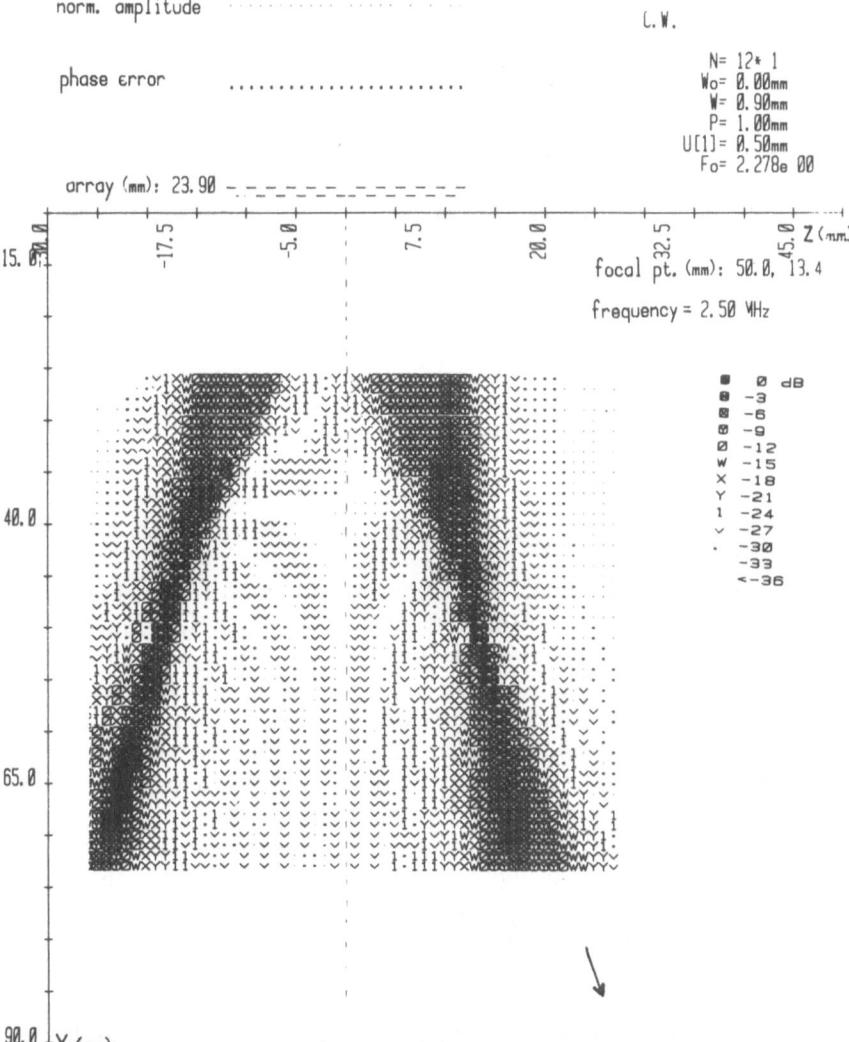

Fig. 2. Modulus of the pressure field in X, Z plane of a 24-element linear array (Periodicity of 1 mm, spacing 0.1 mm) focused at a point $f(50, 13.4$ mm) CW mode.

with a 1 mm periodicity (p). All the transducers are identical, with a width of 0.9 mm. The applied continuous wave (CW) signal on each of the elements is so phased (φ_i) that the focus is located 50 mm in front of the array, and 15° away from the axis. We have visualized the acoustic pressure level (in dB referred to the value at focus) by using a series of letters whose grey scale decreases from the highest value to the lowest one. The amplitude applied to each transducer is uniform. There is no phase error (the phase error being defined as the deviation from the theoretical quadratic law). This result is the well-known focus figure with -13 dB side lobes and grating lobes due to the array periodicity p being greater than wavelength $\lambda (p/\lambda = 1.6)$. These grating lobes, which are only a few dB down as compared with the main lobe, can be eliminated by using higher spatial sampling ($p/\lambda \leqq 1$). In addition, the side lobes can be decreased by using amplitude weighing.

Figure 3 shows the result obtained for a 48-element array with an element spacing of 0.5 mm ($p/\lambda \cong 0.8$). We used a Hamming function for amplitude weighing, as shown at the top of Figure 3.

In order to obtain adequate resolution in the direction of propagation, short pulses have to be used, which allows us to obtain a point pressure distribution in 2 dimensions. Figure 4 shows the point pressure-amplitude distribution visualized for different travel times. Reference time has been taken at the exact time the pulse reaches the focal point. It should be noted that, to go from a CW excitation to a pulsed one, we assumed that the transducers have a bandwidth at least equal to the frequency spectrum of a 1 μsec pulse. We also assumed that the transducer transfer function had a Gaussian form, with a 1 MHz bandwidth at -3 dB.

The transducer arrangement we have just described is optimal, but it is difficult to construct, because a great many independent transmitters with time delay and programmable amplitude are needed, in order to achieve dynamic focusing.

Figure 5 shows the results of a 24-element array excited with short pulses. The element periodicity is, in this case, 1 mm ($p/\lambda \cong 1.6$). The Figure shows that use of a 1 μsec pulse reduces the grating lobe as it is now 15 dB down when compared with the main lobe (it was 3 dB down in the CW case). For a 2 μsec pulse, the grating lobe is 9 dB down and for a 3 μsec pulse it is only 6 dB down. However, the results are better if the focal point is on the axis: with the same periodicity, the grating lobes are then 24 dB down for a 1 μsec pulse duration.

The electronic implementation of phase-delay is simpler than of time-delay, and we will now investigate the differences between the two techniques in order to determine the degradation in phase-delay systems. All the above results were obtained with time-delay, which means that temporal coincidence is achieved at the focal point. In phase-delay, the pulses are simultaneously applied to all transducers, but the phase is delayed for each pulse in order to achieve phase coincidence at the focal point. The limiting condition for phase-delay is that, at the focal point, the transmitted pulses of all elements at least partially overlap in time.

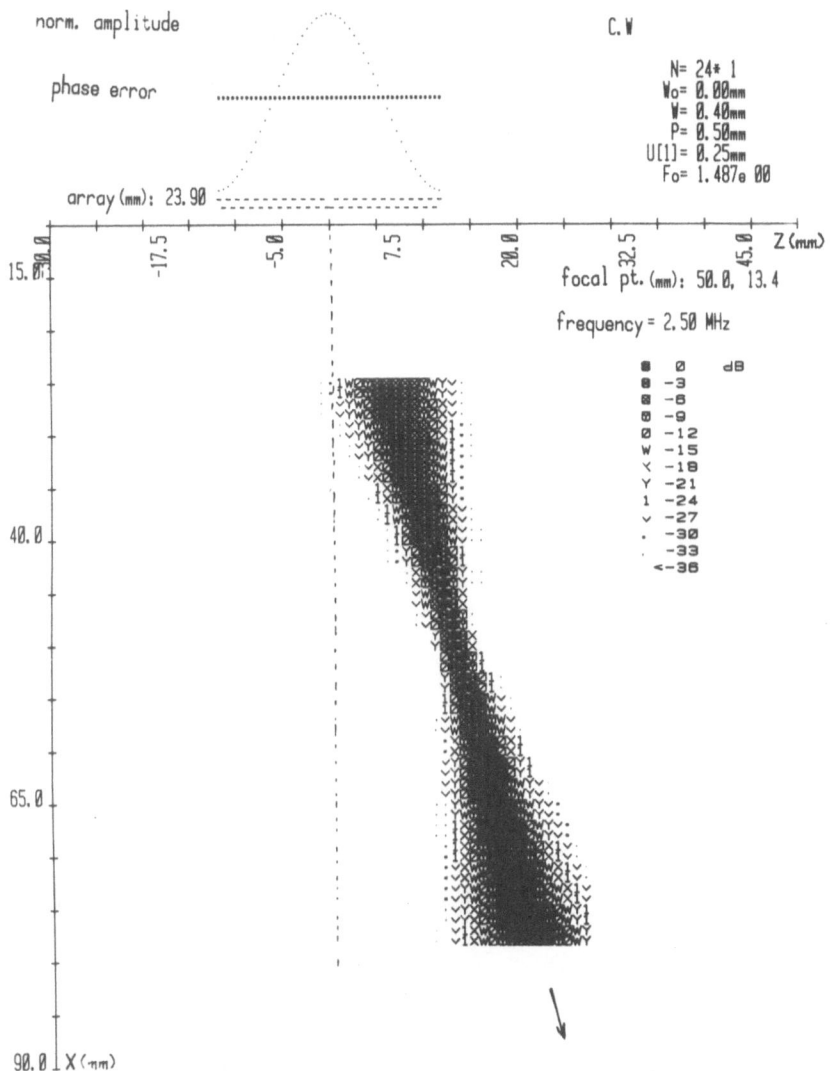

Fig. 3. Modulus of the pressure field in *X, Z* plane of a 48-element linear array (periodicity of 0.5 mm spacing 0.1 mm) focused at a point *f*(50, 13.4 mm) – CW mode.

Figure 6 shows an example of a phase-delay system with a 1 μsec pulse. The parameters are identical to those of Figure 4, but with phase-delay instead of time-delay. At the focal point we can see a widening of the main lobe by a factor of 2 to 3, with a loss in sensitivity of 6 dB (12 dB transmit-receive).

Finally, we investigated the influence of phase and amplitude errors. As a matter of fact, we need to know the tolerances associated with a good response. We introduced random errors in phase and amplitude into the program (3). The maximum distorsion for the phase is about 36° ($\lambda/10$), for

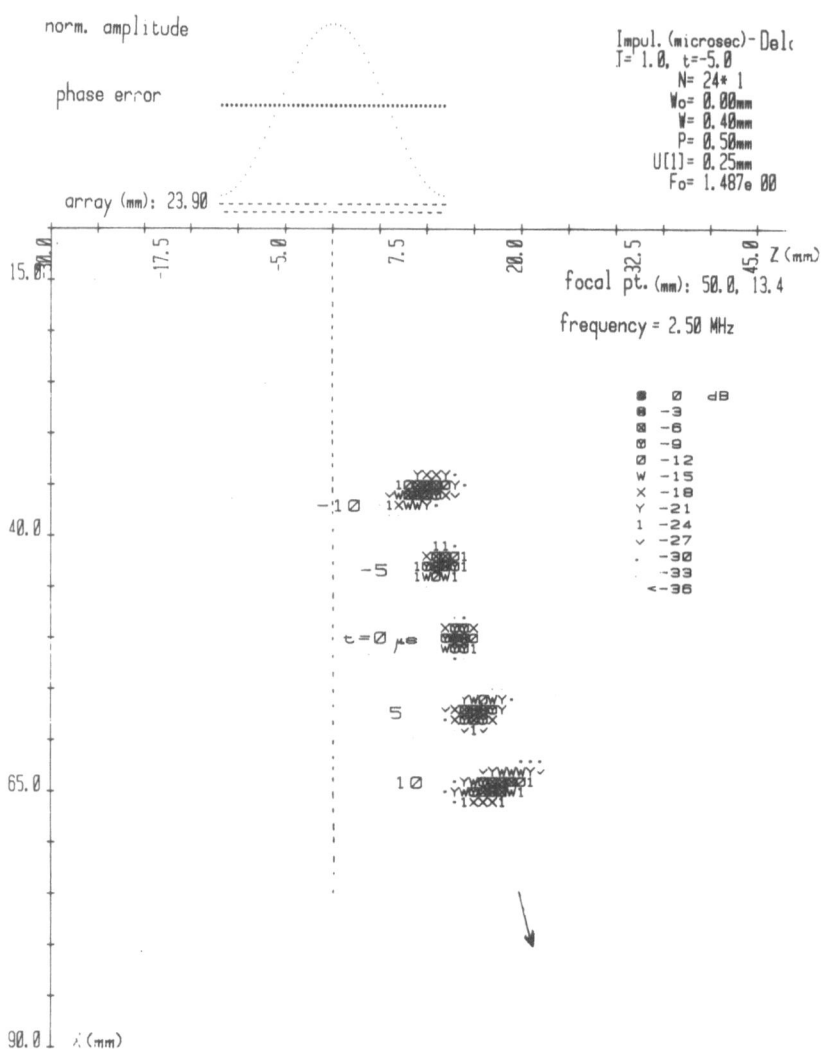

Fig. 4. Modulus of the pressure field in *X, Z* plane at different travel times in pulse mode (same array as Figure 3). Pulse duration is 1 μsec, reference time is taken at focal point.

the amplitude it is ±1.5 dB. In Figure 7 we can see some parasitic signals, 27 dB down in relation to the main lobe.

The main conclusions from this simulation study are:

1. Grating lobe cancellation:
   - Off-axis focusing: $p/\lambda < 1$ is required; $p/\lambda < 0.5$ for large deflection angle ($>45°$)
   - On-axis focusing: $p/\lambda < 2$ could be used; small element spacing is required.
2. Secondary lobe reduction:
   - By amplitude weighing.

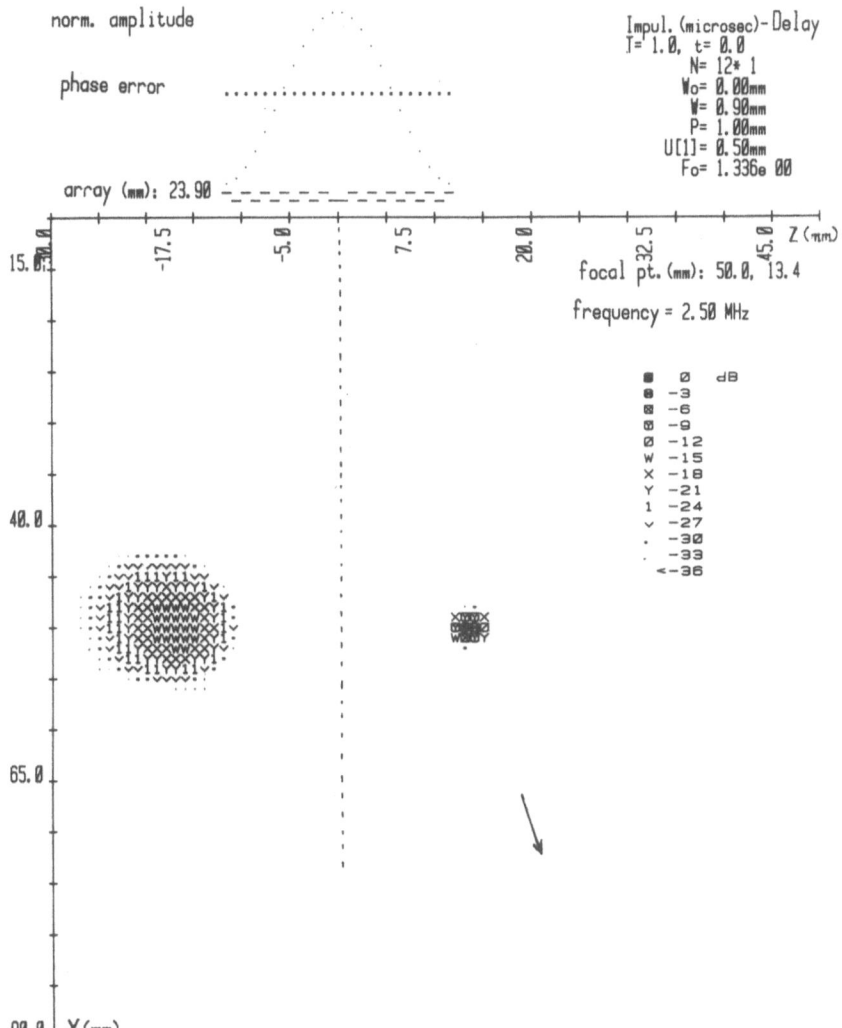

Fig. 5. Modulus of the pressure field impulse mode at focal point travel time (same array as Figure 2 but with amplitude weighing). Pulse duration is 1 μsec.

    – With "Hamming" weighing, secondary lobes are 35 dB below (−70 transmit-receive) the main lobe, increasing the main lobe width by a factor 1.4.

3. Pulse mode:
    – "Phase" system could not be used to design devices having a temporal resolution lower than 4 or 5 wavelengths; in other words, it could only be used with angular aperture $< \pm 5°$ (to obtain range resolution identical to lateral resolution).
    – "Group delay" system must be used for an array with greater aperture.

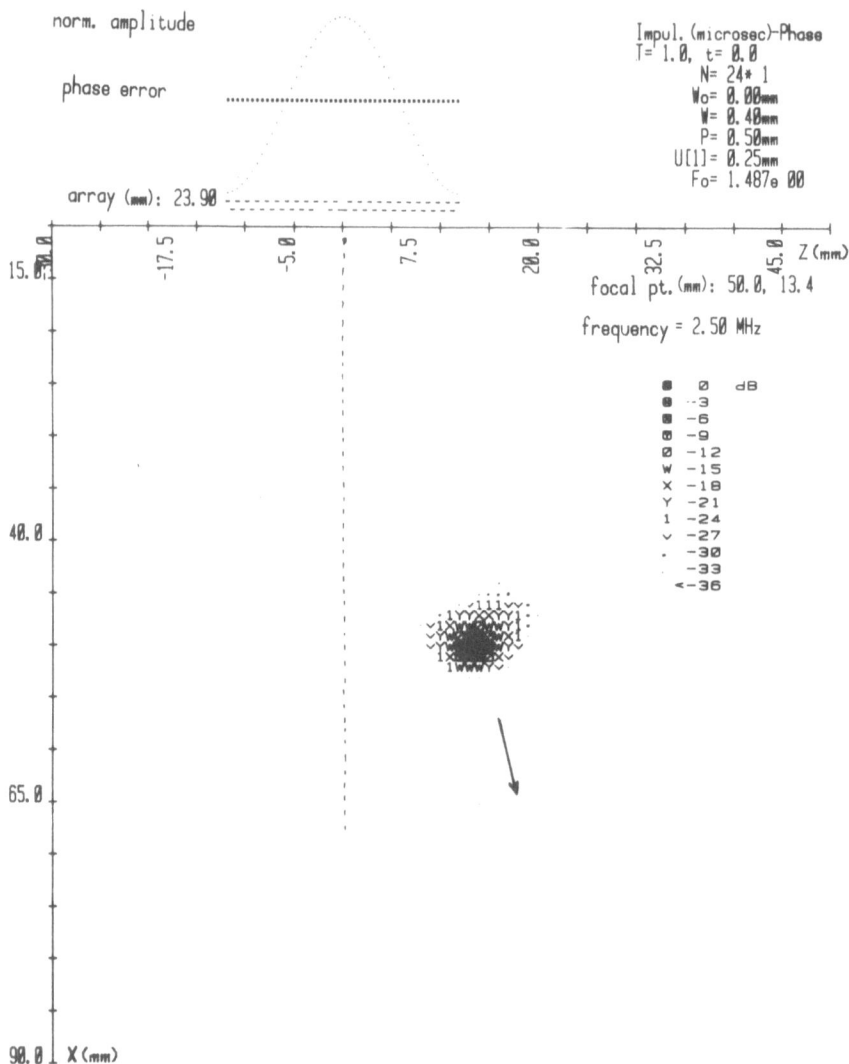

Fig. 6. Modulus of the pressure field in pulse mode at focal point travel time. Same as Figure 4 but with "phase delay" instead of "time delay" driving pulse.

4. Phase and amplitude errors:
   $\Delta\varphi$ of $36°(\lambda/10)$ and ΔA of ± 1.5 dB keep the spurious signals at least of 20 dB below (-40 dB transmit-receive) in CW, lower still in pulse mode (depending on pulse duration).

TRANSIENT RESPONSE OF SINGLE ELEMENT TRANSDUCER

The single transducer used for the previous simulation was a rectangular bar (Figure 8), and we assumed that it acted as a perfect rectangular piston expander source, well coupled to water-load, within which it generated a

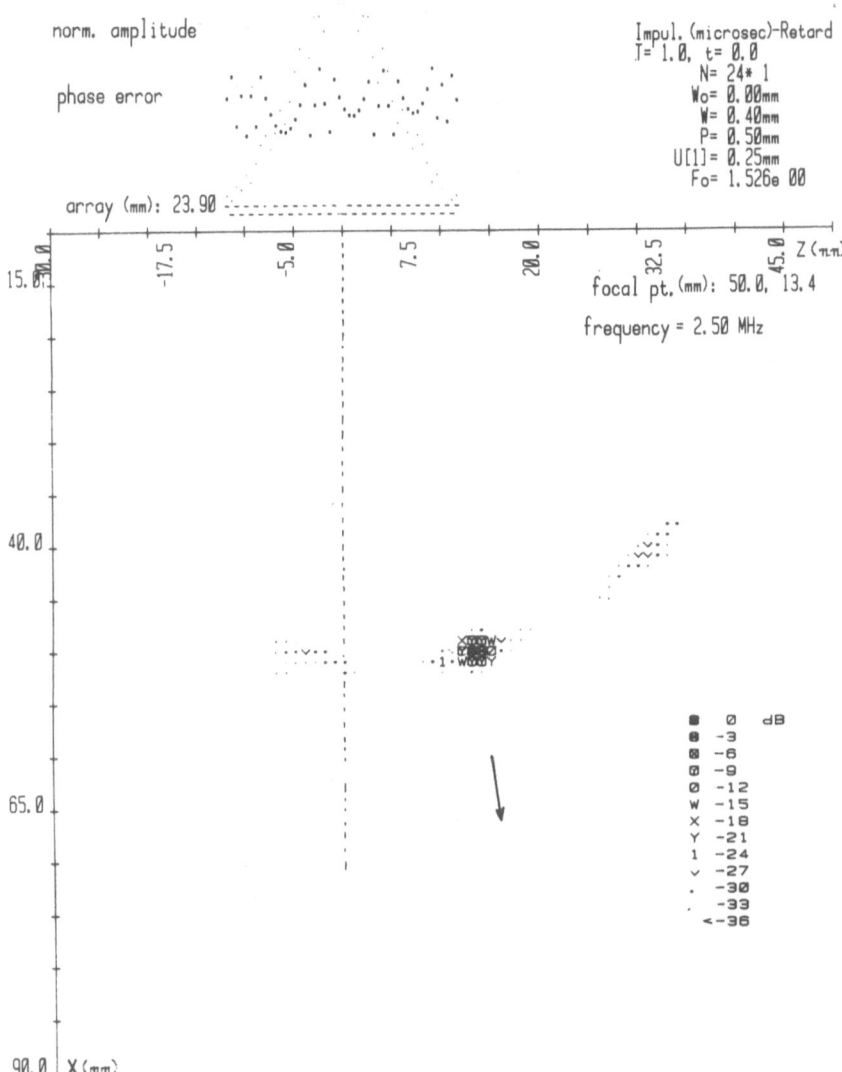

Fig. 7. Modulus of the pressure field in pulse mode at focal point travel time. Same array as Figure 3 but with amplitude and phase error as indicated at the top of the figure.

pressure wave. As a matter of fact, when we drive this structure with a pulse applied to the radiating electrode, the electric field parallel to the thickness gives rise to deformations in three dimensions. We can see in Figure 8 one example of deformation for a normal mode calculated by the FE method (4), in the simple case of a free rectangular ceramic bar. This drawing shows results for two 1/8 segments of the bar, the other sections are obtained by symmetry. Two examples are shown: the first resembles a length plate mode (third harmonic), the second a thickness expansion mode (fundamental), which is the closest mode to the piston mode we need. Anyway, these

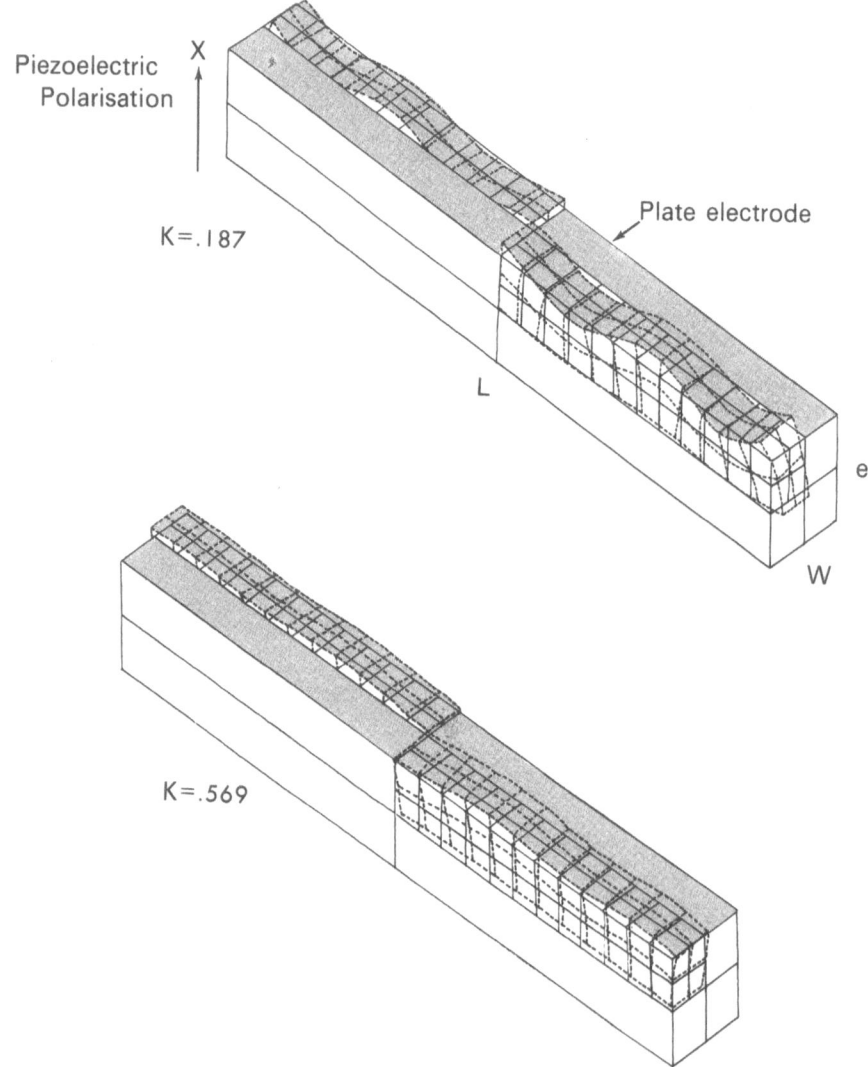

Fig. 8. Two normal modes of vibration calculated by the FE method, for a rectangular PZT ceramic bar with electric field parallel to thickness.

deformations are not very close to the assumption of a perfect rectangular piston expansion source. In fact, the deformation pattern results from reflections appearing on the six fases of the bar. When the length of the bar is large ($L \gg W, e$), as in our case, the reflection on the small bottom faces may be ignored and we can reduce the problem from three to two dimensions. Although this case is simpler, we still have to use the complex time-consuming FE method to obtain the deformation of the structure. The dispersion curves have therefore been plotted experimentally for a PZT ceramic type. These curves show normalized frequencies versus the width to thickness ratio, and we see that the only way to get a non-dispersive expensional mode without lateral modes, is to work with $W/e < 1$ (see Fig. 9). In this case, the front face displacement of the element acts like a perfect piston and all the electrical energy can be transferred to acoustic energy, launched as a pressure wave in the water load. The frequency is independent of width and is now only a function of thickness. So, the problem is reduced to a one-dimensional one and analytical solutions can be derived.

In summary, the "beam" structure, which is defined by the two conditions

$$L \gg W, e$$
$$W/e < 1$$

is a very helpful one for array design because, firstly, it corresponds to a

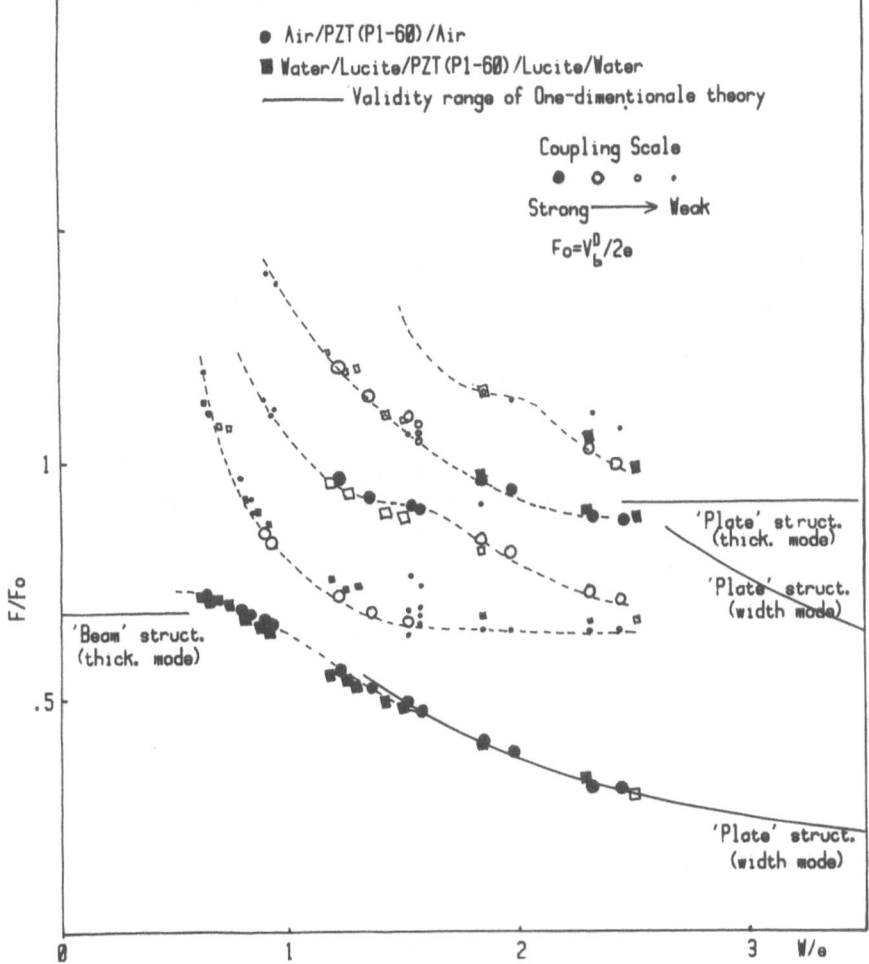

Fig. 9. Transducer normalized frequency versus width to thickness ratio (W/e) for PZT rectangular shaped ceramics.

broad bandwidth, high frequency and broad angular acceptance acoustic
bulk wave generation and, secondly, analytical solutions can be easily
derived. The analysis of this one-dimensional transducer can be made by
following the Mason analysis (5) and the equivalent circuit of Figure 10 can
be derived with the following parameters (6) (7):

$$\varepsilon'_{33} = \varepsilon^T_{33}(1 - K^2_{31})(1 - K'^2_{31})$$

$$K'_{33} = (K_{33} - BK_{31})/\sqrt{(1 - B^2)(1 - K^2_{31})}$$

$$h'_{33} = K'^2_{33}/d_{33} \ (1 - K'^2_{33})(1 - BK_{31}/K_{33})$$

$$v^D_b = 1/\sqrt{ps^E_{33}(1 - B^2)(1 - K'^2_{33})}$$

$$\text{with } B = s^E_{33}/\sqrt{s^E_{11}s^E_{33}}$$

the other parameters having the usual meaning. Front and back layers can be
taken into account in this equivalent circuit in which they act as a transmission line. So, the response of such a structure (transfer function, electrical
impedance ....) can be calculated in the same classical way as a multilayer
plate-mode bulk wave transducer. In particular, broad bandwidth is achieved
using the quarter-wave layer matching technique. We showed (8) that, for a
one layer structure, the optimum acoustic impedance of the layer is:

$$Z = \sqrt[3]{2Z_T Z^2_L}$$

Z_T: transducer impedance and Z_L: load impedance.

For this optimum impedance, the theoretical bandwidth is greater than
50% for a ceramic PZT transducer loaded by water. The high efficiency is
achieved by minimization of the energy lost by the rear face. This has been
done by using an unmatched backing, which could be realized in two ways:

– low impedance backing $Z_B \lesssim 2.10^6$ kg/m²/sec.
– high impedance backing unmatched by a quarter-wave layer.

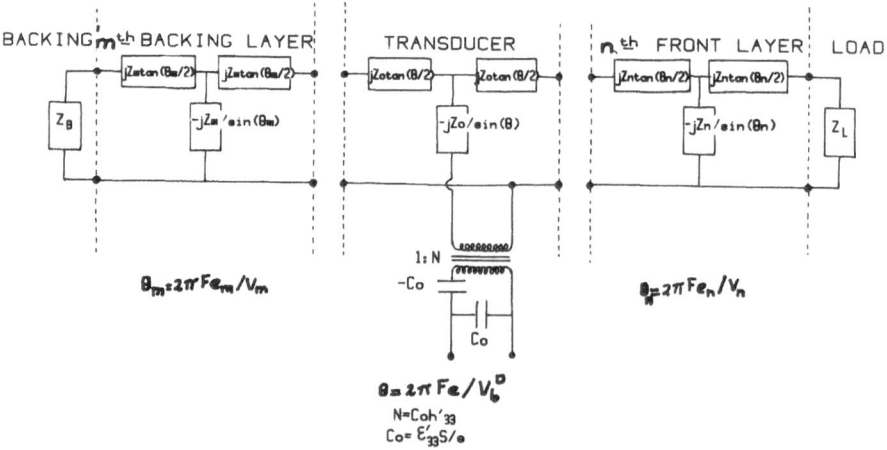

Fig. 10. Multilayer transducer equivalent circuit.

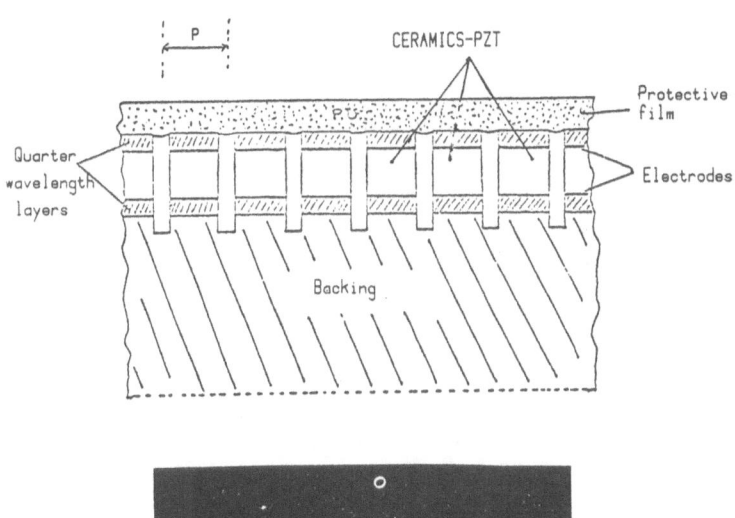

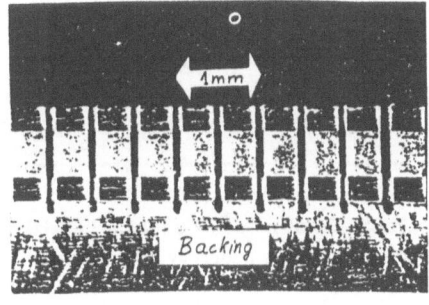

Fig. 11. Schematic arrangement of the "multilayer" multi-element array structure.

These two backing structures are equivalent from the point of view of the transducer efficiency; the choice between the two depends mainly on the availability of suitable materials which also have adequate mechanical rigidity and acoustic absorption in order to eliminate spurious signals caused by reflected energy inside the backing material.

This analysis led us to the design of a multilayer multi-element structure which is shown on Figure 11. The piezoelectric ceramic is coupled to the propagation medium with a quarter-wave layer and a second one decouples the ceramic from a heavy backing. One multilayer structure has been built, bonding two plexiglass layers on each side of a PZT ceramic with a stainless steel backing (photograph of Fig. 11). The cutting of the individual elements uses a multiwire saw, which provides a spacing between elements of about 0.1 mm. The layers are cut, right through as can be seen on Figure 11, and the front face of the structure is then covered with a protective polyurethane film, which traps air between adjacent elements. This technique minimizes electro-acoustic cross-coupling between elements. At 2.5 MHz, the typical dimensions are:

- ceramic thickness $\quad\quad\quad e = 0.56$ mm
- array periodicity $\quad\quad\quad\quad p = 0.50$ mm

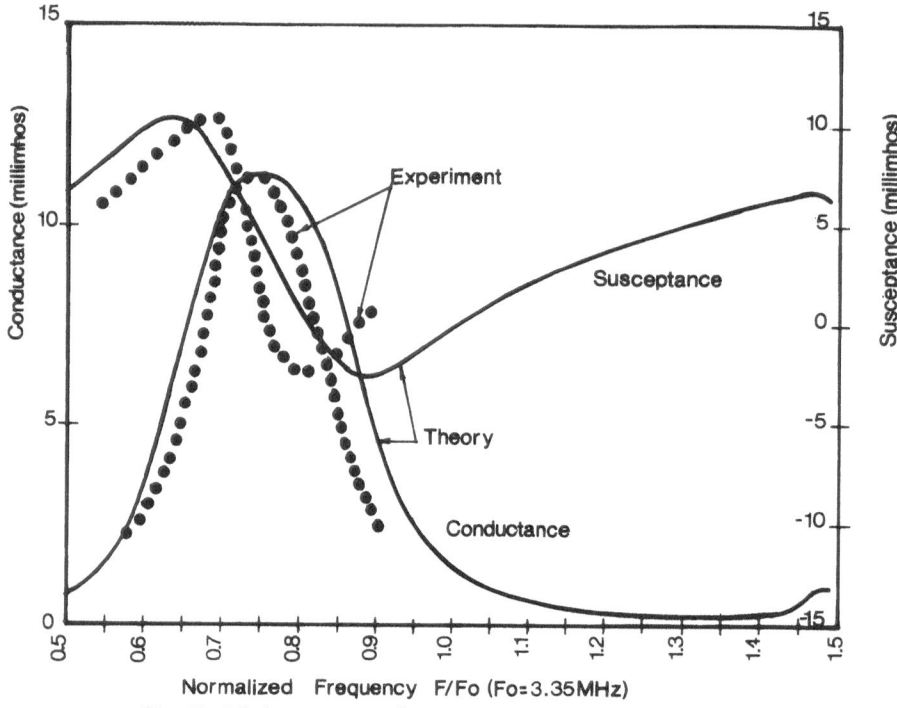

Fig. 12. Admittance versus frequency of one element of the array.

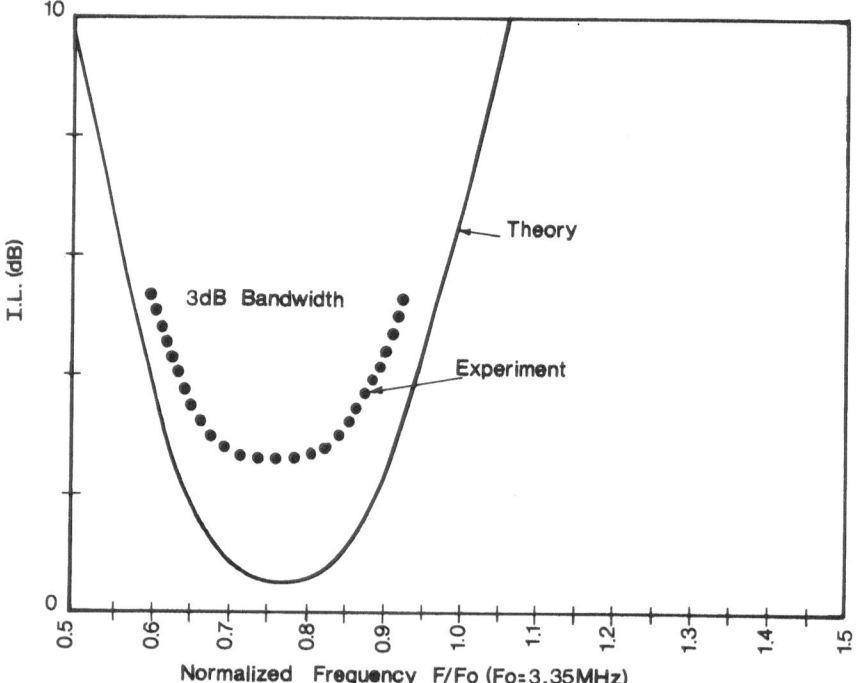

Fig. 13. Conversion loss versus frequency or transfer function modulus of one array's element.

- element width $W = 0.40$ mm
- element length $L = 11$ mm
- quarter-wave thickness $e' = 0.28$ mm
- anti-resonant frequency $F_0 = 3.35\ MHz$

This structure has been tested in water. Figure 12 shows the electrical admittance of one element as a function of frequency. The agreement between theoretical and experimental results is very good. Figure 13 shows the insertion loss as a function of frequency, i.e. the modulus of the transfer function. A low conversion loss ($\cong -3$ dB) can be seen; an absolute bandwidth of 800 kHz (32%) enables us to work with 1.3 μsec short pulses.

As we can see from the formula previously derived, plexiglass ($Z \cong 3.3 \times 10^6$ kg/m^2 sec) is not the optimum material for broad bandwidth. Theoretically, the ideal impedance would here be 5.1×10^6 kg/m^2/sec, but no materials with this impedance are available. Studies on new composite materials, based on epoxy, are in progress. A bandwidth of up to 50% has been obtained with such materials.

ARRAY PERFORMANCES

Arrays have been built with the structure just described. We will now describe results obtained for a 48-element array, working at 2.5 MHz. Figure 14 is a complete view of the array, on which we can see the electrical connections directly bonded onto the printed circuit. This array has been

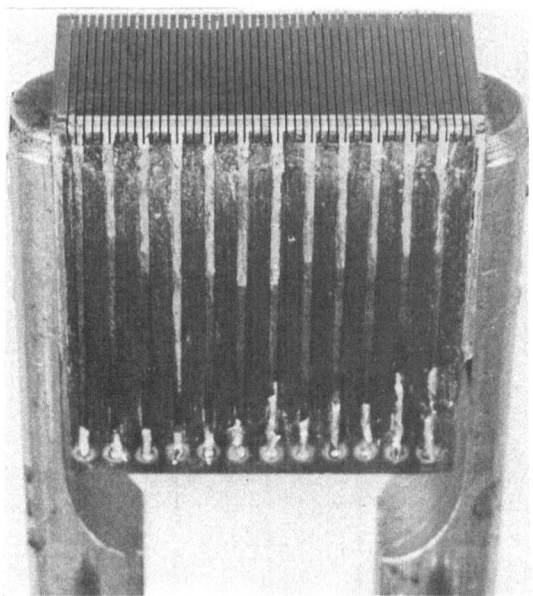

Fig. 14. Top view of the 48 element array.

tested in water with a fixed focus. We used electronic driving circuits for this, enabling us to apply independent pulses to each transducer, whose delays are suitably related, in order to get a focused point at a given distance. The acoustic beam is tested with a point probe (angular aperture: $\pm 20°$, bandwidth: 50%). Pressure profiles are recorded by moving this point probe in front of the array. Figure 15 shows the acoustic beam profile obtained in the focal plane, which is in good agreement with the theory. The slight scale difference may be due to the difference between the real propagation velocity of the medium and the velocity used for computation (1500 m/sec). Figure 16 is a profile obtained in the same experimental conditions, but with an amplitude weighting of the input pulses applied to the various array elements, thus reducing the side lobes. We get a -3 dB beam-width of about 3

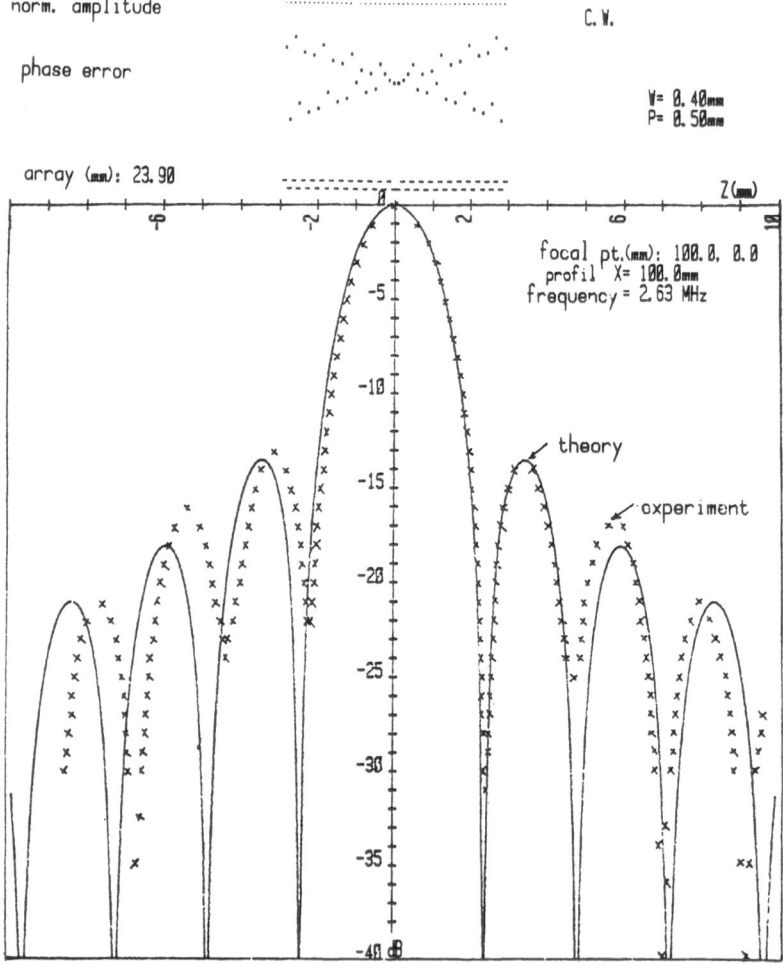

Fig. 15. Pressure beam profile of the array in focal plane (one-axis focusing, $X_0 = 100$ mm).

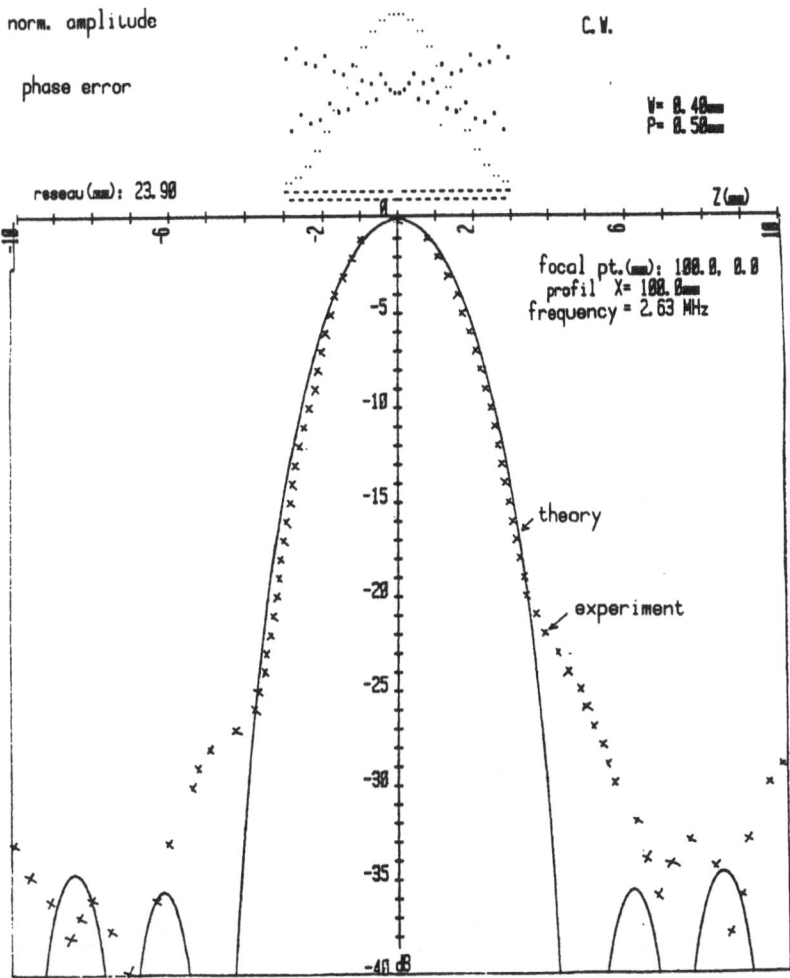

Fig. 16. Same as Figure 13 but with amplitude weighting as indicated at the top of the figure.

mm, with side lobes at −30 dB. Some deviation can be seen between the lateral parts of the measured and the theoretical profiles; this takes place below 20 dB, which shows that the array deviates by less than 10%. Finally, Figure 17 shows the −3 dB acoustic beam-width for various focal points.

CONCLUSIONS

This study enabled us to define a basic array structure working at 2.5 MHz, but which could be extended to use frequencies up to 5 MHz. This structure shows no spurious lobes and no spurious resonant mode with a broad bandwidth (30% now but extended to 50% with new material) and with high

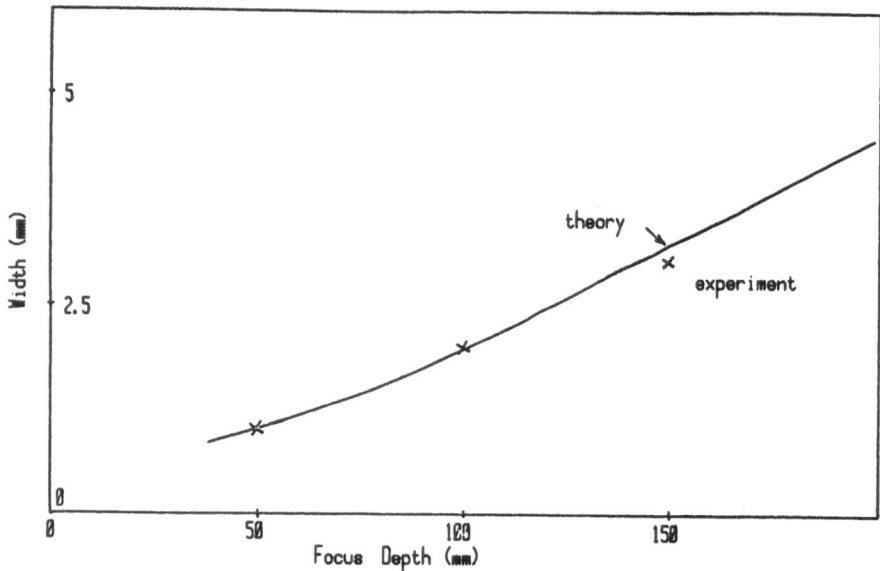

Fig. 17. 3 dB-beam width at different focalization depths.

efficiency. We built a 48-element array which demonstrates the quality of this basic structure, particularly the possibility of obtaining real-time images with a resolution of less than 1 mm in two dimensions. The low loss enables us to work with a better dynamic range, which could be very interesting for image processing.

REFERENCES

1. Defranould Ph, J Souquet: Design of low-loss, wideband ultrasonic arrays for medical imaging. Third International Symposium on Ultrasonic Imaging and Tissue Characterization, NBS Gaithersbury June 5–7, 1978 (to be published in Ultrasonic Imaging).
2. Tancrell RH, J, Callerame, DT Wilson: Near-field, transient acoustic beam-forming with arrays. IEEE Ultrasonics Symposium Philadelphia, Sept. 1978.
3. Beaver WL: Phase error effects in phased array beam-steering. IEEE 1977 Ultrasonics Symposium Proceedings, p. 264–267.
4. Boucher D: Application d'une méthode "éléments finis-perturbation" au calcul des modes de vibration de polyèdres piézoélectriques. Thèse 3éme Cycle, 1979.
5. Mason WP: Physical acoustics, Vol. 1, Part A, New-York, London, Academic Press, 1964.
6. Defranould Ph: Etude des réseaux de transducteurs piézoélectriques pour l'application à l'imagerie ultrasonore médicale. Thomson-CSF, rapport DASM 78/06/146 PhD, fév. 78–80 p.
7. Defranould Ph, J Souquet: Design of a two-dimensional array for B and C ultrasonic system, 1977 IEEE Ultrasonics Symposium Proceedings, p. 259–263.
8. Souquet J, Ph, Defranould, J Desbois: Design of low-loss wide-band ultrasonic transducers for non-invasive medical application. IEEE Sonics and Ultrasonics, March 1979.

POSSIBILITIES AND LIMITATIONS OF PULSED DOPPLER SYSTEMS

A.P.G. HOEKS, R.S. RENEMAN, C.J. RUISSEN, and F.A.M. SMEETS

Pulsed Doppler systems differ from the commonly used continuous wave (CW) Doppler devices in applications and limitations. A pulsed Doppler system enables the instantaneous measurement of the average blood flow velocity relative to the axis of the ultrasound beam in a small sample volume which can be positioned along the ultrasound beam. Contamination by undesired Doppler signals from outside the region of interest can thus be prevented. This feature is particularly useful for studying the behaviour of vessel walls or heart valves, or in situations where blood-vessels are closely spaced, as at the bifurcation of arteries. However, the required depth of investigation sets an upper bound to the maximum velocity which can be detected unambiguously. Moreover, the wide bandwidth of the emitter/receiver section, necessary to achieve a good axial resolution, will increase the noise level, limiting the exploration range. Proper positioning of the sample volume requires some skill, especially if the ultrasound beam is narrow. To reduce this problem, modern pulsed Doppler systems are equipped with some additional features. Either the duration of the sample gate can be altered during positioning, or the pulsed Doppler system is combined with an echo system. Another approach is the development of multi-gate systems, enabling the simultaneous measurement of the instantaneous velocity in a number of adjacent sample volumes. This offers the advantage of easy operation combined with detailed information about the instantaneous velocity distribution over the cross-section of a blood-vessel. The real-time presentation of velocity profiles may cause some problems since they depend on time, depth and velocity.

Quantitative volume flow measurement with pulsed Doppler systems is difficult because this requires the instantaneous measurement of the diameter of the bloodvessel and the velocity averaged over the cross-sectional area, information which cannot be obtained accurately.

The performance and limitations of any pulsed Doppler system are closely related to the design considerations of the apparatus. Before discussing these considerations, a short overview of the basic configuration and operation will be given (Fig. 1). Short bursts of ultrasound, generated by gating the internal master oscillator, are repeatedly transmitted into the tissues by a piezo-electric transducer (3, 9). The transducer then acts as a receiver to pick up the back-scattered echoes returning from various interfaces and particles. In the phase detector the received and amplified echo signal is mixed with two reference signals in quadrature, derived from the master oscillator. The

Charles T. Lancée (ed.), Echocardiology, 413–419. All rights reserved
Copyright © 1979 by Martinus Nijhoff Publishers bv, The Hague/Boston/London

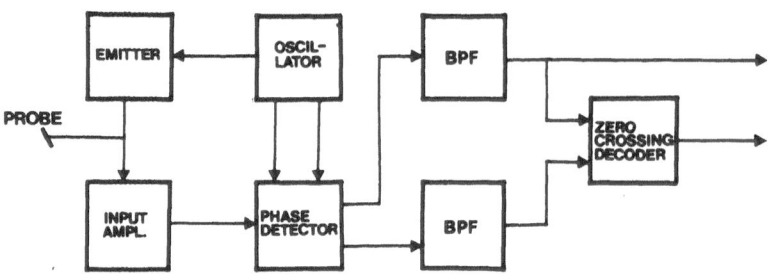

Fig. 1. Block diagram of a pulsed Doppler system. BPF stands for bandpass filter.

outputs of the phase detector, after proper low-pass filtering, reveal the phase relationship between the master oscillator and the echo at each range. After a pre-selected delay with respect to emission, corresponding to the desired depth, both outputs of the phase detector are temporarily stored in "sample and hold" circuits. In each transmit/receive cycle the contents of the sample and hold circuits are updated. The consecutive phase samples constitute the familiar Doppler signals in quadrature in a sampled form, provided that the sampling rate, i.e. the pulse repetition frequency exceeds at least twice the maximum Doppler frequency. To suppress low Doppler frequencies with relatively high amplitude, originating from tissue interfaces, and to eliminate the sampling frequency, both signals are fed into a bandpass filter. With a zero-crossing counter, the average velocity as an instantaneous function of time is determined. Considering the phase relationship between the in quadrature Doppler signals, reveals the direction of the flow (7).

The performance of a pulsed Doppler system in terms of axial resolution and signal to noise ratio of the Doppler signals depends on emission frequency, pulse repetition frequency, duration of emission, width of the ultrasound beam, bandwidth of the transducer and input amplifier and characteristics of the lowpass filter incorporated in the phase detector. All these parameters are interrelated and a particular selection may limit the applicability of the system.

A pulsed Doppler system should combine good axial resolution and a good signal to noise ratio for the Doppler signals. The axial resolution limits the possibility of making a detailed analysis of flow patterns, while a high signal to noise ratio is a prerequisite for proper functioning of the zero-crossing counter. However, these objectives conflict, i.e. improving the axial resolution will affect the signal to noise ratio.

The axial resolution depends on the bandwidth of the transducer and the input amplifier, the width of the ultrasound beam, the duration of emission and the cut-off frequency of the lowpass filter in the phase detector. Increasing the bandwidth of the transducer by proper backing will reduce its efficiency for electro-acoustical conversion (15) and hence the level of the echo, while enlarging the bandwidth of the input amplifier will cause a higher noise level at its output. Shortening the duration of emission will improve the axial resolution but will reduce the signal level. For optimal results the

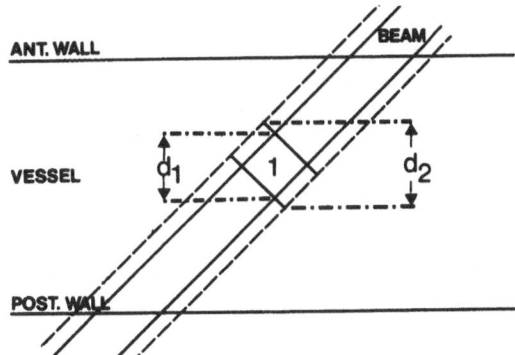

Fig. 2. The effect of an increased width of the ultrasound beam on the axial resolution, indicated by d_1 and d_2, and the sample volume (1).

duration of the sample gate should match the duration of emission (9). The duration of the sample gate is approximately $1/(2f_c)$ where f_c is the cut-off frequency of the lowpass filter in the phase detector (6). Moreover, the axial resolution deteriorates when beam width is increased (Fig. 2). A narrow beam over a long range is only possible at high emission frequencies while a narrow beam can be achieved locally by focusing (15).

The choice of the emission frequency depends on the range of interest and on that velocity range which is to be detected unambiguously. The attenuation of ultrasound is proportional to the square of the emission frequency while the scattering by blood particles is proportional to the fourth power (14), yielding an optimal emission frequency varying with range. The expected velocity range at a given depth of investigation limits the emission frequency, since the depth range sets an upper bound to the pulse repetition frequency (11).

Because of the reciprocal relationships between the basic parameters of a pulsed Doppler system it is impossible to design a system which will function optimally over a wide exploration and velocity range. An axial resolution of less than 1 mm is only possible for short range applications, e.g. directly underneath the skin. For cardiac applications, the resolution is relative poor. Although for these applications the emission frequency is lower, frequency ambiguity may still occur because of the high velocities present in the cardiac cavity and in the arterial system close to the heart.

The velocity waveform, as a function of time, of a pulsed Doppler system is not equivalent to the velocity output of a CW-device, since the latter is supposed to detect the average velocity over the cross-sectional area of a blood-vessel. Real-time estimation of the average flow velocity as an instantaneous function of time with a pulsed Doppler system, requires knowledge about the instantaneous velocity distribution over the cross-section of the blood-vessel.

The size and shape of the sample volume depends on the local beamwidth and the duration of the sample gate. Small sample volumes enable detailed recording of flow patterns but are difficult to position and to maintain at the desired spot. Positioning is facilitated by utilizing the echo-output of a pulsed Doppler device although its quality is poor due to the type of registration used. In measuring velocities relative to the axis of the ultrasound beam most tissue interfaces will not be perpendicular to the beam, causing reduced echolevels. Another method to ease positioning is the incorporation of a sample gate with variable duration. The localization of the blood-vessel can then be performed using a long sample gate duration.

Since pulsed Doppler systems detect the velocity in a small sample volume in comparison to the cross-sectional area of the blood-vessel, the detected velocities will have more or less the same magnitude. Therefore, the band-width of the corresponding Doppler spectrum will be narrow. Hence the inherent error of a zero-crossing counter in determining the average frequency will be small (9). If the sample volume is small, pulsed Doppler systems are well suited for detailed studies of flow patterns at the bifurcation of arteries or distal from stenosis (10). Changes in flow pattern occur at a degree of stenosis where volume flow does not decrease significantly (12, 13). Because contamination by undesired Doppler signals originating from interfaces or particles outside the region of interest is suppressed, pulsed Doppler systems can be employed for such cardiac investigations as heart valve behaviour and heart wall motion (1, 2).

Equipping a pulsed Doppler system with an echo system will provide additional information about the region of interest. In the echo display, the position of the sample gate can be indicated, avoiding uncertainty about the site of velocity detection. Moreover, information is obtained about vessel diameter and the angle under which the velocity is measured. A current drawback of the combined system is the reduced pulse repetition frequency of the Doppler device to allow successive operation of both systems. For reliable velocity measurements the echo system should be switched off as soon as the site of measurement is localized.

Improved orientation can also be established by the extension of the single gate system to a multi-gate system by activating the phase-detector repeatedly in each transmit/receive cycle and performing the required signal processing for each of the sample outputs (filtering and zero-crossing detection). The data-processing can be done in parallel (8, 9) or serially. The last approach looks the most promising, since the required hardware is almost independent of the number of gates (3, 4). With a multi-gate system, the velocity in a number of adjacent sample volumes can be detected simultaneously, enabling the instantaneous measurement of the velocity distribution over the cross-section of a bloodvessel. Recently, a 32-gate pulsed Doppler system with serial data-processing has been completed by the authors. The major characteristics of the system are an emission frequency of 6 MHz, a pulse repetition frequency selectable at 20 and 10 kHz and a duration of emission of 1 or 2 μsec. The axial resolution is in the order of 1 mm. Because the velocity distribution is three-dimensional (velocity, time and depth), its on-line presentation requires another approach as compared to a

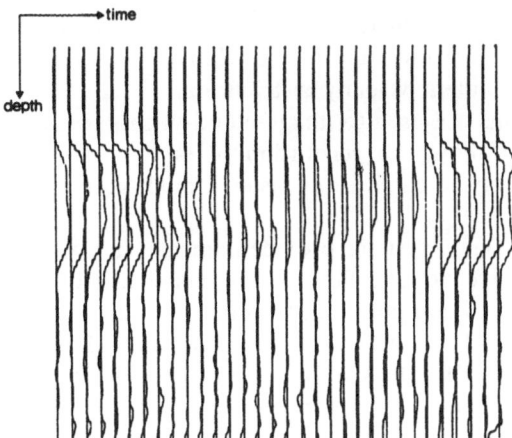

Fig. 3. Velocity profiles as recorded at 25 msec intervals in the common femoral artery. The distance between baselines is equivalent to 1 kHz.

single-gate system. Therefore, the multi-gate system is extended with a digital memory for storage of velocity profiles at a pre-selected rate. The on-line display shows the last recorded velocity distributions, up to a maximum of 256 profiles. The updating of the digital memory can be interrupted by an external trigger command. An off-line plotter output in two modes is provided. In the depth mode, the velocity profiles are presented as recorded (Fig. 3) while the time mode shows the velocity waveforms of the individual gates (Fig. 4). Multi-gate systems offer the possibility to detect relative

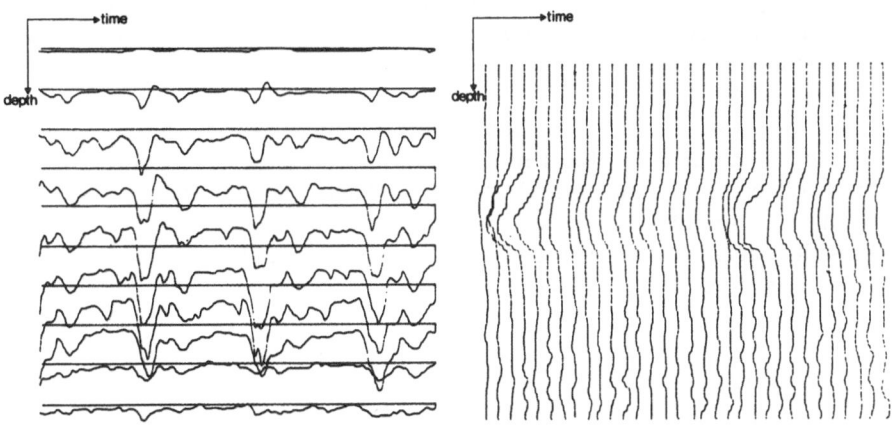

Fig. 4. Velocity distribution as recorded from the common carotid artery as a function of time at 1 mm intervals (left panel) and as a function of depth at 50 msec intervals (right panel). The velocity profiles cover the last 2 cardiac cycles of the velocity waveforms in the left panel. The distance between baselines in both presentations is equivalent to 1 KHz.

changes in the vessel diameter instantaneously. Current research is aimed at the simultaneous determination of the relative excursions of the vessel walls and the time-dependent velocity distribution.

Doppler systems are used to image blood-vessels transcutaneously. Pulsed Doppler devices allow the generation of both cross-sectional and lateral views. Imaging can be carried out faster if multi-gate systems are employed (5).

Although multi-gate systems provide information about the velocity distribution, quantitative volume flow measurement is troublesome since it involves three steps of computation. In order to find the average velocity over the cross-section of an artery, a weighted sum should be made of the velocities found (3, 4), followed by a correction for the angle between flow direction and the axis of the ultrasound beam. The last step is the multiplication of the average velocity by the cross-sectional area of the vessel. Since, with the present state of technology, each step introduces additional errors, the final result is likely to be too unreliable to serve clinical diagnostic purposes.

The basic configuration of a pulsed Doppler system has been discussed. In order to obtain optimal results in terms of axial resolution and signal to noise ratio of the detected Doppler signals the design of a pulsed Doppler system should be tailored to its application since most basic characteristics are conflicting. Single gate pulsed Doppler devices are useful assets, especially in regions where contamination by undesired Doppler signals may easily occur. The positioning of the sample gate can be facilitated by employing a sample gate with adjustable duration, or by the incorporation of a pulse echo system. The echo system will provide additional information about vessel diameter and the angle under which the velocity is detected.

Another approach is the development of multi-gate pulsed Doppler systems. They provide instantaneous information about the velocity distribution over the cross-section of a blood-vessel. Incorporation of a memory circumvents the problems associated with the real-time presentation of velocity profiles.

Although with transcutaneous pulsed Doppler systems valuable information can be assessed, the step to quantitative volume flow measurement in vivo still presents problems. On the other hand the simultaneous measurement of the relative changes in vessel diameter and velocity distribution may provide additional information about the functional state of the major arteries in normal subjects and patients.

REFERENCES

1. Baker D et al.: Pulsed Doppler echocardiography. In: Echocardiology with Doppler applications and real-time imaging, Bom N (ed), The Hague, Martinus Nijhoff, 1977, p 207–221.
2. Barber FE et al.: Duplex scanner II. ULTSYM Proc IEEE Cat 74, CHO 8961, SU, 1974.
3. Brandestini M.: Die signalverarbeitung in perkutanen Ultraschall Doppler Blutfluss Messgeraeten. Dissertation Swiss Federal Institute of Technology (ETH), TH 5711, 1975.

4. Brandestini M: Topoflow, a digital full range Doppler velocity meter. IEEE Trans on Sonics and Ultrasonics, vol. SU-25, Sept. 1978, p 287.
5. Fish PJ: Multichannel, direction-resolving Doppler angiography. Excerpta Medica International Congress Series, no. 363, Excerpta Medica, Amsterdam, 1975, p 153–159.
6. Gabor D.: Theory of communication. IEE 93:429, 1946.
7. McLeod FD: A directional Doppler flowmeter. Proc 7th Int Conf Med Biol Engng, Stockholm, 13–14, 1967.
8. McLeod FD: Multi-channel pulsed Doppler techniques. In: Cardiovascular applications of ultrasound, Reneman RS(ed), Amsterdam, North-Holland Publ. Co., 1974, p 85.
9. Peronneau P et al.: Theoretical and practical aspects of pulsed Doppler flowmetry: real-time application to the measure of instantaneous velocity profiles in vitro and in vivo. In: Cardiovascular applications of ultrasound, Reneman RS (ed), Amsterdam, North-Holland Publ. Co., 1974, p 66.
10. Peronneau P et al.: Bloodflow patterns in large arteries. In: Ultrasound in medicine, White DN (ed), New York and London, Plenum Press Publ., 1977, vol. 3B, p 1193.
11. Reneman RS. A Hoeks: Continuous wave and pulsed Doppler flowmeters – a general introduction. In: Echocardiology with Doppler applications and real-time imaging, Bom N (ed), The Hague, Martinus Nijhoff, 1977, p 189.
12. Reneman RS, MP Spencer: Local Doppler audio spectra in normal and stenosed carotid arteries in man. Ultrasound in Medicine and Biology (in press).
13. Sandmann W et al.: Turbulenzmessung mit dem Doppler-Ultraschallverfahren: eine neue Methode der Qualitatskontrolle in der Arterienchirurgie. In: Ultraschall-Doppler Diagnostik in der Angiologie. Kriesmann A, Bollinger A (eds), Stuttgart, Georg Thieme Verlag, 1978, p. 77.
14. Shung KK et al.: Scattering of ultrasound by blood. IEEE Trans on Biomed Engng. Vol. BME-23, 6, Nov., 1976.
15. Wells PNT: Physical principles of ultrasonic diagnosis. London, Academic Press, 1969.

REAL-TIME BLOOD FLOW IMAGING

L.G. POURCELOT

Vascular visualization is generally made by injection of contrast medium in the vascular system and performing an angiography. This technique is very useful in clinical practice, bus has drawbacks, and is even dangerous, for some applications (carotid angiography, coronary arteriography ...). The goal of many researchers is to detect cardiovascular disease very early and to evaluate the clinical or surgical treatment, without any risk for the patient. It is therefore necessary to develop accurate, non-invasive methods for examination of the cardiovascular system, especially those areas accessible for surgery. Developments of such techniques may reduce the number of useless arteriographies and permit better definition of the indications for arteriography in patients whose clinical signs are not sufficient to directly justify this type of investigation.

Ultrasonic techniques promise to have a great future in this field of diagnosis, both for real-time visualization of cardiac and vascular structures and for blood flow detection. We can distinguish three different methods of echo-Doppler systems:
- the combined use of TM and pulsed Doppler,
- real-time B-scanning, associated with pulsed Doppler,
- Doppler arteriography with a continuous wave or a pulsed wave device.

One of our main projects was to develop a system for real-time, grey-scale Doppler imaging, in order to show the blood circulation and its modification during each cardiac cycle.

I. VASCULAR VISUALIZATION

1. *Real-time B-scan*

The need for real-time imaging of the cardiac and vascular structures has been the cause of much research over the past years. The rapid change in position of the scanning line can be achieved using either a mechanical probe, a multi-transducer array with electronic switching, or a phased-array system. The B-scanning can be linear or sectorial. Current images are of sufficient quality for a good visualization of normal arteries.

In vascular pathology, especially in case of atheromatous plaques, echograms are sometimes difficult to analyse due to the variety of response shown by the plaques:

– soft atherosclerotic lesions, low in calcium, may produce relatively low back-scattering: thus they appear as relatively sonolucent areas like blood on the B-mode scan,

– in other cases, atheromatous plaque is clearly seen, with strong echoes within the arterial lumen (Fig. 1)'

– calcium deposits within plaques or vascular walls do produce an important shadow due to the absorption of ultrasonic energy.

These results demonstrate the interest of Doppler detection for quantitative evaluation of suspected areas and for visualization of the internal vessel diameter. The combined use of real-time B-scanning and pulsed Doppler permits the location of the sample volume within the field of view. This combination could probably, in the future, give sufficient information about the cross-section of the vessel, and the angle between the ultrasonic beam and the flow vector, for the computation of the actual flow.

2. Doppler imaging

The detection of Doppler-shifted ultrasonic waves reflected from moving blood makes it possible to locate, and to visualize, internal sections of vessels in a transcutaneous and atraumatic way. This Doppler angiography can be achieved using either a continuous wave or a pulsed wave apparatus. A probe-position resolver detects the coordinates of the Doppler beam and delivers signals to a storage monitor. Using a continuous wave Doppler system, we get a projection of the vessels, resembling an arteriographic image while, when using a pulsed Doppler, we can generate cross-sectional and lateral views of blood vessels. The dots are intensified and stored on the screen when the Doppler signal is detected. Several minutes are required for

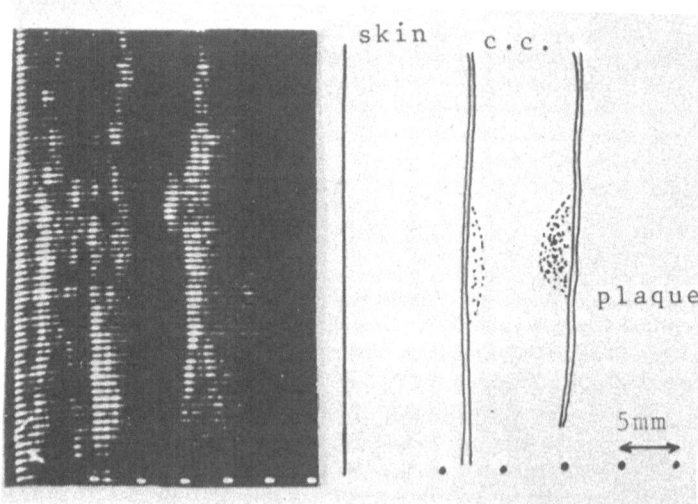

Fig. 1. View of an atheromatous plaque within the lumen of a common carotid artery (5 MHz multitransducer system with dynamic focussing).

each image: this low image-rate is not compatible with routine examination, especially in agitated or uncooperative patients, and does not give direct information about velocity profiles. Doppler tomography can be produced more quickly if we use a multigated system, allowing the simultaneous storage of several separate loci of detected flow.

We tried to drastically increase the Doppler image rate, but that is obviously a complex problem. Indeed, it is necessary to go from a very low image rate (1 image in several minutes) to a much faster one (10 to 15 images/sec). The ratio of these values, around 1000, clearly reveals the encountered difficulties.

II. PRACTICAL DEVELOPMENTS

The instantaneous Doppler imaging system was developed in several stages. We started with the study of a multigated Doppler device in order to detect simultaneous flow signals at several points along the explorating beam. It is well known that Doppler shift can be correctly converted, in terms of velocity and direction of flow, only if the sample time is sufficiently long. Thus, for the computation of blood velocities, it is necessary to study the Doppler shift at one point for at least 1/200 sec. This time is long when compared with that required for amplitude detection in B-scanners. The ratio of these times is around 10,000, that means that we get 10,000 dots on a B-scan for only 1 point on the Doppler scan, if we only use one Doppler channel.

The Doppler prototype we developed uses 10 gates, i.e. 10 simultaneous channels working at a 4 MHz frequency. Figure 2 shows example of velocity

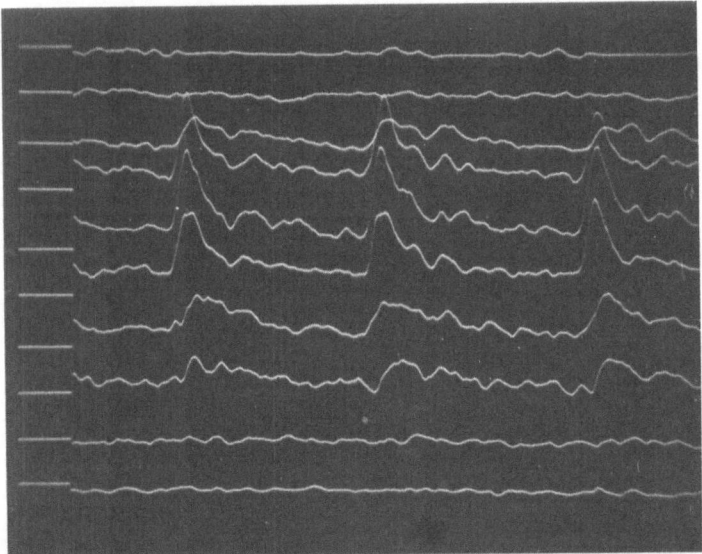

Fig. 2. Common carotid velocity patterns recorded using a multigated Doppler device.

traces simultaneously recorded in' several points across a normal common carotid artery. The proximal wall of the artery is located at the upper part of the picture. The zero lines are shown on the left side of the picture, and the step between each gate corresponds to 1.5 mm.

From the velocity signals we can either display the instantaneous velocity profile through the vessels, or modulate, on a screen, the corresponding Doppler points. This modulation is proportional to the blood velocity and can be directional if required, i.e. we can display arterial and venous flows simultaneously or alternately. On Figure 3, we see discrete values of instantaneous velocity profiles in normal carotid arteries. These profiles have been recorded during one cardiac cycle, only. The maximum amplitude corresponds to the systolic peak velocity, and the lowest amplitude to the diastolic velocity. For reference, the dots at the bottom of each profile correspond to the zero levels. As is well known from continuous wave Doppler studies, this picture confirms that the flow in the common and internal carotids does present a continuous diastolic component, whereas the flow in the external carotid is near zero in diastole. The asymetrical shape of the instantaneous velocity profile at the level of the bulb just before the bifurcation predicts these two different characteristics of the blood circulation in the internal and external carotid arteries.

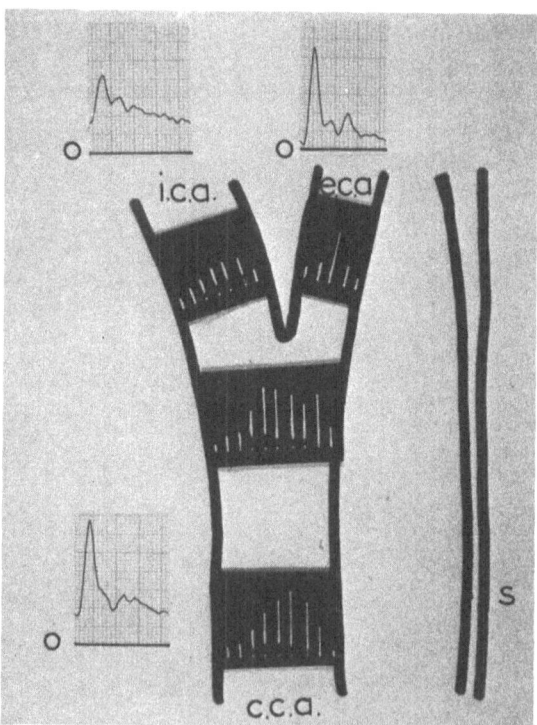

Fig. 3. Velocity profiles in normal carotid arteries.

The second stage of our work was to develop a system for fast translation of the Doppler beam. Mechanical motion does not appear to be suitable for this purpose, due to the fact that it gives a permanent Doppler shift between transmitted and reflected waves. For this reason we used a discontinuous motion of the ultrasonic beam employing an electronic scanning of multi-transducers. The probe is an array of 10 piezo-electric transducers. The switching from one line to the next is done every 5 msec, so that the frame rate is approximately 20 images/sec. For several reasons (data density, switching noise, etc.), the maximum frame rate is 15/sec at present. The dimensions of the area detected are 2×1.5 cm^2. It is easy to decrease this frame rate if necessary or, to pass from Doppler imaging to the display of velocity tracings or profiles along a selected line.

A schematic diagram of the electronic network is shown in Figure 4. A 4 MHz oscillator drives the electronic unit. Ten transmitters are connected to each transducer of the probe; the echo signals detected by each receiver are selected by 10 gates and led to the amplifiers and demodulators. Flow direction is computed in phase detectors and Doppler signals from the 10 selected depths are converted into velocity signals. These signals can be used either for intensity modulation of the Doppler image, or for the instantaneous display of velocity patterns and velocity profile.

RESULTS

In vitro and in vivo studies have enabled determination of possibilities of the multi-transducer, multigated Doppler apparatus. First trials were performed on a cotton thread rotating in a water tank at a speed of 0.15 m/sec. For each

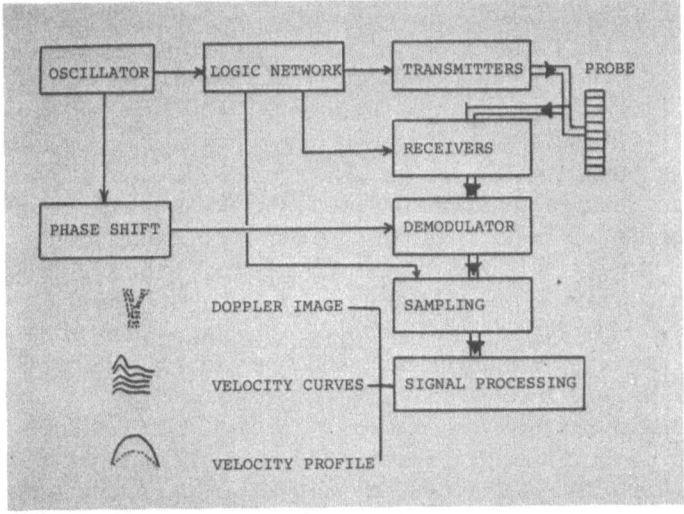

Fig. 4. Schematic diagram of the real-time Doppler imaging system.

point of the picture, we get the direction and the velocity of the reflector and we can display, in real-time on an oscilloscope, either both segments of the thread or only the segment corresponding to the positive or negative Doppler shift. Dot intensity is related to the magnitude of the velocity signal. Figure 5 shows velocity signals versus time for each of the ten Doppler channels, corresponding to the ten different depths. Gate number 6 alternately detects a positive and negative Doppler shift when it intercepts either one or the other segment of the thread. Gates number 1 and 10 detect either a negative or a positive signal only. We can see the progressive transition of velocity signals from the entirely negative to the entirely positive value.

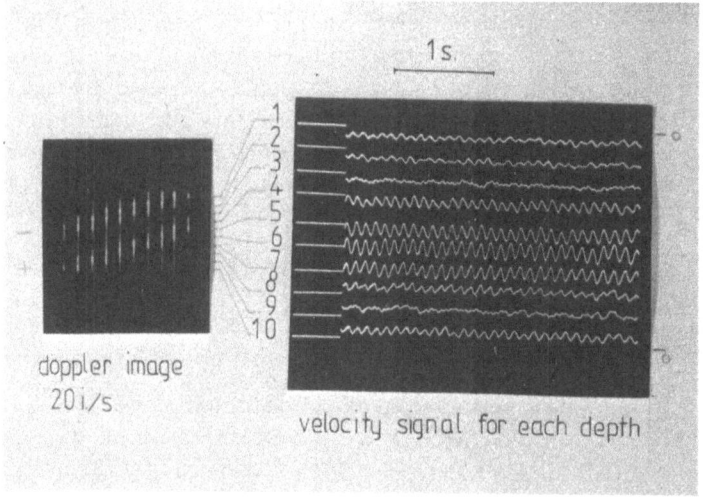

Fig. 5. Instantaneous visualization of a cotton thread rotating in water.

In vivo studies, as reported in this paper, have been performed on normal carotid arteries. With the small-sized probe, longitudinal or transverse cross-sections of these arteries are easily carried out. Doppler arteriographies represent functional images: the velocity grey-scale presentation gives dynamic information about the velocity of the blood at each of the 100 points of the image. It is hoped to increase the number of exploration points to 1000 in the near future. Figure 6 displays longitudinal sections of the same normal carotid bifurcation, obtained using a 5 MHz multi transducer B-scan (left side) and the real-time 4 MHz Doppler imaging system (right side). These cross-sections are complementary and one can easily observe the carotid bifurcation in each case.

Figure 7 shows transverse sections of the carotid arteries, from the lower to the upper part of the neck. Internal and external carotid arteries are clearly differentiated above the bifurcation. The nearly circular section of the common carotid becomes double-lobed at the level of the bulb.

The apparatus is able to separate venous from arterial flow, as de-

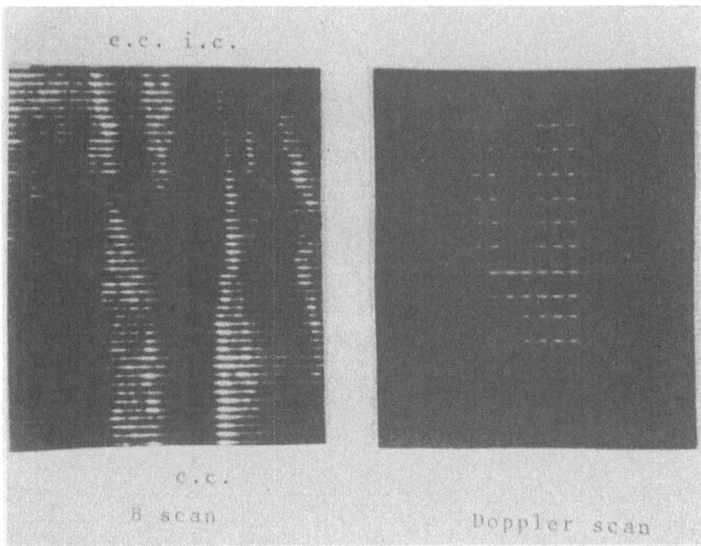

Fig. 6. Comparison of real-time B-scan and real-time Doppler scan of the same normal carotid bifurcation.

monstrated on Figure 8. A transverse cross-section of the common carotid artery and jugular vein is displayed on the central view. On lateral views, the arterial (a) or the venous (v) Doppler signal, only, were used for intensity modulation.

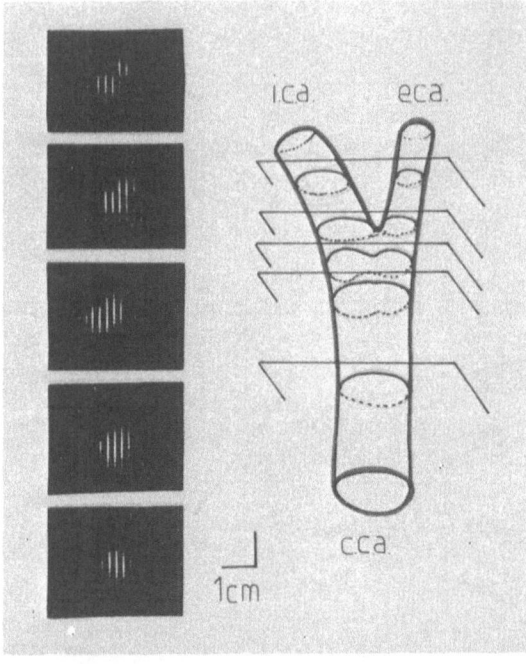

Fig. 7. Transverse cross-sections of normal carotid arteries.

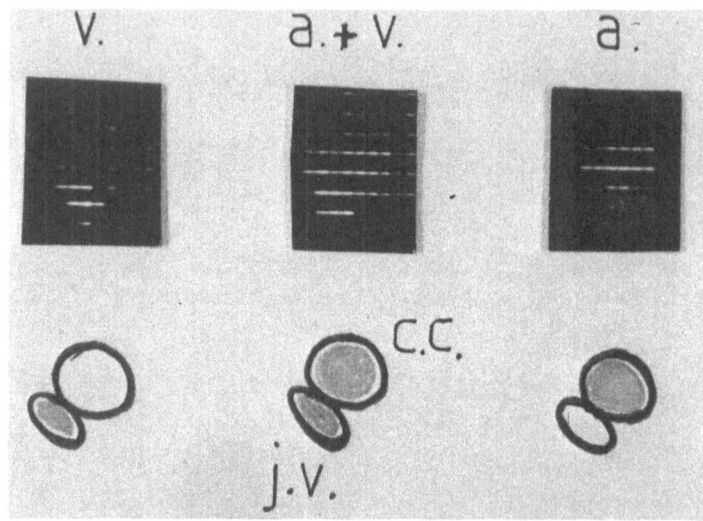

Fig. 8. Real-time Doppler imaging of arterial and venous flow.

CONCLUSIONS

Imaging of vascular walls or atheromatous plaques can be achieved using real-time B-scanner, but the difference in appearance of sonolucent or shadowing calcium deposits has revealed the importance of blood flow detection associated with vascular visualization.

Doppler examination has led to Doppler arteriography using a continuous

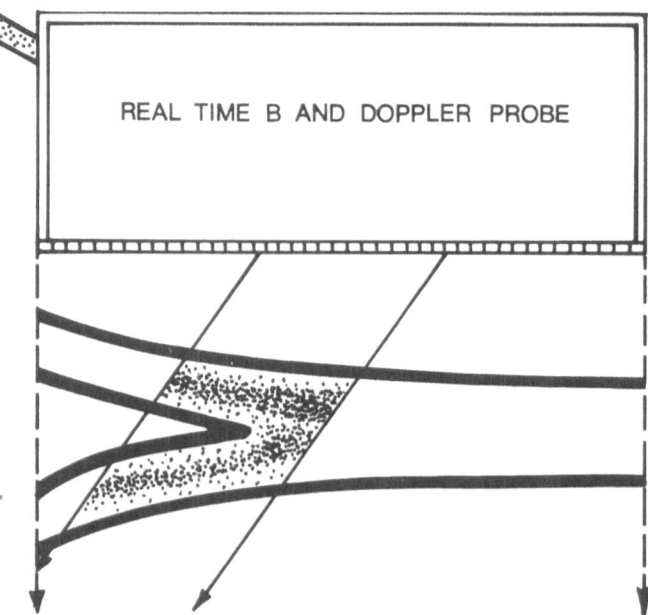

Fig. 9. Combined use of real-time, B- and Doppler scanning.

wave or a pulsed wave system. Several minutes are required for each Doppler arteriograph. In order to increase the frame rate, we developed a new multigated multi-transducer Doppler system, which produces a blood flow map in a very short time. In the current prototype, an instantaneous Doppler tomography of the carotid arteries is displayed at a frame rate of 15/sec.

Our next objective is to couple a fast Doppler imaging system and a dynamic B-scanner in the same probe. By combining these two techniques, we could display, for instance using two different colours, a small Doppler image superimposed on the dynamic B-scan, (Fig. 9) in real-time.

Translation and steering of the Doppler beam could be achieved by electronic switching and phasing. These results would be of the greatest interest for the study of hemodynamic disturbances in carotid and femoral arteries. Congenital cardiopathies seem to be one of the most important fields of application of these new imaging modes. We can expect the development of such techniques to lead to significant reduction in invasive examination procedures in the near future.

ACKNOWLEDGMENTS

We gratefully acknowledge the technical assistance of Dominique Besse.

This work was supported by Grant of the Institut National de la Recherche Médicale: ATP no 35.76.67.

REFERENCES

1. Barber, FE, DW Baker, DE Strandness Jr, GD Mahler: Duplex scanner II: for simultaneous imaging of artery tissues and flow. Ultrasonic Symposium Proceedings IEEE, 1974, cat R74, CHO 896–1 SU.
2. Baker DW, DE Strandness Jr, SL Johnson: Pulsed Doppler techniques: some examples from the University of Washington. Ultrasound Med Biol. 2:251, 1976.
3. Bournat JP, P Peronneau, A Herment: Yes-no ultrasonic Doppler method of detection for vascular imaging. Ultrasound Med Biol 3:105, 1977.
4. Brandestini M: Signalverarbeitung in perkutanen Ultraschall Doppler Blufluss Mess-geräten. Dissertation I.B.T., Zürich, 1976.
5. Fish JP: Multichannel, direction-resolving Doppler angiography. Proceedings of the Second European Congress on ultrasonic in medicine, Münich 12–16 May 1975.
6. Pourcelot L.: Echo Doppler systems. Applications for the detection of cardiovascular disorders. In: Echocardiology, Bom N (ed) The Hague, Martinus Nijhoff, 1977, p 245–256.
7. Pourcelot L, D Besse, C Pejot, Th Planiol: Visualisation du sang circulant par effet Doppler. Proc Biosigma 78:407, Paris, April 1978.
8. Pourcelot L, M Berson, A Roncin: Imagerie ultrasonore en temps réel à haute résolution. Proc Biosigma 78:116, Paris, April 1978.
9. Ramsey Jr SD, JC Taenzer, JF Holzemer, JR Suarez, PS Green: A real time ultrasonic B-scan/Doppler artery-imaging system. Ultrasonics Symposium Proceedings IEEE, 1975, Cat 75, CHO 996–4 SU.
10. Spencer MP, JM Reid, PS Paulson: Diagnosis of carotid artery disease and cerebral vascular insufficiency with Doppler angiography and ophtalmic artery sonography. Ch. 21 in: Cardiovascular applications of ultrasound, Reneman RS (ed), Amsterdam, North-Holland Publ. Co., 1974.
11. Strandness Jr DE, DS Sumner: A new approach to arterial visualization. Ch. 19 in: Cardiovascular applications of ultrasound, Reneman RS (ed), Amsterdam, North-Holland Publ. Co, 1974.

FOCUSSING BY MEANS OF WAVE FIELD EXTRAPOLATION

A.J. BERKHOUT and J. RIDDER

Abstract

Until now, focussing of ultra-sound has always been represented by a summation procedure along wave-fronts. Generally, the summation procedure will be preceded by time correction as in most practical cases the transducers are not situated on a wave-front surface.

In this paper we will introduce a novel approach to focussing which is fundamentally different from the conventional ones. It can be subdivided into two steps:
1. Wave field extrapolation.
   Using the wave equation, the recorded data is transformed into a series of new recordings which represent simulated registrations at new positions of the recording plane.
   Wave field extrapolation can be described by spatial (de)convolution.
2. Imaging.
   The imaging principle formulates that the upper parts of the simulated recordings, related to recording planes inside the medium of investigation, form together the focussed result.

Based on this new concept, it is shown that a recursive focussing technique can be formulated which can handle velocity variations within the aperture. Another interesting conclusion is that for optimum focussing a frequency-dependent weighting function within the aperture should be used.

Finally, it is shown that during the imaging step an operator can be applied to improve the axial resolution as well. It is also shown that recursive focussing is pre-eminently suited to correcting for depth-dependent absorption.

INTRODUCTION

In most dynamically-focussed ultrasonic imaging devices focussing consists of two operations (1, 2):
1. Dynamic time correction
2. Summation

or, in mathematical terms,

$$\langle P(\mathbf{r}_A, \omega) \rangle = \int_{S_0} P(\mathbf{r}_0, \omega) e^{jk\Delta r} \, dS_0, \qquad (1)$$

$\mathbf{r}_0$ defining the points in the receiver plane S_0, $\mathbf{r}_A$ defining the position of the focussed result and $\Delta \mathbf{r} = \mathbf{r}_A - \mathbf{r}_0$.

In general, the focussing operator should be described by a time correction *and* an amplitude correction part (3).

$$\langle P(\mathbf{r}_A, \omega) \rangle = \int_{S_0} A^-(\Delta r, \omega) P(\mathbf{r}_0, \omega) e^{jk\Delta r} \, dS_0. \qquad (2)$$

It will be shown that, with the Kirchhoff diffraction theory, an expression for

$A^-(\Delta r, \omega)$ can be obtained:

$$A^-(\Delta r, \omega) = \frac{\Delta z}{2\pi} \frac{1 - jk\Delta r}{\Delta r^3}. \tag{3}$$

Note from (3) that the amplitude correction part is frequency depdendent.

WAVE FIELD EXTRAPOLATION IN TERMS OF SPATIAL CONVOLUTION

One of the most fundamental expressions in wave theory was published as early as 1883 by Kirchhoff (Fig. 1):

$$P(\mathbf{r}_A, \omega) = -\frac{1}{4\pi} \oint \left[P(\mathbf{r}, \omega) \nabla \left\{ \frac{\exp(-jk\Delta r)}{\Delta r} \right\} \right.$$
$$\left. - \frac{\exp(-jk\Delta r)}{\Delta r} \nabla P(\mathbf{r}, \omega) \right] \cdot \mathbf{n} \, dS \tag{4}$$

with S being a closed surface
    $\mathbf{n}$ representing a unit-vector perpendicular to S
    A is a point inside S
    Δr distance between A and the surface S
    $P(\mathbf{r}, \omega)$ is the pressure distribution on S.

If we choose a plane surface for S it can be derived that (Fig. 2)

$$P(\mathbf{r}_B, \omega) = \frac{\Delta z}{2\pi} \int_{S_1} \frac{1 + jk\Delta r}{\Delta r^3} P(\mathbf{r}_1, \omega) e^{-jk\Delta r} \, dS_1. \tag{5}$$

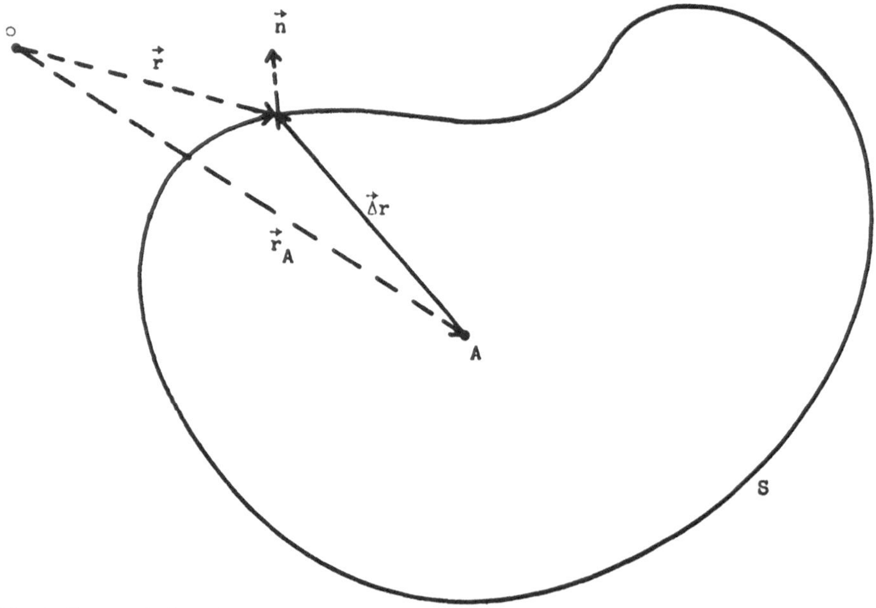

Fig. 1. Geometrical configuration for the Kirchhoff-integral.

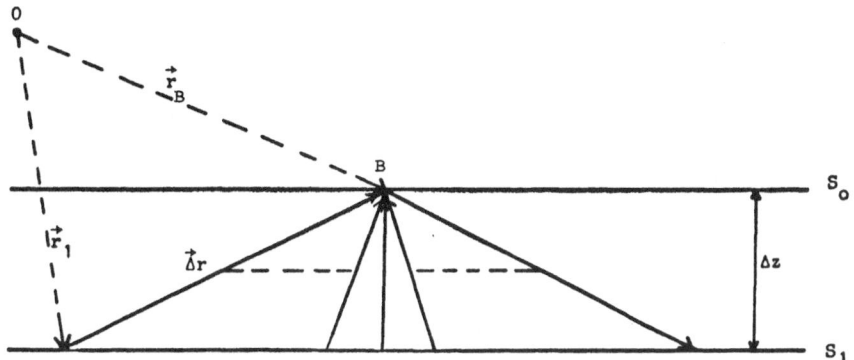

Fig. 2. Geometrical configuration for upward-extrapolation.

Expression (5) is often referred to as the *Rayleigh integral.*

In terms of spatial convolution expression (5) can be written as:

$$P(\mathbf{r}_{B}, \omega) = \int_{S_1} G(\mathbf{r}_B - \mathbf{r}_1, \omega)\, P(\mathbf{r}_1, \omega)\, \mathrm{d}S_1 \tag{6a}$$

with

$$G(\mathbf{r}, \omega) = \frac{z}{2\pi}\frac{1 + jkr}{r^3}\,\mathrm{e}^{-jkr}. \tag{6b}$$

Expression (6a) describes the extrapolation of the wavefield from the *source plane* S_1 to the *recording plane* S_0. This procedure is called *upward extrapolation* and $G(\mathbf{r}, \omega)$ is named the *upward extrapolation operator.*

Taking into account the presence of noise, the total pressure in any point on the recording plane S_0 can be formulated by:

$$P(\mathbf{r}_0, \omega) = \int_{S_1} G(\mathbf{r}_0 - \mathbf{r}_1, \omega)\, P(\mathbf{r}_1, \omega)\, \mathrm{d}S_1 + N(\mathbf{r}_0), \tag{7}$$

where $N(\mathbf{r}_0)$ is the noise contribution.

Similarly, let us introduce the downward extrapolation operator F. The pressure in a point A in source plane S_1 can be *estimated* from the pressure in recording plane S_0 by applying a downward extrapolation step according to

$$\langle P(\mathbf{r}_A, \omega)\rangle = \int_{S_0} F(\mathbf{r}_A - \mathbf{r}_0, \omega)\, P(\mathbf{r}_0, \omega)\, \mathrm{d}S_0. \tag{8}$$

Using (7):

$$\langle P(\mathbf{r}_A, \omega)\rangle = \int_{S_0} F(\mathbf{r}_A - \mathbf{r}_0, \omega)\left[\int_{S_1} G(\mathbf{r}_0 - \mathbf{r}_1, \omega)\, P(\mathbf{r}_1, \omega)\, \mathrm{d}S_1\right]\mathrm{d}S_0$$
$$+ \int_{S_0} F(\mathbf{r}_A - \mathbf{r}_0, \omega)\, N(\mathbf{r}_0)\, \mathrm{d}S_0$$

$$= \int_{S_1} \left[\int_{S_0} F(\mathbf{r}_A - \mathbf{r}_0, \omega) \, G(\mathbf{r}_0 - \mathbf{r}_1, \omega) \, \mathrm{d}S_0 \right] P(\mathbf{r}_1, \omega) \, \mathrm{d}S_1 + N(\mathbf{r}_A). \qquad (9)$$

$$\underbrace{\qquad\qquad\qquad\qquad\qquad\qquad\qquad}_{W(\mathbf{r}_A - \mathbf{r}_1, \omega)}$$

Consequently, for each frequency we may write

$$\langle P(\mathbf{r}_A, \omega) \rangle = \int_{S_1} W(\mathbf{r}_A - \mathbf{r}_1, \omega) \, P(\mathbf{r}_1, \omega) \, \mathrm{d}S_1 + N(\mathbf{r}_A) \qquad (10a)$$

with

$$W(\mathbf{r}, \omega) = \int_{S_0} F(\mathbf{r} - \mathbf{r}_0, \omega) \, G(\mathbf{r}_0, \omega) \, \mathrm{d}S_0. \qquad (10b)$$

From equations (10a) and (10b) we can draw the following conclusions:

1. Downward extrapolation (i.e. focussing) can be formulated in terms of spatial *wavelet deconvolution*, spatial wavelet $G(\mathbf{r}, \omega)$ being given by wave theory.

2. Spatial resolution of focussed data is given by the width of output wavelet $W(\mathbf{r})$. Note that $W(\mathbf{r}, \omega)$ is directly related to the *length* of downward extrapolation operator (i.e. focussing operator) $F(\mathbf{r}, \omega)$ and that the *length* of $F(\mathbf{r}, \omega)$ is determined by the size of the aperture of the recording plane S_0.

3. From the theory of inverse filtering it follows that $W(\mathbf{r}, \omega)$ should represent a *zero-phase* wavelet, whose spatial bandwidth is determined by the noise power spectrum (4).

DOWNWARD EXTRAPOLATION (FOCUSSING) OPERATOR

Because expressions (10a) and (10b) both represent convolutions, these equations can be written in the Fourier domain (Fourier transformation with respect to k_x and k_y) as simple multiplications

$$\langle \tilde{P}(k_x, k_y, \Delta z, \omega) \rangle = \tilde{W}(k_x, k_y, \Delta z, \omega) \, \tilde{P}(k_x, k_y, \Delta z, \omega)$$
$$+ \tilde{N}(k_x, k_y, \Delta z, \omega) \qquad (11a)$$

with

$$\tilde{W}(k_x, k_y, \Delta z, \omega) = \tilde{F}(k_x, k_y, \Delta z, \omega) \, \tilde{G}(k_x, k_y, \Delta z, \omega). \qquad (11b)$$

Now let us consider the above described spatial deconvolution theory in an idealized situation (*noise free*, no limitation on *bandwidth* or *aperture*, *infinitely small* sampling interval). Then we may take, for all frequencies,

$$\tilde{F}(k_x, k_y, \Delta z, \omega) = 1/\tilde{G}(k_x, k_y, \Delta z, \omega) \qquad (12)$$

or, using (11b),

$$\tilde{W}(k_x, k_y, \Delta z, \omega) = 1 \qquad (13a)$$

or

$$W(\mathbf{r}, \omega) = \frac{\delta(\mathbf{r})}{\pi r} = \delta(x)\delta(y). \tag{13b}$$

Hence, applying (10a), we may conclude that in the idealized situation we have no loss of information:

$$\langle P(\mathbf{r}_A, \omega) \rangle = P(\mathbf{r}_A, \omega).$$

If we substitute in (12) the Rayleigh operator (see also Appendix A), then we obtain for the idealized situation:

$$\tilde{F}(k_x, k_y, \Delta z, \omega) = 1/e^{j\Delta z \sqrt{[\omega^2/c^2 - (k_x^2 + k_y^2)]}}$$

$$= e^{j\Delta z \sqrt{[\omega^2/c^2 - (k_x^2 + k_y^2)]}}.$$

Excluding the extreme near field ($k_x^2 + k_y^2 > w^2/c^2$), inverse Fourier transformation of (14) yields the space-frequency version:

$$F(\mathbf{r}, \omega) = \frac{\Delta z}{2\pi} \frac{1 - jkr}{r^3} e^{jkr}. \tag{15}$$

Substitution of this result in (8) yields:

$$\langle P(\mathbf{r}_A, \omega) \rangle = \frac{\Delta z}{2\pi} \int_{S_0} \frac{1 - jk\Delta r}{\Delta r^3} e^{jk\Delta r} P(\mathbf{r}_0, \omega) \, dS_0. \tag{16}$$

Equation (16) describes the downward extrapolation and $F(\mathbf{r}, \omega)$ is called a downward extrapolation (focussing) operator (Fig. 3). Because $F(\mathbf{r}, \omega)$ is derived using the Kirchhoff diffraction theory, expression (16) is known as the *Kirchhoff-summation approach* in seismic literature.

Now, we may draw the following conclusions:

1. The current Kirchhoff-summation approach uses a downward extrapolation operator which assumes an idealized far-field situation (noise-

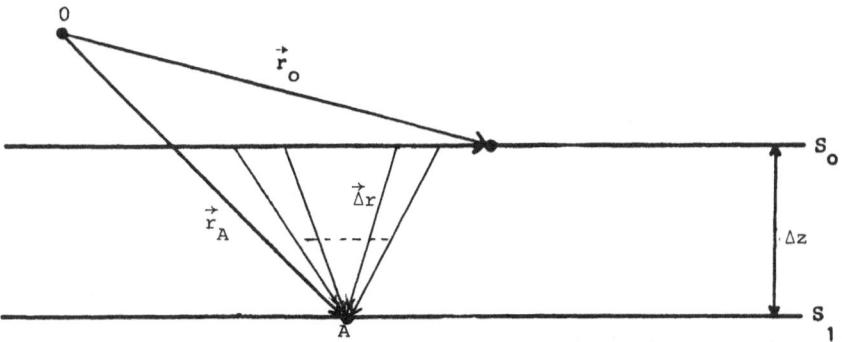

Fig. 3. Geometrical configuration for downward-extrapolation.

free, no limitation on bandwidth and aperture, infinitely small sampling interval).
2. In terms of linear inverse filtering theory, focussing according to
   Kirchhoff summation involves band-limited "Spatial spiking deconvolution", the band limitation given by the absence of the extreme near
   field.

Equation (16) describes downward extrapolation (focussing) in the space-
frequency domain. After every extrapolation step we are interested in
$\langle p(\mathbf{r}_A, t=0)\rangle$ only. So the inverse Fourier transformation of $\langle P(\mathbf{r}_A, \omega)\rangle$ to
the space-time domain reduces to (imaging):

$$\langle p(\mathbf{r}_A, t=0)\rangle = \frac{1}{2\pi} \int_{f_{min}}^{f_{max}} \langle P(\mathbf{r}_A, \omega)\rangle \, d\omega. \tag{17}$$

It is interesting to see that, during inverse transformation, deconvolution for
depth resolution (conventional least-squares inverse filtering) can easily be
applied:

$$\langle p(\mathbf{r}_A, t=0)\rangle = \frac{1}{2\pi} \int_{f_{min}}^{f_{max}} H(\mathbf{r}_A, \omega) \langle P(\mathbf{r}_A, \omega)\rangle d\omega \tag{18a}$$

with (4)

$$H(\mathbf{r}_A, \omega) = \frac{S_{n\Delta z}^*(\omega)}{|S_{n\Delta z}(\omega)|^2 + |N_{n\Delta z}(\omega)|^2}, \tag{18b}$$

where $S_{n\Delta z}(\omega)$ represents the acoustic wavelet at depth $n\Delta z$ and $|N_{n\Delta z}(\omega)|^2$
represents the spatial noise power spectrum.

Note that with each inverse Fourier transformation another deconvolution
filter as given by (18b) can be applied. This means that time-variance can be
realized in a very elegant way.

PROPOSAL FOR A NEW FOCUSSING TECHNIQUE

In the foregoing, we have demonstrated that optimum downward extrapolation can be compared with optimum, finite-duration, wavelet deconvolution in the time domain. For the spatial version, the time coordinate should
be replaced by the spatial coordinate(s) x and/or y, filter duration should be
replaced by aperture and the time wavelet should be replaced by a spatial
wavelet being defined by the *wave theory*. It is important to realize that the
frequency, f, should be considered as a *parameter*.

In the following, we shall propose an alternative focussing technique based
on the following principles:
1. Downward extrapolation is done *recursively* in order compensate for
   lateral velocity variations.

Apart from economical arguments, the step size Δz is determined according to the degree of lateral variations in the velocity (upper limit) and the discretization error (lower limit).

2. Downward extrapolation is carried out in the *frequency domain*. This approach offers significant advantages:

   a. the operator can be optimized per frequency component (as it should be).

   b. application consists of a simple spatial convolution per frequency component.

   Item (b) means that only FFT and convolution routines are needed for the focussing scheme proposed. Application of these routines can be extremely fast as special purpose hardware is available.

3. The optimum amplitudes for the downward extrapolation operator are computed according to a *least-squares criterion*. For the two-dimensional situation this means:

$$\sum_m \left[\sum_{n=-\Delta L}^{\Delta L} F_n G_{m-n} - D_m \right]^2 \text{ is minimum,} \qquad (19)$$

with D_m being the samples of the desired spatial wavelet,

G_m being the samples of the spatial wavelet as given by wave theory:

$$G_m = A_m^+ \, e^{-jk\Delta r_m} \text{ with } \Delta r_m = \sqrt{(m\Delta x)^2 + \Delta z^2},$$

F_n being the samples of the optimum downward extrapolation operator:

$$F_n = A_n^- \, e^{jk\Delta r_n},$$

ΔL defining the operator length.

Differentiating (19) to F_n yields the complex-valued normal equations

$$
\begin{pmatrix}
R(0) & R^*(1)\text{-------}R^*(2N) \\
R(1) & R(0)\text{--------}R^*(2N-1) \\
\vdots & \vdots \\
R(N) & R(N-1)\text{----}R^*(N) \\
\vdots & \vdots \\
R(2N) & R(2N-1)\text{---}R(0)
\end{pmatrix}
\begin{pmatrix}
F(-N) \\
F(-N+1) \\
\vdots \\
F(0) \\
\vdots \\
F(N)
\end{pmatrix}
=
\begin{pmatrix}
X(-N) \\
X(-N+1) \\
\vdots \\
X(0) \\
\vdots \\
X(N)
\end{pmatrix}
\qquad (20)
$$

with

$$R(n) = \sum_m G^*_{m-n} G_m, \quad X(n) = \sum_m G^*_{m-n} D_m$$

and D_m representing the desired spatial wavelet.

For a certain choice of step size Δz and operator length ΔL, the least-squares error is a measure of the accuracy of the extrapolation.

4. After downward extrapolation to depth level $n\Delta z$, the focussed result is given by (imaging):

$$\int_{f_{min}}^{f_{max}} P(\mathbf{r}_n, \omega)\, d\omega. \tag{21}$$

Note that space-variant band-limitation and frequency weighting can be easily applied during the inverse transformation.

CONCLUSIONS

1. Upward extrapolation is presented as a spatial *convolution* procedure for each frequency component, the spatial wavelet being given by the wave theory and the acquisition geometry used. It is shown that downward extrapolation (focussing) should be considered as a wavelet *deconvolution* procedure, the spatial wavelet being given by the upward extrapolation operator.
2. The Kirchhoff summation operator acts as a band-limited spatial spiking deconvolution filter, the band-limitation given by the extreme near field only. This explains the ever-present noise in sections focussed according to the Kirchhoff approach. Therefore, any focussing technique which does not take this property into account may generate excessive spatial noise.
3. A new focussing technique has been proposed, whose main features can be summarized by the following five items:
   a) The method is recursive, in order to compensate for lateral velocity variations: the output of the previous extrapolation step is used as input for the next extrapolation.
   A small extrapolation step size Δz should be selected in the case of fast (lateral) variations in velocity. Spatial sampling imposes a lower limit on Δz.
   b) Downward extrapolation is carried out in the space-frequency domain and is realized by a space-variant convolution for each frequency component, the space-variancy being defined by the lateral velocity variation.
   c) The actual focussing result is obtained by a (weighted) summation over all frequency components. During summation any filtering procedure (e.g. least-squares inverse filtering to improve the depth resolution) can be included.
   d) Focussing in two dimensions involves *single*-channel convolution for each frequency component while for focussing in three dimensions a *two*-channel convolution should be applied. With respect to existing (three-dimensional) focussing techniques this means a significant simplification in data handling.
   e) In the least-squares procedure for the computation of the optimum downward extrapolation (focussing) operator, a desired spatial wavelet

has been introduced which avoids the generation of spatial noise caused by the focussing procedure. The width of this wavelet depends on the frequency component, the size of the aperture and the depth level.

REFERENCES

1. Von Ramm OT, FL Thurstone: Cardiac imaging using a phased array ultrasound system. Circulation 53:258, 1976.
2. Ligtvoet CM, J Ridder, CT Lancée, F Hagemeijer, WB Vletter, WJ Gussenhoven: A dynamically focussed multiscan system, In: Echocardiology with Doppler applications and real time imaging, Bom N (ed), The Hague, Martinus Nijhoff, 1977, p 313–323.
3. Berkhout AJ: Seismic migration – forward and inverse modeling by wave field extrapolation, Amsterdam, Elsevier/North Holland (to appear autumn 1979).
4. Berkhout AJ: Least-squares inverse filtering and wavelet deconvolution. Geophysics 42:1369, 1977.

APPENDIX A

The rayleigh operator

The wave-equation for pressure data is given by:

$$\frac{\partial^2 p}{\partial x^2} + \frac{\partial^2 p}{\partial y^2} + \frac{\partial^2 p}{\partial z^2} = \frac{1}{c^2}\frac{\partial^2 p}{\partial t^2}. \tag{A-1}$$

Applying a triple Fourier transform with respect to x, y and t gives*

$$\frac{d^2\tilde{P}}{dz^2} + \left\{\frac{\omega^2}{c^2} - \left(k_x^2 + k_y^2\right)\right\}\tilde{P} = 0 \tag{A-2}$$

with $\tilde{P} = \tilde{P}(k_x, k_y, z, \omega)$.

The solution of (A-2) is well known:

$$\tilde{P}(k_x, k_y, z, \omega) = \tilde{P}(k_x, k_y, 0, \omega)e^{-jz\sqrt{[\omega^2/c^2 - (k_x^2 + k_y^2)]}}. \tag{A-3}$$

Equation (A-3) formulates a multiplication of two functions in k_x and k_y. Therefore, inverse Fourier transform to the $x-y$ space yields a spatial convolution:

$$P(x, y, z, \omega) = \int\int_{S_1} G(x - x_1, y - y_1, z, \omega)\, P(x_1, y_1, 0, \omega)\, dx_1 dy_1 \tag{A-4}$$

with

$$G(x, y, z, \omega) = \int_{k_x}\int_{k_y} e^{-jz\sqrt{[\omega^2/c^2 - (k_x^2 + k_y^2)]}}\, e^{-j(k_x x + k_y y)}\, dk_x\, dk_y,$$

*Transformation from x, y, z, t-domain (space-time domain) to k_x, k_y, z, ω-domain wavenumber-frequency domain).

and $k_x^2 + k_y^2 \leq \dfrac{\omega^2}{c^2}$.

Now, if we introduce the new variables

$$x = p \cos \phi \qquad y = \rho \sin \phi \qquad r = \sqrt{\rho^2 + z^2}$$
$$k_x = q \cos \theta \qquad k_y = q \sin \theta$$

then we obtain after some manipulations the expression for the operator G:

$$G(x, \ y, \ z, \ \omega) = \frac{z}{2\pi} \ \frac{1 + jkr}{r^3} \ e^{-jkr} \tag{A-5}$$

with $k = \dfrac{\omega}{c}$.

Note that in result (A-5) the extreme near field, defined by $k_x^2 + k_y^2 > \dfrac{\omega^2}{c^2}$, has been deleted.

Comparison of (A-4) and (6) shows that these equations are equivalent. Hence, expression (A-3) describes the upward extrapolation in the k_x, k_y, z, ω-domain. So for the upward extrapolation operator we find

$$G(k_x, \ K_y, \ z, \ \omega) = e^{-jz\sqrt{[\omega^2/c^2 - (k_x^2 + k_y^2)]}}.$$

This operator is also called the *Rayleigh operator*.

M/Q-MODE ECHOCARDIOGRAPHY

The synthesis of conventional echo with digital multigate Doppler**

MARCO A. BRANDESTINI, MARK K. EYER, and JAMES G. STEVENSON

Conventional M-mode techniques provide for dynamic recording of cardiac anatomy. The addition of the flow information gained via pulsed Doppler has proven to be a valuable complement to the echo image. In a prototype unit developed in our laboratories, a high resolution velocity profile has been obtained using a digital multigate Doppler. Using a single transducer, the two processors (Fig. 1) produce an echo and a flow component for every spatial point, resulting in four dimensions of information (echo amplitude, flow velocity, depth and time). Those parameters are displayed in a meaningful way with the aid of digital image storage interfaced to a color television monitor. In the experimental setup, flow, presented in shades of red and blue according to direction and velocity, is distinguished from the echo pattern, which is presented in gray tones.

In initial clinical trials, the detection of flow abnormalities has been most dramatic when marked alterations of flow are present, such as in case of patent ductus arteriosus, ventricular septal defect and valvular insufficiency. Based on these trials, the new device appears to offer the advantage of easier visualization of flow disturbancies and their characteristics over a large area. It is therefore felt, that M/Q techniques increase the sensitivity and specificity of non-invasive ultrasonic diagnosis.

1. SIMULTANEOUS PROCESSING OF ECHO AND DOPPLER INFORMATION

Conventional M-mode has been limited to detection of cardiac structures and their position with respect to time (cardiac phase). In a more technical language this means: Only the *amplitude* of the return signal or the echo information is being processed.* The *phase* of the return signal, so far, has been neglected with a single exception (1). Phase or more precisely, the change of phase versus time is, of course, the well known Doppler shift, that one expects to result from scattering of the incident sound wave by moving blood cells. Regarding the return signal – containing both specular echoes and scattering components – as a complex signal, it seems logical to extract magnitude and phase by a dedicated processor as illustrated in Figure 1. Due

---

*In order to be specific, in this article, the term *return signal* is used as opposed to echo signal (basis for A-, M- and B-Modes), which contains only a portion of the available information.

**Work supported by grant NIH HL-07293.

Charles T. Lancée (ed.), Echocardiology, 441–446. All rights reserved

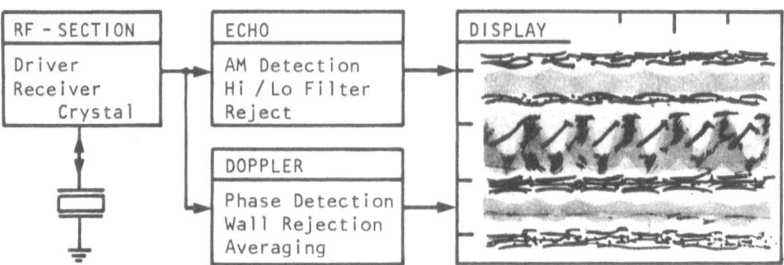

Fig. 1. Simultaneous echo and Doppler processing.

to the complexity of the process, the phase detection had been limited to a single spatial region, called the sample volume. Clinical usefulness of a device equipped with echo and Doppler processing has been reported on many occasions (1) (2), and such a system has been commercially available for some time (3).

Digital processing of the return signal made it possible to detect both echo intensity and velocity of any target along the sound beam of the transducer (4). The spatial velocity profile superimposed on the echo information yields the M/Q display shown in the examples of Figures 2, 3 and 4.

Axial resolution of echo and Doppler are limited by the same constraints (namely system bandwidth) and are on the order of 0.3 mm. Regardless of digital processing, the Doppler detection is affected by range/velocity ambiguity and uncertainty of the velocity- (frequency-) estimate due to the finite observation time.

2. FEATURES OF THE DIGITAL ECHO/DOPPLER INSTRUMENT

The primary goal of the system design has been to add the novel Doppler features to the established echo device in the most logical way. In this regard all common echo modalities (e.g. log. compression, edge enhancement, low amplitude reject etc.) are still found in the digital processor. So is the possibility to acoustically assess the blood flow at any point along the sound beam, which is the standard procedure in Doppler diagnosis (5).

Digital processing combined with microprocessor control allows for further operational convenience. Sweep rate, depth, compression scheme; basically all the controls that do not require a continuous adjustment, are done via a keyboard by single letter commands. The selected parameters appear on the TV monitor for straightforward interaction. Addition of captions and other patient information to the record is a valuable asset, especially for documentation purposes (cf. Figs. 2–4).

3. CLINICAL RESULTS

Initial applications of the M/Q processor have been in areas that are currently evaluated by pulsed Doppler echocardiography, to identify the additional diagnostic contribution of the new device.

Since most patients with congenital heart disease have a marked blood flow abnormality in the heart or great vessels, Doppler exams have had immediate applications for detection of those symptoms.

In cases of ventricular septal defect, the most frequently encountered intracardiac defect, pulsed Doppler examinations have been very useful to identify the jet caused by the VSD (2). In some cases, where the jet is not discrete, its precise localisation has been difficult. On patients with pulmonary hypertension, and less turbulent VSD flow, the jet has also been more difficult to find by probing with the sample volume throughout the ventricles.

The M/Q display provides flow information across the *whole* echo, and as seen in Figure 3, immediately pinpoints the VSD jet, so that the sample volume could then quickly be guided into place.

In cases of patent ductus arteriosus, when examined from a standard precordial approach, the M/Q display demonstrates systolic flow from right ventricle into the pulmonary artery in shades of red, while diastolic flow from aorta through ductus into the pulmonary artery is indicated by blue color. Again, the color presentation of flow across the entire depth of the M-mode tracing quickly identifies any disturbance.

In cases of valvar stenosis, as shown in Figure 4, the turbulent flow pattern is characterized as a mixing of colors, representing all the different velocities and directions of the individual blood cells. This speckly pattern contrasts with the uniform and smooth colors present in areas of normal flow (cf. Fig. 2.).

While Figure 4 is of aortic stenosis, semilunar valvar insufficiency has also been shown with the new device, with the insufficiency jet appearing as mixed color pattern on the ventricular side of the valve, in diastole. It would appear, that the M/Q exam adds substantially to the non-invasive estimation of severity of insufficiency, simply by showing the extent of the insufficiency jet.

4. CONCLUSIONS

The few results, picked from initial trials, should demonstrate the potential for assessing cardiac anatomy and flow simultaneously. The color flow overlay provides a highly intelligible distinction between the different degrees of information and helps the operator to relate the new technique to the more familiar M-mode.

We also believe, that the possibility of recording flow information is a valuable complement to conventional modalities. In fact, several authors have reported on the usefulness of contrast echocardiography – an invasive and less quantitative procedure – for gaining a closer insight into cardiovascular function (7).

Extension of echo/Doppler processing to two-dimensional cross sectional scanning has already been implemented in a peripheral vascular prototype system (8).

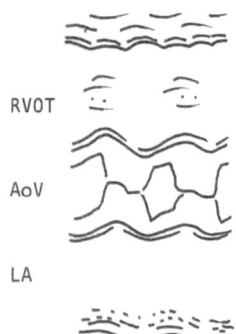

RVOT

AoV

LA

ECG

Sweep rate:
 1/2 sec markers

Depth markers
 1 cm spacing

Mid - record
 indicator (2cm)

Arrow (∧) indi-
cates, that flow
towards the trans-
ducer is blue.

Tonal velocity
scale in red (top)
and blue (bottom)
 11cm/sec / div

Velocities in the
range of ± 6cm/sec
are not displayed
(black threshold)

Horizontal line
indicates, where
flow is acousti-
cally monitored.
(sample volume)

Full size caption
field: ID, date,
vel. scale, title,
fmax, p.r.f.,
ECG delay, crystal,
frame counter.

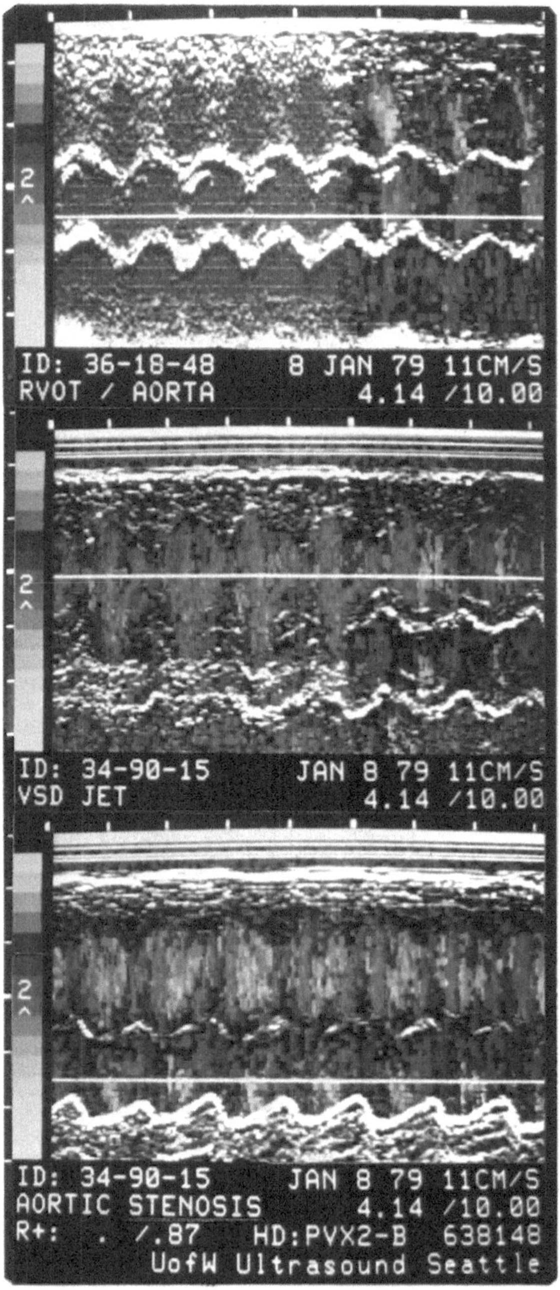

ID: 36-18-48   8 JAN 79 11CM/S
RVOT / AORTA   4.14 /10.00

ID: 34-90-15   JAN 8 79 11CM/S
VSD JET   4.14 /10.00

ID: 34-90-15   JAN 8 79 11CM/S
AORTIC STENOSIS   4.14 /10.00
R+:   . /.87   HD:PVX2-B   638148
              UofW Ultrasound Seattle

Fig. 2. Representative M/Q display.

From a standard precordial approach, the right ventricular outflow tract, aortic valve and left atrium are seen in standard fashion. (The displayed image has been digitized to 160×192 pixels, each being either 16 shades of grey or colors, M-mode quality may thus be inferior to state of the art techniques).

The record has been arranged to show echo features on one half and flow velocity patterns on the other.

Note how the flow is uniform throughout the cardiac cycle in this normal subject.

Fig. 3. M/Q trace from patient with ventricular septal defect.

From a precordial approach, the right ventricular outflow tract with sample volume line, is at the top. The aortic root and valve leaflets are seen at the right, while a sweep has been made from the ventricles to the left. The ventricular septum is continuous with the anterior aortic root. The scattered blue colors indicate the position of the VSD jet as it flows from left ventricle, through septum, into the right ventricle, giving disturbed flow to right ventricle. This figure vividly illustrates how the jet is localized within the septum, and how its extent and velocity components can immediately be estimated.

Fig. 4. M/Q record in patient with aortic stenosis.

On the top is right ventricular outflow tract, next posterior is aortic root with sample volume line within and a portion of left atrium at the bottom of the record. While the normal RVOT flow is biphasic (clearly divided red and blue areas), the flow signal in the aortic root is composed of many colors, representing turbulent flow caused by aortic stenosis.

The authors hope, that the novel M/Q technique described in this report, will find further clinical acceptance as a helpful complement to the present echo/ultrasound diagnosis.

REFERENCES

1. Baker DW, SA Rubenstein, GS Lorch: Pulsed Doppler echocardiography: Principles and applications. Am J Med 63:69, 1977.
2. Stevenson JG, I Kawabori, T Dooley, WG Gunteroth: Diagnosis of ventricular septal defect by pulsed Doppler echocardiography. Circulation 58:322, 1978.
3. Advanced Technology Laboratories: Mark IV System. Bellevue, Wash.
4. Brandestini MA, FK Forster: Blood flow imaging using a discrete-time frequency meter. IEEE ULTSYM Proc. Cat 78 CH 1344-1SU p 348.
5. Part V in: Cardiovascular application of ultrasound. Reneman RS (ed), North Holland/ American Elsevier, 1974.
6. Stevenson JG, T Dooley, I Kawabori: Patent ductus arteriosus in a neonatal intensive care unit. Circulation 58 (supp II):110, 1978.
7. Hagemeijer F, PW Serruys, WG van Dorp: Contrast echocardiology. In: Echocardiology, Bom N (ed), Martinus Nijhoff, 1977, p 147.
8. Eyer MK, MA Brandestini, DJ Phillips, DW Baker: Color digital echo/Doppler image presentation. Article submitted to UMB, 1979.

ULTRAFAST ELECTRONICAL IMAGE RECONSTRUCTION DEVICE

B. DELANNOY, R. TORGUET, C. BRUNEEL, and E. BRIDOUX

The motion of the cardiac valves is very fast, so that a very high acoustic image rate is required for their observation. A slow motion picture system enables a quantitative study of these valves to be made during all phases of the cardiac cycle.

A prototype cardiac imaging apparatus was built, where the ultrasonic images are reconstructed using optical techniques. The final images appear in optical form, at rates up to 1000 per second, and may be recorded on film using a cine camera. Such a solution proved very unsatisfactory, owing to the time needed for film development, and a magnetic record on tape would be more satisfactory. The quasi-real-time examination of the observed tomograph resulting in rapid diagnosis would then be possible. The matching of a magnetic recording system to the optical imaging apparatus would require the fast conversion of optical images into video-frequency electrical signals using a camera, whose characteristics would need to be well above the current technological limits. Another solution has therefore been tested, which consists of a purely electronic reconstruction of the acoustic images, thus giving the necessary video-frequency electrical signals directly. The problems encountered with the fast magnetic recording on a standard video tape recorder are examined, and a possible solution is given for our particular case, whereby the information may be expanded in time, during two consecutive images.

ELECTRONIC PROCESSING IMAGING APPARATUS

The magnetic tape recording of an optical image, using a camera, may be performed using, either a photo-diode array with very fast multiplexing, or else a "Fanworth"-type image dissector. The electronic image reconstruction scheme enables a real image to be obtained using a group of N piezoelectric transducers (Fig. 1) without the need for any intermediate optical system. In each group, the electrical signals issuing from the different transducers of the acoustical-field sampling array are so phased as to sum constructively for the signals arising from a point source lying on the axis of symmetry of the group, and destructively for off-axis point sources.

The reconstruction of the whole image requires a number of groups equal to the number of lines in the image. Each group is shifted from its neighbours by the spatial period of the array and all groups work in parallel, thus

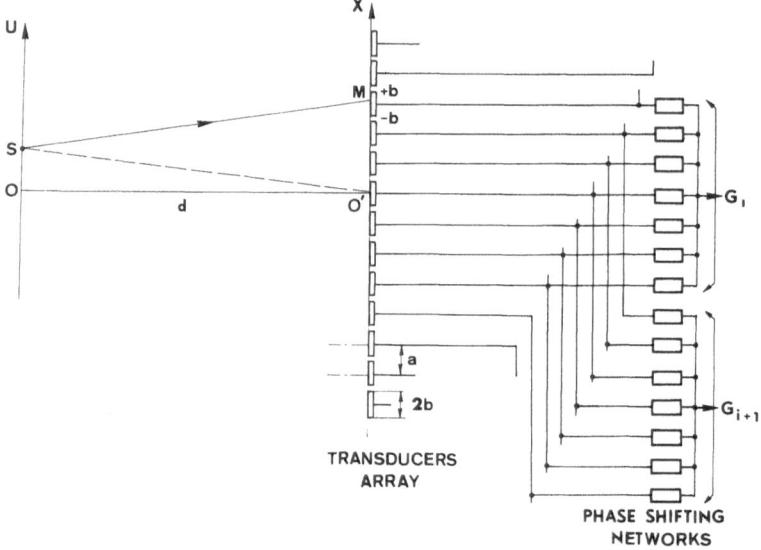

Fig. 1. Receiving array and transducer group connections.

enabling very high image rates to be obtained. The amplitude level of the first order parasitic images introduced by the spatial sampling process is related to the aperture of each group of N transducers, by the analytical relation:

$$\frac{I_1}{I_0} = \frac{\mathrm{Si}\left[\frac{\pi b}{\lambda a}(Wa + 2\lambda)\right] + \mathrm{Si}\left[\frac{\pi b}{\lambda a}(Wa - 2\lambda)\right]}{2\,\mathrm{Si}\left[\frac{\pi b}{\lambda a}Wa\right]},$$

where Si is the Sine Integral function, b the half width of each transducer, λ the radiated acoustic wavelength, a the spatial sampling period and W is the angular aperture of each group given by:

$$W = Na/d$$

if d is the observation distance.

In Figure 2, the first order parasitic image relative amplitude level versus the product $W \cdot a$ is shown for the values $\lambda = 0.5$ mm and $2b/a = 0.9$.

The system was designed to retain a constant angular aperture when the observation distance is varied. In this way, the parasitic image level is limited to a known fixed value. The moving focus feature is performed by varying the phase delays when the source distance changes, in order to get a zoom effect. The fast multiplexing of the group output signals gives the video-frequency signal, which is visualized, using a suitable monitor, at rates up to 1000 images per second, or else recorded, using a video tape recorder, after processing. The performance rated for this imaging device is comparable with

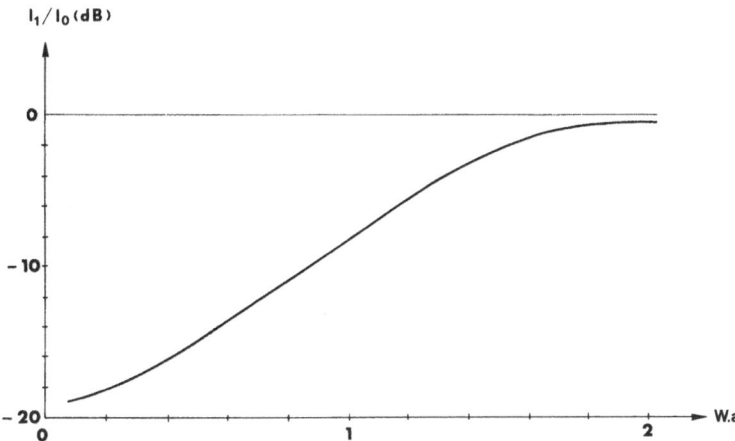

Fig. 2. First-order, secondary image level predicted for the experimental system for $\lambda = 0.5$ mm and $2b/a = 0.9$.

that of the acoustico-optical processing system. The spatial resolution is nearly equal to 4 mm, if a 4 dB criterion is assumed and the apparatus has 20 processing channels and a spatial sampling period equal to 2 mm.

In order to increase the resolution without raising the parasitic image level, the reduction of the spatial sampling period, a, is necessary. This in turn must be accomplished while keeping the product "angular aperture W and spatial period a" constant. The number of transducers per group is then multiplied by a factor inversely proportionnel to a^2, and W by a factor inversely proportional to a.

VIDEO-FREQUENCY SIGNAL PROCESSING

The cardiac ultrasound image corresponds to a maximum exploration depth of 15 cm and may be produced in 200 μsec with a frame rate of 1000 per second. The mean data rate for this type of echocardiographic imaging is given by 1000 frames per second, with 40 lines of 100 image points per line, giving 4×10^6 image points per second. The data rate is therefore lower than that for standard television, where frames of 625 lines with 830 image points per line and a frame rate of 25 per second gives 12×10^6 image points per second. The acoustic image points are not, however, uniformly time-distributed but are concentrated in the 200 μsec image format time. Thus the instantaneous data rate is as high as 20×10^6 image points per second, requiring a minimum bandwidth of 10 MHz, and thus exceeding current technical capabilities. This problem may be solved by temporarily storing the data in buffer memories and then processing it before re-recording, using a constant 1 msec frame time. This then requires a minimum bandwidth of 2 MHz, which is available as a standard option.

RECORDING ON A STANDARD VIDEO TAPE RECORDER

The reduction of the required bandwidth by buffering enables a standard video tape recorder to be used as the recording device, even for a 40-channels imaging device, which seems to be the current technological limit imposed by the electronics needed for the reconstruction system and by the construction of the sampling transducer array. This technique has some definite advantages related to the helical scan used on the magnetic tape: a great quantity of data may be stored on reasonable lengths of tape and slow-motion observation is possible, while fixed head rotation speed enables frequency-modulated recording and provides good fidelity at the reading stage.

CONCLUSION

In order to retain the advantages of the high image rate capability of some imaging devices, a recording and slow-motion picture system must be added to them. The recording may be performed using a cine camera and magnetic tape recording for the acousto-optic processing imaging system, but only if the optical images are rapidly converted into video-frequency signals. With the purely electronic reconstruction system, currently developed in our laboratory, the optical-electronic conversion is bypassed and direct recording of the output video-frequency signals onto magnetic tape is possible, using time expansion of the information-carrying signals after buffering. Moreover, a standard video tape recorder may be used for this purpose, with only a few technical modifications being then required in order to meet our recording and slow-motion picture observation criteria. In the medical field, this device could not only provide as useful information as that to be obtained from a TM scanner but would provide this data for the whole cardiac valve instead for a single isolated point on the valve.

REFERENCES

1. Torguet R, C Bruneel, E Bridoux, JM Rouvaen: Acoustical image reconstruction devices. In: Echocardiology, Bom N. (ed), p. 299–304. The Hague, Martinus Nijhoff, 1977, p 299–304.
2. Delannoy B, R Torguet, C Bruneel, E Bridoux: Traitement analogique électronique d'images ultrasonores à grande cadence. Biosigma, Paris avril 1978. p 128–133.
3. Delannoy B, R Torguet, C Bruneel, E Bridoux, JM Rouvaen, H Lasota: Acoustical image reconstruction in parallel-processing analog electronic system. J Appl Phys, to be published March 1979.

NEW SECTOR-SCAN ECHOGRAPHIC IMAGING DEVICES

F. HAINE, R. TORGUET, G. BRUNEEL, E. BRIDOUX, and C. THOMIN

INTRODUCTION

The main advantage of sector-scan imaging devices over their linear scanning counterparts, is their capability to produce images through observation windows of very small area. Structures situated behind ultrasound opaque substances may therefore be visualized. Such a feature seems to be highly appreciated by users and, consequently, many sector-scan imaging instruments are now under development. A number of techniques may be used for sector-scanning and a distinction can be made between mechanical and electronic scanning devices.

PERFORMANCE AND LIMITATIONS OF EXISTING DEVICES

i. *Mechanical devices*

The mechanical scan devices make use of a rotating or oscillating transducer. The angular aperture of the sector explored in generally greater than 30 degrees, but the image rate is usually low, of the order of 20–30 images per second. The focusing of the acoustic beam, when available at all, is fixed.

The spatial resolution of these devices is not usually very good, being mostly in the 5–10 mm range. Other specific drawbacks concern the probe itself and its manipulation. The probe contains moving parts and may be rather bulky and awkward to handle. It may also be subject to vibration and mechanical wear (1, 2).

ii. *Electronic devices*

The general characteristics of electronic scan devices make them potentially more attractive. The moving (mechanical) parts are no longer necessary and the probe dimensions are greatly reduced. Moreover, a moving focus over the whole exploration depth becomes feasible. The operating principle is analogous to that of a radar array antenna; each elementary transducer of a linear array is driven by a suitably delayed signal, in order to synthesize a wave front tilted with respect to the normal axis of the front face of the transducer. The viewing direction is altered by varying the delays. In devices implemented, the delays are varied between 0 and about 10 μsec, using programmable tapped delay lines, controlled by a computer or a microprocessor. A very fine delay adjustment is necessary for building up an acoustic beam converging in the viewing direction. The design complexity is mainly due to the high number of intermediate taps e.g. 64, needed for the delay lines. A limited number of elements normally leads to a restriction in the number of fundamentally distinct viewing lines, often 16 or 32 (3, 4, 5).

A NEW PROPOSED DEVICE

Our aim was to substitute the digital control of the electronic sector-scan systems described earlier by what we hope will prove a less expensive, less complicated analog processor. This has the additional advantage of increasing the number of scan directions by a factor of 2–4.

Basically the system consists of a circular array of small emitter-receiver, piezoelectric elements, and an electronic lens. This lens is made up of linear sampling array, followed by delay lines and a third array, which is simply the probe contacting the medium to the analyzed. By separating the scanning and focusing functions, the long delays required for scanning can be synthesized using a very simple, cheap analog processor. The focusing of the re-emitted beam is performed by the set of miniature delay lines, with a maximum delay of 500 nsec. This relatively short delay is sufficient since the delay distribution is independent of the viewing angle (see Fig. 1).

By sequentially switching the transducers of the circular array, one obtains a point source, moving in a circle, whose emission reaches the lens with a variable angle of incidence, The re-emitted beam is deflected through an angle θ', which is proportional to θ. In the reception mode, the electronic lens' moving focus permits the image points to be projected in focus onto the first circular array. The latter is connected to the electronic receiving system. The emitting and receiving paths in the processor are separated, therefore different fixed delay line sets may be used for emission and reception and different focal lengths may also be chosen for the emission and reception paths. Thus, good spatial resolution may then be kept over the whole observation depth.

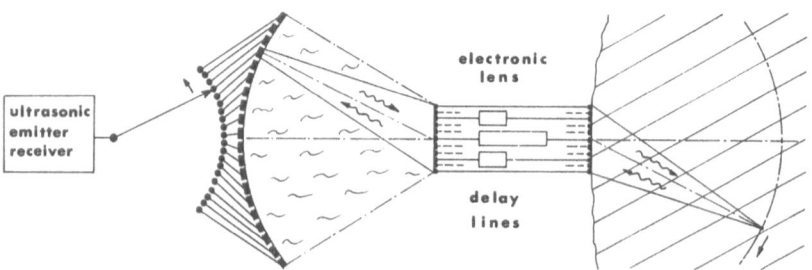

Fig. 1. Principle of the electronic sector-scan.

EXPERIMENTAL RESULTS

Experimental set-up

A simplified diagram of the imaging device is given in Figure 2. The active probe area is equal to 15×15 mm². It consists of either 2 arrays of 21 transducers each with a spatial period of one wavelength, or of 41 transducers with a spatial period of one half-wavelength, that is 0.75 mm at a 2 MHz working frequency. The acoustic beam width is approximately 5 mm at a 100 mm distance from the probe, this figure being solely determined by the probe dimensions and the wavelength. Visual inspection of the beam, by means of a Schlieren optical system, was used to monitor the correct operation of the system, that is the focusing and the maximum scanning angle, at present equal to 55 deg (see Fig. 3).

Surface-wave device

Standard photolithographic and micro-welding techniques may be used for the development of surface wave analog processors, leading to automated fabrication. The bulk acoustic-wave processors are then replaced by their acoustic surface Rayleigh wave counterparts. Only the re-emitting array uses the bulk acoustic wave mode. The angle θ of the incident beam and θ' of the

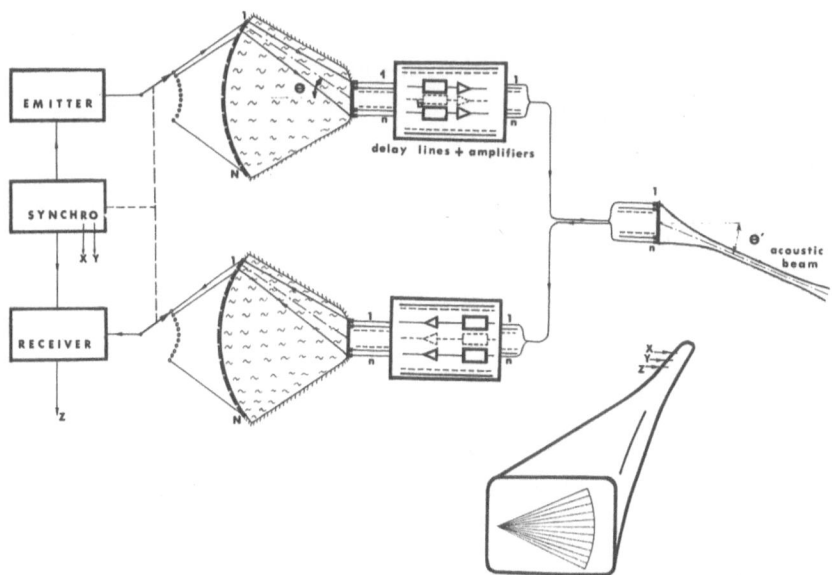

Fig. 2. Block diagram of the experimental set-up.

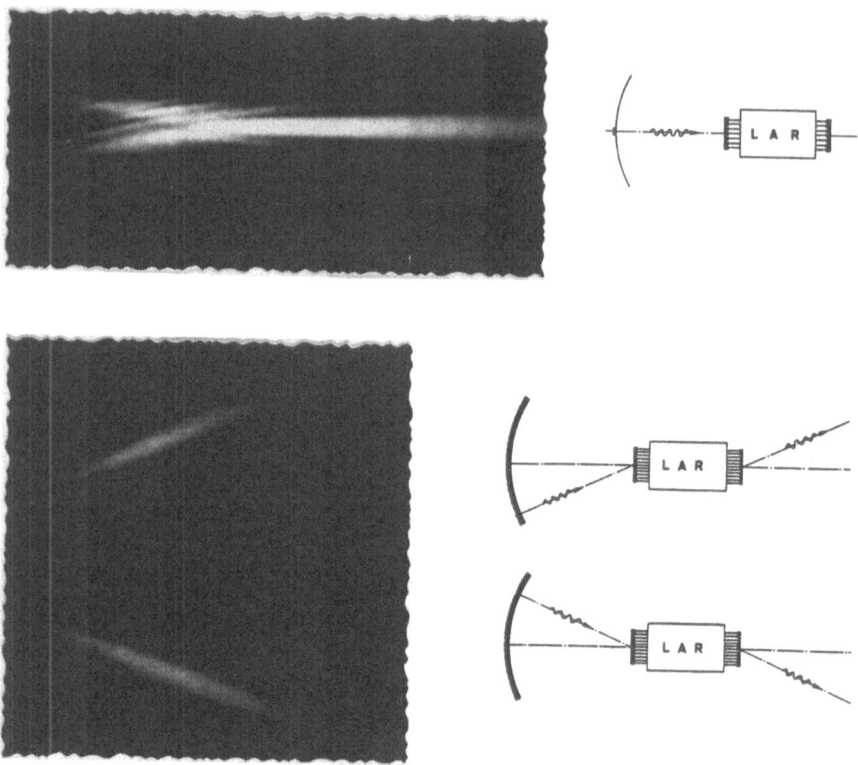

Fig. 3. Schlieren images of the acoustic beams. LAR = delay lines (lignes à retard).

exploration beam are related by the equation

$$\sin \theta' = \frac{\lambda'}{\lambda} \cdot \frac{a}{a'} \cdot \sin \theta,$$

The re-emitted bulk wave wavelength λ' being higher than that (λ) of the surface waves (typically, λ'/λ is close to 3), the angle θ' is higher than θ (6), for an aperture ratio $a/a' \cong 1$.

Results

The visualization of test objects has been used as an initial test of the usefulness of our system for imaging applications. The images obtained were always very close to the original objects. An example can be seen in Figure 4, where the image of 8 bars equally spaced on a circle is given. The bars were in cross-section with a 2 mm diameter. The supplementary arcs of circle are given for showing the sector-scanning. Matching the system to biomedical imaging application requirements, and more specifically to those in the cardiologic field, is now in progress.

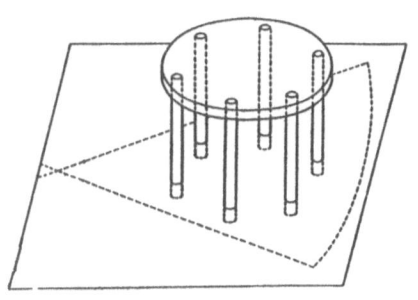 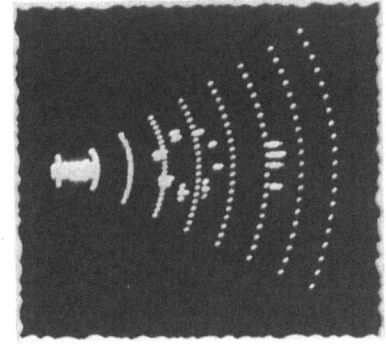

Fig. 4. Sector scan of model targets.

CONCLUSION

The results obtained with our new imaging devices are very encouraging. The spatial resolution is comparable to that given by the digital computer driven systems, but with a more straightforward design. The number of transducers in the probe may therefore be increased, together with the useful angular scanning angle, without adding too much complexity to the system design and construction tasks.

REFERENCES

1. Holm HH, JK Kristensen, JF Pedersen, S Hanche, A Northeved: A new mechanical real time ultrasonic contact scanner. Ultrasound Med Biol 2:19, 1975.
2. Shaw A, JS Paton, NL Gregory, DJ Wheatley: A real time 2-dimensional ultrasonic scanner for clinical use. Ultrasonic 14:35, 1976.
3. Somer JC: Phased array systems. In: Echocardiography, Bom N (ed), The Hague, Martinus Nijhoff, 1977, p 325–333.
4. Thurstone FL, OT von Ramm: A new ultrasound imaging technique employing two-dimensional electronic beam steering. In: Acoustical Holography Vol. 5, Proceedings of the fifth international symposium, Booth Newell (ed), New York and London, Plenum Press, 1973, p 249–259.
5. von Ramm OT, FL Thurstone, J Kisslo: Cardiovascular diagnosis with real–time ultrasound imaging. In: Acoustical Holography, Vol. 6, Proceedings of the sixth international symposium, Booth Newell (ed), New York and London, Plenum Press, 1975, p 91–102.
6. Cauvard P, P Hartemann, C Bruneel, F Haine: Ultrasound beam scanning driven by surface-acoustic-waves. IEEE ultrasonic symposium, September 25-27, 1978, Cherryville U.S.A.

STRUCTURE RECOGNITION AND DATA EXTRACTION IN TWO-DIMENSIONAL ECHOCARDIOGRAPHY

J.A. VOGEL, O.L. BASTIAANS, J. ROELANDT, and J. HONKOOP

INTRODUCTION

In the last years many methods have been developed for computerized analysis of M-mode echocardiograms obtained with a single element system (1–7). In a real-time, two-dimensional system, time motion data, as well as cross-sectional information, are available for further analysis.

A processing system has been developed for the digitization of complete series of echocardiographic cross-sections (8, 9). Acquisition of these two-dimensional echocardiographic data requires a substantially more complex system than is needed for M-mode. System design considerations may limit the suitability for clinical use.

When processing the echocardiographic data, attention is directed to recording the motion of cardiac structures. Use of semi-automated techniques for analysing the images may improve the applicability of the system. Employing a method for segmentation of cardiac structures allows the presentation of these structures in space-time display. Data-processing results in graphic presentation of a two-dimensional structure in motion and in the visualization of the two-dimensional amplitude spectrum of the movement of a structure. These methods combine structure and dynamic information in one image.

This paper will discuss acquisition methods for time-series of cross-sectional data, processing of these data and presentation techniques for derived diagnostic information.

ACQUISITION OF ECHOCARDIOGRAPHIC DATA

A system for the acquisition of real-time series of two-dimensional echocardiographic images must meet a number of requirements. Practical design considerations may lead to functional and technical limitations of the system. The system uses a PDP-11/10 minicomputer and 2.5 Mb disk with a maximum data-transfer rate of 125 kb/sec; digitized images are stored on the disk under computer control. The basic concepts and design of the acquisition methodology will therefore be discussed in terms of these constraints and of the clinical requirements; namely, that the system should be able to record and replay moving images as seen during the diagnostic routine. Clinical experience with video recording has shown that a recording period of several heart cycles and a recording speed of 50 images per second is sufficient to obtain the necessary visual information. Two methods have been developed for storage of analog echo data in the computer system.

ON-LINE DIGITIZATION

The first method requires fast analog-to-digital conversion as the sequential two-dimensional images are digitized on-line during the clinical investigation. The system is used in combination with a 20-element linear array system. The echo-amplitude information is converted into 16 intensity levels, providing 4 data bits per sample point. Since only the envelope of the RF signal is used, the depth resolution needed requires a 1 MHz sampling frequency.

On-line, real-time acquisition has been proposed by many other authors in the echographic field (10–16). An on-line system preserves all echo-information and offers optimum possibilities for signal processing. Some recent techniques, such as dynamic focussing and beam-steering, need both processing of the RF signal itself and increased ultrasound image line density, requiring a complex, digital system; whereas, since the information in the envelope of the signal is sufficient for image processing, a relatively simple hybrid system can be used. In day-to-day clinical practice, the images to be processed, whether M-mode or two-dimensional are selected from a large time-series of recordings.

VIDEO-DIGITIZATION

The second method for digitization is based on images preserved as video recordings. Due to the distinct advantages of recording ultrasound data on magnetic video tape, video registration was selected for our general clinical practice. Useful images for processing are selected from the complete video recordings of a patient.

A real-time digitizer is available for digitizing into a video-scanned memory. The digitizing level is computer-controlled and can be selected from 256 different values. A block diagram of the system is shown in Figure 1.

Processing starts with automatic determination of maximum (white) and minimum (black) intensity in the grey-scale image. The resulting intensity range is divided into 16 digitizing levels. For a standard echocardiogram, this division is based on equidistant levels.

Video recordings of echographic images of any format can be digitized with up to 256 video lines, 256 points per line and 256 possible digitizing levels. A dedicated sync-separating unit allows correct video-scanning for any video recorder signal. The video-scanned RAM memory also allows display of processed images on a standard TV monitor. Data reduction is accomplished by automatic rejection of TV lines without echo information. The images are stored on the digital disk. The method described requires po-

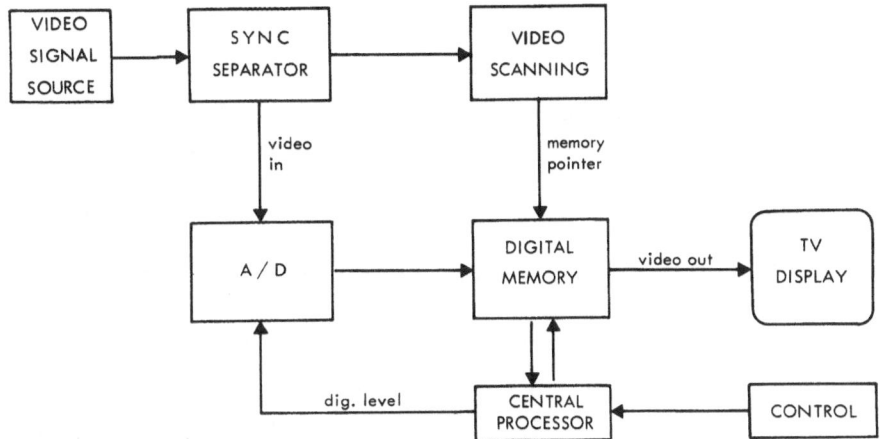

Fig. 1. Block diagram of the video digitizer. The sync separation unit allows correct video scanning for any video recorder signal.

Video images can be digitized with up to 256 video lines, 256 points per line and 256 digitizing levels. Digitized images are displayed via a video scanned digital memory.

sitioning of each sequential image as a still frame for processing purposes. The full digitization process can take several minutes for each patient.

PROCESSING OF ECHOCARDIOGRAPHIC IMAGES

Two-dimensional, real-time systems that allow the study of cross-sections of the heart are now widely used in cardiology. On video recordings of the generated echocardiographic images, cardiac motion and correct geometry of cardiac structures can be studied afterwards. Structures in two-dimensional images are recognized by their motion in time.

In still video-frames, information from motion is lost and recognition and quantitation of structures are often incorrect. Reliable quantitative analysis of motional information is usually carried out on time-motion recordings, obtained with a single element system.

M-MODE RECONSTRUCTION

Digitization of the sequential cardiac images with the equipment described has resulted in a combination of two-dimensional information with time-motion relationships. Registration of the movement of structures is made possible by a time-motion reconstruction technique. The M-mode can be reconstructed along any video line in an echocardiographic two-dimensional cross-section, by extracting this line from the successive images. Reconstructed M-modes are displayed in grey-scale.

INTERACTIVE SEGMENTATION

An interactive technique has been developed for the segmentation of cardiac structures in a series of one hundred successive images (corresponding to two seconds real-time). The method is based on structure recognition in the M-mode images successively reconstructed for each line from top to bottom, of the two-dimensional images.

The operator selects the required structure in the first M-mode (corresponding to the top of the two-dimensional image) and traces it with a light-pen. On moving to the next M-mode in the sequence, the computer uses the traced line as a first approximation in its search for the structure. The new line is then displayed to the operator, who may accept it or may correct the line, using the light-pen. Line sections redrawn by the operator replace corresponding sections of the computed "best line" and, if necessary, the whole tracing can be replaced in this way. The new line is then used as a first approximation for the next M-mode and so on until all M-modes have been segmented and the last line of the two-dimensional images has been reached. The segments found are then rearranged for imaging purposes and Figure 2 shows how the outline of a structure, which is not easily identified in the original two-dimensional cross-section on the left, can now be clearly seen in the view on the right, where the data from the M-mode segmentation has been superimposed. The new data is now available for use with clinical programs.

The method used by the computer program to make estimations of tracings, can be demonstrated with the aid of Figure 3. An M-mode reconstruction is shown together with two Amplitude-modes. The upper A-mode represents the indicated line in the M-mode, the amplitudes are stored in array A_1, the lower A-mode corresponds to the same line in the next M-mode, its amplitudes are stored in array A_2.

Due to tracing of a structure in the M-mode as shown in Figure 3, one of the points in array A_1 of the upper A-mode has been marked as the actual position of the traced structure. This point is called C_1. It may be marked because of any property, such as maximum grey-level, edge, or even more complex grey pattern. The program now has to find the point C_2 in array A_2 of the lower A-mode, with the same property as C1 by a matching algorithm. For this, LW successive array elements, with array element C_1 as center, are shifted along element A_2 in order to determinate the position of best match. To eliminate redundant calculations, an expectation window is centered in the array element of A_2 which directly corresponds to the position of C_1. The point C_2 is defined as the x-position within the expectation window where the match function

$$M_{1,2}(x) = \sum_{i=0}^{LW-1} \left| A_2\left(x - \frac{LW}{2} + i\right) - A_1\left(C_1 - \frac{LW}{2} + i\right) \right|$$

is minimal. These calculations are carried out for each line in the M-mode

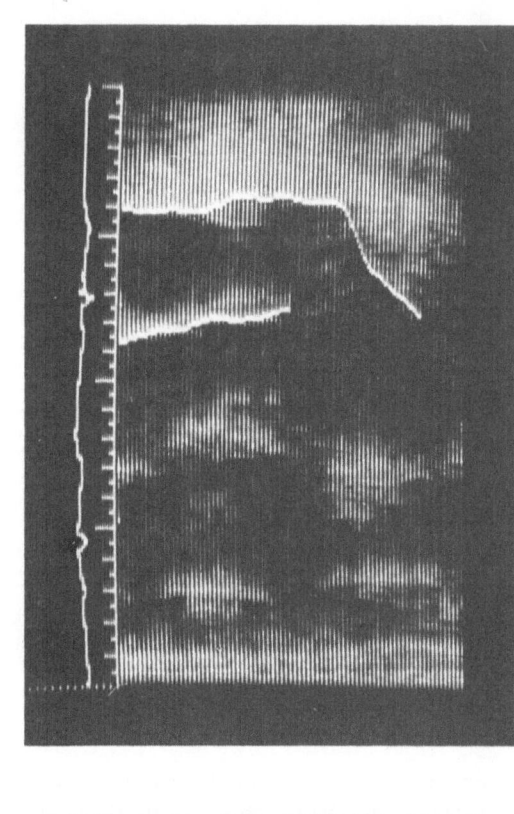

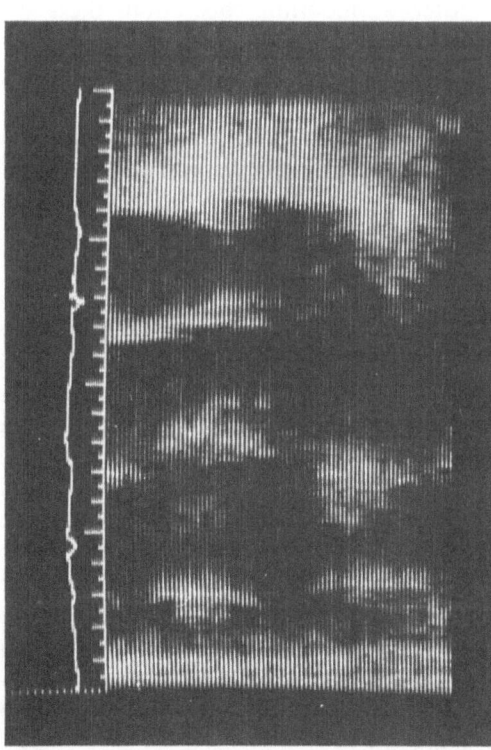

Fig. 2. An original cross-section is shown to the left. Superimposing of detected data for two structures is shown to the right.

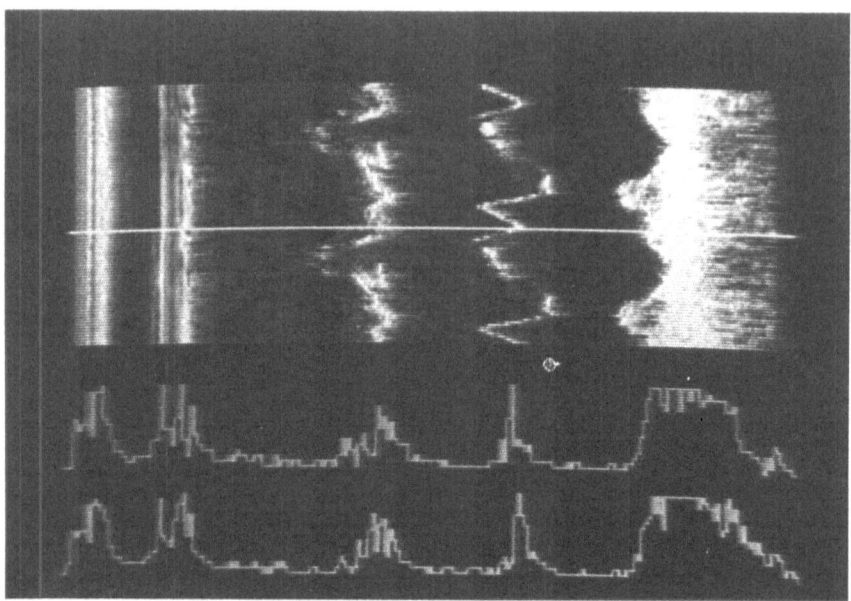

Fig. 3. Reconstructed M-mode together with the Amplitude-mode along the corresponding lines of two successive M-modes of the time series of echograms.

and its corresponding line in the next M-mode. In this way one hundred points C_2 are found. After a smoothing operation, these points are the estimation for the tracing in the next M-mode. In the interactive system, the operator is requested to accept, reject or improve the tracing. Improvement of the detection algorithm by using filtering methods before matching has been omitted because of their heavy processing time requirements. In an interactive system, the response time is an important factor for system efficiency.

DISPLAY TECHNIQUES

After the traced structure has been rearranged into the correct time and space positions, a time-series of cross-sectional line figures is available. Display of motional and structural information, such as that available in the time-series, requires a three-dimensional display technique. In Figure 4 the endocardium of the left ventricular posterior wall is displayed as a function of time. From top to bottom, the right outline of the figure represents the endocardium from the aortic area down to the apex, i.e. to the segmentated endocardium of the left ventricular posterior wall shown in Figure 2. Subsequently, the results of segmentation are displayed for the complete time-series to the left of the original line. The structure is therefore displayed from lower right to upper left, as a function of time. Grey-scale is calculated by a gradient technique to simulate light shining on this quasi three-dimensional object.

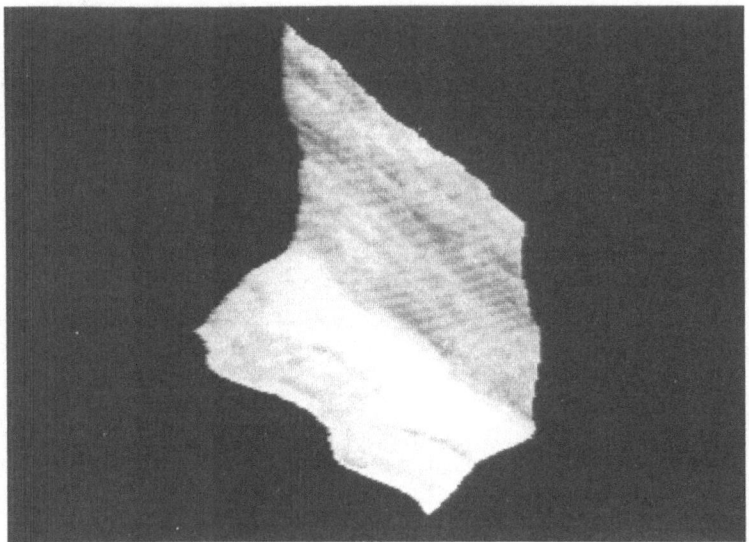

Fig. 4. The endocardium of the left ventricular posterior wall displayed as function of time (see text for details).

Similar reconstructions have been made for the other cardiac structures. Mitral dynamics can be studied and quantified in this way and visualization of the interventricular septum allows the study of septal contraction as a wave sequence from the aorta to the apex. Thickening and motion pattern of the septum can be calculated at any desired level. An overall picture of regional wall and structure movement throughout the cardiac cycle is obtained in a two-dimensional amplitude spectrum. An example of this imaging technique is given in Figures 5, 6 and 7. Time is represented on the horizontal axis; two seconds of information are displayed from left to right. The cardiac structure is represented on the vertical axis. From top to bottom on the vertical axis the structure is displayed in the direction from the aortic region towards the apex. The position of structures is converted into amplitude information, for which several methods of presentation exist. In black/white pictures where the information is presented in line figures, contours of equal amplitude are drawn at linear intervals. An example of this type of display is given by Gibson (17) for processed X-ray images.

In grey-scale pictures, amplitude information is incorporated in the grey levels. For a ventricular study, the inward movement of a structure represents a change in grey level from black to white, along any horizontal line, while outward movement is represented by darkening of the pixels of the picture. Optimum use of grey-scale information is obtained by histogram-equalization. Resulting images are shown in Figure 5, 6 and 7. A grey-scale display matching the distance scale on the axis relates each grey-level to a distance between transducer and structure. As shown in these figures, grey-scale can also be converted to colour in order to emphasize the equal

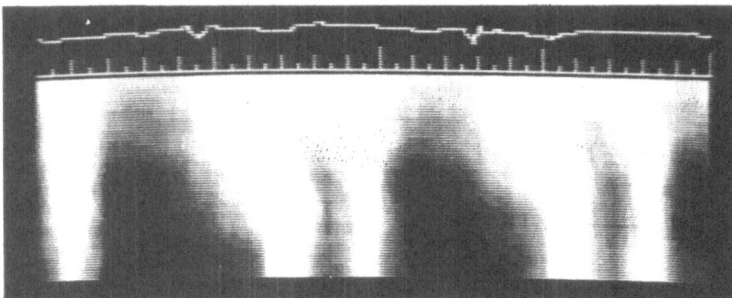

Fig. 5. Two-dimensional amplitude spectrum of motion of the anterior mitral valve leaflet of a patient with a normally functioning left ventricle (see text for details).

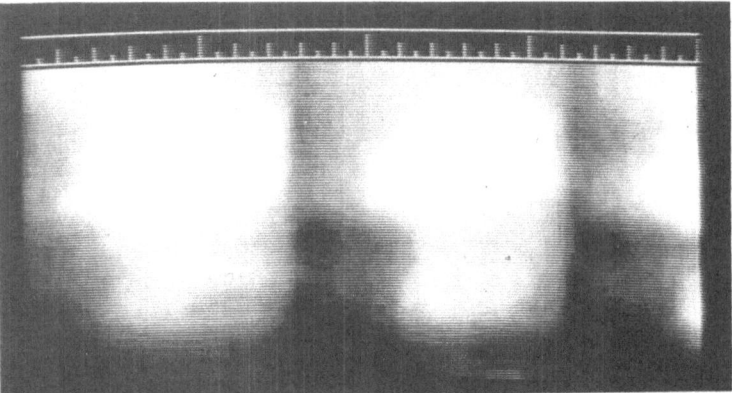

Fig. 6. Amplitude spectrum of motion of the anterior mitral valve leaflet of a patient with mitral stenosis (see text for details).

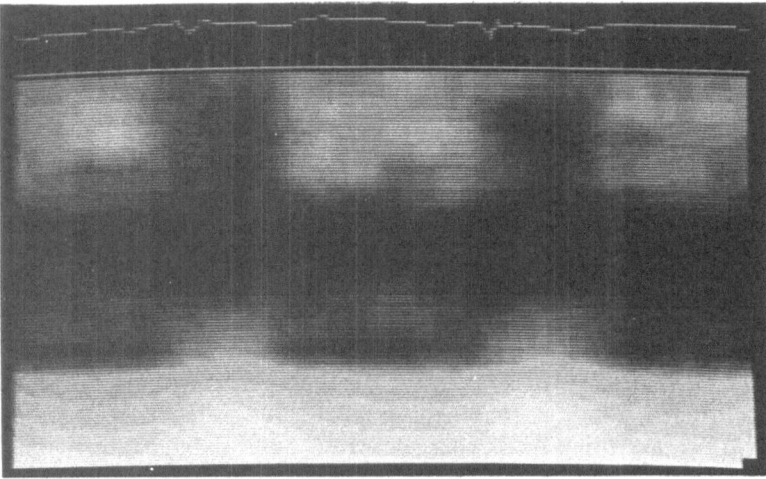

Fig. 7. Motion pattern of the posterior wall from atrial region down to the apex for a patient with a normal left ventricle (see text for details).

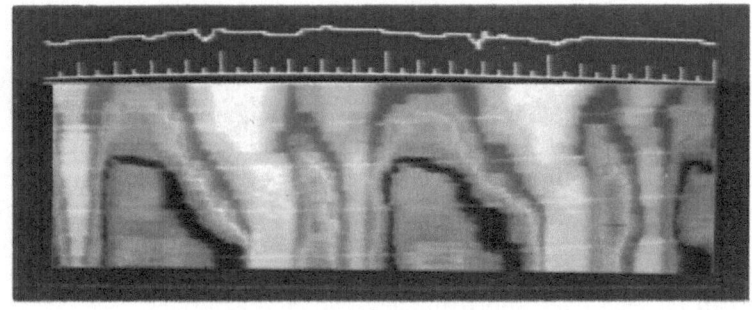

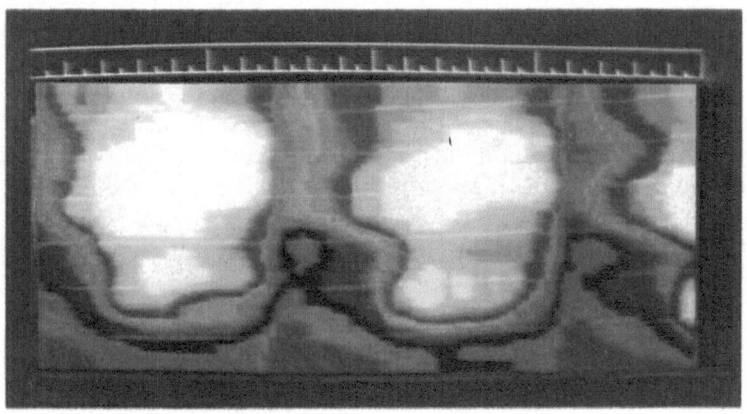

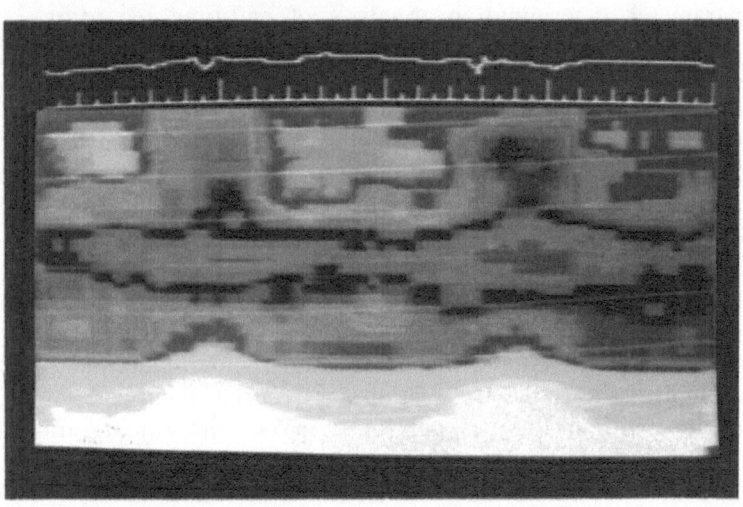

amplitude contours in the image. The images can be completed by adding the ECG and patient-information.

The movement of the anterior mitral valve leaflet of a patient with a normally-functioning left ventricle is shown in Figure 5. The dynamic events of the leaflet are clearly demonstrated in this figure. The higher part of the image illustrates the movement of the annulus, and the lowest part of the image the movement of the free edge of the valve leaflet. Systolic closure. opening in early diastole anteriorly towards the septum, partial closure of its neutral position in mid-diastole and re-opening during atrial systole of the leaflet can be seen over approximately two cardiac cycles.

For a patient with mitral stenosis, the change in the echocardiographic pattern of the mitral valve is shown in Figure 6. The typical, M-shaped, motion pattern of the leaflet is replaced by a "square wave" pattern, which is directly related to the hemodynamics of this disease. Two-dimensional studies of mitral valve dynamics are also reported by Brun (18).

In Figure 7, the motion pattern of the posterior wall from the atrial region down to the apex is shown for the patient with the normally-functioning left ventricle. After the QRS complex, anterior motion of the left ventricular wall together with posterior motion of the atrial region of the wall is demonstrated. It is important to realize that motion patterns in the images discussed are the result both of motion of the structure itself and of movement of the heart as a whole.

DISCUSSION

Echocardiographic data-processing is directed towards proper presentation and efficient handling of diagnostic information by means of display methods and parameter determination. Analysis of real-time recordings of two-dimensional images combines structural information with the dynamic information in time-motion relations. A systematic approach for quantification is obtained by using a time-motion reconstruction technique and semi-automatic segmentation of the structures. This approach permits rapid calculation of, hitherto difficult to acquire, diagnostic information, such as volume-time diagrams, ventricular-mass estimates and the display methods described in this paper.

Some processing work done in the echocardiographic field suggests that it may be possible to automate the structure detection completely and thus reduce the processing time. (15, 16, 19) However, our experience has shown that, up till now, the complexity of the echocardiographic images does not allow completely automated detection on a routine basis.

The processing techniques developed in our laboratory, and partially described in this article, allow the assessment of information on regional and overall ventricular function and the measurement of left ventricular dimension, mitral valve opening and posterior wall dynamics. The results described have been obtained from experience with a small selection of patients. The equipment and software package have now reached the stage at which processing of recordings can be carried out for larger groups of patients on a more routine basis.

REFERENCES

1. Upton MT, DG Gibson, DJ Brown: Instantaneous mitral valve leaflet velocity and its relation to left ventricular wall movement in normal subjects. 38:51, 1976.
2. Van Zwieten G, JA Vogel, AHA Bom, H Rijsterborgh: Computer assisted analysis of M-mode echocardiograms. Proc. "Computers in Cardiology", 1977.
3. Brower RW, WC van Dorp, JA Vogel, JR Roelandt: An improved method for the quantitative analysis of M-mode echocardiograms. European J Cardiol 313:171, 1975.
4. Teichholz Louis E, Gray R, Caputo, Jose Meller, Norman Kashdan, Diane LeBlanc, Michael v. Herman: Computer-assisted interactive interpretation of clinical echocardiograms. Computers in Cardiology 1977, IEEE Cat. no. 77CH 1254-2C.
5. Pai AG, NS Cahill, BA Dubroff, HA Fozzard, HC Brooks: Digital computer analysis of M-scan echocardiograms. J Clinical Ultrasound 4:173, 1976.
6. Decoodt PR, DG Mathey, HJC Swan: Automated analysis of left ventricular diameter time course from echocardiographic recordings. Computers in Biomedical Research 9:549, 1976.
7. Saffers, SLV Nixon, DJ Mishelevich: A simple method for computer aided analysis of echocardiograms. Am J Cardiol 38:34, 1976.
8. Vogel JA, CM Ligtvoet, N Bom, G van Zwieten, PG Hugenholtz: Processing equipment for two-dimensional echocardiographic data. Ultrasound in Med Biol, Pergamon Press (1975).
9. Vogel JA, RW Brower, N Bom, G van Zwieten, J Roelandt: Automation in processing of echocardiographic data. Computers in Cardiology (1975).
10. Waag RC, R Gramiak: Methods for ultrasonic imaging of the heart. Ultrasound in Med & Biol 147-1:8 (1976.
11. Gramiak R, RC Waag: Cardiac reconstruction imaging in relation to other ultrasound systems and computer tomography. Am J Röntgenol 127:91, 1976.
12. McSherry DH: Computer processing of diagnostic ultrasound data. IEEE Trans Sonics & Ultrasonics 21:91, 1974.
13. Matsumoto M, H Matsuo, A Kitabatake, M Inque, Y Hamanaka, S Tamura, K Tanaka, H Abe: Three-dimensional echocardiograms and two-dimensional echocardiographic images at desired planes by a computerized system. Ultrasound in Med & Biol 3:163, 1977.
14. Romic CA, AD Hagan: Automated echocardiogram analysis, Proc. San Diego Biomedical Symposium, 145 (1974).
15. Hirsch M, WJ Sanders, RL Popp, DC Harrison: Computer processing of ultrasonic data from the cardio-vascular system. Comp Bio-Med Res 6:336 (1973).
16. Robison EP, TA Pryor, SJ Willard, DS Jones, JD Ridges: Recognition of left ventricular borders using two-dimensional echocardiographic images. Comp Bio-Med Res 9:247, (1976).
17. Upton MT, DG Gibson: The study of left ventricular function from digitized echocardiograms. Progress in Cardiovascular Diseases 20, No. 5, 1978.
18. Brun Ph, C Oddou, A Kulas, F Laurent: Small computer development of echocardiographic information related to left ventricle and mitral valve in diastole. Comp Cardiol. 267–274, 1977.
19. Kuwahara M, S Eiho, H Kitagawa, K Minato, N Mike: Computer analysis of ultrasonic echocardiogram. Proc. of U.S.-Japan Seminar on Image Analysis, Oct. 31–Nov. 4, 1978, Tokyo.

VIDEO TRACING OF M-MODE ECHOCARDIOGRAMS

G. VAN ZWIETEN, O.L. BASTIAANS, J. HONKOOP, and J.A. VOGEL

1. INTRODUCTION

Various computer-based systems for deriving LV function parameters from M-mode echocardiograms are in use to-day. They are mainly based on manual digitizing of structures of interest with the aid of a digitizing tablet (1, 2, 3, 4). Our experience with such a system indicates that, for large series of heartbeats, this is still a cumbersome procedure. It is the purpose of this paper to present a new development in further automation of digitizing large numbers of M-mode echocardiograms.

Accurate analysis of echocardiograms can only be carried out by a physician or cardiologist experienced in echocardiography. Since the actual digitizing of echocardiograms is often performed by personnel with less experience in interpreting echocardiograms, the echocardiogram is first traced with an ordinary lead pencil by the echocardiographer responsible for the interpretation. We have developed a method of digitizing a pre-traced echocardiogram directly, with a TV camera, which overcomes the need to retrace the recordings on a digitizing tablet.

2. HARDWARE

The hardware employed consists of a PDP 11/10 minicomputer with 32 Kbyte main memory, a 2.4 Mbyte disc and a Decwriter. In addition to the standard configuration we have a 8 Kbyte TV scanned memory (Fig. 1). This part of memory is directly accessible by the Central Processor. It is also equipped with real-time A/D and D/A converters so as to fill or display this memory as a 256×256 point image, 1 bit per point. The threshold level of the A/D converter is under program control. The scanning of the TV memory is synchronized with the camera signal, which allows us to mix the camera and the memory images for operator judgement. A simple data-entry keyboard is added for control of the digitizing program (Fig. 2).

3. PREPARATION OF RECORDINGS

The recordings to be digitized (on Kodak direct print paper) must be pre-traced with an ordinary lead pencil in a prescribed manner, as indicated in

Charles T. Lancée (ed.), Echocardiology, 469–475. All rights reserved

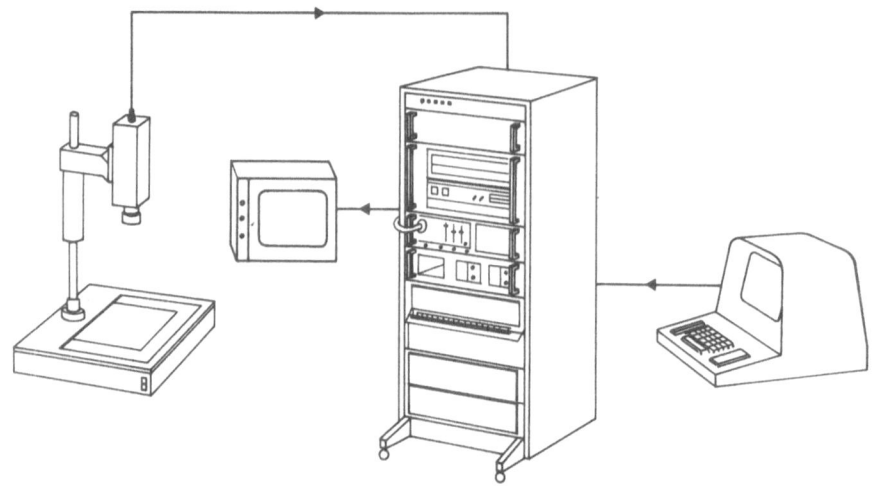

Fig. 1. System configuration.

Figure 3. At the start of a recording, the time and distance calibration has to be indicated. This is done in such a fashion that automatic recognition is easy. The structures of interest have to be pre-traced as continuous lines. In addition, time events (such as R-waves) have to be indicated as vertical lines at the bottom of the recording, not intersecting the indicated structures.

After this preparation, the recording is placed under the TV-camera. By through illumination, a good contrast between the marked structures and the background is obtained. The orientation of the recording is such that the

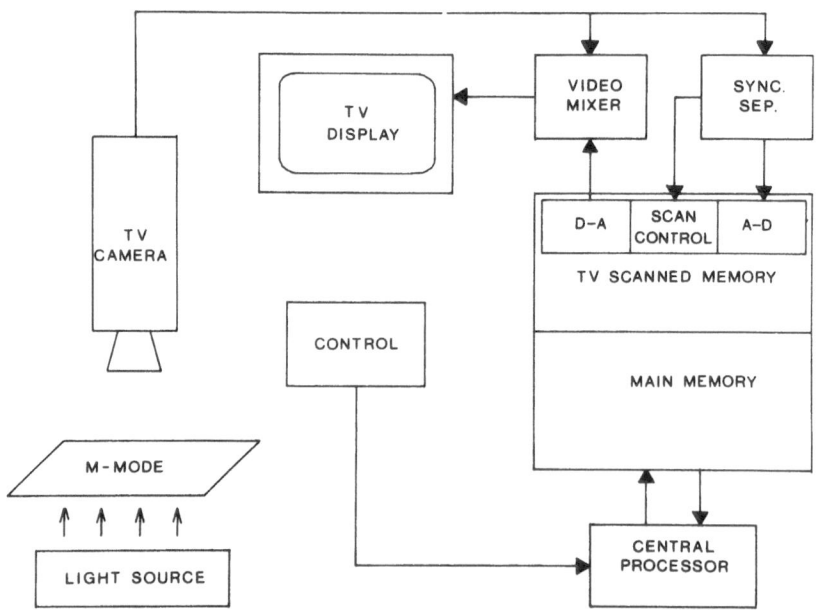

Fig. 2. Block diagram of video-digitizing system.

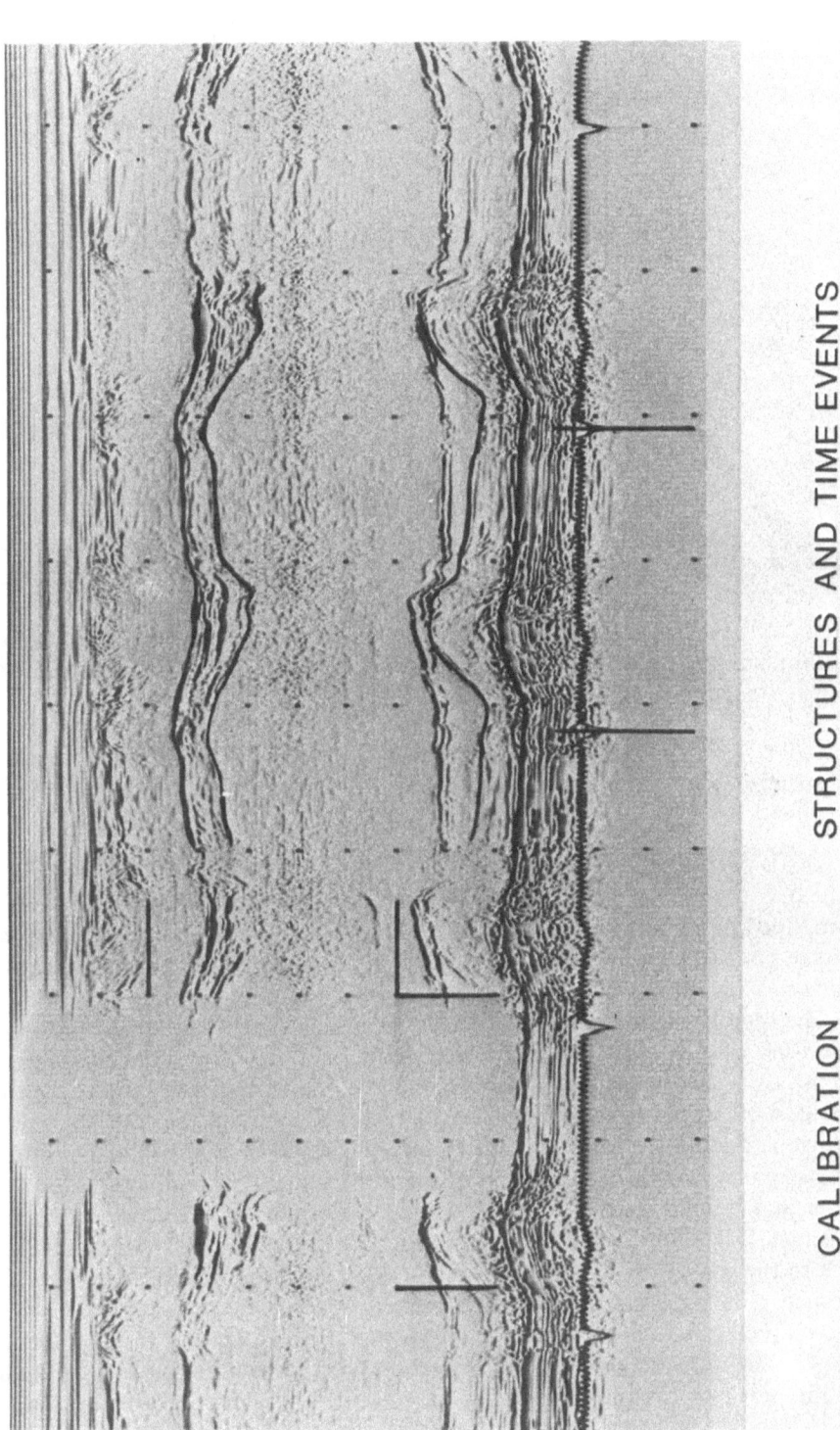

Fig. 3. Example of pencil-marked M-mode recording.

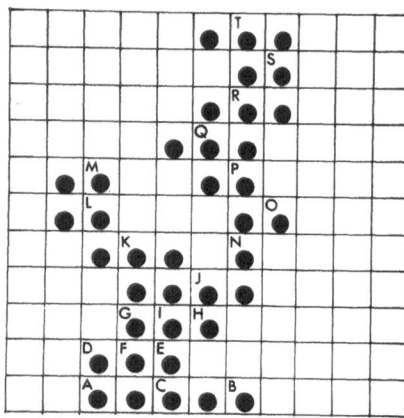

Fig. 4. Simplified diagram of thresholded image. For explanation see text.

time axis of the recording is perpendicular to the TV scanning lines. Consequently, the structures to be found will run from the bottom to the top of the image.

4. SOFTWARE

1. *Line search algorithm*

The most important part of the software is the line search algorithm. A simplified diagram of an image is shown in Figure 4. Each box represents an image point. The marked boxes were below the threshold level and digitized as zeroes (displayed black) the others as ones (displayed white).

The search starts at the lower left-hand corner of the image and proceeds from left to right until a single black point, or a group of adjacent ones, is found (A to B). From this group, the middle one is marked as belonging to the desired structure (point C). Then a search is made in the line above the previous one for a group of black points connected to group A-B i.e. group D-E. Again the middle one is marked (point F). On the next line we find group G-H and point I is marked. This process is repeated until the upper line is reached. When a branch occurs, the branch point is retained. If a branch ends before the top of the image is reached, the algorithm jumps back to the last branch point and the other branch is tried. When the upper line is reached the marked points are declared as a structure. If there are more structures to be searched for, the procedure is repeated at the bottom line just to the right of the previous starting group. Typically a structure is digitized in less than 1 sec.

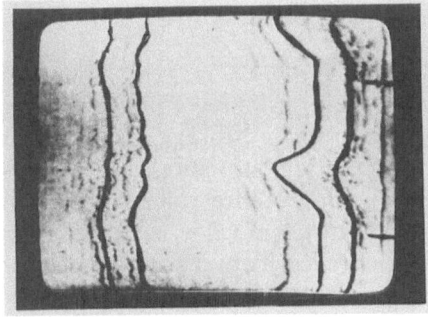 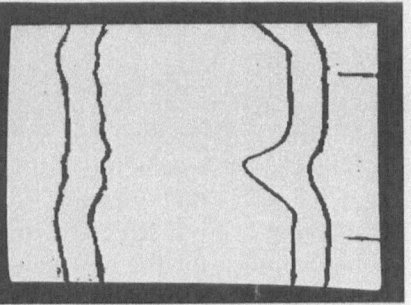

Fig. 5a. Pencil-marked M-mode recording with back-illumination as seen by TV camera.

Fig. 5b. Thresholded image.

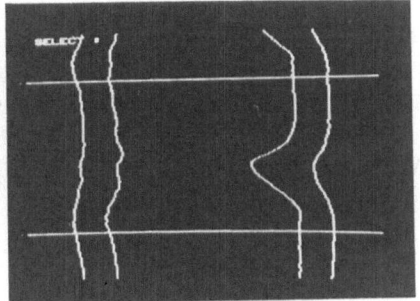 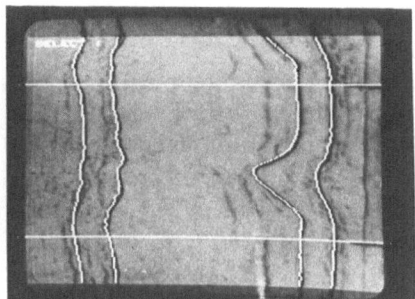

Fig. 5c. Structures and time events detected.

Fig. 5d. Result superimposed on original image.

2. Control program

The line search algorithm is incorporated in the control program. The digitizing starts with a request for an initial video threshold level to be adjusted by the operator. This level is used by the digitizing sub-programs, with automatic adjustment when needed.

At first the calibration part is placed under the TV camera. After successful calibration the first heartbeat is placed under the camera (Fig. 5a) and thresholded (Fig. 5b). Digitizing of the structures is then performed as described above (Fig. 5c). In addition, the time events are found from the right side of the image. The result is displayed superimposed on the camera image (shown in Fig. 5d) for operator acceptance. When accepted, the co-ordinates are stored on disk. This process is repeated for as many heartbeats as needed. The speed of digitizing is such that, for example, a recording of 100 consecutive beats from a patient with atrial fibrillation was digitized in 20 min.

3. *Data compression*

Since the system is intended for digitizing large series of recordings, we use a simple data compression technique for co-ordinate storage. Due to the perpendicular TV scanning method, the digitized structures are already sampled at equal time intervals, so that only the distance values need to be stored. From a given structure, only the first distance value is stored as an absolute number; for the next points, the differences between the point itself and its predecessor are stored. Four difference values are encoded in one 16 bit word. This results in a compression ratio of almost 4:1.

5. ACCURACY

When we consider an area of 7.5 by 7.5 cm, which is usually adequate for digitizing one beat from a LV echocardiogram, a 256×256 point digitizing results in a resolution of 0.3 mm. This is the same resolution as that obtained with manual digitizing using a tablet of 1024×1024 points on a 30×30 cm surface. Due to non-linearity of the deflection of the TV camera, this will be worse at the boundaries of the image. Worst case accuracy will then be 0.9 mm. However, the actual manual digitizing accuracy will also be worse, due to tracing errors.

6. DISCUSSION

Recognition of structures by an experienced echocardiographer is a rather complex process. Even in average quality echocardiograms, adequate structure recognition is often possible. Although in selected echocardiograms automatic detection is possible (5, 6, 7), in our experience automatic detection in large series of average quality echocardiograms leads to a high failure rate. Therefore, it was decided not to incorporate automatic detection in the system presented here.

Our system clearly separates the three phases of analyzing echocardiograms, namely: 1) interpretation. 2) digitizing and 3) computation. The pencil marking of the recordings can be performed by the investigator responsible, at leisure. The digitizing is performed without any additional manual digitizing errors. This is especially advantageous when processing large series of echocardiograms. The separation of digitizing and computation allows another computer to be used for calculating the desired parameters, while the digitizing is performed with a small dedicated computer with the special hardware required for the method described.

7. CONCLUSION

We have developed a system for automatic digitizing of pre-traced, M-mode echocardiograms with the aid of a regular TV camera. The system allows us to perform large scale studies which would otherwise be impractical to do. It has been used successfully in a number of studies requiring digitization of hundreds of heartbeats.

REFERENCES

1. Gibson DG, DJ Brown: Assessment of left ventricular systolic function in man from simultaneous echocardiographic and pressure measurements. Brit Heart J 38:8, 1976.
2. Decoodt PR, DG Mathey, HJC Swan: Automated analysis of the left ventricular diameter time curve from echocardiographic recordings. Computers and Biomed Res 9:549, 1976.
3. Teichholz LE, GR Caputo, J Meller, N Kashdan, D LeBlanc, MV Herman: Computer-assisted interactive interpretation of clinical echocardiograms. Computers in cardiology 1977, IEEE Cat. no. 77CH 1254-C.
4. Van Zwieten G, JA Vogel, AHA Bom, H Rijsterborgh: Computer-assisted analysis of echocardiograms. Computers in cardiology 1977, IEEE Cat. no. 77CH 1254-C.
5. Ledley FD, JB Wilson: Computer Analysis of Ultrasoundcardiograms. Computers in Biol and Med 4:27, 1974.
6. Hirsh M, WJ Sanders, RL Popp, DC Harrison: Computer processing of ultrasonic data from the cardiovascular system. Computers and Biomed Res 6:336, 1973.
7. Kuwahara M, S Eiho, H Kitagawa, K Minato, N Miki: Computer analysis of ultrasonic echocardiogram. Proc U.S.-Japan Seminar on image analysis, 1978.

AUTHORS AND SUBJECT INDEX

ERRATA

Page x,   line 8, P. MACKINTOSH should read P. MACINTOSH

Page x,   line 12 from bottom, G. DROBINSKY should read
               G. DROBINSKI

Page xii,   top line, E. ORZAN should read F. ORZAN

Page xii,   line 17 from bottom, Y. PARK should read Y.-D. PARK

Page xiii,   line 14, H. HOFFMAN should read H. HOFFMANN

Page 73,   title, ECHOCARDIOGRAPY should read
               ECHOCARDIOGRAPHY

Page 131,   line 4, HIROSHI SAKAKIBARAT should read
               HIROSHI SAKAKIBARA

Page 237,   title, DILATION should read DILATATION

Page 400,   Figure 4, top right, Delc should read Delay